OXFORD
AMERICAN
HANDBOOK
OF CLINICAL
MEDICINE

MW00328533

Published and forthcoming Oxford American Handbooks

OXFORD AMERICAN HANDBOOK OF CLINICAL MEDICINE

EDITED BY

JOHN A. FLYNN, MD, MBA
GENERAL INTERNAL MEDICINE
JOHNS HOPKINS UNIVERSITY

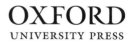
OXFORD
UNIVERSITY PRESS

OXFORD
UNIVERSITY PRESS

Great Clarendon Street, Oxford OX2 6DP

Oxford University Press is a department of the University of Oxford.
It furthers the University's objective of excellence in research, scholarship,
and education by publishing worldwide in

Oxford New York

Auckland Cape Town Dar es Salaam Hong Kong Karachi
Kuala Lumpur Madrid Melbourne Mexico City Nairobi
New Delhi Shanghai Taipei Toronto

With offices in
Argentina Austria Brazil Chile Czech Republic France Greece
Guatemala Hungary Italy Japan South Korea Poland Portugal
Singapore Switzerland Thailand Turkey Ukraine Vietnam

Oxford is a registered trade mark of Oxford University Press
in the UK and in certain other countries

Published in the United States
by Oxford University Press Inc., New York

© Oxford University Press, 2007

British Library Cataloguing in Publication Data
Data available

Library of Congress Cataloging in Publication Data
Data available

Flynn, John A., MD
  Oxford American Handbook of Clinical Medicine / John Flynn.
    p. cm.—(Oxford American Handbooks)
  Adapted from: Oxford Handbook of Clinical Medicine/Murray Longmore,
  Ian B. Wilkinson, Supraj R. Rajagopalan. 6th ed. 2004.

  Includes bibliographical references and index.
  ISBN-13: 978-0-19-518849-3 (flexicover book : alk. paper)
  ISBN-10: (invalid) 0-19-518849-3 (flexicover book : alk. paper)
  1. Clinical medicine–Handbooks, manuals, etc. I. Longmore, J. M. (J. Murray).
Oxford Handbook of Clinical Medicine. II. Title. III. Series.

  [DNLM: 1. Clinical Medicine--Handbooks. WB 39 F648o 2007]
  RC55.F53 2007
  616—dc22   2006103201

Typeset by Newgen Imaging Systems (P) Ltd., Chennai, India
Printed in China
on acid-free paper by
Phoenix Offset

10 9 8 7 6 5 4

Preface

Often during the many weekend and evening hours spent working on this text, I would look directly out of my office window at the façade of the Johns Hopkins Administration building. In a room of this building William Osler completed his work, *The Principles and Practice of Medicine*, over one hundred years ago. This Magnum opus was written to provide current information regarding the clinical management of patients based on known scientific principles of the time. It also included sage advice on the art of compassionate care-giving that a capable physician should provide to their patients. Just as we do now, physicians-in-training then worked assiduously to learn both the art and science of clinical medicine. While the science has moved forward at breakneck speed providing us with new discoveries that may directly enhance our patients' health, much of the essentials of the art of care-giving have stayed the same, though their practice is threatened by the pace and challenges within today's environment of health care delivery.

This book is intended for physicians-in-training: medical students and those in their residency. It aims to present both the science and art of patient management. Upon entrance to the clinical years, the medical student is challenged not only to remember and assimilate an enormous volume of information but also to synthesize this material within the context of their work with patients on the wards. This is an iterative process where your learning will come in many forms and from many sources. This book is one of those sources. It is designed as a reference to be used when considering symptoms and medical conditions that your patients present to you. While designed to fit into your pocket, it is formatted to accommodate the growth and development of your knowledge. To do this, you are encouraged to make notes on the blank spaces provided. Another great source of learning will be the many patients that you care for over the years of your training. As you see each patient, there will always be questions that arise. Use each such experience as a stimulus for your learning. Let your patients become foundations for this knowledge base as you progress in your transition to becoming an experienced physician. Gaudete itinerem; aevum permanebit. (Latin translation for 'Relish the journey; it will last a lifetime').

John A. Flynn

Oxford University Press makes no representation, express or implied, that the drug dosages in this book are correct. Readers must therefore always check the product information and clinical procedures with the most up to date published product information and data sheets provided by the manufacturers and the most recent codes of conduct and safety regulations. The authors and the publishers do not accept responsibility or legal liability for any errors in the text or for the misuse or misapplication of material in this work.

Acknowledgments

Since becoming a physician and an educator over two decades ago, I can honestly say there is no finer work in the world. I have been privileged to be surrounded by the most inquisitive of students, the most supportive of colleagues, and the most sincere of mentors. My special thanks to the many medical students at Hopkins and the members of the Osler housestaff (especially the Barker Firm) that I have had the privilege of training. I thank you for your thirst for knowledge, your passion, and your tireless efforts on behalf of your patients. It is your growth and development that I have delighted in over so many years.

I am deeply grateful for my many colleagues within the Division of General Internal Medicine. You have always been there to provide clinical advice as well as guidance in conducting the affairs of our large and noteworthy enterprise. It is more than a team of professionals—it is a family. I have been fortunate to have a long line of ardent supporters in my role as an academic clinician-educator in the Department of Medicine at Johns Hopkins. These include Mary Betty Stevens, Jack Stobo, Dave Hellmann, Ed Benz, Mike Klag, Bill Schlott, David Levine, Fred Brancati, and Mike Weisfeldt. You have each allowed me to do what I love doing, and helped to build a like-minded group of physicians.

I extend my deepest appreciation to each of the section editors who so bravely stepped forward and took ownership of this project and who demonstrated such pride in its development, I am so honored to be your associate. To William Lamsback and the entire staff of the Oxford University Press who have given me tremendous support, encouragement, and advice throughout the development of this text. To my many patients who have allowed me to become part of their lives in the role of healer, caregiver, and comforter.

I would like to thank the many students and residents who participated in the review of the text and suggested many valuable revisions. I would like to particularly thank Chrissy Kistler, MD, at the University of Michigan, and Shantanu Agrawal, MD, at the University of Pennsylvania for proofreading the entire text and suggesting additions and modifications. Thanks also go to the participants of our ongoing medical student focus groups held at Johns Hopkins and Thomas Jefferson University. The students in these lively groups provided frank assessments of the handbook and offered many insights that helped us shape the material into a book that would address their needs on the wards and beyond.

To my family—Emilee, John, Sarah, Jayne, Christian, Patrick, and W. Andrew. You provide me with such joy and immense pride in all of your accomplishments and your care for one another. To my father, the greatest man I have ever known.

I dedicate this book to my wife—my life—Monica. For nearly three decades, she has been my source of unconditional support and love and endless patience. All I am is because of you.

John A. Flynn,
Johns Hopkins University
2007

Contents

List of Contributors

John G. Bartlett, M.D.
Johns Hopkins University
Infectious Disease

Ari M. Blitz, M.D.
Johns Hopkins University
Radiology

Jonathan Buscaglia, M.D.
Johns Hopkins University
Gastroenterology

Arjun S. Chanmugam, M.D.
Johns Hopkins University
Emergency Medicine

Michael J. Choi, M.D.
Johns Hopkins University
Renal Medicine

Colleen Christmas, M.D.
Johns Hopkins University
Geriatric Medicine

John A. Flynn, M.D., M.B.A.
Johns Hopkins University
Rheumatology

Susan L. Gearhart, M.D.
Johns Hopkins University
Surgery

Benjamin Greenberg, M.D., M.H.S.
Johns Hopkins University
Neurology

Mark T. Hughes, M.D., M.A.
Johns Hopkins University
Thinking About Medicine

Lisa Jacobs, M.D.
Johns Hopkins University
Surgery

Sanjay Jagannath, M.D.
Johns Hopkins University
Gastroenterology

Mathew Kim, M.D.
Johns Hopkins University
Endocrinology

Daniel Laheru, M.D.
Johns Hopkins University
Oncology

Katarzyna Macura, M.D.
Johns Hopkins University
Radiology

Jeffrey L. Magaziner, M.D.
Johns Hopkins University
Clinical Skills

Alison R. Moliterno, M.D.
Johns Hopkins University
Hematology

Albert J. Polito, M.D.
Mercy Medical Center
Pulmonary Medicine

Gregory P. Prokopowicz, M.D., M.P.H.
Johns Hopkins University
Epidemiology

Stuart Russell, M.D.
Johns Hopkins University
Cardiovascular Medicine

Lisa A. Simonson, M.D.
Johns Hopkins University
Symptoms and Signs

Stephen D. Sisson, M.D.
Johns Hopkins University
Biochemistry

C. Matthew Stewart, M.D., Ph.D.
Johns Hopkins University
Practical Procedures

Rosalyn W. Stewart, M.D., M.S.
Johns Hopkins University
Practical Procedures

Neel Vibhaker, M.D.
Johns Hopkins University
Emergency Medicine

Clifford R. Weiss, M.D.
Johns Hopkins University
Radiology

Symbols and abbreviations

1°	Primary
2°	Secondary
♂:♀	male-to-female ratio (♂:♀ = 2.1 means twice as common in males)
∵ ~	on account of (∴ means *therefore*; ~ means *approximately*)
–ve; +ve	negative and positive, respectively
↑; ↓; ↔	increased, decreased, and normal, respectively (eg serum level)
Δ	diagnosis
ΔΔ	differential diagnosis
A₂	aortic component of second heart sound
A2A	angiotensin-2 receptor antagonist (AT-2, A2R, and AIIR)
Ab	antibody
ABC	airway, breathing, and circulation: basic life support
ABG	arterial blood gas measurement (P_aO_2, P_aCO_2, pH, HCO_3^-)
ABPA	allergic bronchopulmonary aspergillosis
ac	*ante cibum* (before food)
ACE(i)	angiotensin-converting enzyme (inhibitors)
ACTH	adrenocorticotrophic hormone
ADH	antidiuretic hormone
Ad lib	ad libitum; as much/as often as wanted (Latin for *at pleasure*)
ADL	activities of daily living
AF	atrial fibrillation
AFB	acid-fast bacillus
AFP	(and α-FP) alpha-fetoprotein
Ag	antigen
AIDS	acquired immunodeficiency syndrome
alk phos	alkaline phosphatase (also ALP)
ALL	acute lymphoblastic leukemia
AMA	antimitochondrial antibody
AMP	adenosine monophosphate
ANA	antinuclear antibody
ANCA	antineutrophil cytoplasmic antibody
APTT	activated partial thromboplastin time
AR	aortic regurgitation
ARB	angiotensin receptor blocker
ARDS	acute respiratory distress syndrome
ARF	acute renal failure
ART	anti-retroviral therapy
AS	aortic stenosis
ASD	atrial septal defect
ASO(T)	antistreptolysin O (titer)
AST	aspartate transaminase
AT-2	angiotensin-2 receptor blocker (also AT-2, A2R, and AIIR)
ATN	acute tubular necrosis
ATP	adenosine triphosphate
AV	atrioventricular
AVM	arteriovenous malformation(s)
AXR	abdominal x-ray (plain)
azt	zidovudine
Ba	barium
BAL	bronchoalveolar lavage
BID	*bis die* (twice a day)
BKA	below-knee amputation
BP	blood pressure

bpm	beats per minute (eg pulse)
ca	carcinoma
CABG	coronary artery bypass graft
cAMP	cyclic adenosine monophosphate (AMP)
CAPD	continuous ambulatory peritoneal dialysis
CBC	complete blood count
CBD	common bile duct
CC	creatinine clearance
CCU	coronary care unit
CHB	complete heart block
CHD	coronary heart disease (related to ischaemia and atheroma)
CHF	congestive heart failure (ie left and right heart failure)
CI	contraindications
CK	creatine (phospho)kinase (also CPK)
CLL	chronic lymphocytic leukemia
CML	chronic myeloid leukemia
CMV	cytomegalovirus
CNS	central nervous system
COPD	chronic obstructive pulmonary disease
CPAP	continuous positive airways pressure
CPR	cardiopulmonary resuscitation
CRF	chronic renal failure
CRP	C-reactive protein
CSF	cerebrospinal fluid
CT	computer tomography
CVP	central venous pressure
CVS	cardiovascular system
CXR	chest x-ray
d	day(s) (also expressed as ×/7)
DC	direct current
DIC	disseminated intravascular coagulation
DIP	distal interphalangeal
dL	deciliter
DM	diabetes mellitus
DU	duodenal ulcer
D&V	diarrhea and vomiting
DVT	deep venous thrombosis
EBM	evidence-based medicine
EBV	Epstein–Barr virus
ECG	electrocardiogram
Echo	echocardiogram
EDTA	ethylene diamine tetraacetic acid (eg in a CBC bottle)
EEG	electroencephalogram
EGD	esophagogastro-duodenoscopy
ELISA	enzyme linked immunosorbant assay
EM	electron microscope
EMG	electromyogram
ENT	ear, nose, and throat
ERCP	endoscopic retrograde cholangiopancreatography
ESR	erythrocyte sedimentation rate
ESRD	end-stage renal disease
EUA	examination under anesthesia
FB	foreign body
FDP	fibrin degradation products
FEV_1	forced expiratory volume in first second

FFP	fresh frozen plasma
F_iO_2	partial pressure of O_2 in inspired air
FROM	full range of movements
FSH	follicle-stimulating hormone
FUO	fever of unknown origin
FVC	forced vital capacity
g	gram
GA	general anesthetic
GB	gall bladder
GC	gonococcus
GCS	Glasgow coma scale
GFR	glomerular filtration rate
GGT	gamma glutamyl transpeptidase
GH	growth hormone
GI	gastrointestinal
G6PD	glucose-6-phosphate dehydrogenase
GTT	glucose tolerance test (also OGTT: oral GTT)
GU	genitourinary
h	hour
HAART	highly active anti-retroviral therapy
HAV	hepatitis A virus
Hb	hemoglobin
HBsAg/HBV	hepatitis B surface antigen/hepatitis B virus
HCC	hepatocellular cancer
Hct	hematocrit
HCV	hepatitis C virus
HDL	high-density lipoprotein
HDV	hepatitis D virus
HHT	hereditary hemorrhagic telangiectasia
HIDA	hepatic immunodiacetic acid
HIV	human immunodeficiency virus
HOCM	hypertrophic obstructive cardiomyopathy
HONK	hyperosmolar nonketotic (diabetic coma)
HRT	hormone replacement therapy
HSV	Herpes simplex virus
ICP	intracranial pressure
ICU	intensive care unit
IDA	iron-deficiency anemia
IDDM	insulin-dependent diabetes mellitus
IFN-α	alpha interferon
IE	infective endocarditis
Ig	immunoglobulin
IHD	ischemic heart disease
IM	intramuscular
INR	international normalized ratio (prothrombin ratio)
IPPV	intermittent positive pressure ventilation
ITP	idiopathic thrombocytopenic purpura
iu	international unit
IVC	inferior vena cava
IVDU	intravenous drug user
IV(I)	intravenous (infusion)
IVU	intravenous urography
JVP	jugular venous pressure
K	potassium
kg	kilogram

L	liter
LAD	left axis deviation on the ECG
LBBB	left bundle branch block
LDH	lactate dehydrogenase
LDL	low-density lipoprotein
LFT	liver function test
LH	luteinizing hormone
LLQ	left lower quadrant
LMN	lower motor neuron
LP	lumbar puncture
LTOT	long term oxygen therapy
LUQ	left upper quadrant
LV	left ventricle of the heart
LVF	left ventricular failure
LVH	left ventricular hypertrophy
µg	microgram
MAI	*Mycobacterium avium intracellulare*
MAOI	monoamine oxidase inhibitors
MC & S	microscopy, culture and sensitivity
MCV	mean cell volume
MDMA	3,4-methylenedioxymethamphetamine
MET	maximal exercise test
mg	milligram
MI	myocardial infarction
min(s)	minute(s)
mL	milliliter
mmHg	millimeters of mercury
MND	motor neuron disease
MRI	magnetic resonance imaging
MRSA	methicillin-resistant *Staphylococcus aureus*
MS	multiple sclerosis (do not confuse with mitral stenosis)
MSU	midstream urine
NAD	nothing abnormal detected
ND	notifiable disease
ng	nanogram
NG(T)	nasogastric (tube)
NIDDM	noninsulin-dependent diabetes mellitus
NMDA	*N*-methyl-*D*-aspartate
NNT	number needed to treat, for 1 extra satisfactory result
NPO	nothing by mouth
NR	normal range—the same as reference interval
NSAIDs	non-steroidal anti-inflammatory drugs
NTG	nitroglycerin (also TNG)
N&V	nausea and/or vomiting
OD	overdose
OGTT	oral glucose tolerance test
OP	opening pressure
OPD	out-patients department
ORh–	blood group O, Rh negative
OT	occupational therapist
P_2	pulmonary component of second heart sound
P_aCO_2	partial pressure of carbon dioxide in arterial blood
PAN	polyarteritis nodosa
P_aO_2	partial pressure of oxygen in arterial blood
PBC	primary biliary cirrhosis

PCR	polymerase chain reaction (DNA diagnosis)
PCV	packed cell volume
PE	pulmonary embolism
PEEP	positive end-expiratory pressure
PERLA	pupils equal and reactive to light and accommodation
PEF(R)	peak expiratory flow (rate)
PFT	pulmonary function tests
PID	pelvic inflammatory disease
PIP	proximal interphalangeal (joint)
PMH	past medical history
PND	paroxysmal nocturnal dyspnoea
PO	*per os* (by mouth)
PPF	purified plasma fraction (albumin)
PPI	proton pump inhibitor, eg omeprazole, lansoprazole, etc.
PR	*per rectum* (by the rectum)
PRN	*pro re nata* (as required)
PSA	prostate specific antigen
PTH	parathyroid hormone
PTT	prothrombin time
qd	each day
qid	*quater in die* (4 times a day); qqh: *quarta quaque hora* (every 4h)
R	right
RA	rheumatoid arthritis
RAD	right axis deviation on the ECG
RBBB	right bundle branch block
RBC	red blood cell
RF	renal failure
RLQ	right lower quadrant
RUQ	right upper quadrant
RV	right ventricle of heart
RVF	right ventricular failure
RVH	right ventricular hypertrophy
Rx	*recipe* (treat with)
s or sec	second(s)
S1, S2	first and second heart sounds
SBE	subacute bacterial endocarditis (IE, *infective endocarditis*, is better)
SC	subcutaneous
SCD	spontaneous compression device
SD	standard deviation
SE	side-effect(s)
SL	sublingual
SLE	systemic lupus erythematosus
SOB	short of breath
SR	slow-release (also called modified-release)
stat	*statim* (immediately; as initial dose)
STD/STI	sexually-transmitted disease or sexually-transmitted infection
SVC	superior vena cava
sy(n)	syndrome
$T°$	temperature
$t_{\frac{1}{2}}$	biological half-life
T3	triiodothyronine
T4	thyroxine
TB	tuberculosis
TFTs	thyroid function tests (eg TSH)
TIA	transient ischemic attack

TIBC	total iron binding capacity
tid	*ter in die* (3 times a day)
TPR	temperature, pulse, and respirations count
TRH	thyroid-releasing hormone
TSH	thyroid-stimulating hormone
U	units
UC	ulcerative colitis
U&E	urea & electrolytes & creatinine in plasma, unless stated otherwise
UMN	upper motor neuron
URT	upper respiratory tract
URTI	upper respiratory tract infection
US(S)	ultrasound (scan)
UTI	urinary tract infection
VDRL	venereal diseases research laboratory
VF	ventricular fibrillation
VMA	vanillyl mandelic acid (HMMA)
V̇/Q̇	ventilation/perfusion ratio
VSD	ventriculo-septal defect
VT	ventricular tachycardia
WBC	white blood cell
WCC	white cell count
wk(s)	week(s)
WR	Wassermann reaction
yr(s)	year(s)
ZN	Ziehl–Neelsen (stain for acid-fast bacilli, eg mycobacteria)

Other abbreviations are given on pages where they occur: consult the *index*.

Thinking about medicine

Mark T. Hughes, M.D., M.A.

Contents

Ideals

Decision and *intervention* are the essence of action: Reflection and conjecture are the essence of thought: The essence of medicine is combining these realms of action and thought in the service of others. We offer these ideals to stimulate both thought and action: Like the stars, these ideals are hard to reach—but they serve for navigation during the night.

- *Remember the goal of healing is to make the person whole:* This applies whether the aim is cure, relief of symptoms in an acute or chronic illness, prevention of complications in a chronic disease, or comfort in an incurable disease.
- *Do not blame the sick for being sick:* They come to you for help. You are there for them, not the other way around.
- *If the patient's wishes are known, comply with them.*
- *Work for your patients, not your attending.*
- *Use ward rounds to boost the patient's morale,* not your own.
- *Treat the whole patient,* not the disease.
- *Admit people*—not 'strokes', 'infarcts', or 'gomers'.
- *Spend time with the bereaved;* you can help them shed their tears.
- *Question your conscience*—however strongly it tells you to act.
- *The nurses know the patient and are usually right;* respect their opinions.
- *Be kind to yourself*—you are not an inexhaustible resource.
- *Give the patient (and yourself) time:* Time to ask questions, time to reflect, time to allow healing to take place, and time to gain autonomy.
- *Give the patient the benefit of the doubt.* If you can, *be optimistic:* Patients want physicians to be realistic but also to instill hope.

Ideal and less than ideal methods of care

The story of Ivan Ilyich illustrates the options: 'Special foods were prepared for him on the doctor's orders, but these became more and more unpalatable, more and more revolting... Special arrangements, too, were made for his bowel movements. And this was a regular torture—a torture because of the filth, the unseemliness, the stench, and the knowledge that another person had to assist him... Yet it was precisely through this unseemly business that Ivan Ilyich derived some comfort. The pantry boy, Gerasim, always came to carry out the chamber pot. Gerasim was a clean, ruddy-faced young peasant who was thriving on town food. He was always bright and cheerful... "Gerasim," said Ivan Ilyich in a feeble voice... "This must be very unpleasant for you. You must forgive me. I can't help it."... "Oh no, sir!" said Gerasim as he broke into a smile, his eyes and strong white teeth gleaming. "Why shouldn't I help you? You're a sick man."... Ivan Ilyich had Gerasim sit down and hold his legs up, and he began talking to him. And, strangely enough, he thought he felt better while Gerasim was holding his legs... After that, Ivan Ilyich would send for Gerasim from time to time and have him hold his feet on his shoulders. And he loved to talk to him. Gerasim did everything easily, willingly, simply, and with a goodness of heart that moved Ivan Ilyich. Health, strength, and vitality in other people offended Ivan Ilyich, whereas Gerasim's strength and vitality had a soothing effect on him.'[1]

It was the pantry boy who was his true healthcare provider and caregiver, who took him on his own terms, cared for him, and gave him time and dignity. While Ivan Ilyich's physicians and others cooperated in the "lie" that he was ill but not dying, "Gerasim was the only one who understood and pitied him." Gerasim did not find his work burdensome, because he understood he was doing it for a dying man. As TS Eliot said, *'there is, at best, only a limited value in the knowledge derived from experience'*—eg the knowledge encompassed in this book. The pantry boy had the innate understanding and the natural compassion that we all too easily lose amid the science, the knowledge, and our stainless steel universe of organized healthcare.

1 Leo Tolstoy 1981 from *The Death of Ivan Ilyich.* Bantam Books.

The bedside manner and communication skills

Our bedside manner matters because it indicates to patients whether they can *trust* us. Where there is no trust, there can be little healing. A good bedside manner is not static: It develops in coordination with the patients' needs, but it is grounded in the timeless clinical virtues of honesty, humor, and humility in the presence of human weakness and human suffering.

The following are examples from an endless variety of phenomena which arise whenever doctors meet patients. One of the great skills (and pleasures) in medicine is to learn how our actions and attitudes influence patients, and how to take this knowledge into account when assessing the validity and significance of the signs and symptoms we elicit. The information we receive from our patients is not 'hard evidence', but a much more plastic commodity, molded as much by the doctor's attitude and the hospital or consulting room environment as by the patient's own hopes and fears. It is our job to adjust our attitudes and environment, so that these hidden hopes and fears become manifest and the channels of communication are always open.

Anxiety reduction or intensification Simple explanation of what you are going to do often defuses what can be a highly charged affair. With children, try more subtle techniques, such as examining the abdomen using the child's own hands, or examining their teddy bear first.

Pain reduction or intensification Compare: 'I'm going to press your stomach. If it hurts, cry out' with 'I'm going to touch your stomach. Let me know what you feel'. The examination can be made to sound frightening, neutral, or joyful, and the patient will relax or tense up accordingly.

The tactful or clumsy invasion of personal space The physical examination can involve close contact with the patient that is normally not acceptable as part of usual social interaction. Acknowledging this to the patient can set both parties at ease. For example, during ophthalmoscopy, simply explain 'I need to get very close to your eyes for this'.

The use of distraction to gather information The skilful practitioner palpating the painful abdomen will start away from the part that hurts. They will watch the patient's face while talking about a hobby or the patient's family while he presses as hard as they need to. If the patient stops talking and frowns only when the doctor's hand is over the right lower quadrant, the doctor will already have found out something useful.

Communication Your skills are useless unless you communicate well. Be simple, and direct. Avoid jargon: 'Remission' and 'growth' are frequently misunderstood. Give the most important details first. Be specific. 'Drink 6 cups of water per day' is better than 'Drink more fluids'. Provide written information with easy readability. Aim for a sixth grade reading level—more like the *Reader's Digest* than the *Wall Street Journal*. If possible, show videos for patient education. Do not assume your patient can read. Naming the pictures but not the words on our visual test chart (p69) helps find this out tactfully.

Inquire about your patient's views of what should be done. Patient-centered care improves provider–patient interactions and patient satisfaction. Find goals of care that can be mutually agreed upon. Learn more about the patient's values. We often talk of *compliance* with our regimens, when what we should talk of is *concordance*, for concordance recognizes the central role of patient participation in all good plans of care.

What is the mechanism? Finding narrative answers

Like toddlers, we should always be asking '*Why?*'—not just to find ultimate causes, but to enable us to choose the simplest level for intervention. Some simple change early on in a chain of events may be sufficient to bring about a cure, whereas later on in the chain such opportunities may not arise.

For example, it is not enough for you to diagnose heart failure in your breathless patient. Ask: '*Why is there heart failure?*' If you do not, you will be satisfied with giving the patient an anti-failure drug, and any side-effects from these, such as uremia or incontinence induced by diuretic-associated polyuria, will be attributed to an unavoidable consequence of necessary therapy. If only you had asked '*What is the mechanism of the heart failure?*' you might have found an underlying cause, eg anemia coupled with ischemic heart disease. You cannot cure the latter, but treating the anemia may be all that is required to cure the patient's breathlessness. But do not stop there. Ask: '*What is the mechanism of the anemia?*' You find a low serum ferritin and you might be tempted to say to yourself, I have the root cause.

Wrong! Put aside the idea of prime causes, and go on asking '*What is the mechanism?*' Return to the patient (never think that the process of history-taking is over). Retaking the history reveals that the patient has a very poor diet. '*Why is the patient eating a poor diet?*' Is he ignorant or too poor to eat properly? You may find the patient's wife died a year ago, he is sinking into a depression, and cannot be bothered to eat. He would not care if he died tomorrow.

You now begin to realize that simply treating the patient's anemia may not be of much help to him—so go on asking '*Why?*': 'Why did you bother to go to the doctor at all if you are not interested in getting better?' It turns out that he only went to see the doctor to please his daughter. He is unlikely to take your treatment unless you really get to the bottom of what he cares about. His daughter is what matters and, unless you can enlist her help, all your therapeutic initiatives will fail. Talk with his daughter, offer help for the depression, teach her about iron-rich foods and, with luck, your patient's breathlessness may gradually begin to disappear. Even if it does *not* start to disappear, you may perhaps have forged a friendship with your patient which can be used to enable him to accept help in other ways—and this dialogue may help you to be a more humane and a kinder doctor, particularly if you are feeling worn out and assaulted by long lists of technical tasks which you must somehow fit into impossibly overcrowded days and nights.

Constructing imaginative narratives yielding new meanings Doctors are often thought of as being reductionist and over-mechanistic. The above shows that always asking 'why' can sometimes enlarge the scope of our inquiries rather than narrowing the focus. Another way to do this is to ask *What does this symptom mean?*—for this person, their family, and our world. For example, a limp might mean a neuropathy, or inability to meet mortgage repayments (if you are a dancer)—or it may represent a medically unexplained symptom which subtly alters family hierarchies both literally (during family walks through the country) and metaphorically. Science is about clarity, objectivity, and theory in modeling our external world. But there is another way of modeling the external world which involves subjectivity, emotion, ambiguity, and the seeking of arcane relationships between apparently unrelated phenomena. The medical humanities explore the latter—and have been burgeoning during the last decade—leading to the existence of two camps—humanities and science. If, while reading this you are getting impatient to get to the real nuts and bolts of technological medicine, you are in the latter camp. We are not suggesting that you leave it—only that you learn to operate out of both. If you do not, your professional life will be full of failures (of which you may deny or remain ignorant). If you do straddle both camps, there will also be failures—but you will realize what these failures mean, and you will know how to transform them.

Always remember that medicine is both an art and a science. The physician must have the technical skill and knowledge to ply their craft, but they need the artistry to practice it with compassion in the context of a patient's life.

Asking questions

No class of questions is 'correct'. Sometimes you need to ask one type of question; sometimes another. The good clinician can shift from one kind to another, in order to use the most effective questions for each individual patient. The aim of asking questions is to *describe*, to find a shared world between the doctor and patient. Questions provide the means to offer practical help: Once the illness is described, a diagnosis can be made and a possible cure offered. If not curable, the experience can at least be shared, mitigated, and so partially overcome. Different kinds of questions either throw light on the experience, or obscure it, as in the examples below.

Leading questions On seeing a bloodstained handkerchief you ask: 'How long have you been coughing up blood?' '6wks, doctor' so you assume hemoptysis for 6wks. In fact, the stain could be due to an infected finger, or to epistaxis. On finding this out later (and perhaps after expensive and unpleasant investigations), you will be upset, but the patient was politely trying to give the sort of answer you were obviously expecting. With such leading questions as these, the patient is not given an opportunity to deny your assumptions.

Questions suggesting the answer 'Was the vomit red, yellow, or black—like coffee grounds?'—the classic description of vomited blood. 'Yes, like coffee grounds, doctor.' The doctor's expectations and hurry to get the evidence into a pre-determined format have so tarnished the story as to make it useless.

Open-ended questions The most open is 'How are you?' This suggests no particular answer, so the direction a patient chooses offers valuable information. Other examples are gentle imperatives such as 'Tell me about the vomit' 'It was dark' 'How dark?' 'Dark with little chunks in it' 'Like…?' 'Like bits of soil in it.' This information is pure gold, although it is not cast in the form of 'coffee grounds'.

Patient-centered questions 'What do you think is wrong?' 'Are there any other aspects of this we might explore?' 'Are there any questions you want to ask?' (a closed question). Better still, try 'What are the other things on your mind?' How is this affecting you? What is the worst thing? It makes you feel…' (The doctor is silent.) Becoming patient-centered gives you a better chance of healing the whole person, and the patient may be more satisfied as a result.

Framing questions in the context of the family This is particularly useful in revealing if symptoms are caused or perpetuated by psychosocial factors. Family-oriented questions probe the network of causes and enabling conditions which allow nebulous symptoms to flourish in a person's life. Who else is important in your life? Are they worried about you? Who really understands you? Until this sort of question is asked, illness may be refractory to treatment. Eg: 'Who is present when your headache starts? Who notices it first—you or your wife? Who worries about it most (or least)? What does your wife do when (or before) you get it?' The spouse's view of the symptoms may be the best predictor of outcome for the patient.

Framing questions in the context of culture In medicine, we may encounter patients from diverse backgrounds, sometimes quite different from our own. The skillful clinician will be self-aware enough to recognize any biases they may have based on their own cultural identity. To be culturally competent, the clinician should be open to exploring the patient's health beliefs from the patient's cultural perspective. Admitting ignorance of the patient's culture in an inquiring, respectful manner may provide clues as to how best help the patient within their worldview.

Echoing Try repeating the last words said as a route to new intimacies, otherwise inaccessible, as you fade into the distance, and the patient soliloquizes

'…I've always been suspicious of my wife.' 'Wife…' 'My wife… and her boss working late at night together.' 'Together…' 'I've never trusted them together.' 'Trusted them together…' 'No, well, I've always felt I've known who my son's real father was… I can never trust those two together.' Without any questions you may unearth the unexpected, important clue which throws a new light on the history.

Empathic opportunities Remember that the purpose of the medical interview is not just to gain information, but to develop a relationship. Are you asking questions in a respectful way that validates the patient's emotional experience? After getting facts about the illness experience, ask the follow-up question, 'How did you feel about that?' and acknowledge the emotions reported. Be attentive to nonverbal communication, which may shed light on the patient's underlying feelings and ↑ the yield of the information. Match body language to build rapport and make it more likely that the patient will be open to answering questions.

The value of silence Sometimes not asking a question will give the patient the opportunity to share important information. There is value in the pregnant pause…

If you only ask questions, you will only receive answers in reply. If you interrogate a robin, he will fly away: Treelike silence may bring him to your hand.

Health and medical ethics

Medicine has its own internal morality. This derives from a patient's illness and their subsequent vulnerability, coupled with the physician's intent to help the patient improve. Each time a physician asks of the patient, "How can I help you?" there is an implicit understanding that the physician will use their expertise to serve the best interests of the patient.

As members of a profession, physicians declare publicly that they will put aside their self-interest in the service of others. While society grants physicians certain privileges, it also expects certain duties of the profession, namely to be the stewards of valuable societal resources.

In the sphere of ethics, physicians are called upon to lead as often as to follow. To do this, we need to return to basic principles, and put society's expectations temporarily on one side.

Our analysis starts with our aim: To do good by promoting people's health. *Health* entails being sound in body and mind, and having powers of growth, development, healing, and regeneration. *How many people have you made healthy (or at least healthier) today? Good* is the most general term of commendation, and entails four chief duties:

Not doing harm (non-maleficence). We owe this duty to all people, not just our patients.

Doing good by positive actions (beneficence). We particularly owe this to our patients. There are four ways by which the patient's good can be defined: (1) the ultimate good, that which has the highest meaning for the patient; (2) the biomedical good, obtained by treatment of the disease; (3) the patient's perception of the good based on their life plan; and (4) the good of the patient as a person, deserving respect and the freedom to make reasoned choices.[1]

Respecting autonomy or respecting the person. Autonomy (self-determination) is not universally recognized; in some cultures facing starvation, it may be irrelevant, or even be considered subversive. But respecting persons and their inherent dignity is to be found across cultures. This is manifested in medicine by upholding patients' rights to be informed, to be offered all the options, to be told the truth, and to have their confidentiality protected.

Promoting justice—distributing scarce resources fairly and treating people fairly, such as when we respect their legal rights.

The point of having these guiding principles is to provide a context for our negotiations with patients. If we want to be better doctors, a good starting point is trying to put these principles into action. Inevitably, when we try to, there are times when the principles seem to conflict with each other. What should guide us when these principles conflict? It is not just a case of deciding off the top of one's head. It requires further inquiry, deliberation, and aspiring to a *synthesis*—if you have the time (time will so often be what you do *not* have; but, in retrospect, when things have gone wrong, you realize that they would not have done so if you had *made* time).

Synthesis When we must act in the face of 2 conflicting duties, one of the duties will take precedence. How do we tell which one? Trying to find out involves getting to know our patients, and asking some questions:
- Are the patient's wishes being complied with?
- What do the patient's loved ones (family and/or friends) think? First ask the patient's permission to speak to the loved ones. Do the patient's loved ones have his or her best interests at heart?
- What do colleagues think? Often having the input of other clinicians can help sort out the complexities of a difficult case.

1 Edmund D. Pellegrino and David C. Thomasma 1988. *For the Patient's Good: The Restoration of Beneficence in Healthcare.* Oxford University Press.

- Is it desirable that the reason for an action be universalizable? (That is, if I say this person is too old for such-and-such an operation, am I happy to make this a general rule for everyone?—Kant's 'law'.)[1]
- What would the man on the street say? These opinions are valuable as they are readily available and they can stop decision-making from becoming dangerously medicalized.
- If an investigative journalist were to sit on a sulcus of mine, having full knowledge of my thoughts and actions, would she be bored or would she be composing vitriol for tomorrow's newspapers? If so, can I answer her, point for point? Am I happy with my answers? Or are they tactical cerebrations designed to outwit her?
- What would I do if nobody were watching? Would I act the same way if there were no consequences in terms of public scrutiny? Will I be able to face myself in the mirror the next morning?
- Do I need the input of the hospital ethics committee? In some cases, ethics consultants can help to facilitate discussion among interested parties, sort out the ethical issues at stake, and provide an opinion about ethically permissible options for resolution of the problem.

1 There are problems with universalizability: sometimes only intuition can suggest how to resolve conflicts between competing universal principles. Universal principles work in the abstract but have drawbacks when applied to real life situations. Also, there is a sense in which all ethical dilemmas are unique—they *cannot* be universal. This leads some ethicists to favor case-based reasoning, ie casuistry.

Medicine, art, and the humanities

Let us start with an elementary observation: The most famous doctors are those immortalized in literature—eg Dr Watson, Dr Zhivago, Dr Frankenstein, and Dr Faustus.[1] Hereby we demonstrate the power of the written word. And it *is* an extraordinary power. When we curl up in an armchair and read for pleasure, we open the portals of our minds because we are alone. While we are reading, there is no point in dissembling. We confront our subject matter with a steady eye because we believe that, while reading to ourselves, we cannot be judged. Then, suddenly, when we are at our most open and defenseless, literature takes us by the throat—and that eye which was so steady and confident a few minutes ago is now perhaps misting over, or our heart is missing a beat, or our skin is covered in a goose-flesh more popular than ever a Siberian winter produced. Once we have been on earth for a few decades, not much in our mundane world sends shivers down our spines, but the power of worlds of literature and art to do this ever grows.

There are, of course, doctors who are quite well known as literary artists: Arthur Conan Doyle, William Carlos Williams, Somerset Maugham, and Anton Chekhov. What about Sigmund Freud? Here is the exception which proves the rule—proves in the sense of testing, for he is not really an exception. We can accept him among the great only in so far as we view his collection of writings as an artistic oeuvre, rather than as a scientific one. Science has progressed for years without Freud, but, as art, his work and insights will survive: And survival, as Bernard Shaw pointed out, is the only test of greatness.

The reason for the ascendancy of art over science is simple. We scientists, in our humble way, are only interested in explaining reality. Artists are good at explaining reality too: But they also *create* it. Our most powerful impressions are produced in our minds not by simple sensations but by the association of ideas. It is a pre-eminent feature of the human mind that it revels in seeing something as, or through, something else: Life refracted through experience, light refracted through jewels, or a walk through the woods transmuted into a pastoral symphony. Ours is a world of metaphor, fantasy, and deceit.

What has all this to do with the day-to-day practice of medicine? The answer lies in the word 'defenseless' above. When we read alone and for pleasure, our defenses are down—and we hide nothing from the great characters of fiction. This openness to the story of another helps to keep us connected with our patients. So often, a professional detachment is all that is left after all those years inured to the foibles, fallacies, and frictions of our patients' tragic lives. It is at the point where art and medicine collide, that doctors can re-attach themselves to the human race and re-feel those emotions which motivate or terrify our patients. Art and literature can cultivate our empathy, so that, at some level, there can be truth to the statement, 'I understand what you're going through,' even though we ourselves may not have had to endure the illness experience of the patient.

We all have an Achilles heel: That part of our inner self which was not rendered forever invulnerable to mortal cares when we were dipped in the waters of the river Styx as it flowed down the wards of our first disillusion. Art and literature, among other things, may enable this Achilles heel to be the means of our survival as thinking, sentient beings, capable of maintaining a sympathetic sensibility to our patients.

Narrative medicine allows us to see *the patient as text*, and thereby foster ethical reasoning and speculation about the patient's worldview of illness. No matter his or her specialty, each physician should recognize that in the practice of medicine, *every* contact with a patient has an ethical and artistic dimension, as well as a technical one.

---

1 Of course Dr Faust, that famous charlatan, necromancer, and quack from medieval Germany, did have a real existence. In fact, there may have been two of them, who together gave rise to myth of devil-dealing, debauchery, and the undisciplined pursuit of science, without the constraints of morality.

Prescribing drugs

Consult the *Physicians' Desk Reference* (PDR) or your local equivalent before prescribing any drug with which you are not thoroughly familiar.

Before prescribing, ask if the patient is allergic to anything. The answer is often 'Yes'—but do not stop here. Find out what the reaction was, or else you run the risk of denying your patient a possibly life-saving and very safe drug, such as penicillin, because of a mild reaction like nausea. Is the reaction a *true allergy* (anaphylaxis, p688 or a rash?), a *toxic effect* (eg ataxia is inevitable if given large quantities of phenytoin), a *predictable adverse reaction* (eg GI bleeding from aspirin), or an *idiosyncratic reaction*?

Remember *primum non nocere*: First do no harm. The more minor the complaint, the more weight this dictum carries. The more serious the complaint, the more its antithesis comes into play: *Nothing ventured, nothing gained.*

Ten commandments These should be written on every tablet.

1 Explore any alternatives to a prescription. Prescriptions lead to doctor-dependency, which in turn frequently leads to bad medicine and drives up the expense of healthcare. There are 3 places to find alternatives:

The kitchen: Lemon and honey for sore throats, rather than penicillin.

The blackboard:—eg education about the self-inflicted causes of esophagitis. Rather than giving expensive drugs, advise against too many big meals, eating close to bedtime, smoking and alcohol excess, or wearing over-tight garments.

Lastly, look to yourself. Giving a piece of yourself, some real empathy, is worth more than all the drugs in your pharmacopoeia to patients who are frightened, bereaved, or weary of life.

2 Find out if the patient wants to take a drug. Are you prescribing for some minor ailment because you want to solve every problem? Patients may be happy just to know the ailment *is* minor. If they know what it is, they may be happy to live with it. Some people do not believe in drugs, and you must find this out.

3 Decide if the patient is responsible. If they now swallow *all* the acetaminophen with codeine pills that you have prescribed for their acute pain at one time, death will be swift.

4 Know of other ways your prescription may be misused. Perhaps the patient, whose 'insomnia' you so kindly treated is actually grinding up your prescription for injection in order to get a fix. Will you be suspicious when they return to say they have lost your prescription?

5 Address these questions when prescribing:
• How many daily doses are there? 1–2 is much better than 4.
• How many other drugs are to be taken? Can they be reduced?
• Can the patient read the instructions on the bottle—and can they open it?
• Is the patient agreeable to enlisting the help of a loved one or caretaker to ensure that they remember to take the pills?
• Is the patient taking the medication properly? Check by counting the remaining pills at the next visit.
• How will the patient refill their prescription?
• How will you know and what will you do if the patient does not come for a follow-up visit?

6 List the potential benefits of the drug for *this* patient.

7 List the risks (side-effects, contraindications, interactions, risk of allergy). Of any new problems, always ask yourself: *Is this a side-effect?*

8 Try to ensure there is true concordance between you and your patient on the risk:benefit ratio's favorability. Document your discussion.

9 Record how you will review the patient's need for each drug and quantify progress (or lack thereof) towards specified, agreed goals, eg pulse rate to mark degree of beta-blockade; or peak flow reading to guide steroid use in asthma.

10 Make a record of all drugs taken. Offer the patient a copy.

The art and science of diagnosing

The central processes of medicine are: Relieving symptoms, providing reassurance and prognostic information, and lending a sympathetic ear. But it is very difficult to do this well, and to ↑ your rapport with your patient, unless you have a working diagnosis. How is this achieved?

We diagnose, it is held, by a 3-stage process: We take a history, we examine, and we do tests. We then collate this information, by a process which is never explained, and compare it with features of diseases we know. We then find the best match, and call this the diagnosis. Other nearly matching diseases then form the differential diagnosis. This model ignores two factors: (1) Often no match can be found. (2) Doctors, in practice, hardly ever work like this. So how *are* diagnoses made?

Diagnosing by recognition For students, this is the most irritating method. You spend an hour asking all the wrong questions, and in waltzes a doctor who names the disease, and sorts it out before you have even finished taking the pulse. This doctor has simply recognized the illness like they recognize an old friend (or enemy). But don't worry: You too will soon reach this position, if you spend enough time at bedsides with other doctors—and you too will just as effortlessly make all the errors that this approach is prone to.

Diagnosing by probability theory Over our clinical lives we unconsciously build up a personal database of diagnoses and outcomes, and associated pitfalls. We unconsciously run each new 'case' through this personal and continuously developing fine-grained probabilistic algorithm—eventually with amazing speed and effortlessness.

Diagnosing by hypothesizing We formulate a hypothesis and then try to disprove or prove it. The generation of a hypothesis can start with the chief complaint. Our subsequent questions in history-taking, the focus of our physical exam, and/or our selection of tests provide the data to prove or disprove our original hypothesis, or to formulate a new one.

Diagnosing by reasoning Like Sherlock Holmes, we exclude each differential diagnosis, and then, whatever is left, *however unlikely*, must be the culprit. This process presupposes that our differential does include the culprit, and that we have methods for *absolutely* excluding diseases. All tests are statistical, rather than absolute—which is why the Holmes technique is, at best, fictional.

Diagnosing by a 'wait and see' approach Some doctors (and patients) need to know immediately and definitively what the diagnosis is, while others can tolerate more uncertainty. With practice, one can sense that the dangers and expense of exhaustive tests can be obviated by the skillful use of time. This cough *might* represent pneumonia, but I may choose not to get a chest x-ray or sputum culture. Rather, I may say 'take this antibiotic if you get a fever—but you probably don't need it, and you'll get better on your own: Wait and see'.

Diagnosing by selective doubting Traditionally, patients are 'unreliable', signs are objective, and lab tests virtually perfect. When diagnosis is difficult, try inverting this hierarchy. The more you do so, the more you realize that there are no hard signs or perfect labs. But the game of medicine is unplayable if you doubt everything, so doubt selectively.

Diagnosing by computer Computing power is the only way of fully mapping the interrelatedness of diseases—eg hyponatremia with eosinophilia points to *Addison's disease*, but if there is oliguria too, a doctor with no computer may have to posit an unrelated disease; but the computer 'knows' that oliguria is a feature of shock, and shock is a complication of Addison's.

Diagnosis by iteration and reiteration

A brief history suggests looking for a few signs, whose assessment leads you to ask further questions, and do a few tests. These results lead to further questions and tests. The process of taking a history never ends on this view, and as this process reiterates, various diagnostic possibilities crop up, and receive more or less confirmation. 'I feel my heart racing'—and the doctor immediately puts his finger on the pulse, and feels it to be irregularly irregular, and infers atrial fibrillation (AF, p120). He wants to know *why* there is AF, so he asks about weight loss and heat intolerance. This suggests hyperthyroidism (p280) as the cause of the AF. While he takes the pulse he notices clubbing of the fingers, so he makes a mental note to do a chest x-ray to see if there are signs of cancer (could this cause the AF?—yes). This reminds him to ask about smoking: While inquiring about habits, he asks about alcohol, and elicits excessive drinking. 'Why now?' 'Because I lost my job.' 'Who cares about this more? You or your husband?' In the time it takes to assess the pulse, the doctor has many promising leads to follow, and is starting to formulate a diagnosis in 3 dimensions: Physical, psychological, and social. The patient's palms are clammy, and the pulse is weak, so the doctor knows he must be prompt and decisive, and gently explains that admission for various tests is needed. Whereupon the patient, who has been holding back tears, now weeps. Now holding her hand, as well as continuing to take her pulse, the doctor becomes aware of a change in rhythm. Is this sinus rhythm, brought on by the Valsalva-like maneuver of weeping? So the doctor now says 'Well... let's see how you get on over the next hour—you'll feel better for crying.' 'Yes, you're right, I feel better already.'

This is a microcosm of the intuitive world of medicine which the systematic (or *only* systematic) doctor never knows. He would come on to the pulse only after a 'full history'—and would have missed everything. The doctor who is prepared to appear muddled, and who can work on many different levels simultaneously, will often be the first to know the diagnosis.

Prevention

Two mottos: *'The only good medicine is preventive medicine'* and *'If preventable…why not prevented?'* During life on the wards you will have many opportunities for preventive medicine, and unconsciously you will pass most of them over, in favor of more glamorous tasks such as diagnosis, and clever interventions, involving probes, scalpels, and imaging. But if we imagine a ward where scalpels remain sheathed and the only thing being probed is our commitment to health, then preventive medicine comes to the forefront, and it is our contention that such a ward might produce more health than some entire hospitals.

Ways of thinking about prevention Preventing a disease (eg by vaccination) is *primary prevention*. Controlling disease in an early form (eg carcinoma-in-situ) is *secondary prevention*. Preventing complications in those already symptomatic is *tertiary prevention*.

The best way of thinking about prevention is *"What can I do now with this patient in front of me?"* On the wards this will often be secondary or tertiary prevention—eg blood pressure screening in diabetes, or colonoscopy in ulcerative colitis (looking for colon cancer), or endoscopic screening for esophageal cancer in Barrett's esophagus.

The first step in prevention is to motivate your patient to take steps to benefit their own health by asking Socratic questions. 'Do you want to smoke?' 'What does your family think about smoking' 'Do you want your children to smoke?' 'Would there be any advantages in giving up?' 'Why is your health important to you?' 'Is there anything more important we can help with?' 'How would you spend the money you might save?' These types of questions along with specific strategies in prevention (p87) are more likely to produce change than withering looks and lectures on lung cancer. In summary: In any preventive activity, get the patient on your side—make them want to change. Once you have done this, preventive activities you might promote include:

1° and 2° disease prevention:	General health:	Cancer screening:
Vaccination (eg flu shot if >65yrs)	Healthy eating	Colon cancer screening
Aspirin if vascular disease	Regular exercise	Pap smears
Cardiovascular risk reduction	Advice on smoking and alcohol	Mammography and annual breast exam
Osteoporosis prevention if on steroids or post-menopausal (calcium, vitamin D, ± bisphosphonate)	House and car dangers: Seatbelts, accidents, falls, gun safety	Genetic counseling, eg if family history positive in two 1st degree relatives

Sometimes referral to other agencies is needed—eg for genetic counseling, contraception, and pre-conception advice.

Concentrate on those preventive activities which are simple, cheap, and have a complication rate approaching zero. When considering a more complicated or 'high-tech' preventive procedure, be on guard for unintended consequences, such as colon perforation in colonoscopy. When risk is involved with the preventive strategy, weigh the procedure in light of the patient's history and other medical problems. Get the patient's input about whether the preventive measure is right for them.

Individualized risk communication When counseling a patient about screening tests, communication should be based on a person's individual risk factors for a condition (eg age, family history, smoking status, cholesterol level). With some conditions, this can be achieved with decisional aids or using formulae. A Cochrane meta-analysis suggests this kind of individualized approach will 'not necessarily' change behavior, although uptake of screening tests *is* improved. At least this technique promotes dialogue, and dialogue opens doors, minds, and possibilities for choice. *Informed participation* is the aim, not passive acceptance of advice. Improved knowledge, beliefs, and risk perceptions can be achieved with this approach. How clinical evidence is presented can make a difference in certain patient populations. Participatory decision-making is facilitated when the physician:

• Understands the patient's experience and expectations.
• Builds partnership.
• Provides evidence, including a balanced discussion of uncertainties.
• Checks for understanding and agreement.
• Presents recommendations informed by clinical judgment and patient preferences.

Difficult patients

'Unless both the doctor and the patient become a problem to each other, no solution is found.'

Jung's aphorism is untrue for half our waking lives: For an anesthesiologist, there is no need for the patient to become a problem in order for the anesthetic to work. But, as with all the best aphorisms, being untrue is the least of their problems. Great aphorisms signify because they unsettle. Our settled and smug satisfaction at finishing a rotation without any problems is so often a sign of failure. We have kept the chaos at bay, whereas, if we were greater men or women, we would have embraced it. Half our waking professional lives we spend as if asleep, on automatic, following protocols or guidelines to some trite destination—or else we are dreaming of what we could do if we had more time, proper resources, and perhaps a different set of colleagues. But if we had Jung in our pockets, he would be shaking us awake, derailing our guidelines, and saluting our attempts to risk genuine interactions with our patients, however much of a mess we make of it, and however much pain we cause and receive. (Pain, after all, is the inevitable companion to lives led authentically.[1]) To the unreflective doctor, and to all average minds, this interaction is anathema, to be avoided at all costs, because it leads us away from anesthesia, to the unpredictable, and to destinations which are unknown.

So, every so often, try being pleased to have difficult patients: Those who question us, those who do not respond to our treatments, or who complain when these treatments do work. Very often, it will seem that whatever you say, it is wrong: Misunderstood, misquoted, and mangled by the mind you are confronting—perhaps because of fear, loneliness, or past experiences which you can only guess at. If this is happening, shut up—but don't give up. Stick with your patient. Listen to what he or she is saying and not saying. And when you have understood your patient a bit more, negotiate, cajole, and even argue—but don't bully or blackmail ('If you do not let your daughter have the operation she needs, I'll tell her just what sort of a mother you are…'). When you find yourself turning to walk away from your patient, turn back and say, 'This is not going very well, is it? Can we start again?' And don't hesitate to call in your colleagues' help: Not to win by force of numbers, but to see if a different approach might bear fruit. By this process, you and your patient may grow in stature. You may even end up with a truly satisfied patient. And a satisfied **patient is worth a thousand protocols**.

---

1 'Some say that the world is a vale of tears. I say it is a place of soul making'—John Keats—the first medical student to formulate these ideas about pain. They did not do him much good, because he died shortly after expressing them. But his ideas can do us good—perhaps if each day we try at least once for authentic interactions with a patient, unencumbered by professional detachment, research interests, defensive medicine, a wish to show off to our peers, or to get though the day with the minimum of fuss.

Is this new treatment any good?
(Analysis & meta-analysis)

This question frequently arises when reading journals. Not only authors, but *all* clinicians, have to decide what new treatments to recommend, and which to ignore. Evidence-based medicine recognizes two fundamental principles: (1) the physician must assess the strength and validity of the evidence for the new treatment based on a hierarchy; (2) Decision makers must consider the patient's values and trade off the benefits, risks, inconvenience, and costs of alternatives.

Users' Guides to the Medical Literature have been created to help the clinician decide whether the results of a research study will help in the care of their patients. In assessing the use of research, ask the following:

1 Are the results valid? Much must be taken on trust as many statistical analyses depend on sophisticated computing. Few papers, unfortunately, present 'raw' data. Look out for obvious faults by asking:

2 Were comparison groups (experimental and control groups) similar in terms of prognosis and clinical characteristics at the start of the study?

3 Were patients randomized to the comparison groups? Did randomization produce groups that were well matched? Were the treatments being compared carried out by practitioners equally skilled in each treatment?

4 Was the study placebo-controlled? Good research can go on outside the realm of double-blind, randomized trials, but you need to be more careful in drawing conclusions—eg for intermittent symptoms, a bad time (prompting a consultation) is followed by a good time, making any treatment given in the bad phase appear effective. *Regression towards the mean* occurs in many areas, eg repeated BP measurement: Because of transitory or random effects, most people having a high value today will have a less high value tomorrow—and most of those having a low value today will have a less extreme value tomorrow. This concept works at the bedside: If someone who is drowsy after a head injury has a high bp, and the next measurements are higher still, ie no regression to the mean, then this suggests a 'real' effect, such as ↑ ICP.

5 Was the study blinded? In a double blind study, both patients and doctors are unaware of which treatment the patient is having. Could patients, doctors, or those assessing outcome have told which treatment was given, eg by the metabolic effects of the drug?

6 Is the sample large enough to detect a clinically important difference, say a 20% drop in deaths from disease X? If the sample is small, the chance of missing such a difference is high. In order to reduce this chance to less than 5%, and if disease X has a mortality of 10%, >10,000 patients would need to be randomized. If a small trial that lacks power (the ability to detect true differences) does give 'positive' results, the size of the difference between the groups is likely to be exaggerated. This is type I error; a type II error applies to results that indicate that there is no effect, when in fact there is. So beware of quite big trials that purport to show that a new drug is equally effective as an established treatment.

7 How large was the treatment effect and how precisely was it measured?

8 Does the study give a clear, clinically significant answer as well as a statistically significant answer in patients similar to those I treat? Are the likely treatment benefits worth the potential risks and costs if applied in the clinical setting?

9 Is the journal peer reviewed? Experts vet the paper before release (an imperfect process, as they have unknown axes to grind ± competing interests).

10 Has time been allowed for criticism of the research to appear in the correspondence columns of the journal in question?

11 If I were the patient, would I want the new treatment?

12 What have the Centers for Disease Control (CDC) or professional organizations said? Have clinical guidelines been developed as a result of the research findings?

Meta-analyses Systematic merging of similar trials can help resolve contentious issues and explain data inconsistencies. It is quicker and cheaper than doing new studies, and can establish generalizability of research. *Be cautious!* In one study looking at recommendations of meta-analyses where there was a later 'definitive' big trial, it turned out that meta-analyses got it wrong 30% of the time, and 20% of even good meta-analyses fail to avoid bias. Bias can result from pharmaceutical funding or from the meta-analyst's own assumptions about the topic under study.

A well-planned large trial may be worth centuries of uncritical medical practice; but a week's experience on the wards may be more valuable than years reading journals. This is the central paradox in medical education. How can we trust our own experiences knowing they are all anecdotal; how can we be open to novel ideas but avoid being merely fashionable? A stance of wary open-mindedness may serve us best.

Resource allocation and QALYs

Resource allocation: How to decide who gets what There is a perception in the United States that healthcare resources are scarce. When one looks at the availability of organ transplants, critical care beds, home care services, and other potentially beneficial treatments, this appears to be true. Resource allocation is about cutting the healthcare cake—the size of which is *given* based on how much society is willing to expend on healthcare as opposed to other societal priorities.

Making the cake Focusing on how to cut the cake diverts attention from the central issue: How large should the cake be? The answer may be that more needs to be spent on our healthcare services, not at the expense of some other health gain, but at the expense of something else.

Slicing the cake In their daily practices, the majority of physicians will not have to contemplate about the larger picture of how society spends its healthcare dollars. They will have to worry about whether the patient can afford the medication just prescribed, whether a proposed treatment will be covered by the insurance plan, where their patient is on the transplant waiting list, etc. How much the everyday clinician needs to factor allocation of resources into treatment recommendations (ie bedside rationing) is a controversial topic. The physician must resist the temptation to live by the dictum *primum non expendere*, and should stay focused on serving the best interests of the patient. However, it must be recognized that in deciding how to slice the healthcare cake, methods have been developed to find a rational basis for allocating resources. One method used by health economists is the QALY.

What is a QALY? The essence of a QALY (Quality Adjusted Life Year) is that it takes a year of healthy life expectancy to be worth 1, but a year of unhealthy life expectancy is regarded as <1. Its exact value is lower the worse the quality of life of the unhealthy person. If a patient is likely to live for 8yrs in perfect health on an old drug, he gains 8 QALYs; if a new drug would give him 16yrs but at a quality of life rated by him at only 25% of the maximum, he would gain only 4 QALYs. The dream of health economists is to buy the most QALYs for his budget. QALYs *are* helpful in guiding rationing, but problems include accurate pricing, the invidiousness of choosing between the welfare of different patients—and the problem of QALYs not adding up: If a vase of flowers is beautiful, are 10 vases (or QALYs) 10 times as beautiful—or might the scent be overpowering?

The inverse care law and distributive justice

Availability of good medical care tends to vary inversely with the need for it in the population served. This operates more completely where medical care is most exposed to market forces...The market distribution of medical care exaggerates maldistribution of medical resources.

There is much evidence in support of this thesis formulated by Tudor Hart, and there is no doubt that if one wants to make a positive contribution to health, it is no good just discovering pathways, blocking receptors, and inventing drugs. The more this is done, the more urgent the need for distributive justice—that unyielding and perpetually problematic benchmark against which all civilizations must, sometime or other, come to measure themselves.

Psychiatry on medical and surgical wards

Psychopathology is common in colleagues, patients, and relatives.

Current mental state Gently probe a patient's thoughts, as you might explore a new garden. What is in bloom now? Where do those paths lead? What is under that stone? *Focus on:* Appearance; speech (rate; content); affect (withdrawn? anxious? suspicious?); mood; beliefs; hallucinations; orientation; memory (recall of current events, president's name); concentration. Note the patient's insight and degree of your rapport. Observe non-verbal behavior.

Depression This is common, and often ignored, at great cost to well-being. 'I would be depressed in her situation…', you say to yourself, and so you do not think of offering treatment. The usual biological guides (early morning awakening, change in appetite, loss of weight, fatigue, and loss of energy) are common on general wards. *Screening questions for major depression are: 'Are you depressed?'* If so, the follow up question, *'Have you found that you aren't enjoying activities that you normally enjoy doing, or that you have lost interest in doing much?'* If yes to both questions, there is a 95% chance the patient has depression. There may also be guilt and feelings of worthlessness. Do not neglect to ask the patient if they have thought about suicide or have passive death wishes. *Don't think it's not your job to recognize and treat depression.* It is as important as pain. Try to arrange activities to boost the patient's morale and confidence, and encourage social interaction. Communicate your thoughts to other members of the team: Nurses, physical and occupational therapists—as well as the patient's loved ones (if the patient wishes). Among these, your patient may find a kindred spirit who can give insight and support. Counseling, psychotherapy, and/or anti-depressants may be appropriate in some patients. If in doubt, try an antidepressant, and see if it helps.

Alcohol This is a common cause of problems on the ward (both the results of abuse and the effects of withdrawal). P214.

The violent patient Ensure your own and others' safety. Do not try to physically restrain violent patients until adequate help is available (eg hospital security guards). Prevent violence by being aware of its early signs, eg restlessness, earnest pacing, clenched fists, morose silences, chanting, or shouting. Try to keep your own intuitions alert to developing problems. Common causes: *Alcohol intoxication, drugs* (recreational or prescribed), *hypoglycemia, acute confusional states* (p323). Once help arrives, try to talk with the patient to calm them—and to gain an understanding of their mental state. Find a nurse who knows the patient. Assess for causes of delirium by measuring oxygen saturation level and blood glucose, or give IV dextrose stat (p726). If not hypoglycemic, before further investigation is possible, drugs may be needed, eg haloperidol ~2mg IM; monitor vital signs closely.

If a rational adult refuses vital treatment, it may be as well to respect this decision, provided they are 'competent', ie they are able to understand the consequences of their actions and what you are telling them, they are able to retain this information, and they can form the belief that it is true. Decision-making capacity is rarely all or nothing, so don't hesitate to get the opinion of an attending physician or psychiatric consultant. Enlist the persuasive powers of someone the patient respects and trusts.

Physical restraints Familiarize yourself with hospital policies, local procedures, and laws pertaining to the use of physical restraints. Consider sitters and chemical restraints before resorting to physical restraints. A confused, violent patient may need to be physically restrained to prevent harm to themselves or others. Reevaluate the need for restraints periodically.

Death: Diagnosis and management

Death is Nature's master stroke, albeit a cruel one, because it allows geno-
types space and opportunity to try on new phenotypes. Our bodies and
minds are these perishable phenotypes—the froth, on the wave of our genes.
These genes are not really our genes. It is us who belong to them for a few
decades. As our neurofibrils begin to tangle, and a neonate walks to a wis-
dom that eludes us, we are forced to give Nature credit for her daring idea.
Of course, Nature, in her haphazard way, can get it wrong: People often die
in the wrong order (one of our chief roles is to prevent this misordering of
deaths, not the phenomenon of death itself).

Causes of death Homicide, suicide, accident, or natural causes.

Diagnosing death The pronouncement of death is an important responsibility of the physician. The physical exam done to diagnose death is a key
symbolic ritual that brings closure to the patient's life and closure for the
physician, members of the healthcare team, and most especially the patient's
family. Death is determined by the absence of pulse and respirations, no
auscultated heart sounds, and fixed pupils.

If a patient is on a ventilator, brain death may be diagnosed even if the heart
is still beating, via *brain death criteria* which entail the irreversible absence of
brain function, particularly in the brainstem. Death of the brainstem is recognized by establishing the absence of cranial nerve and respiratory reflexes.
The Uniform Determination of Death Act recognizes that death can be
diagnosed by neurologic criteria. In addition to evidence of a catastrophic
brain injury, the following prerequisite criteria must be met:

　Deep coma with absent respirations (hence on a ventilator).
　The absence of drug intoxication and hypothermia (<32°C).
　The absence of hypoglycemia, acidosis, hepatic failure, and electrolyte
　imbalance.

Tests: For determination of brain death, the following tests should be performed by qualified personnel. Repeat the tests after a suitable interval—at
least 6h, although sometimes 12–24h is required to confirm irreversibility of
the coma. It is often recommended that a neurologist perform the confirmatory tests.

- Tests to establish that brainstem reflexes are absent:
  - Unreactive pupils. Absent corneal response.
  - No oculocephalic reflex (Doll's eye test).
  - No vestibulo-ocular reflexes, ie no eye movement occurs after or during
    slow injection of 60mL of ice-cold water into each ear canal in turn. Visualize
    the tympanic membrane first to eliminate false negative tests, eg due to wax.
  - No motor response within the cranial nerve distribution should be elic-
    ited by adequate stimulation, eg absent facial grimacing when pressing on
    supraorbital ridge.
  - No gag reflex or response to bronchial stimulation with a catheter to the
    level of the carina.
- Additional tests:
  - No spontaneous or reflex motor responses to noxious stimuli. There
    should also be no autonomic response to noxious stimuli or vagal stimula-
    tion. Spinal reflexes are not relevant to the diagnosis of brain death.
  - Positive Apnea test: No respiratory effort in response to hypercarbia. A
    tube is inserted through the endotracheal tube to the level of the carina in
    order to deliver continuous oxygen at a rate of 2–4L/min. The ventilator is
    disconnected, allowing P_aCO_2 to rise to ≥60mmHg or more (for patients
    with COPD, a rise of 20mmHg above their baseline). P_aCO_2 typically rises at
    a rate of 3mmHg per minute. Patients should be monitored for any hemo-
    dynamic instability during the test, and the test should be stopped if SBP falls
    by ≥20%, cardiac arrhythmias emerge, or the patient becomes hypoxic.

Other considerations: Ancillary studies may be needed when the prerequisite criteria cannot be met, eg the patient is receiving sedative or anesthetic infusions. An EEG recording is not a standard requirement, unless brain death is to be diagnosed within 6h of apparent cessation of brain activity. Cerebral blood flow studies, eg with isotope angiography, are helpful when the patient is receiving treatments that suppress cerebral metabolic activity.

Organ donation: The point of diagnosing brain death is partly that this allows organs (kidney, liver, cornea, heart, or lungs) to be donated and removed with as little damage from hypoxia as possible. Do not avoid the topic with loved ones. Many are glad to give consent and to think that some good can come after the death of their relative, that some part of the relative will go on living, giving a new life to another person.

After death Inform the patient's attending and consultants. Meet with the patient's next of kin and offer emotional support. Ask if they want an autopsy. Autopsy permission may be granted (in order of priority) by: Spouse, adult child, parent, sibling. Sign death certificates promptly. If DOA or within 24h of admission, or the cause is violence, trauma, accident, neglect, surgery, anesthesia, therapeutic mishap, drug/alcohol overdose, suicide, poisoning, or is unknown or suspicious, inform the Coroner/Medical Examiner.

Facing death

People imagine that they are not afraid of death when they think of it while they are in good health (Marcel Proust). So, to get into the mood, as a thought experiment, place a finger in your left supraclavicular fossa, and feel there the craggy node of Virchow, telling of some distant gastric malignancy, as if it were your death warrant. Perhaps you have just 4 months left. Live with this 'knowledge' for the rest of the day, or rest of the week, and see how it changes your attitude to family and friends on the one hand, and the million irrelevances which clutter our minds on the other. As the week unfolds, you may experience thoughts and feelings that are new to you, but all too familiar to your patients. And as the months and years roll by, and you find yourself sitting opposite certain patients, put that finger once more on that metaphorical node and turn it over in your mind, and it will turn you, so you are sitting not opposite your patient but beside him. There is only so much comfort you can bring in this way, as, in the end, you cannot tame death.

Whenever you find yourself thinking *it is better for them not to know,* suspect that you mean: *It is easier for me not to tell.* We find it hard to tell for many reasons: It distresses patients; it may hold up a ward round; we do not like acknowledging our impotence to alter the course of diseases; telling reminds us of our own mortality and may unlock our previous griefs. We use many tricks to minimize the pain: *Rationalization* ('They would not want to know'); *intellectualization* ('Research shows that 37% of people at stage 3 survive 2 years...'); *brusque honesty* ('You are unlikely to survive 1 month' and, so saying, the doctor rushes off to more vital things); *inappropriate delegation* ('The nurse will explain it all to you when you are calmer').

Why it may help the patient to be told:
- The patient already half knows but everyone shies away so they cannot discuss their fears (of pain, or that their family will not cope).
- There may be many affairs for the patient to put in order.
- To enable them to judge if unpleasant therapy is worthwhile.

Most patients are told less than they would like to know.

Breaking bad news Being able to deliver bad news compassionately and effectively is one of the most important skills of the physician. While each discussion must be individualized to the particular patient, some general principles have been recommended. These have been encapsulated in the mnemonic SPIKES[1]:
- *Setting the stage:* Sit down. Arrange for privacy. Avoid interruptions.
- *Patient's perceptions:* What does the patient know about the situation?
- *Invitation for information:* How does the patient want to be given information? Patients may either desire or shun information.
- *Knowledge:* Giving a warning shot before providing information, '*I'm sorry to tell you that ...*' Use language that the patient can understand.
- *Emotions:* Acknowledge emotions and offer empathetic statement, '*I can see that this is upsetting to you.*'
- *Summary and strategy:* Review discussion and set agenda based on goals of care. Address any lingering misunderstanding, uncertainty, or fears.

What are the patient's worries likely to be? Put yourself in the patient's place.
- Give some information, and then the opportunity to ask for more.
- Be sensitive to hints that they may be ready to learn more. 'I'm worried about my son'. 'What is worrying you most?' 'Well, it will be a difficult time for him, (pause) starting school next year.' Silence, broken by the doctor 'I get the impression there are other things worrying you.' The patient now has the opportunity to proceed further, or to stop. Ensure that the patient's personal physician and the nurses know what you have and have not said. Also make sure that this is written in the notes.

1 Baile WF, Buckman R, Lenzi R 2000 *Oncologist* **5** 302–11.

Stages of acceptance Accepting death takes time, and may involve passing through 'stages' on a path. It helps to know where your patient is on this path (but progress is rarely orderly and need not always be forward: The same ground often needs to be covered many times). At first there may be *shock* and *numbness*, then *denial* (which reduces anxiety), then *anger* (which may lead you to dislike your patient, but anger can have positive attributes, eg in energizing people—and it can trump fear and pain; it is different from hostility), then *grief*, and then, perhaps, *acceptance*. Finally there may be intense longing for death as the patient moves beyond the reach of worldly cares.[1]

Living wills/advance directives If a patient has the capacity to make their own decisions, then they should be asked directly what their treatment preferences are. If a patient lacks capacity and their views are known, comply with them. Some patients spell out their views in a written document. But these views change, are ambiguous, or are hard to interpret, even if a living will exists. Living wills only take effect when the patient is terminally ill. In many cases, there can be uncertainty or disagreement about whether to invoke the living will because it is not clear that the patient is 'absolutely, hopelessly ill'.

If a patient desires to complete an advance directive, it is often more preferable to have the patient designate a durable power of attorney for healthcare or healthcare agent—a person who will speak for the patient if the patient is too ill to speak for himself. Designation of a healthcare agent can also be fraught with difficulties, especially if the named surrogate has not had a prior discussion with the patient about their wishes.

Perhaps the best strategy is to focus less on completion of the advance directive form and more on the discussion involved in advance care planning. This will be an ongoing process with the patient, reviewing the goals of care in light of the changing clinical situation and the patient's hopes, fears, prognosis, quality of life, loved ones' wishes, and underlying values.

---

1 JS Bach 1727 *Ich habe genug*, Cantata No. 82 composed for the Feast of the Purification.

Surviving residency

If some fool or visionary were to say that our aim should be to produce the greatest health and happiness for the greatest number of our patients, we would not expect to hear cheering from the tattered ranks of midnight housestaff: Rather, our ears are detecting a decimated groan—because these men and women know that there is something at stake in a housestaff training program far more elemental than health or happiness: Namely survival. Here we are talking about our own survival, not that of our patients. It is hard to think of a greater peacetime challenge than these first months on the wards. Within the first weeks, however brightly your armor shone, it will now be smeared and splattered, if not with blood, then with the fallout from very many decisions that were taken without sufficient care and attention. Not that you were lazy, but *force majeure* on the part of Nature and the exigencies of ward life have, we are suddenly stunned to realize, taught us to be second-rate: For to insist on being first-rate in all areas is to sign a kind of death warrant for many of our patients, and, more pertinently for this page, for ourselves. Perfectionism cannot survive in our clinical world. To cope with this fact, or, to put it less depressingly, to flourish in this new world, don't keep repolishing your armor (what are the 10 causes of atrial fibrillation—or are there 11?), rather furnish your mind—and nourish your body (regular food and drink make those midnight groans of yours less intrusive). Do not voluntarily deny yourself the restorative power of sleep.

We cannot prepare you for finding out that you do not much like the person you are becoming, and neither would we dream of imposing on our readers a recommended regimen of exercise, diet, and mental fitness. Finding out what can lead you through adversity is the art of living. What will you choose: Physical fitness, music, martial arts, poetry, the sermon on the mount, juggling, meditation, yoga, a love affair—or will you make an art form out of the ironic observation of your contemporaries?

Many nourish their inner person through a religious belief, and attend mosque, church, synagogue, or temple. A multicultural society provides diversity and room for all branches of expression. Bear in mind not to compare yourself with your contemporaries. Those who make the most noise are often *not waving but drowning*. Plan your recreation in advance. Start thinking about what you will do after your training and seek out an advisor and mentor in the specialty you select. Such inquiries supply energy to get you through the long, though now limited, hours of residency, and may motivate you if the going gets tough. Not that this is any guarantee that the plans will work, but if your yoga, your sermons, and your fitness regimens turn to ashes in your mouth, then at least you will know the direction in which to spit.

Residency is not just a phase to get through and to enjoy where possible (there are frequently *many* such possibilities); it is also the anvil on which we are beaten into a new and perhaps rather uncomfortable shape. Luckily not all of us are made of iron and steel so there is a fair chance that, in due course, we will spring back into something resembling our normal shape, and, in so doing, we may come to realize that it was our weaknesses, not our strengths, which served us best.

Residency can encompass tremendous up-and-down swings in energy, motivation, and mood, which can be precipitated by small incidents. If you are depressed for more than a day, speak to a sympathetic friend, partner, or counselor to help you put it in perspective. Seek help for your own problems. Find professional help if needed. You are not the best person to plan your assessment, treatment, and referral. When in doubt, communicate.

On being busy: Corrigan's secret door

Unstoppable demands, ↑ expectations as to what medical care should bring, the rising number of elderly patients, coupled with the introduction of new and complex treatments all conspire, it might be thought, to make doctors ever busier. In fact, doctors have always been busy people. Sir Dominic Corrigan was so busy 150yrs ago that he had to have a secret door made in his consulting room so that he could escape from the ever-growing waiting room of eager patients.

We are all familiar with the phenomenon of being hopelessly over-stretched—and of needing Corrigan's secret door. Competing, urgent, and simultaneous demands make carrying out any task left but impossible: The resident is trying to put up an intravenous infusion on a hypotensive patient when his pager goes off. On his way to the phone a patient is falling out of bed, being held in, apparently, only by his visibly lengthening catheter (which had taken the house officer an hour to insert). He knows he should stop to help but, instead, as he picks up the phone, he starts to tell the nurse about 'this man dangling from his Foley' (knowing in his heart that the worst will have already happened). But he is interrupted by a thud coming from the bed of the lady who has just had her occluded left anterior descending artery attended to: However, it is not her, but her visiting husband who has collapsed and is now having a seizure. At this moment a Code Blue is called, summoning him to some other patient. In despair, he turns to the nurse and groans: 'There must be some way out of here!' At times like this we all need Corrigan to take us by the shadow of our hand, and walk with us through his metaphorical secret door, into a calm inner world. To enable this to happen, make things as easy as possible for yourself.

First, however lonely you feel, you are not alone. Do not pride yourself on not asking for help. If a decision is a hard one, share it with a colleague. Second, take any chance you get to sit down and rest. Have a cup of coffee with other members of the staff, or with a friendly patient (patients are sources of renewal, not just devourers of your energies). Third, do not miss meals. If there is no time to go to the cafeteria, ensure that food is put aside for you to eat when you can: Hard work and sleeplessness are twice as bad when you are hungry. Fourth, avoid making work for yourself. It is too easy for physicians in training, trapped in their image of excessive work and black-mailed by misplaced guilt, to remain on the wards following up on patients, rewriting notes, or rechecking lab results at an hour when the priority should be caring for themselves. Fifth, when a bad part of the rotation is looming, plan a good time for when you are off duty, to look forward to during the long nights.

Finally, remember that however busy the call day (and night), your period of duty will end. For you, as for Macbeth:

Come what come may,
Time and the hour runs through the roughest day.

Epidemiology

Gregory P. Prokopowicz, M.D., M.P.H.

Contents

Why epidemiology is relevant to the practicing physician

Epidemiology is the study of the distribution of clinical phenomena in human populations. Clinical epidemiology is the application of epidemiologic methods to the care of the patient. The fruits of clinical epidemiology include: Identification of the causes of disease, prediction of the development of disease and its clinical outcomes, rational use of clinical tests, assessment of the risks and benefits of therapies, and evaluation of screening technologies.

Identification of causes of disease Epidemiologic methods enable one to determine the *risk factors* responsible for disease. The association of smoking with lung cancer, dyslipidemia with coronary artery disease, and hypertension with stroke are examples of the valuable findings of epidemiology with relevance for the practitioner. Novel risk factors, such as C-reactive protein for coronary artery disease and homocysteine for stroke, continue to be identified. The up-to-date physician should have an awareness of how such associations are derived and whether they are likely to be important for clinical care.

Prediction of disease and its clinical outcomes By identifying risk factors, the physician can predict which of his or her patients is most likely to develop disease. Mathematical models, such as the Framingham risk score, can be used to calculate the risk of clinical outcomes in a given patient, and thereby to guide the choice of therapy.

Rational use of clinical tests Laboratory and radiographic tests are a daily part of clinical practice, but few tests provide totally unambiguous results. Quantification of test performance, using sensitivity, specificity, positive and negative predictive values, and likelihood ratios facilitates appropriate selection and interpretation of tests.

Assessment of risks and benefits of therapy Quantitative measures of effect, such as the *number needed to treat*, enable the clinician to accurately weigh the benefits of therapy against any harms, and to compare the cost effectiveness of competing therapies.

Evaluation of screening technologies An ↑ number of investigations may be performed on the healthy patient with the intent of detecting early disease. Emerging technologies, such as multi-slice spiral computed tomography and genetic testing with single nucleotide polymorphisms, will reveal new abnormalities of uncertain significance. Appropriate counseling of the patient with respect to such screening tests requires an understanding of the issues involved.

Evidence-based medicine

This is the conscientious and judicious use of current best evidence from clinical research in the management of individual patients.

The problem Traditionally, the teaching and practice of medicine has relied largely on three sources of knowledge: Pathophysiology, expert opinion, and personal clinical experience. Important limitations have become apparent in these sources of information. Predictions from pathophysiology may not hold in clinical practice; for example, suppression of ventricular ectopy following myocardial infarction with encainide or flecainide led to a surprising ↑ in mortality. Expert opinion may be out of date or biased due to conflict of interest. And personal experience is likely to be unduly influenced by striking clinical outcomes, such as a rare but devastating side effect in a generally safe drug.

The solution Evidence-based medicine (EBM) directs the physician to be aware of the quality of the information on which his or her practice is based, and to conscientiously choose the most reliable sources. This presupposes a *hierarchy of evidence*, ie a ranking of types of information according to susceptibility to bias and chance effects. Such hierarchies generally place RCTs at the highest tier, followed by observational studies, then unsystematic clinical observations, pathophysiologic reasoning, and expert opinion. *Meta-analyses* and *systematic reviews* are often given even greater credence than RCTs, although this depends on the quality of the review.

27

The four steps of EBM *Formulate the clinical question.* The first step is to focus our sometimes vague uncertainty into a question that can be answered. The acronym PICO may be of help: What sort of *Patient* are we considering; what is the *Intervention* we are contemplating; to what alternative can we *Compare* the intervention, and what *Outcomes* are important for our patient? *Search the literature.* The practice of EBM optimally requires access to computerized literature sources such as PubMed. Time spent learning appropriate search techniques, eg by using the tutorials, will pay off with better results. *Appraise the literature that you have found.* Here we are interested in the validity of the study, the results of the study, and the applicability to our patient. *Apply the findings to the individual patient.* In applying the findings to our particular patient we must consider our patient's unique clinical characteristics and values.

Criticisms of EBM Searching the primary literature and assessing its validity in the context of a busy clinical practice is difficult. In response, proponents of EBM have suggested the use of *pre-appraised literature sources*, such as ACP PIER, Clinical Evidence, Up-To-Date, and the journals *Evidence-Based Medicine* and *ACP Journal Club*. These resources provide clinically relevant summaries of the primary literature and obviate the laborious critical appraisal of individual papers by the clinican. In addition, tools for winnowing out the clinically useful articles from the morass of medical literature have been developed; these including literature filters and selective email notification services.

The suggestion has been made that EBM is primarily a means of controlling costs by denying what would otherwise be considered appropriate care. While certain techniques of EBM may be used to this end, the principles of EBM do not require that the least expensive alternative be chosen, and evidence-based practice guidelines have not invariably resulted in lower costs. Perhaps the most significant criticism of EBM is that it has never itself been subject to the sort of rigorous evaluation that it espouses for other therapies. Specifically, we do not know if physicians who adhere closely to the principles of EBM have better patient outcomes than those who do not. Proponents of EBM point to studies showing that expert opinions voiced in traditional review articles may lag behind evidence from the latest studies, and that patients receiving therapies for which there is good evidence do better than those who do not. But these are indirect measures of the effectiveness of EBM; direct comparisons of EBM practitioners with non-EBM practitioners, either in the form of RCTs or observational studies, are lacking.

Associations and causality

Association Epidemiological research is concerned with comparing rates of disease in populations with different exposures, eg rates of lung cancer in a population of men who smoke, compared with men who do not. A difference in rates suggests an *association* between the disease and the exposure (in this case, smoking). The search for meaningful associations may be complicated by the presence of *confounders*, ie factors that are related to both the exposure and the disease. For example, an apparent association between alcohol use and lung cancer may simply reflect the fact that both are related to tobacco use. Associations may also be due simply to chance. The strength of an association is expressed as the *risk ratio*, ie the risk of developing the disease among those with the exposure, divided by the risk of developing the disease among those without the exposure.

Prevalence and incidence In order to compare rates of disease between groups, standard measures of disease occurrence are used. *Prevalence* is the number of cases of disease present in a defined population divided by the total number of people in that population. Since it is not usually practical to count an entire population at once, the *period prevalence* is often given, indicating that the measurement took place over a period of time. For example, the prevalence of obesity in the US (BMI > 30) during the 1999–2002 NHANES survey period was 30%. *Lifetime prevalence* is the proportion of a population that has *ever* experienced the condition of interest, and *point prevalence* is the proportion with the condition at a given point in time. For example, the lifetime prevalence of headache in women has been reported at 99%, and the point prevalence at 22%.

Incidence is the number of new cases occurring in a defined population that is initially free of the disease, over a specified time period, eg the incidence of breast cancer among U.S. women from 1998–2002 was 134 per 100,000 (SEER cancer statistics review).

Observational studies Associations are often discovered using *observational studies*. Such studies are distinguished from experimental studies or *clinical trials* in that the investigator does not control the exposure; she or he merely observes the subjects who are exposed and those who are not and records the outcomes occurring in each group. Observational studies usually take one of three forms:

1 *Cohort (prospective) studies:* The group, or cohort, consisting of subjects exposed to the suspected causal factor (eg smoking) is followed alongside a control group consisting of subjects not exposed. The incidence of the disease is compared between the groups over the duration of the study. Because the exposure information is recorded as it occurs, cohort studies do not have recall bias. However, they can be very expensive and time-consuming, particularly for diseases with low incidence rates.

2 *Case-control (retrospective) studies:* The study group consists of those with the disease (eg lung cancer); the control group consists of those without the disease. The previous occurrence of the exposure (eg smoking) is compared between each group. Case–control studies are particularly useful for the investigation of rare diseases, but they suffer from recall bias: Inaccuracy in the subjects' reporting of the exposure (eg smoking).

3 *Cross-sectional studies:* The population of interest is surveyed for the presence of both the exposure and the disease at the same time. This design is usually quick and inexpensive, and provides prevalence data, but it may not enable the investigator to determine whether the exposure preceded development of the disease, since both are measured at the same time.

Establishing causality The finding of an association between an exposure and a disease does not prove that the exposure causes the disease. Reports abound in the media of supposed links between various foods and worsened or improved health; which will turn out to be valid? Sir Austin Bradford Hill, a British epidemiologist, recognized this problem in the context of evaluating occupational hazards, and proposed nine criteria for establishing causality. These are:

1 *Strength of the association* Does the disease occur *much* more frequently among the exposed than among the unexposed, such as with lung cancer, or is it only slightly more common?

2 *Consistency* Does the relation hold across different studies in different populations?

3 *Specificity* Is the exposure the only potential cause of the disease, or vice versa? This is not required for causality, but when present it strengthens the argument.

4 *Temporality* Does the cause precede the effect?

5 *Dose response* Does a greater exposure lead to a greater risk of disease?

6 *Plausibility* Is there a plausible biologic mechanism to explain the causality?

7 *Coherence* Does the cause-and-effect relation fit with histopathology and other information about the disease?

8 *Experiment* Does alteration of the exposure, if possible, result in a change in frequency of outcome?

9 *Analogy* Is there a similar disease known to be caused by a similar exposure?

Risk of disease and its outcomes

As physicians, we are frequently called upon to prognosticate. Our patients want to know: Should I be worried about this cough? Is my cholesterol low enough? How long am I going to be in the hospital? Application of epidemiologic principles can help answer these questions.

Which is more likely: An uncommon manifestation of a common disease or a common manifestation of an uncommon disease? When we consider the significance of a new symptom reported by a patient, we are engaging in a process of risk stratification. Is the sudden, stabbing mid-back pain reported by this 65-year-old diabetic with hypertension likely to be from muscle strain? Myocardial infarction? Aortic dissection? In formulating a diagnosis, we estimate the likelihood of various diseases in our patient and also consider how commonly each disease would present with the symptoms we see in front of us. Proper use of epidemiology can guide our application of this information to the patient. Consider the development of angioedema in a person taking an ACE inhibitor. Angioedema is a rare symptom with ACE inhibitor use (seen in 0.1–0.2% of patients), but is commonly seen in patients with C1 inhibitor deficiency (perhaps 90% of such patients). C1 inhibitor deficiency itself is rare, occurring in only about one in 50,000 in the general population. If a patient on an ACE inhibitor develops angioedema, should we check for C1 inhibitor deficiency? We may intuitively feel that it is a reasonable part of a comprehensive evaluation of angioedema. However, the probability of our patient having ACE-inhibitor induced angioedema is 0.1–0.2%, whereas the probability that he or she has C1 inhibitor is 0.9 × 1/50,000 or 0.0018%. It is thus 50–100 times more likely that our patient's angioedema is due to the ACE inhibitor.

Doctors as gamblers Medical decision making can be seen as a form of gambling. For example, a busy physician might see 20 patients in an afternoon session. How should she or he decide which symptoms to monitor expectantly and which to investigate until a cause is found? Some patients may offer 5 separate symptom groups in the course of a single visit. Full elucidation of these symptoms might reveal additional complaints, leading to a potentially endless cycle of investigation. Certainly some of these complaints might not seem too serious ('this pain in my toe…'). But on reflection, even toe pain might be dangerous if caused by emboli or osteomyelitis. Similarly, fingernail problems with a slight rash might mean arsenic poisoning, lethargy may mean cancer, and so on. Since almost any symptom can be seen as a manifestation of some fatal illness, an attitude of excessive pessimism is to be avoided, as it would lead to many sleepless nights for the doctor and much excessive testing for the patient. On the other hand, an attitude of complacency or blind optimism would be no better and might be worse, resulting in missed diagnoses. Rather, **the physician should be a shrewd gambler,** able to use subtle clues to change his or her outlook from pessimism to optimism and vice versa. Sometimes the approach is scientific, relying on quantitative estimates of the probability of disease just as the poker player calculates the probability of filling an inside straight. But sometimes it is intuitive, as when the gambler reads the face of his opponent, or the physician relies on her gut sense that something is 'not right' about the appearance of a patient, a sense that may be invaluable even if it cannot be expressed in words or numbers.

Calculation of the risk of disease outcomes

Epidemiologic investigations have enabled the practitioner to calculate a patient's overall risk based on the presence or absence of several individual risk factors. For example, the **Framingham Risk Calculator** permits an assessment of cardiac risk. It uses age, total cholesterol, HDL cholesterol, blood pressure, diabetes, and smoking status to calculate the 10-year risk of coronary heart disease.

Patient 62-year-old smoker with total cholesterol of 242, HDL cholesterol of 41, BP 148/90, not diabetic.

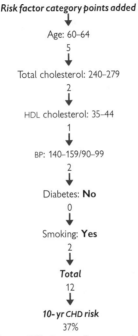

Risk factor category points added
↓

Age: 60–64

5
↓

Total cholesterol: 240–279

2
↓

HDL cholesterol: 35–44

1
↓

BP: 140–159/90–99

2
↓

Diabetes: **No**

0
↓

Smoking: **Yes**

2
↓

Total

12
↓

10- yr CHD risk

37%

This patient thus has a 37% chance of coronary heart disease (stable angina, unstable angina, myocardial infarction, and coronary heart disease death).

http://hin.nhlbi.nih.gov/atpiii/calculator.asp

31

Evaluation of diagnostic tests

Only rarely does a single test provide a definitive diagnosis. More often, tests alter our assessment of the likelihood of a condition being present. When taking a history and examining patients, we estimate (consciously or unconsciously) how likely various diagnoses are. The results of testing modify those estimates. A test is worthwhile if it alters the post-test probability (ie the likelihood that a patient has disease, given the test results), and if the results affect our management of the patient.

Basic test statistics All tests have false positives and false negatives, as summarized below:

	Patient has the condition	Patient does not have the condition
Test result is positive	True positive (*a*)	False positive (*b*)
Test result is negative	False negative (*c*)	True negative (*d*)

For tests with a dichotomous outcome (ie positive or negative), the following statistics are commonly used:

Sensitivity: The proportion of people with disease who test positive: (a/a+c).

Specificity: The proportion of people without disease who test negative: (d/d+b).

Positive predictive value: The proportion of people testing positive who have the disease: (a/a+b).

Negative predictive value: The proportion of people testing negative who do not have the disease: (c/c+d).

In addition to the above, the *likelihood ratio* (LR) is quite useful, because it does not require that the test have a dichotomous outcome (ie be limited to one of two values).

Likelihood ratio: The likelihood of having the given test result if the patient *has* disease, divided by the likelihood of having the same result if the patient *does not have* disease. The mnemonic WOWO (With Over WithOut) may be helpful. For example, the likelihood ratio for iron deficiency anemia with a serum ferritin of 15–24 is 8.8. This means that the likelihood of seeing a ferritin in the range of 15 to 24 is 8.8 times greater in patients with iron deficiency than in those without. Furthermore, the likelihood ratio for a ferritin of 45–99 is 0.54. This means that it is almost 50% *less* common to obtain a ferritin of 45–99 in a patient with iron deficiency than in a patient without iron deficiency.

Advantages of the likelihood ratio (LR) There are two major advantages to using likelihood ratios. The first is that they enable us to take into account the exact value of a test result, rather than simply classifying it as positive or negative. This is in accord with how we practice medicine. For example, a patient with chest pain and a troponin I of 20ng/mL will certainly get our attention more than one with a troponin of 0.6ng/mL, despite the fact that both would be reported as 'positive' in a lab that uses a cutoff value of 0.5. In this case, the LR for myocardial infarction associated with a troponin of 20ng/mL would be much higher than the LR for a troponin of 0.5ng/mL. The traditional test statistics (sensitivity, specificity, and positive and negative predictive values) treat all tests as either positive or negative and lose the important information carried by extreme values.

The second advantage to LRs is that they can be used to calculate a post-test probability, even when multiple tests are used in sequence. This uses the formula:

Pre-test odds × LR(test result) = post-test odds

To use this formula, one must convert between probability and odds using the formulas:

Odds = probability/(1−probability)
Probability = odds/(1+odds)

Handy pocket-card nomograms are available to apply these formulas without having to do the actual calculations.

Using likelihood ratios Assume you are faced with a patient with ascites and abdominal discomfort. You are considering the diagnosis of spontaneous bacterial peritonitis (SBP). After examining the patient, you estimate the chance that she has SBP to be low, about 20%. You perform a paracentesis, and find 600 PMNs/uL. How does this affect the likelihood that she has SBP?

Number of PMNs in ascitic fluid	Likelihood ratio
>1000	22.3
501–1000	2.78
251–500	1.14
0–250	0.08

Pre-test odds = 0.2/(1− 0.2) = 0.25
Post-test odds = 0.25 × 2.78 = 0.695

Post-test probability = 0.695/(1 + 0.695) = 0.41

Thus, our new estimate is that she has about a 40% probability of SBP. Had the fluid shown >1000 PMNs, the post-test probability would have been 85%.

The effectiveness of therapy

While some therapies have gained general acceptance through dramatic uncontrolled demonstrations, eg insulin for diabetes or penicillin for streptococcal infection, most modern therapies require a comparison with a control group to demonstrate safety and effectiveness. This can sometimes be accomplished using an observational study, such as a cohort study. However, to minimize bias, *controlled clinical trials* are preferred.

Experimental studies In contrast to observational studies, *experimental studies* or *clinical trials* involve active assignment by the investigator of subjects to the treatment under consideration.

Randomized controlled trials (RCTs): Assignment to the treatment and control groups is performed randomly to avoid selection bias and help ensure that the two groups do not differ with respect to confounding factors. This is generally felt to be the optimal design for assessing the effect of therapeutic interventions.

Comparability of groups In both cohort studies and RCTs, it is desirable that the two groups be similar to one another with respect to all factors that could affect the outcome, except for the intervention being studied. In large RCTs, random assignment makes this likely to occur, but the reader should still check to see that the two groups are comparable. If they are not, adjustment procedures such as matching, stratification, or multivariate analysis may be used.

Allocation concealment In RCTs, assignment to treatment or control is done without advance knowledge by the investigator or the subject

Blinding Following randomization, it is often desirable to prevent the subjects and members of the study team from knowing who is receiving treatment and who is receiving placebo. This helps minimize bias in the measurement of the outcome, and equalizes the placebo effect between the two groups.

Outcome measures If the risk of dying from an MI after 'standard treatment' is 10%, and a new treatment reduces this to 8%, then the relative risk is 0.8, ie 8/10 and the relative risk reduction is 20% [(10 – 8/10) × 100%]. While this may sound impressive, it is important to also consider the absolute risk reduction (ARR), which is 10% – 8% = 2%. Thus, if 100 people with MI receive the drug, only ~2 would be expected to derive benefit. This may also be expressed as the number needed to treat, which is calculated as (1/ARR), with ARR expressed as a fraction rather than a percent. In this example the NNT would be 1/0.02 = 50; thus, one would need to treat 50 people to prevent one death from MI.

If the outcome being studied is rare, the NNT may be quite high. For example, in some preventive studies of mild hypertension in the young, ~800 people may need to be treated to prevent one stroke. Furthermore, if one were to compare a new antihypertensive regimen to an older one, with the NNT for the older treatment being 800 and the new treatment only marginally better, the NNT to prevent one death or stroke *by adopting the new regimen in place of the old* might be several thousand. The implication is that adoption of the new treatment, if it is more expensive than the old, is not likely to be cost-effective.

Intention-to-treat analysis Despite the best efforts of the investigators, some subjects inevitably fail to follow the study protocol. What should be done with patients assigned to the control group who wind up taking the treatment, and vice versa? One option is to analyze the subjects according to what they actually did in the study, ie if a subject did not adhere to the treatment plan, they should be lumped in with the control group. Similarly, if a subject who was assigned to control opted to use the therapy, they should be analyzed as part of the treatment group. This is called *on treatment analysis*, and it has a certain plausibility. However, it is now common practice to analyze subjects according to the group to which they were randomized, regardless of whether they stuck with the study plan. This is known as *intention-to-treat analysis*, and offers the following advantages:

• The initial comparability of groups produced by randomization is preserved.
• The results reflect imperfect adherence and are therefore more like what will happen when the intervention is used in actual practice.
• Outcomes such as death which may or may not be due to the therapy or control will not be overlooked.

Examples of NNTs

Study	Outcome	NNT
Statins for 1° prevention	Death (MI)	931 (78) for 5yrs
Statins for 2° prevention	Death (MI)	30 (15) for 5.4yrs
Mild hypertension	Stroke	850 for 1yr
Systolic hypertension in elderly	Stroke	43 for 4.5yrs
Aspirin in acute MI	Death	40
Streptokinase in acute MI	Death	40
ACE-i for CHF (NYHA class IV)	Death	6 for 1yr

Screening

Screening is defined as the application of a test to detect a potential disease or condition in a person who has no known signs or symptoms of that disease, so that treatment might be more effective, less expensive, or both; or with the aim of identifying and modifying risk factors to prevent disease.[1]

Because screening is applied to a generally healthy population, most of whom will not benefit from the screening (because they would not have developed the disease regardless), extra care must be taken to ensure that the screening is worthwhile.

Wilson and Jungner criteria for screening[2]

1 The condition being sought should be an important health problem, for the individual and the community.
2 There should be an acceptable form of treatment for patients with identified disease.
3 The natural history of the condition, including its development from latent to declared disease, should be adequately understood.
4 There should be a recognizable latent or early symptomatic stage.
5 There should be a suitable screening test or examination for detecting the disease at the latent or early symptomatic stage, and this test should be acceptable to the population.
6 The facilities required for diagnosis and treatment of patients revealed by the screening program should be available.
7 There should be an agreed policy on whom to treat as patients.
8 Treatment at the pre-symptomatic, borderline stage of a disease should favorably influence its course and prognosis.
9 The cost of case-finding (which would include the cost of diagnosis and treatment) needs to be economically balanced in relation to possible expenditure on medical care as a whole.
10 Case-finding should be a continuing process, not a 'once and for all' project.

Biases Assessment of screening programs may reveal the following problems:

Lead-time bias Patients who are screened for asymptomatic disease may simply find that they are being diagnosed earlier, even if the early diagnosis does nothing to improve their ultimate prognosis. If the success of the screening program is measured in 5-yr survival from the time of diagnosis, one may get the incorrect impression that screening is helping patients when it is not.

Length bias Cases of indolent disease, such as slow-growing prostate cancers, are more likely to be discovered on routine screening, because they remain in the population for a longer time. Because such cases have a generally better prognosis, studies that use survival from time of diagnosis as the outcome will find benefit among patients who are screened over those who are not.

Overdiagnosis bias In the extreme case, some patients may harbor cancers (eg of the prostate, kidney, or thyroid) that would never have caused symptoms during their natural life. Identification and removal of such 'cancers' is not helpful to the patient and may cause harm.

1 Modified from Eddy D 2004 How to Think About Screening. *In Screening for Diseases: Prevention in Primary Care.* ACP Press.
2 Wilson JMG, Jungner G 1968 *Principles and Practice of Screening for Disease.* World Health Organisation, Geneva.

Examples of effective screening	Unproven/ineffective screening
Papanicolau smears for cervical cancer	Chest radiograph for lung cancer
Mammography for breast cancer	Urinalysis for diabetes or kidney disease
Colonoscopy for colorectal adenomas	Digital rectal exam and PSA for prostate cancer
Blood pressure for hypertension	Total body CT scanning

NB: Screening for cervical cancer and mammography (p386) are far from perfect—both are susceptible to false negatives, and a negative result might lead that patient to take risks or be inattentive to signs of disease occurring between screenings.

Clinical skills

Jeffrey L. Magaziner, M.D.

Contents

The way to learn physical signs is at the bedside, with guidance from an experienced colleague. This chapter is not intended as a substitute for this process: It is simply an aid.

We ask questions to get information to help with differential diagnosis. But we also ask questions to find out about the inner life and past exploits of our patients so that we can respect them as individuals and understand them as a whole. The patient is likely to notice and reciprocate this respect, and this reciprocation is the foundation of most of our therapeutic endeavors. The message is not that special people should get special services: Rather that it is easy to like, and hence promote the interests of, patients with whom you can identify. The challenge is to identify with as broad a range of humanity as possible, without getting exhausted by this task.

Principle sources: *Clinical Examination*: A systematic guide to physical diagnosis, 5ᵗʰ edn, NJ Talley and S O'Connor (2005) London: Elsevier, *Aids to Undergraduate Medicine*, 6ᵗʰ edn, JL Burton and BJL Burton (1997), Churchill Livingstone.

The patient now waiting for you in room 9...

The first news of your next patient will often be via a phone call 'There's an MI on the way in'—or 'There's someone delirious in room 9'—or 'Can you take the overdose in room 12?' On hearing such sanitized dehumanized descriptions, our minds will start painting pictures, and the tone of these messages have the habit of coloring these pictures. So when we arrive at the bedside, our mind is far from a *tabula rasa* or blank canvas on which the patient can paint his woes.

The mind is always painting pictures, filling in gaps—and falling into traps. Perception is an active process, for, as Marcel Proust, that life-long all-knowing patient, observed[1]:

> We never see the people who are dear to us save in the animated system, the perpetual motion of our incessant love for them, which before allowing the images that their faces present to reach us catches them in its vortex, flings them back upon the idea that we have always had of them, makes them adhere to it, coincide with it.

So if you want to know your patient, take snapshots of him from various angles, and briefly contemplate him in the round before Proust's vortex whisks you off track. You can prepare for these snapshots in the blink of an eye, saying to yourself: 'When I open my eyes I'm going to see my patient face to face' and in that clinical blink, divest yourself of those prejudices and expectations which all good diagnosticians somehow ignore. When you open your eyes you will be all set for a Gestalt recognition of incipient myxedema (the cause of the delerium in room 9), jaundice, anemia, or, perhaps more importantly, the recognition that the person in front of you is frightened, failing, or dying.

---

1 *The Guermantes Way* **i** p187 trans. CK Scott Moncrieff.

Taking a history

Taking (or receiving) histories is what most of us spend most of our professional life doing: It is worth doing it well. An accurate history is the biggest step in making the correct diagnosis. History-taking, examination, and treatment of a patient begin the moment one reaches the bedside. (The divisions imposed by our page titles are somewhat misleading.) Try to put the patient at ease: A good rapport may relieve distress on its own. It often helps to shake hands. Please do so gently, for if they have an underlying arthritis a 'normal' grasp may be quite uncomfortable. Always introduce yourself. Check whether the patient is comfortable. Be conversational rather than interrogative in tone. General questions (age, occupation, marital status) help break the ice and help assess mental functions.

Chief complaint (CC) 'What has been the trouble recently?' Record the patient's own words rather than medical shorthand, eg short of breath rather than 'dyspnea'.

History of presenting illness (HPI) When did it start? What was the first thing noticed? Progress since then? Ever had it before? **PQRST Questions:** Provocative/palliative factors, Quality of pain (sharp/burning/deep/aching), Region/radiation, Severity (scale of 1 to 10, 10 being childbirth), Timing (duration and sequence with other symptoms).

Style of questioning At first, questions should be open-ended. Once a differential diagnosis begins to crystallize, specific directed questions about the diagnoses you have in mind (+ its risk factors, eg travel—p502) and a review of the relevant system can be asked.

Past medical history (PMH) Ever hospitalized? Illnesses? Operations? Ask specifically about diabetes, asthma, hypertension, heart disease, stroke, epilepsy, peptic ulcer, anesthetic problems.

Drug history (DH) Any tablets, injections? Any 'over-the-counter' drugs? Herbal remedies, oral contraceptives? Ask the features of allergies; it may not have truly been one.

Family history (FH) Age, health, and cause of death, if known, of parents, siblings, and children; ask about TB, diabetes, and other relevant diseases. Areas of the FH may need detailed questioning, eg to determine if there is a significant FH of heart disease you need to ask about the health of the patient's grandfathers and siblings, smoking, hypertension, hyperlipidemia, and peripheral vascular disease before they were 60yrs old, as well as ascertaining the cause of death.

Social history (SH) Probe without prying. 'Who else is there at home?' Job, marital status, spouse's job and health. Housing—any stairs at home? Who visits—relatives, neighbors, visiting nurse? Mobility—any walking aids needed? Who does the cooking and shopping? What can the patient not do because of the illness? The SH is all too often seen as a dispensable adjunct, eg while the patient is being rushed to the OR. But vital clues may be missed about the quality of life and it is too late to ask when the surgeon's hand is deep in the belly and he or she is wondering how radical a procedure to perform.

Alcohol, recreational drugs, tobacco How much? How long? When stopped? The CAGE questionnaire is useful as a screening test for alcoholism (p67). Quantify smoking in terms of *pack-years*: 20 cigarettes smoked per day for 1yr equals 1 pack year. Don't make assumptions about substance use based on age or other demographic information: All patients should be screened.

Review of systems (ROS) To uncover undeclared symptoms. Some of this may already have been incorporated into the history.

Don't hesitate to retake the history after a few days: Recollections change.

Drawing family trees to reveal dominantly inherited disease

Advances in genetics are touching all branches of medicine. It is increasingly important for doctors to identify patients at high risk of genetic disease, and to make appropriate referrals. The key skill is drawing a family tree to help you structure a family history as follows:

1 Start with your patient. Draw a square for a male and a circle for a female. Add a small arrow (►see below) to show that this person is the *propositus* (the person through whom the family tree is ascertained).

2 Add your patient's parents, brothers, and sisters. Record basic information only, eg age, and if alive and well (a&w). If dead, note age and cause of death, and pass an a diagonal line through that person's symbol.

3 Ask the key question 'Has anybody else in your family had a similar problem as yourself?', eg heart attack/angina/stroke/cancer. Ask only about the family of diseases that relate to your patient's main problem. Do not record a full medical history for each family member: Time is too short.

4 Extend the family tree upwards to include grandparents. If you haven't revealed a problem by now, go no further—you are unlikely to miss important familial disease. If your patient is elderly it may be impossible to obtain good information about grandparents. If so, fill out the family tree with your patient's uncles and aunts on both the mother's and father's sides.

5 Shade those in the family tree affected by the disease. ● = an affected female; ■ = an affected male. This helps to show any genetic problem and, if there is one, will help demonstrate the pattern of inheritance.

6 If you have identified a familial susceptibility, or your patient has a recognized genetic disease, extend the family tree down to include children, to identify others who may be at risk, and who may benefit from screening. You must find out who is pregnant in the family, or may soon be, and arrange appropriate genetic counseling.

The family tree below shows these ideas at work and indicates that there is evidence for genetic risk of colon cancer.

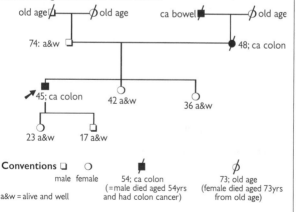

Conventions

□ male   ○ female

■ 54; ca colon
(=male died aged 54yrs
and had colon cancer)

⌀ 73; old age
(female died aged 73yrs
from old age)

a&w = alive and well

This page owes much to Dr Helen Firth, who we thank

41

Review of systems

The review of systems often seems like an endless list of questions when one is first learning how to take a history. However, it is an important safety net to identify issues the clinician may have forgotten to ask about or the patient forgot to mention. With increasing experience, the review of systems can often be parsed down and greatly expedited.

General questions may be the most significant, eg in identifying TB, endocrine problems, or cancer: • Weight loss • Night sweats • Any lumps • Fatigue • Sleeping pattern • Appetite • Fevers • Itch • Recent trauma.

Cardiorespiratory symptoms Chest pain. Exertional dyspnea (=breathlessness; quantify exercise tolerance *and how it has changed*: Eg stairs climbed, or distance walked, before onset of breathlessness). Paroxysmal nocturnal dyspnea. Orthopnea, ie breathlessness on lying flat (a symptom of left ventricular failure: Quantify in terms of number of pillows the patient must sleep on to prevent dyspnea). Edema. Palpitations (awareness of heartbeats). Cough. Sputum. Hemoptysis (coughing up blood). Wheezing.

Gut symptoms Abdominal pain (constant or colicky, sharp or dull; site; radiation; duration; onset; severity; relationship to eating and bowel action; alleviating/exacerbating, or associated features). Other questions—think of symptoms throughout the GI tract, from mouth to anus:

- Swallowing
- Indigestion
- Nausea/vomiting
- Bowel habit
- Stool:
  - color, consistency, blood
  - difficulty flushing away
  - tenesmus or urgency

Tenesmus is the feeling that there is something in the rectum which cannot be passed (eg due to a tumor). Hematemesis is vomiting blood. Melena is altered (black) blood passed PR, with a characteristic smell.

Genitourinary symptoms Incontinence (stress or urge). Dysuria (painful micturition). Hematuria (bloody urine). Nocturia (needing to urinate at night). Frequency (frequent urination) or polyuria (passing excessive amounts of urine). Hesitancy (difficulty starting urination). Terminal dribbling.

Vaginal discharge. Menses: Frequency, regularity, heavy or light, duration, painful. First day of last menstrual period (LMP). Number of pregnancies. Menarche. Menopause. Any chance of pregnancy now?

Neurological symptoms *Special senses:* Sight, hearing, smell, and taste. Seizures, fainting. Headache. 'Pins and needles' (paresthesiae) or numbness. Weakness ('Do your arms and legs work?'), poor balance. Speech problems. Sphincter disturbance. Higher mental function and psychiatric symptoms. The important thing is to assess function: What the patient can and cannot do at home, work, etc.

Musculoskeletal symptoms Pain, stiffness, swelling of joints. Diurnal variation in symptoms (ie with time of day). Functional deficit.

Thyroid symptoms *Hyperthyroidism:* Prefers cold weather, ill-tempered, sweaty, diarrhea, oligomenorrhea, weight loss (though often ↑ appetite), tremor, palpitations, visual problems. *Hypothyroidism:* Depressed, slow, tired, thin hair, hoarseness, heavy periods, constipation, dry skin, prefers warm weather.

History-taking may seem deceptively easy, as if the patient knew the hard facts and the only problem was extracting them; but what a patient says is a mixture of hearsay ('she said I looked very pale'), innuendo ('you know, doctor, down below'), legend ('I suppose I bit my tongue; it was a real seizure, you know'), exaggeration ('I didn't sleep a wink'), and improbabilities ('The Pope put a transmitter in my brain'). The great skill (and pleasure) in taking a history lies not in ignoring these garbled messages, but in making sense of them.

Physical examination

With a few exceptions (eg BP), physical examination is not a good screening test for detecting undisclosed disease. Plan your examination to emphasize the areas that the history suggests may be abnormal. A few well-directed, problem-orientated minutes can save hours of fruitless, but very thorough, physical examination. You will still be expected to examine all 4 major systems (cardiovascular, respiratory, abdominal, and neurological), but with time you will be adept at excluding any major undisclosed pathology. Practice is the key.

Look at your patient as a whole to decide how sick he or she seems to be. Do they appear well or *in extremis*? Try to decide *why* you think so. Are they in pain and does it make them lie still (eg peritonitis) or writhe about (eg colic)? Is breathing labored and rapid? Are they obese or cachectic? Is behavior appropriate? Can you detect any unusual **smell** eg hepatic fetor, cigarettes, alcohol?

Specific diagnoses can often be made from **the face and body habitus** and these may be missed unless you stop and consider them: Eg acromegaly, thyrotoxicosis, myxedema, Cushing's syndrome, or hypopituitarism. Is there an abnormal distribution of body hair (eg bearded ♀, or hairless ♂) suggestive of endocrine disease? Is there anything to trigger thoughts about Paget's disease, Marfan's, myotonia, and Parkinson's syndrome? Look for rashes, eg the malar flush of mitral disease and the butterfly rash of lupus.

Assess the degree of **hydration** by examining the skin turgor, the axillae, and mucus membranes. Sunken orbits may also occur in dehydration. Check peripheral perfusion. Record the temperature, and BP (lying and standing may be compared to identify postural hypotension, a sign of volume depletion).

Check for **cyanosis** (central and peripheral, p72). Is the patient **jaundiced**? Yellow skin is unreliable and may resemble the lemon tinge of uremia, pernicious anemia, or carotenemia (sclerae are not yellow). The sign of jaundice is yellow sclerae seen in good daylight. **Pallor** is a nonspecific sign and may be racial, familial, or cosmetic. **Anemia** is assessed from the palmar skin creases and conjunctivae—usually pale if Hb <8–9g/dL: You cannot conclude anything from *normal* conjunctival color; but if they are pale, the patient is probably anemic. Koilonychia and stomatitis (redness around the mouth, particularly at its lateral edge) suggest iron-deficiency. Anemia with jaundice suggests malignancy or hemolysis. Pathological **hyperpigmentation** is seen in Addison's, hemochromatosis (slate-grey) and amiodarone, gold, and minocycline therapy.

Palpate for **lymph nodes** in the neck (from behind), axillae, groins, epitrochlear region, and abdomen. Any **subcutaneous nodules** (p78)?

Don't forget to look at the results of **urinalysis** and **urine output charts** where indicated. Look at the **temperature chart**. Average temperature values are 36.8°C (mouth), 36.4°C (axilla), 37.3°C (rectum). *Hypothermia* is defined as a temperature <35°C; special thermometers may be needed to measure temperatures below this level. A morning[1] temperature ≥37.3°C (mouth) or >37.7°C (rectum) constitutes a *fever*. Note the periodicity of any fever. Do not always believe the temperature chart—if you suspect that the patient has a fever (eg by back-of-the-hand on the forehead), take the temperature yourself.

---

[1] The nadir is at 6 AM; with a zenith at 6 PM; the mean amplitude of variability is 0.5°C.

The hands

A wealth of information can be gained from gently shaking hands and rapidly examining the hands of the patient. Are they warm and well-perfused? Warm, sweaty hands may signal hyperthyroidism while cold, moist hands may be due to anxiety. Are the rings tight with edema? Lightly pinch the dorsum of the hand—persistent ridging of the skin suggests loss of tissue turgor ie dehydration. Are there any nicotine stains? Does the patient have difficulty shaking your hand (rheumatoid arthritis, p368)? Reluctance to let go is also a sign of loneliness.

Nails *Koilonychia (spoon-shaped nails)* suggests iron deficiency (also fungal infection or Raynaud's). *Onycholysis (destruction of nails)* is seen with hyperthyroidism, fungal nail infection, and psoriasis. *Beau's lines* are transverse furrows that signify temporary arrest of nail growth and occur with periods of severe illness. As nails grow at ~0.1mm/d, by measuring distance from the cuticle it may be possible to date the stress. *Mees' lines* are single white, transverse bands sometimes seen in arsenic poisoning or renal failure. *Muehrcke's lines* are paired white, parallel transverse bands sometimes seen in hypoalbuminemia. *Terry's nails:* Proximal portion of nail is white/pink, nail tip is red/brown (causes: Cirrhosis, chronic renal failure). *Pitting* is seen in psoriasis & alopecia areata.

Splinter hemorrhages are fine longitudinal hemorrhagic streaks (under nails), which in the febrile patient may suggest infective endocarditis. They may be normal—being caused, eg by gardening, when their subconjunctival correlates will be *absent*.

Nail-fold infarcts are characteristically seen in vasculitic disorders.

Clubbing of the nails occurs with many disorders p72. There is an exaggerated longitudinal curvature and loss of the angle between the nail and the nail-fold (ie no dip). Also the nail feels 'boggy'. The cause is unknown but may be due to ↑ blood flow through multiple arteriovenous shunts in the distal phalanges.

Chronic paronychia is a chronic infection of the nail-fold and presents as a painful swollen nail with intermittent discharge. Treatment: Keep nails dry; antibiotics, eg erythromycin 250mg/6h PO and nystatin ointment.

Changes occur in **the hands** in many diseases. *Palmar erythema* is associated with cirrhosis, pregnancy, and polycythemia. *Pallor* of the palmar creases suggests anemia. *Pigmentation* of the palmar creases is normal in Asians and Blacks but is also seen in Addison's. An odd rash on the knuckles (Gottron's papules) with dilated end-capillary loops at the nail-fold suggests dermatomyositis (p376). *Dupuytren's contracture* (fibrosis and contracture of palmar fascia) is seen in liver disease, trauma, epilepsy, and ageing. Swollen proximal interphalangeal (PIP) joints with distal (DIP) joints spared suggests rheumatoid arthritis; swollen DIP joints suggests osteoarthritis, gout, or psoriatic arthritis. Look for *Heberden's* (distal) and *Bouchard's* (proximal) 'nodes' (osteophytes—bone overgrowth at a joint—seen with osteoarthritis).

45

The cardiovascular system

History Ask about age, occupation, hobbies, sport, and ethnic origin.

Presenting symptoms	*Risk factors for CVD*
Chest pain	Smoking
Dyspnea—exertional?	Hypertension
orthopnea? PND?	Diabetes mellitus
Ankle swelling	Hyperlipidemia
Palpitations; dizziness; blackouts	Family history[1] (cardiovascular disease)
Past history	*Past tests and procedures:*
Angina or MI	ECG Echocardiography
Rheumatic fever	Angiograms Stress tests
Intermittent claudication	Angioplasty/stents CABG (bypass grafts)

Appearance Ill or well? In pain? Dyspneic? Are they pale, cold, and clammy? Is there corneal arcus or xanthelasma (hyperlipidemia)? Is there a malar flush (mitral stenosis, low cardiac output)? Are there signs of Graves' disease (bulging eyes, goiter—p280)? Is the face dysmorphic, eg Down's syndrome, Marfan's syndrome—or Turner's, Noonan's, or William's syndromes? Can you hear the click of a prosthetic valve?

Hands Finger clubbing occurs in congenital cyanotic heart disease and endocarditis. Splinter hemorrhages, Osler's nodes (tender nodules in finger pulps) and Janeway lesions (red macules on palms) are signs of infective endocarditis. If found, examine the fundi for Roth's spots (retinal infarcts). Are there nail-fold infarcts (vasculitis) or nailbed capillary pulsation (Quincke's sign, aortic regurgitation)? Is there arachnodactyly (Marfan's) or polydactyly (ASD)? Are there tendon xanthomata (hyperlipidemia)?

Pulse see p48

Blood pressure The *systolic* blood pressure is the pressure at which the pulse is first heard as the cuff is deflated; the *diastolic* is when the heart sounds disappear (Korotkov sound K5) or become muffled (K4—use, eg in the young who often have no K5; state which you use). The *pulse pressure* is defined as the difference between systolic and diastolic. It is narrow in aortic stenosis and wide in aortic regurgitation. Examine the fundi for hypertensive changes. *Shock* may occur if systolic <100mmHg. *Postural hypotension* is defined as a drop in systolic >15mmHg or diastolic >10mmHg on standing.

Jugular venous pressure see p48

Precordium Inspect for *scars*: Median sternotomy (CABG or valve replacement). Inspect for any pacemakers. Palpate the *apical beat*. Normal position: 5th intercostal space in the mid-clavicular line. Is it displaced laterally? Is it abnormal in nature: *Heaving* (mitral or aortic regurgitation, VSD), *thrusting* (aortic stenosis), *tapping* (mitral stenosis), *diffuse* (LV failure, dilated cardiomyopathy) or *double impulse* (HOCM)? Is there dextrocardia? Feel for *left parasternal heave* (RV enlargement eg in pulmonary stenosis, cor pulmonale, ASD) or *thrills* (transmitted murmurs).

Auscultating the heart see box OPPOSITE.

Lungs Examine the lung bases for crackles and pleural effusions, indicative of cardiac failure.

Edema Examine the ankles, legs, sacrum, torso for pitting edema.

Abdomen Hepatomegaly and ascites may occur in right-sided heart failure. Pulsatile hepatomegaly occurs with tricuspid regurgitation. Splenomegaly may occur with infective endocarditis.

Peripheral pulses Palpate radial, brachial, carotid, femoral, popliteal, dorsalis pedis, and posterior tibial pulses. Feel for *radio-femoral* (coarctation of the aorta) and radio-radial delay (eg from aortic arch aneurysm). Auscultate for *bruits* over the carotids and elsewhere, particularly if there is inequality between pulses or absence of a pulse. Causes: Atherosclerosis (elderly), vasculitis.

---

1 1st degree relative <60yrs of age.

Auscultating the heart

If you spend time listening to the history, and feeling pulses, auscultation should hold few surprises: You will often already know the diagnosis.

- Listen with bell and diaphragm at the apex (mitral area). Identify 1st and 2nd *heart sounds*: Are they normal? Listen for *added sounds* (p50) and *murmurs* (p52). Repeat at lower left sternal edge and in aortic and pulmonary areas (right and left of manubrium)—and in both the left axilla (radiation of mitral regurgitation) and over the carotids (radiation of aortic stenosis).
- Reposition the patient in the left lateral position: Again feel the apical beat (is it tapping, as in mitral stenosis?) and listen specifically for a diastolic rumble of mitral stenosis. Sit the patient up and listen at the lower left sternal edge for the blowing diastolic sound of aortic regurgitation—accentuated at the end of expiration.

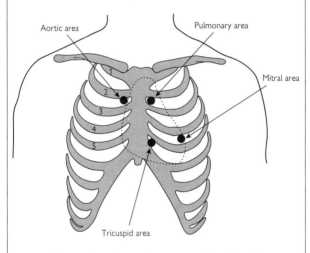

Locations for auscultating heart valve murmurs. After *Clinical Examination* 4th edn, N Talley and S O'Connor (2002), Blackwell Science.

The jugular venous pressure

The internal jugular vein acts as a manometer of right atrial pressure. Observe two features: The *height* (jugular venous pressure, JVP) and the *waveform* of the pulse. JVP observations are often difficult. Do not be downhearted if the skill seems to elude you. Keep on watching necks, and the patterns you see may slowly start to make sense.

The height Observe the patient at 45°, with his head turned slightly to the left. Look for the right internal jugular vein, which passes just medial to the clavicular head of sternocleidomastoid up behind the angle of the jaw to the ear lobes. The JVP is the vertical height of the pulse above the sternal angle. It is raised if >5cm. Pressing on the liver normally produces a transient rise in the JVP. If the rise persists throughout a 15sec compression, it is a *positive hepatojugular reflux sign* (or abdominojugular reflux when pressure is applied to the center of the abdomen) This is a sign of right ventricular failure, reflecting inability to eject the ↑ venous return.

The jugular venous waveform See BOX.

Abnormalities of the JVP

Raised JVP with normal waveform: Fluid overload, right heart failure.

Raised JVP with absent pulsation: SVC obstruction.

Large a wave: Pulmonary hypertension, pulmonary stenosis.

Cannon a wave: When the right atrium contracts against a closed tricuspid valve, large 'cannon' *a* waves result. *Causes:* Complete heart block, atrial flutter, single chamber ventricular pacing, ventricular arrythmias/ectopics.

Absent a wave: Atrial fibrillation.

Large systolic v waves: Tricuspid regurgitation—look for earlobe movement.

Constrictive pericarditis: High plateau of JVP (which rises on inspiration—Kussmaul's sign) with deep x and y descents.

Pulses

Assess the radial pulse to determine *rate* and *rhythm*. *Character* and *volume* are best assessed at the brachials or carotids. A *collapsing pulse* may also be felt at the radials when the patient's arm is elevated above his head.

Rate Is the pulse tachycardic (>100bpm) or bradycardic (<60bpm)?

Rhythm An irregularly irregular pulse occurs in AF or multiple ectopics. A regularly irregular pulse occurs in 2° heart block and ventricular bigeminy.

Character and volume

Bounding pulses are caused by CO_2 retention, liver failure, and sepsis.

Small volume pulses occur in aortic stenosis, shock, and pericardial effusion.

Collapsing pulses are caused by aortic incompetence, AV malformations, hyperdynamic circulation and patent ductus arteriosus.

Anacrotic (slow-rising) pulses occur in aortic stenosis.

Bisferiens pulses occur in combined aortic stenosis and regurgitation.

Pulsus alternans (alternating strong and weak beats) suggests LVF, cardiomyopathy, or aortic stenosis.

Jerky pulses occur in HOCM.

Pulsus paradoxus (systolic pressure weakens in inspiration by >10mmHg) occurs in severe asthma, pericardial constriction, or cardiac tamponade.

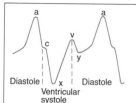

• a wave:	atrial systole
• c wave:	closure of tricuspid valve, not normally visible
• x descent:	fall in atrial pressure during ventricular systole
• v wave:	atrial filling against a closed tricuspid valve
• y descent:	opening of tricuspid valve

The jugular venous pressure wave. After *Clinical Examination* 4th edn, ed Macleod, Churchill Livingstone.

Distinguishing arterial and venous pulses

In distinguishing venous from arterial pulses, note that the venous pulse:
• Is not usually palpable.
• Is obliterated by finger pressure on the vein.
• Rises transiently following pressure on the abdomen (*abdominojugular reflux*) or on the liver (*hepatojugular reflux*).
• Alters with changes in posture and respiration.
• Usually has a double pulse for every arterial pulse.

Arterial pulse waveforms

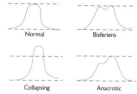

Typical arterial pulse waveforms. After *Aids to Undergraduate Medicine* 6th edn, J Burton, Churchill Livingstone.

Measuring blood pressure

• Use the correct size cuff. The width of the cuff should be at least 40% of the arm circumference. The bladder should be centered over the brachial artery, and the cuff applied snugly. Support the arm in a horizontal position at mid-sternal level.
• Inflate the cuff while palpating the brachial artery, until the pulse disappears. This provides an estimate of systolic pressure.
• Inflate the cuff until 30mmHg above systolic pressure, then place stethoscope over the brachial artery. Deflate the cuff at 2mmHg/s.
• *Systolic pressure:* The appearance of sustained repetitive tapping sounds (Korotkoff I).
• *Diastolic pressure:* Usually the disappearance of sounds (Korotkoff V). However, in some individuals (eg pregnant women) sounds are present until the zero-point. In this case, the muffling of sounds, Korotkoff IV, should be used.

The heart sounds

Listen systematically: Sounds then murmurs. While listening, palpate the carotid artery: S_1 is synchronous with the upstroke.

The heart sounds The 1st and 2nd sounds are usually clear. Confident pronouncements about other sounds and soft murmurs may be difficult. Even senior colleagues disagree with one another about the more difficult sounds and murmurs.

The 1st heart sound (S_1) represents closure of mitral (M_1) and tricuspid (T_1) valves. Splitting in inspiration may be heard and is normal.

In mitral stenosis, because the narrowed valve orifice limits ventricular filling, there is no gradual decrease in flow towards the end of diastole. The valves are therefore at their maximum excursion at the end of diastole, and so shut rapidly leading to a loud S_1 (the 'tapping' apex). S_1 is also loud if diastolic filling time is shortened eg if the P–R interval is short, and in tachycardia.

S_1 is soft if the diastolic filling time is prolonged eg if the P–R interval is long, or if the mitral valve leaflets fail to close properly (ie mitral regurgitation). The intensity of S_1 is variable in AV block, atrial fibrillation, and nodal or ventricular tachycardia.

The 2nd heart sound (S_2) represents aortic (A_2) and pulmonary valve (P_2) closure. The most important abnormality of A_2 is softening in aortic stenosis. A_2 is said to be loud in tachycardia, hypertension, and transposition, but a loud A_2 is probably not a useful clinical entity.

P_2 is loud in pulmonary hypertension and soft in pulmonary stenosis. *Splitting* in inspiration is normal and is mainly due to the variation with respiration of right heart venous return, causing the pulmonary component to move. *Wide splitting* occurs in right bundle branch block, pulmonary stenosis, deep inspiration, mitral regurgitation, and VSD. *Wide fixed splitting* occurs in ASD. *Reversed splitting* (ie splitting ↑ on expiration) occurs in left bundle branch block, aortic stenosis, PDA (patent ductus arteriosus), and right ventricular pacing. A single S_2 occurs in Tetralogy of Fallot, severe aortic or pulmonary stenosis, pulmonary atresia, Eisenmenger syndrome, large VSD, hypertension. NB: Splitting is heard best in the pulmonary area.

A *3rd heart sound (S_3)* may occur just after S_2. It is low pitched and best heard with the bell of the stethoscope. S_3 is pathological over the age of 30yrs. A loud S_3 occurs in a dilated left ventricle with rapid ventricular filling (mitral regurgitation, VSD) or poor LV function (post MI, dilated cardiomyopathy). In constrictive pericarditis or restrictive cardiomyopathy it occurs early and is more high pitched ('pericardial knock').

4th heart sound (S_4) occurs just before S_1. It represents atrial contraction against a ventricle made stiff by any cause, eg aortic stenosis, or hypertensive heart disease.

Triple and gallop rhythms A 3rd or 4th heart sound occurring with a sinus tachycardia may give the impression of galloping hooves. An S_3 gallop sounds like 'Ken-tucky', whereas an S_4 gallop sounds like 'Tenne-ssee'. When S_3 and S_4 occur in a tachycardia, eg with pulmonary embolism, they may summate and appear as a single sound, a summation gallop.

An *ejection systolic click* is heard early in systole with bicuspid aortic valves, and if BP↑. The right heart equivalent lesions may also cause clicks.

Mid-systolic clicks occur in mitral valve prolapse.

An *opening snap* precedes the mid-diastolic murmur of mitral stenosis. It indicates a pliable (noncalcified) valve.

Prosthetic sounds are caused by nonbiological valves, on opening and closing. *Rumbling sounds* usually indicate ball and cage valves (eg Starr–Edwards); *singing clicks* usually indicate tilting disc valve (eg single disc: Bjork Shiley; bileaflet: Jude—usually quieter).[1]

---

1 Prosthetic mitral valve clicks occur in time with S_1, aortic valve clicks in time with S_2.

The cardiac cycle

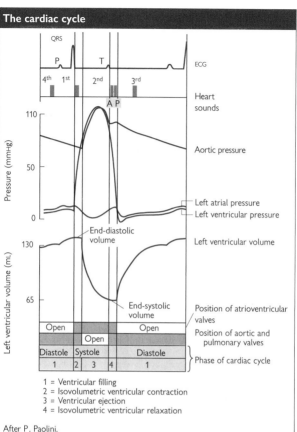

QRS

P   T

ECG

4th 1st   2nd   3rd   Heart sounds

A P

Aortic pressure

Left atrial pressure
Left ventricular pressure

End-diastolic volume   Left ventricular volume

End-systolic volume   Position of atrioventricular valves

Open | Open   Position of aortic and pulmonary valves

Open

Diastole | Systole | Diastole   Phase of cardiac cycle

1 | 2 | 3 | 4 | 1

1 = Ventricular filling
2 = Isovolumetric ventricular contraction
3 = Ventricular ejection
4 = Isovolumetric ventricular relaxation

After P. Paolini.

51

Cardiac murmurs

Always consider other symptoms and signs before auscultation and think: What do I expect to hear? However, don't let your expectations determine what you hear.

Use the stethoscope correctly. The bell is good for low-pitched sounds (eg mitral stenosis) and should be applied gently to the skin. The diaphragm filters out low pitches, making higher pitched murmurs easier to detect (eg aortic regurgitation). NB: A bell applied tightly to the skin becomes a diaphragm.

Consider any murmur in terms of *character, timing, loudness, area where loudest, radiation,* and *accentuating maneuvers*.

When in doubt, rely on echocardiography rather than disputed sounds.

Character and timing A *systolic-ejection murmur* (SEM, crescendo–decrescendo) usually originates from the outflow tract and waxes and wanes with the intraventricular pressures. SEMs may be innocent and are common in children and high output states (eg tachycardia, pregnancy). Organic causes include aortic stenosis and sclerosis, pulmonary stenosis, and HOCM.

A *pansystolic murmur* (PSM) is of uniform intensity and merges with S_2. It is usually organic and occurs in mitral or tricuspid regurgitation (S_1 may also be soft in these), or a ventricular septal defect. Mitral valve prolapse may produce a late systolic murmur ± midsystolic click.

Early diastolic murmurs (EDM) are high pitched and easily missed: Listen for the 'absence of silence' in early diastole. An EDM occurs in aortic and, though rare, pulmonary regurgitation. If the pulmonary regurgitation is secondary to pulmonary hypertension, which is itself due to mitral stenosis, then the edm is called a Graham Steell murmur.

Mid-diastolic murmurs (MDM) are low pitched and rumbling. They occur in mitral stenosis (accentuated presystolically if heart still in sinus rhythm), rheumatic fever (Carey Coombs' murmur: Due to thickening of the mitral valve leaflets), and aortic regurgitation (Austin Flint murmur: Due to the fluttering of the anterior mitral valve cusp caused by the regurgitant stream).

Intensity Systolic murmurs are graded on a scale of 1–6 (see BOX). Diastolic murmurs, being less loud, are graded 1–4. Intensity is a poor guide to the severity of a lesion—an esm may be inaudible in severe aortic stenosis.

Area where loudest Though an unreliable sign, mitral murmurs tend to be loudest over the apex, in contrast to the area of greatest intensity from lesions of the aortic (right 2nd intercostal space), pulmonary (left 2nd intercostal space) and tricuspid (left sternal edge) valves.

Radiation The SEM of aortic stenosis classically radiates to the carotids, in contrast to the PSM of mitral regurgitation which radiates to the axilla.

Accentuating maneuvers *Movements* that bring the relevant part of the heart closer to the stethoscope accentuate murmurs (eg leaning forward for aortic regurgitation, left lateral position for mitral stenosis).

Expiration ↑ blood flow to the left-side of the heart and therefore accentuates left sided murmurs; *inspiration* has the opposite effect.

The *Valsalva maneuver* (forced expiration against a closed glottis) ↓ systemic venous return, accentuating mitral valve prolapse and HOCM, but softening mitral regurgitation and aortic stenosis. Squatting has exactly the opposite effects. *Exercise* accentuates mitral stenosis.

Non-valvular murmurs A *pericardial friction rub* may be heard in pericarditis. It is a superficial scratching sound, not confined to systole or diastole. *Continuous murmurs* are present throughout the cardiac cycle and may occur with a patent ductus arteriosus, arteriovenous fistula, or ruptured sinus of Valsalva.

Common heart murmurs

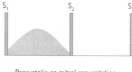

– Ejection-systolic eg aortic stenosis

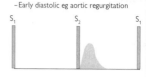

– Early diastolic eg aortic regurgitation

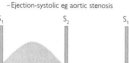

– Pansystolic eg mitral regurgitation

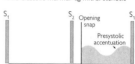

– Mid-diastolic murmur eg mitral stenosis

Opening snap
Presystolic accentuation

Grading intensity of heart murmurs

The following grading is commonly used for systolic murmurs:

Grade 1/6:   Very soft, only heard after listening for a while
Grade 2/6:   Soft, but detectable immediately
Grade 3/6:   Clearly audible, but no thrill palpable
Grade 4/6:   Clearly audible, palpable thrill
Grade 5/6:   Audible with stethoscope only partially touching chest
Grade 6/6:   Can be heard without placing stethoscope on chest

The respiratory system

History Age, race, occupation.

Presenting symptoms
- *Cough:* Duration? Character (eg brassy/barking/hollow)? Nocturnal
  (see box) (asthma)? Exacerbating factors? Sputum/hemoptysis?
- *Dyspnea* Duration? Steps climbed/distance walked before onset? NYHA
  classification (p127)? Diurnal variation (≈asthma)?
- *Hoarseness* • eg due to laryngitis, recurrent laryngeal nerve palsy, singer's
  nodules, or laryngeal tumor.
- *Fever/night sweats* (p75) • *Chest pain* (p88) • *Wheeze* (p56) • *Stridor* (p81)

Past history Pneumonia/bronchitis? TB? Atopy (asthma/eczema/hay fever)?
Previous CXR abnormalities? Lung surgery?

Family history Atopy? Emphysema? TB?

Social history Quantify smoking in terms of pack-years (20 cigarettes/day
for 1yr = 1 pack-year). Occupational exposure (farming, mining, asbestos
exposure)? Animals at home (eg birds)? Recent travel/TB contacts?

Drug history Respiratory drugs (eg steroids, bronchodilators)? Any other
drugs, especially those with respiratory side-effects (eg ACE inhibitors, cytotoxics, beta-blockers, amiodarone)?

Examination Undress to the waist, and sit patient on the edge of the bed.

Inspection Assess *general health*: Are they diseased? Cachectic? Using accessory muscles of respiration, eg sternocleidomastoids, platysma, and strap
muscles of the neck (infrahyoid)? Are there signs of respiratory distress? Is
there stridor (p81)? Count the *respiratory rate* and note *breathing pattern*. Is
there Kussmaul's (rapid, deep respiration, p77) or Cheyne–Stokes (apnea
alternating with hyperpnea, p71) breathing? Look for *chest wall deformities*.
Inspect the chest for scars of past surgery, chest drains, or radiotherapy (skin
thickening and tattoos demarcating the field of irradiation). Note *chest wall
movement*: Is it symmetrical? If not, pathology is on the restricted side. Is
there paradoxical respiration (abdomen sucked in with inspiration; seen in
diaphragmatic paralysis)?

Examine the hands for *clubbing* (p72), peripheral cyanosis, nicotine staining, and wasting/weakness of the intrinsic muscles—seen in T1 lesions (eg
Pancoast, p166). Palpate the wrist for tenderness (hypertrophic pulmonary
osteoarthropathy, HPOA, from lung cancer). Check for *asterixis* (CO_2 retention flap). Palpate the pulse for obvious *paradox* (weakens in inspiration;
quantify in mmHg by measuring BP in inspiration and expiration).

Inspect the face Check for the ptosis and constricted pupil of Horner's syndrome (eg Pancoast). Are the tongue and lips bluish (central cyanosis)?

Feel the trachea in the sternal notch (it should pass just to the right).
If deviated, concentrate on the upper lobes for pathology. Note the presence
of *tracheal tug* (descent of trachea with inspiration, suggesting severe airflow
limitation). Palpate for *cervical lymphadenopathy* from behind, with the
patient sitting forward.

Examining the chest If an abnormality is detected, try to localize it to the
likely segment (see BOX).

Further examination Look at the JVP (p48) and examine the heart for signs
of *cor pulmonale* (p188). Look at *temperature charts*. Inspect the *sputum* (see
BOX). Check peripheral O_2 saturation.

Respiratory distress occurs when high negative intrapleural pressures are
needed to generate air entry. Signs include: Tachypnea, nasal flaring, tracheal
tug, the use of accessory muscles of respiration, intercostal, subcostal, and
sternal recession, and pulsus paradoxus (fall in systolic BP by >10mmHg during
inspiration).

Characteristic coughs

Coughing is a relatively nonspecific symptom, resulting from irritation anywhere from the pharynx to the lungs. The character of a patient's cough may, however, give some clues as to the underlying cause:

Loud, brassy coughing suggests pressure on the trachea eg by a tumor.

Hollow, 'bovine' coughing is associated with recurrent laryngeal nerve palsy.

Barking coughs occur in acute epiglottitis.

Chronic cough: Think of pertussis, TB, foreign body, asthma (eg nocturnal).

Dry, chronic coughing may occur following acid irritation of the lungs in esophageal reflux, and as a side-effect of ACE inhibitors.

Do not ignore a change in character of a chronic cough; it may signify a new problem eg infection, malignancy.

Sputum examination

Always inspect any sputum produced. Send suspicious sputum for microscopy (Gram stain) culture, and cytology.

Black carbon specks in the sputum suggests smoking, the most common cause of ↑ sputum production.

Yellow/green sputum suggests infection eg bronchiectasis, pneumonia.

Pink frothy sputum suggests pulmonary edema.

Bloody sputum (hemoptysis) may be due to malignancy, TB, infection, or trauma, and requires investigation for these causes.

Clear sputum is probably saliva.

The respiratory segments supplied by the segmental bronchi

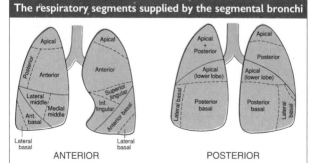

Examining the chest

Inspection Look for deformities of the spine (kyphoscoliosis) or chest wall (pectus excavatum or carinatum, p71), or scars from surgery. Count respiratory rate, note use of accessory muscles of respiration.

Palpation *Lymphadenopathy:* Check for cervical lymphadenopathy from behind, with the patient sitting forward. *Tracheal position:* Is it central or displaced to one side (towards an area of collapse, away from a large pleural effusion or tension pneumothorax; slight deviation to the right is normal). *Expansion:* Use both hands to compare chest expansion on both sides; expansion <5cm on deep inspiration is abnormal. Reduced expansion implies pathology on that side. Test *tactile fremitus* by asking the patient to repeat '99' while palpating the chest wall over different respiratory segments, comparing similar positions over each lung in turn. ↑ tactile fremitus implies consolidation, but is less sensitive than vocal resonance (p83).

Percussion Percuss symmetrical areas of the anterior, posterior, and axillary regions of the chest wall. When percussing posteriorly, move the scapulae out of the way by asking the patient to move his elbows forward across his chest. Do not forget to percuss the supraclavicular fossa (lung apices). *Causes of a dull percussion note:* Collapse, consolidation, fibrosis, pleural thickening, or pleural effusion (classically stony dull). The *cardiac dullness* is usually detectable over the left side of the chest. The *liver dullness* usually extends up to the fifth rib, right mid-clavicular line; if the chest is resonant below this level, it is a sign of lung hyperexpansion (eg asthma, emphysema). *Causes of a hyperresonant percussion note:* Pneumothorax or hyperinflation (COPD).

Auscultation Listen with the diaphragm over symmetrical areas of the anterior, posterior, and axillary regions of the chest wall, and use the bell to auscultate over the supraclavicular fossae. Consider breath sounds in terms of *quality, intensity*, and the *presence of additional sounds*.

Quality and intensity Normal breath sounds have a rustling quality and are described as vesicular. *Bronchial breathing* has a hollow quality; there may be a gap between inspiration and expiration. Bronchial breath sounds occur where normal lung tissue has become firm or solid, eg consolidation, localized fibrosis, above a pleural effusion, or next to a large pericardial effusion (Ewart's sign). It may be associated with ↑ tactile fremitus, vocal resonance, and whispering pectoriloquy (p83). *Diminished breath sounds* occur with pleural effusions, pleural thickening, pneumothorax, bronchial obstruction, asthma, or COPD. *The silent chest* occurs in life-threatening asthma and is due to severe bronchospasm which prevents adequate air entry into the chest.

Added sounds *Wheezes* are caused by air passing through narrowed airways. They may be monophonic (a single note, signifying a partial obstruction of one airway, eg tumor) or polyphonic ('My chest sounds like a load of cats'—multiple notes, signifying widespread narrowing of airways of differing caliber, eg asthma, COPD). Wheezes may also be heard in left ventricular failure ('cardiac asthma'). *Crackles (crepitus, rales)* are caused by the reopening, during inspiration, of the small airways which have become occluded during expiration. They may be fine and high pitched if coming from distal air spaces (eg pulmonary edema, fibrosing alveolitis) or coarse and low pitched if they originate more proximally (eg bronchiectasis). The timing of crackles is important; early crackles suggest small airways disease (eg COPD), whereas late/paninspiratory crackles suggest disease confined to the alveoli. Crackles that disappear on coughing are insignificant. *Rhonchi* are low pitched variable sounds that can be heard in a wide variety of pulmonary pathology and are therefore nonspecific. *Pleural rubs* are caused by movement of the visceral pleura over the parietal pleura, when both surfaces are roughened, eg by an inflammatory exudate. Causes include adjacent pneumonia, pulmonary infarction. *Pneumothorax click* is produced by shallow left pneumothorax between the 2 layers of parietal pleura over-lying the heart and is heard during cardiac systole.

Specialized Maneuvers *Egophony* The patient says 'e' and in listening to the chest wall the sound produced is 'a'. Caused by consolidation resulting in alteration of frequency of transmitted sounds to the chest wall *Bronchophony* is intensification of volume of spoken words in areas of consolidation. *Whispered pectoriloquy* is similar to bronchophony, but the patient whispers and the words are audible only over areas of consolidation.

Gastrointestinal history

Presenting symptoms
Abdominal pain
Nausea, vomiting, hematemesis
Dysphagia (p194)
Indigestion (dyspepsia, p196)
Recent change in bowel habit
Diarrhea or constipation
Rectal bleeding (p80) or melena
Appetite, weight change
Mouth ulcers; jaundice (p202)
Pruritus; Dark urine, pale stools
Social history
Smoking, alcohol
Overseas travel, tropical illnesses
Contact with jaundiced persons
Occupational exposures
Sexual orientation.

Past history
Peptic ulcer
Carcinoma
Jaundice, hepatitis
Blood transfusions, tattoos
Previous operations
Last menstrual period, LMP
Past treatment
Steroids, the Pill
NSAIDs; antibiotics
Dietary changes
Family history
Irritable bowel disease
Inflammatory bowel disease
Peptic ulcer
Polyps, cancer
Jaundice.

Examining the gastrointestinal system

Inspect (and smell) for signs of chronic liver disease:
- Hepatic fetor on breath (p210)
- Purpura (purple stained skin)
- Spider nevi
- Leuconychia (hypoalbuminemia)
- Gynecomastia
- Scratch marks
- (pruritus)
- Palmar erythema
- Clubbing (rare)
- Muscle wasting
- Jaundice
- Liver flap (asterixis, a coarse irregular tremor seen in hepatic failure)

Inspect for signs of malignancy, anemia, jaundice, hard Virchow's node in left supraclavicular fossa. Look at the abdomen. Note:
- Visible pulsation (aneurysm)
- Striae (stretch marks, eg pregnancy)
- Peristalsis
- Distension
- Scars
- Genitalia
- Masses
- Hernia.

If abdominal wall veins look dilated, assess *direction of flow*. In inferior vena caval (IVC) obstruction, flow below the umbilicus is up; in portal hypertension (*caput medusae*), it is down. *The cough test:* While looking at the face, ask the patient to cough. If this causes abdominal pain, flinching, or a protective movement of hands towards the abdomen, suspect peritonitis.

Genitourinary history

Presenting symptoms
Fever, groin pain, dysuria, hematuria
Urethral/vaginal discharge
Sex—any problems? Painful intercourse
  (dyspareunia)
Menses: Menarche, menopause, length of
  periods, amount, pain? intermenstrual
  loss? 1st day of last period (LMP)?

Past history
Urinary tract infection
Renal colic
DM, BP↑, gout, analgesic use
Previous operations.
Social history
Smoking
Sexual orientation.

Detecting outflow obstruction (eg from prostatic hypertrophy). Ask:
When you want to urinate, is there delay before you start? (*Hesitancy*)
Does the flow stop and start? Do you go on dribbling when you think you've stopped, even after giving it a good shake? (*Terminal dribbling*)
Is your stream getting weaker? Can you hit the wall OK? (*Poor stream*)
Do you ever urinate when you do not want to? (*Incontinence*)
Do you feel the bladder is not empty after urinating? On feeling an urge to urinate, do you have to go at once? (*Urgency*) Do you urinate often at night? (*Nocturia*) In the day? How often? (*Frequency*).

Palpating and percussing the abdomen

Adjust the patient so that he or she is lying flat, with their head resting on only 1 pillow, and their arms at their side. Make sure that the patient and your hands are warm.

Palpation While palpating, be looking at their face to assess any pain. First palpate gently through each quadrant, starting away from the pain. Note tenderness, guarding (involuntary tensing of abdominal muscles because of pain or fear of it), and rebound tenderness (greater pain on removing hand than on gently depressing abdomen: It is a sign of peritoneal inflammation); Rovsing's sign (appendicitis).

Palpating the liver: Begin in the right iliac fossa with the patient breathing deeply. Use the radial border of the index finger to feel the liver edge, moving up 2cm at a time at each breath. Assess its size (causes of hepatomegaly—p76), smoothness, and tenderness. Is it pulsatile (tricuspid regurgitation)? Confirm the lower border and define the upper border by percussion (normal upper limit is in 5th intercostal space): It may be pushed down by emphysema. Listen for an overlying bruit. *The scratch test* is an alternative method of identifying the lower liver edge. Start with the diaphragm of the stethoscope over the right costal margin. Gently scratch the abdominal wall, starting in the right lower quadrant and working up towards the liver edge. A sharp increase in transmission of the scratch will be heard when the lower border of the liver is reached.

Palpating the spleen: Start in the periumbilical region, moving towards the left upper quadrant with each respiration. *Features of the spleen differentiating it from kidney* one cannot get above it (ribs overlie its top); overlying percussion note is dull; it moves more with respiration—towards the umbilicus; it may have a palpable notch on its medial side. If you suspect splenomegaly but cannot detect it, assess the patient in the right lateral position with your left hand pulling forwards from behind the rib cage. Is the percussion note dull in the mid-axillary line in the 10th intercostal space (if it is, it implies splenomegaly)?

Palpating the kidneys: Try bimanually with the left hand under the patient to push it up in the renal angle. Attempt to ballot the kidney (ie bounce it gently but decisively between a hand applied to the flank and the other applied opposite, anteriorly). It moves only slightly with respiration. However, the kidneys are not palpable in the vast majority of patients.

Percussion If this induces pain, there may be peritoneal inflammation below (eg an inflamed appendix). Some experts use percussion first, before palpation, because even anxious patients do not expect this to hurt—so, if it does hurt, this is a very valuable sign. Percuss for the shifting dullness of ascites: The level of right-sided flank dullness increases by lying on the right, and vice versa on lying on the left. Ultrasound is a more reliable way of detecting ascites.

Auscultation Bowel sounds: Absence implies ileus; they are enhanced and tinkling in bowel obstruction. Listen for bruits.

Examine Mouth, tongue, rectum, genitalia, urine, as appropriate.

Order of the examination during abdominal exams: It can be useful to auscultate before palpation/percussion, as bowel sounds can be stimulated by palpation and may mask vascular bruits (you should not palpate deeply in the vicinity of bruits lest you damage an aneurysm)—and this is the preferred order in many places.

The neurological system

History This should be taken from the patient and if possible, from a close friend or relative as well. The patient's memory, perception, or speech may be affected by the disorder making the history difficult to obtain. Note the progression of the symptoms and signs: Gradual deterioration (eg tumor) vs intermittent exacerbations (eg multiple sclerosis) vs rapid onset (eg stroke). Ask about age, occupation, ethnic origin. Right- or left-handed?

Presenting symptoms

- *Headache:* (p320) Different from usual headaches? Acute/chronic? Speed of onset? Single/recurrent? Unilateral or bilateral? Associated aura (migraine, p322)? Any meningismus (p336)? Worse on waking (↑ICP)? ↓ conscious level?
- *Weakness:* Speed of onset? Muscle groups affected? Sensory loss? Any sphincter disturbance? Loss of balance? Associated spinal/root pain?
- *Visual disturbance:* Eg blurring, double vision (diplopia), photophobia, visual loss. Speed of onset? Any preceding symptoms? Pain in eye?
- *Special senses:* Hearing, smell, taste.
- *Dizziness:* (p324) Illusion of surroundings moving (vertigo)? Hearing loss/tinnitus? Any loss of consciousness?
- *Speech disturbance:* Difficulty in expression, articulation, or comprehension? Sudden onset or gradual?
- *Dysphagia:* Solids and/or liquids? Intermittent or constant? Difficulty in coordination? Painful (odynophagia)?
- *Involuntary movements:* (p348) Frequency? Duration? Mode of onset? Preceding aura? Loss of consciousness? Tongue biting? Incontinence? Any residual weakness/confusion? Family history?
- *Skin sensation disturbance:* Eg numbness, 'pins & needles' (paresethesia), pain, odd sensations. Distribution? Speed of onset? Associated weakness?
- *Tremor:* (p348) Rapid or slow tremor? Present at rest? Worse on deliberate movement? Taking β-agonists? Any thyroid problems? Any family history?

Cognitive state If there is any doubt about the patient's cognition, an objective measure is performance in a cognitive test such as the mini-mental state examination (MMSE)

Past medical history Ask about meningitis/encephalitis, head/spine trauma, seizures, previous operations, risk factors for vascular disease (AF, hypertension, hyperlipidemia, diabetes mellitus, smoking), and recent travel. Is there any chance that the patient is pregnant (preeclampsia)?

Drug history Any anticonvulsant/antipsychotic/antidepressant medication? Any psychotropic drugs (eg ecstasy)? Any medication with neurological side-effects (eg isoniazid)?

Social and family history What can the patient do and not do? Any neurological or psychiatric disease in the family? Any consanguinity?

Examining the neurological system

The neurological system is usually the most daunting examination to learn, but the most satisfying once perfected. Learn at the bedside from a senior colleague, preferably a neurologist. There is no substitute for practice. Be aware that books present ideal situations: Often one or more signs are equivocal or even contrary to expectation; don't be put off, consider the whole picture, including the history; try re-examining the patient.

Higher mental function Conscious level (Glasgow coma scale, p684), orientation in time, place, and person, memory (short- and long-term).

Speech Is there alteration in the sound of the voice (dysphonia eg in laryngitis, recurrent laryngeal nerve palsy, or vocal cord tumor)? Dysphagia, dysarthria.

Skull and spine Malformation. Signs of injury. Palpate scalp. If there is any question of spinal injury, *do not move the spine*. Is there meningismus (p336)? Auscultate for carotid/cranial bruits.

Motor system (upper or lower limb) It is essential to discriminate whether weakness is upper (UMN) or lower (LMN) motor neuron (p310).

Inspect for posture abnormality (eg 'pyramidal' posture of UMN lesions), or involuntary movement, wasting, or fasciculation (muscle twitching, not moving the limb)?

Drift: Patient sitting, arms outstretched, eyes closed. Do arms drift downwards (termed pronator drift)? Unequal drift is a valuable sign of subtle focal motor deficits, occurring in UMN weakness, cerebellar disease, and loss of proprioception (pseudoathetosis). Then:

Tone: Look for *hypotonia* (floppy) or *spasticity* (pressure fails to move a joint until it gives way, like a clasp-knife), rigidity (lead pipe), rigidity + tremor = cogwheeling. Is there *clonus* (=rhythmic muscle 'beats' on sudden stretching, eg gastrocnemius on ankle dorsiflexion) at the wrist, patella, or ankle?

Strength: Oppose each movement. Ascertain the distribution of any weakness—which movements/nerve roots are affected (myotomes, p316)? Quantify strength of each movement.

Reflexes: Brisk in UMN lesions, reduced/absent in LMN lesions. Biceps reflex: (C5–6), triceps (C7–8), brachoradialis (C5–6), knee (L3–4 ± L2), ankle (S1–2), abdominals (lost in UMN lesions), plantars (up-going in UMN lesions). Test *Hoffman's reflex* (flicking a finger may cause neighboring digits to flex—may be positive in UMN lesions).

Coordination: Finger–nose (touch nose with a finger), rub heel up and down shin, rapid alternating movements (eg rapidly pronate and supinate hand on dorsum of other hand; clumsiness in this (dysdiadochokinesis) occurs in cerebellar lesions). Is there apraxia?

Gait: Have patient walk: Normally; heel-to-toe; on heels; then on toes. Observe standing feet together ± squatting. If balance is worse on shutting the eyes, Romberg's test is positive, implying abnormal joint position sense. If they cannot perform this even with eyes open, this may be cerebellar ataxia, but is not Romberg's positive.

Sensation Light touch (cotton wool), pain (pin-prick), vibration (128Hz tuning fork), joint position sense. Testing temperature sensation is not usually required, but can be performed with test tubes filled with hot and cold water. Determine if any sensory loss is below a spinal cord level (eg cord compression), or in a glove and stocking distribution (eg peripheral neuropathy)?

Cranial nerves see p62

Cranial nerve examination

Approach to examining the cranial nerves Where is the lesion? Think systematically. Is it in the brainstem (eg MS), or outside, pressing on the brainstem? Is it the neuromuscular junction (myasthenia) or the muscles (eg a dystrophy)? Cranial nerves may be affected singly or in groups.

Face the patient (helps spot asymmetry). For causes of lesions, see BOX.

I *Smell:* Test ability of each nostril to differentiate familiar smells.

II *Acuity* in each eye separately, and its correctability with glasses or pin-hole. *Visual fields:* Compare during confrontation with your own fields or formally. Any losses/inattention? Sites of lesions. *Pupils:* (p79) size, shape, symmetry, reaction to light (direct and consensual), and accommodation if reaction to light is poor. *Ophthalmoscopy:* Darken the room. Instill tropicamide 0.5%, 1 drop, if needed. Select the focusing lens for the best view of the optic disc (pale? swollen?). This is found when the ophthalmoscope's dot of light is reflected from the cornea at 9 o'clock (right disc) or 3 o'clock (left disc). Follow vessels outwards to view each quadrant; look back through the lenses to inspect lens and cornea. If the view is obscured, examine the red reflex, with your focus on the margin of the pupil, to look for cataract. You will get a view of the fovea if you ask the patient to look at the ophthalmoscope's finest beam (after drops) Pathology here merits prompt ophthalmic referral.

III, IV, and VI: *Eye movements. III palsy:* Ptosis, large pupil, eye down and out. *IV palsy:* Diplopia on looking down and in (often noticed on descending stairs)—head tilting compensates for this (ocular torticollis). *VI nerve palsy:* Horizontal diplopia on looking out. *Nystagmus* is involuntary, often jerky, eye oscillations. Horizontal nystagmus is often due to a peripheral (ie vestibular) lesion. However, cental nervous system lesions can cause horizontal nystagmus.If it is more in whichever eye is abducting, MS may be the cause (internuclear opthalmoplegia). If there is associated deafness or tinnitus, suspect a peripheral cause (eg CNVIII lesion, barotrauma, Ménière's). If it varies with head position, suspect benign positional vertigo (p324). Vertical nystagmus is often from a central etiology. Nystagmus lasting 2 beats or less is normal, as is brief nystagmus at the extremes of gaze.

V *Motor palsy:* 'Open your mouth': Jaw deviates to side of lesion.
Sensory: Corneal reflex lost first; check all 3 divisions.

VII *Facial nerve lesions* cause droop and weakness. As the forehead has bilateral representation in the brain, only the lower two-thirds is affected in UMN lesions, but all of one side of the face in LMN lesions. Ask to: 'raise your eyebrows'; 'show me your teeth'; 'puff out your cheeks'. Test taste (rarely done) with salt/sweet solutions.

VIII *Hearing:* (p326) Ask patient to repeat a number whispered in an ear while you block the other. Perform Weber's and Rinne's tests. *Balance.*

IX and X *Gag reflex:* Touch the back of the palate with a cotton tip applicator to elicit a reflex contraction. The afferent arm of this reflex involves IX, the efferent arm involves X. X lesions will also cause the palate to be pulled to the normal side on say 'Ah'.

XI *Trapezii:* 'Shrug your shoulders' against resistance.
Sternocleidomastoid: 'Turn your head to the left/right' against resistance.

XII *Tongue movement:* Deviates to the side of the lesion.

Causes of cranial nerve lesions

Any cranial nerve may be affected by diabetes mellitus; stroke; MS; tumors; sarcoidosis; vasculitis, eg polyarteritis (p378), lupus; syphilis. Chronic meningitis (malignant, TB, or fungal) tends to pick off the lower cranial nerves one-by-one.

I Trauma; respiratory tract infection; frontal lobe tumor; meningitis.

II *Field defects* may start as small areas of visual loss (*scotomas*, eg in glaucoma). *Monocular blindness:* Lesions of one eye or optic nerve, eg MS, giant cell arteritis. *Bilateral blindness:* Methanol, tobacco amblyopia; neurosyphilis. Field defects—*Bitemporal hemianopia:* Optic chiasm compression, eg pituitary adenoma, craniopharyngioma, internal carotid artery aneurysm. *Homonymous hemianopia:* Affects half the visual field contralateral to the lesion in each eye. Lesions lie beyond the chiasm in the tracts, radiation, or occipital cortex, eg stroke, abscess, tumor.

Optic neuritis (mild pain on moving eye, loss of central vision, afferent pupillary defect, disc swelling from papillitis). *Causes:* Demyelination (eg MS); rarely sinusitis, syphilis, collagen vascular disorders.

Ischemic papillopathy: Swelling of optic disc due to ischemia of the posterior ciliary artery (eg in giant cell arteritis).

Papilledema (swollen discs): (1) ↑ICP (tumor, abscess, encephalitis, hydrocephalus, benign intracranial hypertension); (2) retro-orbital lesion (eg cavernous sinus thrombosis, p334).

Optic atrophy (pale optic discs and reduced acuity): MS; frontal tumors; Friedreich's ataxia; retinitis pigmentosa; syphilis; glaucoma; Leber's optic atrophy; optic nerve compression.

III alone Diabetes; giant cell arteritis; syphilis; posterior communicating artery aneurysm; idiopathic; ↑ICP (if uncal herniation through the tentorium compresses the nerve). Third nerve palsies without a dilated pupil are typically 'medical' (eg diabetes; BP↑). Early dilatation of a pupil implies a compressive lesion, from a 'surgical' cause (tumor; aneurysm).

IV alone Rare and usually due to trauma to the orbit.

VI alone MS, Wernicke' encephalopathy, false localizing sign in ↑ICP, pontine stroke (presents with fixed small pupils ± quadriparesis).

V *Sensory:* Trigeminal neuralgia (pain but no sensory loss), herpes zoster, nasopharyngeal cancer, acoustic neuroma (p324). *Motor:* Rare.

VII *LMN:* Bell's palsy (p354), polio, otitis media, skull fracture, cerebellopontine angle tumors eg acoustic neuroma, parotid tumors, herpes zoster (Ramsay Hunt syndrome). *UMN:* (spares the forehead—bilateral innervation) Stroke, tumor.

VIII Noise, Paget's disease, Ménière's disease, herpes zoster, acoustic neuroma, brainstem CVA, drugs (eg aminoglycosides).

IX, X, XII Trauma, brainstem lesions, neck tumors.

XI Rare. Polio, syringomyelia, tumors near jugular foramen, stroke, bulbar palsy, trauma, TB.

Groups of cranial nerves VIII, then V ± VI: Cerebellopontine angle tumors, eg acoustic neuroma (p324; facial weakness is, surprisingly, not a prominent sign). V, VI (Gradenigo's syndrome): Lesions within the petrous temporal bone. III, IV, VI: Stroke, tumors, Wernicke's encephalopathy, aneurysms, MS. III, IV, V$_a$, VI: Cavernous sinus thrombosis, superior orbital fissure lesions (Tolosa–Hunt syndrome). IX, X, XI: Jugular foramen lesion. *Other differential diagnoses:* Myasthenia gravis, muscular dystrophy, myotonic dystrophy, mononeuritis multiplex (p350).

Speech and higher mental function

Aphasia (Impairment of language caused by brain damage.) *Assessment:*

1 If speech is fluent, grammatical and meaningful, aphasia is unlikely.

2 *Comprehension:* Can the patient follow one, two, and several step commands? (touch your ear, stand up then close the door).

3 *Repetition:* Can the patient repeat a sentence?

4 *Naming:* Can the patient name common and uncommon things (eg parts of a watch)?

5 *Reading and writing:* Normal? They can be affected like speech in dysphasia.

Classification: Broca's (expressive) anterior phasia: Non-fluent speech produced with effort and frustration with malformed words, eg 'spoot' for 'spoon' (or 'that thing'). Reading and writing are impaired but comprehension is relatively intact. Patients understand questions and attempt to convey meaningful answers. *Site of lesion:* Infero-lateral dominant frontal lobe.

Wernicke's (receptive) posterior aphasia: Empty, fluent speech, like talking ragtime with phonemic *(flush* for *brush)* and semantic *(comb* for *brush)* paraphasias/neologisms (may be mistaken for psychotic speech). The patient is oblivious of errors. Reading, writing, *and* comprehension are impaired (replies are inappropriate). *Site of lesion:* Posterior superior temporal lobe (dominant).

Conduction aphasia: *(Traffic between Broca's and Wernicke's area is interrupted.)* Repetition is impaired; comprehension and fluency less so.

Anomic aphasias: Naming is affected in all aphasias, but in anomic aphasia, objects cannot be named but other aspects of speech are normal. This occurs with dominant posterior temporoparietal lesions.

Mixed aphasias are common. Discriminating features take time to emerge after an acute brain injury. Consider speech therapy (of variable use).

Dysarthria Difficulty with articulation due to incoordination or weakness of the musculature of speech. Language is normal (see above).

Assessment: Ask to repeat 'baby hippopotamus'.

Cerebellar disease: Ataxia speech muscles cause slurring (as if drunk) and speech irregular in volume and scanning or staccato in quality.

Extrapyramidal disease: Soft, indistinct, and monotonous speech.

Pseudobulbar palsy: Spastic dysarthria *(upper motor neuron).* Speech is slow, indistinct, and effortful ('Donald Duck' or 'hot potato' voice from bilateral hemispheric lesions, MND, or severe MS.

Bulbar palsy: Lower motor neuron (eg facial nerve palsy, Guillain–Barré, MND—any associated palatal paralysis gives speech a nasal character.

Dysphonia Difficulty with speech volume due to weakness of respiratory muscles or vocal cords (Myasthenia, p356; Guillain–Barré syndrome, p352). Parkinson's gives a mixed picture of dysarthria and dysphonia.

Apraxia (poor performance of complex movements despite ability to perform each individual component) Test by asking the patient to copy unfamiliar hand positions, or mime an object's use, eg a comb. Can they do familiar gestures, eg a salute? The term 'apraxia' is used in 3 other ways:

- *Dressing apraxia:* The patient is unsure of the orientation of clothes on his body. Test by pulling one sleeve of a sweater inside out before asking the patient to put it back on (mostly nondominant hemisphere lesions).
- *Constructional apraxia:* Difficulty in assembling objects or drawing—a 5-pointed star (nondominant hemisphere lesions, hepatic encephalopathy).

Gait apraxia: More common in the elderly; seen with bilateral frontal lesions, lesions in the posterior temporal region, and hydrocephalus.

The mini-mental state examination (MMSE)

(*Kafka's law*: 'In youth we take examinations to get into institutions. In old age to keep out of them.') The MMSE is often used to test memory and cognition, but it isn't all that reliable. Tester variability means that a 2–3 point improvement (eg on starting some new treatment) may go undetected.

- *What day of the week is it?* [1 point]
- *What is the date today? Day; Month; Year* [1 point each]
- *What is the season?* Allow flexibility during times of seasonal change [1 point]
- *Can you tell me where we are now? What country are we in?* [1 point]
- *What is the name of this town?* [1 point]
- *What are two main streets nearby?* [1 point]
- *What floor of the building are we on?* [1 point]
- *What is the name of this place?* (or *what is this address?*) [1 point]
- Read the following, then offer the paper: '*I am going to give you a piece of paper. When I do, take the paper in your right hand. Fold the paper in half with both hands and put the paper down on your lap.*' [Give 1 point for each of the three actions]
- *Show a pencil and ask what it is called.* [1 point]
- *Show a wristwatch and ask what it is called.* [1 point]
- Say (once only): '*I am going to say something and I would like you to repeat it after me: No ifs, ands, or buts.*' [1 point]
- Say: '*Please read what is written here and do what it says.*' Show card with: CLOSE YOUR EYES written on it. Score only if action is carried out correctly. If respondent reads instruction but fails to carry out action, say: 'Now do what it says' [1 point]
- Say: '*Write a complete sentence on this sheet of paper.*' Spelling and grammar are not important. The sentence must have a verb, real or implied, and must make sense. 'Help!', 'Go away' are acceptable [1 point]
- Say: '*Here is a drawing. Please copy the drawing.*' [See drawing below] Mark as correct if the 2 figures intersect to form a 4-sided figure and if all angles are preserved [1 point]
- Say: '*I am going to name 3 objects. After I have finished saying all three I want you to repeat them. Remember what they are because I am going to ask you to name them again in a few minutes.*' Name 3 objects taking 1s to say each, eg APPLE; TABLE; PENNY. Score first try [1 point each object] and repeat until all are learned.
- Say: '*Now I would like you to take 7 away from 100. Now take 7 away from the number you get. Now keep subtracting until I tell you to stop.*' Score 1 point each time the difference is 7 even if a previous answer was incorrect. Go on for 5 subtractions (eg 93, 86, 79, 72, 65) [5 points]
- Say: '*What were the three objects I asked you to remember a little while ago?*' [1 point each object]

Interpreting the score The maximum is 30; 28–30 does not support the diagnosis of dementia. A score 25–27 is borderline; <25 suggests dementia but consider also *acute confusional state* and *depression*. ~13% of over 75s in the general population have scores <25

Close your eyes

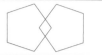

Psychiatric assessment

Introduce yourself, ask a few factual questions (precise name, age, marital status, job, and who is at home). These will help your patient to relax.

Presenting problem Then ask for the main problems which have led to this consultation. Sit back and listen. Don't worry whether the information is in a convenient form or not—this is an opportunity for the patient to come out with his or her worries unsullied by your expectations. After 3–5min you should have a list of all the problems (each sketched only briefly). Read them back to the patient and ask if there are any more. Then ask about:

History of presenting problem For each problem obtain details, both current state and history of onset, precipitating factors, and effects on life.

Check of major psychiatric symptoms Check those which have not yet been covered: *Depression* (low mood, anhedonia (inability to feel pleasure), thoughts of worthlessness/hopelessness, sleep disturbance with early morning waking, loss of weight and appetite). Ask specifically about *suicidal thoughts and plans*: 'Have you ever been so low that you thought of harming yourself?', 'What thoughts have you had?'. *Hallucinations* ('Have you ever heard voices when there hasn't been anyone there, or seen visions?'), and *delusions* ('Have you ever had any thoughts or beliefs which have struck you afterwards as bizarre?'); *anxiety* and *avoidance behavior* (eg avoiding shopping because of anxiety or phobias); *obsessive thoughts* and *compulsive behavior*, *eating* disorders, *alcohol* (CAGE questionnaire—see BOX) and *other drugs*.

Present circumstances Housing, finance, work, marriage, friends.

Family history Ask about health, personality, and occupation of parents and siblings, and the *family's medical and psychiatric history*.

Background history Try to understand the presenting problem.

Biography (relationships with family and peers as a child; school and work record; sexual relationships and current relationships; and family). Previous ways of dealing with stress and whether there have been problems and symptoms similar to the presenting ones.

Premorbid personality (mood, character, hobbies, attitudes, and beliefs).

Mental state examination This is the state *now*, at the time of interview.
- *Observable behavior:* Eg excessive slowness, signs of anxiety.
- *Mode of speech:* Include the rate of speech, eg retarded or garbling (pressure of speech). Note its content.
- *Mood:* Note thoughts about harming self or others. Gauge your own responses to the patient. The laughter and grandiose ideas of manic patients are contagious, as to a lesser extent is the expression of thoughts from a depressed person.
- *Beliefs:* Eg about one's self, their own body, about other people, and the future. Note abnormal beliefs (delusions), eg that thoughts are overheard, and abnormal ideas (eg persecutory, grandiose).
- *Unusual experiences or hallucinations:* Note modality, eg visual.
- *Orientation:* In time, place, and person. What is the date? What time of day is it? Where are you? What is your name?
- *Short-term memory:* Give a name and address and test recall after 5min. Make sure that they have the address clear before waiting for the 5min to elapse.
- *Long-term memory:* Current affairs recall. Name of current political leaders. This tests many other CNS functions, not just memory.
- *Concentration:* Months of the year backwards.
- Note the patient's *insight* and the degree of your *rapport*.

Nonverbal behavior Gesture, gaze and mutual gaze, expressions, tears, laughter, pauses (while listening to voices?), attitude (eg withdrawn).

Screening tests for alcoholism

The CAGE questionnaire has long been used as a screening test for alcoholism; two or more positive answers suggests an alcohol problem:
• Have you ever felt you should cut down on your drinking?
• Have you ever been annoyed at others' concerns about your drinking?
• Have you ever felt guilty about drinking?
• Have you ever had alcohol as an eye-opener in the morning?

Another test, that has been shown to be more sensitive than CAGE in some populations (eg pregnant ♀), is the TWEAK questionnaire. The test is based on a 7-point scale (2 points for a +ve reply to either of the first 2 questions, 1 point for each of the remaining questions), with ≥2 points suggesting an alcohol problem:
• Have you an ↑ tolerance of alcohol?
• Do you worry about your drinking?
• Have you ever had alcohol as an eye-opener in the morning?
• Do you ever get amnesia after drinking alcohol?
• Have you ever felt the need to cut down on your drinking?

Method and order for routine examination

We all have our own system, but sometimes containing elements unique to each doctor, arising from his or her own interaction with countless past patients and their eccentricities. This fact is one reason why it is often so helpful to ask for second opinions: The same field may be ploughed again but yield quite a different harvest.

1 Look at the patient. Healthy, unwell, or *in extremis*? Skill in this vital Gestalt comes only with time. *Beware those who are sicker than they look*, eg cardiogenic shock; cord compression; nonaccidental injury.

2 Pulse, BP; T°.

3 Examine nails, hands, conjunctivae (anemia), and sclera (jaundice). Consider: Paget's, acromegaly, endocrine disease (thyroid, pituitary, or adrenal hypo-/hyper-function), body hair, abnormal pigmentation, skin.

4 Examine mouth and tongue (*cyanosed; smooth; furred; beefy*, ie rhomboid area denuded of papillae by *Candida*, eg after much steroid inhaler use).

5 Examine the neck from behind: Nodes, goiter.

6 Make sure the patient is at 45° to begin CVS examination in the neck: JVP; feel for character and volume of carotid pulse.

7 The precordium. Look for abnormal pulsations. Feel the apical beat (character; position). Any parasternal heave or thrill? Auscultate (bell & diaphragm) apex in the left lateral position, then the other 3 areas (p46) and carotids. Sit the patient forward: Listen during expiration.

8 Sit patient forward to find sacral edema; look for ankle edema.

9 Begin the respiratory examination with the patient at 90°. Observe (and count) respirations; note posterior chest wall movement and feel for tactile fremitus. Assess expansion, then percuss and auscultate the chest with the bell.

10 Sit the patient back. Feel the trachea. Inspect again. Assess expansion of the anterior chest. Percuss and auscultate again.

11 Examine the breasts (if indicated) and axillary nodes.

12 Lie the patient flat with only one pillow. Inspect, palpate, percuss, and auscultate the abdomen.

13 Look at the legs: Perfusion, pulses, edema?

14 CNS exam: *Cranial nerves*: Pupil responses; fundi, EOMI, visual fields. Do corneal reflexes. 'Open your mouth; stick your tongue out; scrunch up your eyes; show me your teeth; raise your eyebrows'. *Peripheral nerves*: Look for wasting and fasciculation. Test tone in all limbs. Stength in all large muscle groups of extremities. Reflexes at biceps, brachioradialis, knees, and ankle. 'Hold your hands out with your palms towards the ceiling and fingers wide. Now shut your eyes'. Watch for pronator drift. 'Keep your eyes shut and touch your nose with each index finger'. 'Lift your leg straight in the air. Keep it there. Put your heel on the opposite knee (eyes shut) and run it up your own shin'. You have now tested power, coordination, and joint position sense. Tuning fork on toes and index fingers to assess sensation.

15 Examine the gait and the speech.

16 Any abnormalities of higher mental function to pursue?

17 Consider rectal and vaginal examination. Is a chaperone needed?

Remember the need for a chaperone when conducting intimate examinations. In general, go into detail where you find (or suspect) something to be wrong.

He moved

all the brightest gems

faster and faster towards the

ever-growing bucket of lost hopes;
had there been just one more year

of peace the battalion would have made
a floating system of perpetual drainage.

A silent fall of immense snow came near oily
remains of the recently eaten supper on the table.

We drove on in our old sunless walnut. Presently
classical eggs ticked in the new afternoon shadows.

We were instructed by my cousin Jasper not to exercise by country
house visiting unless accompanied by thirteen geese or gangsters.

The modern American did not prevail over the pair of redundant bronze puppies.
The worn-out principle is a bad omen which I am never glad to ransom in August.

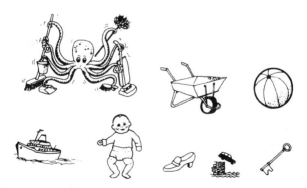

Record the smallest type (eg N. 12 left eye, N. 6 right eye, spectacles worn) or object accurately read or named at 30cm

Symptoms and signs

Lisa A. Simonson, M.D.

Symptoms are features which patients report. *Physical signs* are elicited at the bedside. Together, they constitute the features of the condition in that patient. Their evolution over time, and interaction with the physical, psychological, and social spheres comprise the natural history of any disease. Here we discuss symptoms in isolation. This is unnatural—but a necessary first step in learning how to diagnose. All doctors have to know about symptoms and their relief: This is what doctors are *for*.

This chapter is disappointing in trying to explain *combinations* of symptoms, as illnesses often do not fit into the 80-or-so features given below. It is hard to compare one list with others on separate pages—and the lists are not exhaustive. Do not expect too much from this chapter: Just a few common causes of common symptoms and signs.

Abdominal distension

Causes: The famous five Fs—*fat, fluid, feces, fetus,* or *flatus*. Also *food* (eg in malabsorption). Specific groups:

Air:	Ascites:	Solid masses:	Pelvic masses:
Gastrointestinal	Malignancy	Malignancy	Bladder: Full or Ca
obstruction	Hypoproteinemia	Lymph nodes	Fibroids; fetus
(incl. fecal)	(eg nephrotic)	Aorta aneurysm	Ovarian cyst
Aerophagia	R heart failure	Cysts: Renal,	Ovarian cancer
(air swallowing)	Portal hypertension	pancreatic	Uterine cancer

Air is resonant on percussion. *Ascites* (free fluid in peritoneal cavity): Signs: Shifting dullness (p59); fluid wave (place patient's hand firmly on his abdomen in sagittal plane and flick one flank with your finger while your other hand feels on the other flank for a fluid wave). The characteristic feature of *pelvic masses* is that you cannot palpate below them (ie their lower border cannot be defined). Causes of *right iliac fossa masses:* Appendix mass or abscess (p442); kidney mass; cecal cancer; a Crohn's or TB mass; intussusception; amoebic abscess or any pelvic mass (above).
Causes of *ascites with portal hypertension:* p212 See causes of *hepatomegaly* (p76), *splenomegaly*.

Abdominal pain

varies greatly depending on the underlying cause. Examples include: Irritation of the mucosa (acute gastritis), smooth muscle spasm (acute enterocolitis), capsular stretching (liver congestion in CHF), peritoneal inflammation (acute appendicitis), direct splanchnic nerve stimulation (retroperitoneal extension of tumor). The *character (constant or colicky, sharp or dull), duration,* and *frequency* depend on the mechanism of production. The *location* and *distribution* of referred pain depend on the anatomical site. *Time of occurrence* and *aggravating or relieving factors* such as meals, defecation, and sleep also have special significance related to the underlying disease process. The site of the pain may provide a clue as to the cause.

Amaurosis fugax

see p330.

Anemia

may be assessed from the skin creases and conjunctivae (pale if Hb<9g/dL). Koilonychia and stomatitis (p45) suggest iron deficiency. Anemia with jaundice suggests malignancy or hemolysis. p557.

Apex beat

This is the point furthest from the manubrium where the heart can be felt beating—normally the 5th intercostal space in the mid-clavicular line (5th ICS MCL). Lateral displacement may be from cardiomegaly or mediastinal shift. Assess character using your palm: A *pressure loaded* apex is a forceful, sustained undisplaced impulse (BP ↑ or aortic stenosis causing LV hypertrophy with unenlarged cavity). A *volume overloaded* (hyperdynamic) apex is forceful, unsustained, and displaced down and laterally (eg cavity enlargement from aortic or mitral incompetence). It is *tapping* in mitral stenosis (palpable 1st heart sound); *dyskinetic* after anterior MI or with LV aneurysm; *double* or *triple impulse* in HOCM (p144).

Athetosis This is due to a lesion in the putamen, which causes slow sinuous writhing movements in the hands, which are present at rest. *Pseudoathetosis* refers to athetoid movements in patients with severe proprioceptive loss.

Backache p366. **Breathlessness (dyspnea)** p73.

Breast pain Often this is premenstrual (*cyclical mastalgia*)—but the patient is often worried that she has breast cancer. So examine carefully (p466) and refer for mammography as appropriate. If there is no sign of breast pathology, and it is not cyclical, think of:

- Tietze syndrome
- Bornholm disease
- Gallstones
- Pulmonary embolus
- Angina
- Cervical radiculopathy
- Estrogens (HRT)

If none of the above, *wearing a firm bra* all day may help, as may NSAIDs.

Cachexia Severe generalized muscle wasting implying malnutrition, neoplasia, CHF, Alzheimer's disease, hyperthyroidism, prolonged inanition, or infection—eg TB, enteropathic AIDS ('slim disease', eg from *Cryptosporidium*, p501).

Carotid bruits may signify stenosis (>30%) often near the internal carotid origin. Heard best behind the angle of jaw. Usual cause: Atheroma. A key question is: *Is he/she symptomatic?* With *symptomless* bruits, risk of stroke is too small (<3% over 3yrs for non-fatal strokes, and ~0.3% for fatal strokes) to justify risk of endarterectomy. If symptomatic, consider Doppler + surgery if stenosis ≥70%, and *possibly* if ≥50%.[1] In anyone with a carotid bruit, consider aspirin prophylaxis. Ask a neurologist's advice.

Chest deformity *Barrel chest:* AP diameter↑, tracheal descent and expansion↓, seen in chronic hyperinflation (eg asthma/COPD). *Pigeon chest (pectus carinatum):* Prominent sternum with a flat chest, seen in chronic childhood asthma and rickets. *Funnel chest (pectus excavatum)* (PLATE 10): Developmental defect involving local sternum depression (lower end). *Kyphosis:* 'Humpback' from ↑thoracic spine curvature. *Scoliosis:* Lateral curvature; both may cause restrictive ventilatory defect.

Chest pains see p88

Cheyne–Stokes respiration Breathing becomes progressively deeper and then shallower (±episodic apnea) in cycles. Causes: Brainstem lesions or compression (stroke, ICP↑). If the cycle is long (eg 3min), the cause may be a long lung-to-brain circulation time (eg in chronic pulmonary edema, poor cardiac output). It is enhanced by narcotics.

Chorea means dance—a continuous flow of jerky movements, flitting from one limb or part to another. Each movement looks like a fragment of a normal movement. *Cause:* Basal ganglia lesion: Huntington's; Sydenham's (p134); SLE (p374); Wilson's (p278); kernicterus; polycythemia vera (p585); neuroacanthocytosis (a familial association of acanthocytes in peripheral blood with chorea, oro-facial dyskinesia, and axonal neuropathy); thyrotoxicosis (p280); drugs (L-dopa, contraceptive steroids). Early stages of chorea may be detected by feeling fluctuations in muscle tension while the patient grips your finger. Treat the underlying cause; reserve drugs (dopamine depletors, ie tetrabenazine, or dopamine receptor blockers) for severe cases. Ask a neurologist for help.

Chvostek's sign Tapping on the facial nerve causes a facial twitch in hypocalcemia, due to nerve hyperexcitability.

---

1 21% reduction in 5yr risk of stroke or surgical death if stenosis ≥70%; 5.7% reduction if 50–70% stenosis; below 50% stenosis surgery is unhelpful/harmful. See PM Rothwell 2003 *Stroke* **34** 514.

Clubbing–Cyanosis

Clubbing Finger nails have exaggerated longitudinal curvature + loss of angle between nail and nail-fold, and the nail-fold feels boggy.

Thoracic causes:
- Bronchial carcinoma (usually *not* small cell)
- Chronic lung suppuration
  - empyema, abscess
  - bronchiectasis
  - cystic fibrosis
- Fibrosing alveolitis
- Mesothelioma

GI causes:
- Inflammatory bowel (especially Crohn's disease)
- Cirrhosis
- GI lymphoma
- Malabsorption, eg celiac

Rare:
- Familial
- Thyroid acropachy
- Unilateral clubbing, from:
  - axillary artery aneurysm
  - brachial arterio-venous malformations

Cardiac causes:
- Cyanotic congenital heart disease
- Endocarditis
- Atrial myxoma

How to test for finger clubbing

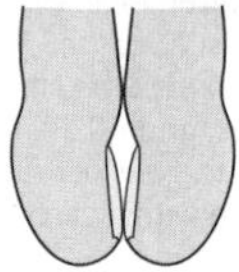

The dorsal aspect of 2 fingers, side by side with the nails touching. Normally, you should see a kite-shaped gap. If not, there is clubbing.

Fig. 1a

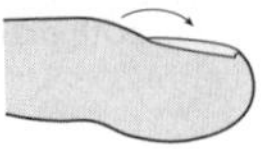

Fig. 1b

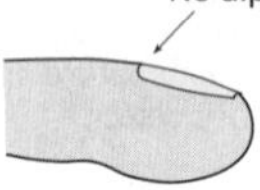

No dip—therefore clubbing

Fig. 1c

Constipation see p200

Cough. p54 See also **Hemoptysis** (p76).

Cramp (Painful muscle spasm.) Cramp in the legs is common, especially at night. It may also occur after exercise. It only occasionally indicates a disease, in particular: Salt depletion, muscle ischemia, or myopathy. Forearm cramps suggest motor neuron disease. Night cramps in the elderly may respond to quinine bisulfate 300mg at night PO twice weekly, or intermittent nightly use until cramps resolve for several days. Writer's cramp is a focal dystonia causing difficulty with the motor act of writing. The pen is gripped firmly, with excessive flexion of the thumb and index finger (± tremor). There is normally no CNS deficit. Oral drugs or psychotherapy rarely help, but botulinum toxin often helps, sometimes dramatically (but it has side-effects). Similar specific dystonias may apply to other tasks.

Cyanosis Dusky blue skin (*peripheral*, eg of the fingers) or mucosae (*central*, eg of the tongue, representing ≥2.5g/dL of Hb in its reduced form, hence it occurs more readily in polycythemia than anemia). Causes:

1 Lung disease resulting in inadequate oxygen transfer (eg COPD, severe pneumonia)—often correctable by ↑ the inspired O₂.

2 Shunting from pulmonary to systemic circulation (eg R–L shunting VSD, patent ductus arteriosus, transposition of the great arteries)—cyanosis is *not* reversed by ↑ inspired oxygen.

3 Inadequate oxygen uptake (eg met-, or sulf-hemoglobinemia).

Acute cyanosis is a sign of impending emergency. Is there asthma, an inhaled foreign body, a pneumothorax (X-RAY PLATE 6), or LVF? p126

Peripheral cyanosis will occur in causes of central cyanosis, but may also be induced by changes in the peripheral and cutaneous vascular systems in patients with normal oxygen saturations. It occurs in the cold, in hypovolemia, and in arterial disease, and is therefore not a specific sign.

Deafness p326. **Dehydration** p616. **Diarrhea** p198.

Dizziness is a trinity: (1) *Vertigo* (p324) is the illusion of rotation as if one just stepped off a merry-go-round. (2) *Imbalance* (ie difficulty in walking straight) eg from peripheral nerve, posterior column, cerebellum or other central pathway failure. (3) *Faintness* (sense of collapse) eg seen in anemia, BP↓, hypoglycemia, carotid sinus hypersensitivity, and epilepsy. 1–3 may coexist.

Dysarthria p64.

Dyspepsia and **indigestion** These are broad terms, used often by patients to signify epigastric or retrosternal pain (or discomfort) which is usually related to meals. Find out exactly what your patient means. 30% have no real abnormality on endoscopy. Of positive findings:

Esophagitis alone	24%	Gastritis	9%	≥2 'lesions'	23%
Duodenal ulcer (DU)	17%	Duodenitis	6%	Bile reflux	0.7%
Hiatus hernia	15%	Gastric ulcer	5%	Gastric cancer	0.2%

Can one avoid endoscopy for dyspepsia in those with *Helicobacter pylori*-induced peptic ulcers with non-invasive tests for *H. pylori*? Non-invasive tests include the ^{13}C-urea breath test, serological tests, and stool antigen tests. One study found that the ^{13}C-urea breath test could safely replace endoscopy in patients under 55yrs with dyspepsia but no sinister symptoms (weight↓, vomiting, hematemesis, dysphagia), no FH of upper GI malignancy, and no past history of NSAID use or gastric surgery. Stool antigen tests and laboratory-based serological tests have a similar sensitivity and specificity to the ^{13}C-urea breath test, but bedside serological tests yield inconsistent results. Some tests are not quick, cheap, or accurate enough for general use. 1999 PCSG guidelines say that testing is not needed for the *first* presentation of dyspepsia: Do endoscopy if there are 'alarm' symptoms (>45yrs, weight↓, vomiting, hematemesis, anemia, dysphagia). Otherwise, try H2 blocker or PPI, and if symptoms recur, test for *H. pylori*; only endoscope if -ve.

Dysphasia p54. **Dysphonia** p54.

Dyspnea (p679) is the subjective sensation of shortness of breath, often exacerbated by exertion. Try to quantify exercise tolerance (eg dressing, distance walked, climbing stairs, NYHA classification—p127). May be due to:

• *Cardiac*—eg mitral stenosis or left ventricular failure of any cause; LVF is associated with *orthopnea* (dyspnea worse on lying; 'how many pillows?') and *paroxysmal nocturnal dyspnea* (PND; dyspnea waking one up). There may also be ankle edema. Any patient who is in shock may also be dyspneic—and this may be shock's presenting feature.

• *Lung*—both airway and interstitial disease. May be hard to separate from cardiac causes; asthma may also wake the patient as well as cause early morning dyspnea and wheeze. Focus on the circumstances in which dyspnea occurs (eg on exposure to an occupational allergen).

• *Anatomical*—ie diseases of the chest wall, muscles, or pleura.

• *Others*—thyrotoxicosis, ketoacidosis, aspirin poisoning, anemia, psychogenic. Look for other clues: Dyspnea at rest *unassociated with exertion* may be psychogenic; look for respiratory alkalemia (peripheral ± perioral paresthesiae ± carpopedal spasm). Speed of onset helps diagnosis:

Acute	Subacute	Chronic
Foreign body	Asthma	COPD and chronic
Pneumothorax (PLATE 6)	Parenchymal disease	parenchymal diseases
Acute asthma	eg alveolitis	Non-respiratory causes
Pulmonary embolus	effusions	eg cardiac failure
Acute pulmonary edema	pneumonia	anemia

Dyspraxia p54.

Dysuria is painful micturition (from urethral or bladder inflammation typically from infection; also urethral syndrome, p240).

Edema. *Causes:* ↑*Venous pressure* (eg DVT or right-heart failure) or *lowered intravascular oncotic pressure* (plasma proteins↓, eg cirrhosis, nephrosis, malnutrition, or protein-losing enteropathy (here water moves down the osmotic gradient into the interstitium to dilute the solutes there). On standing, venous pressure at the ankle rises due to the height of blood from the heart (~100mmHg). This is short-lived if leg movement pumps blood through valved veins; but if venous pressure rises, or valves fail, capillary pressure rises, fluid is forced out (edema), PCV rises locally, and microvascular stasis occurs. *Pitting edema; nonpitting edema:* (ie non-indentible) ≈ poor lymph drainage (lymphedema), eg primary (Milroy's syndrome) or secondary (radiotherapy, malignant infiltration, infection, filariasis). The mechanism is complex.

74

Epigastric pain *Acute causes:* Peritonitis; pancreatitis; GI obstruction; gall bladder disease; peptic ulcer; ruptured aortic aneurysm; irritable bowel syndrome. Referred pain: Myocardial infarct, pleural pathology. Psychological causes are also important. *Chronic causes:* Peptic ulcer; gastric cancer; chronic pancreatitis; aortic aneurysm; nerve root pain.

Facial pain This can be neurological (eg trigeminal neuralgia) or from any other pain-sensitive structure in the head or neck (SEE BOX). *Postherpetic neuralgia:* This nasty burning-and-stabbing pain (eg ophthalmic division of V) all too often becomes chronic and intractable. Skin previously affected by zoster is exquisitely sensitive. Treatment is difficult. Give strong psychological support whatever else is tried. Transcutaneous nerve stimulation, capsaicin ointment, and infiltration of local anesthetic may be tried. Amitriptyline eg 10–25mg/24h at night may help, as may carbamazepine (NNT ≈ 4). NB: Meta-analyses indicate that famciclovir and valaciclovir given in the acute stage may ↓duration of neuralgia.

Non-neurological causes of facial pain

Neck	Cervical disc pathology
Sinuses	Sinusitis; neoplasia
Eye	Glaucoma; iritis; eye strain
Temporomandibular joint	Arthritis
Teeth	Caries; abscess; malocclusion
Ear	Otitis media; otitis externa
Vascular	Giant cell arteritis

NB: When all causes are excluded, a group which is mostly young and female remains ('atypical facial pain') who complain of unilateral pain deep in the face or at the angle of cheek and nose, which is constant, severe, and unresponsive to analgesia. Do not dismiss these as psychological: Few meet criteria for hysteria or depression. Do not expose these patients to the risks of destructive surgery; while many are prescribed antidepressants, some neurologists advocate no treatment.

Fecal incontinence This is common in the elderly. Be sure to find out who does the washing: They may be under particular stress, and benefit from assistance at home. The cause may disappear if constipation (p200) is treated (='overflow incontinence'/diarrhea). Do a rectal exam. *Other GI causes:* Rectal prolapse; sphincter laxity; severe hemorrhoids. Others: See BOX.

Non-gastrointestinal causes of fecal incontinence	
Neurological	Spinal cord compression, Parkinson's disease, stroke, epilepsy
Endocrinological	Diabetes mellitus (autonomic neuropathy), myxedema
Obstetric	Damage to puborectalis (or nerve roots) at child-birth

NB: Treatment is directed to the cause if possible. Avoid dehydration. Be sure to do a rectal exam to exclude overflow incontinence. If all sensible measures fail, try the brake-and-accelerator approach: Enemas to empty the rectum (eg twice weekly) and codeine phosphate eg 15mg/12h PO on non-enema days to constipate. This is not a cure, but makes the incontinence predictable.

Fatigue This feeling is so common that it is a variant of normality. Only 1 in 400 episodes leads to a consultation with a doctor. Do not miss depression which often presents in this way. Even if the patient is depressed, a screening history and examination is important to rule out chronic disease. *Tests* should include CBC, ESR, chemistry panel, TFTS ± CXR. Arrange follow-up to see what develops, and to address any emotional problems that develop.

Fever and night sweats While moderate night sweating is common in anxiety states, drenching sweats requiring several changes of night-clothes is a more ominous symptom associated with infection (eg TB), lymphoproliferative disease, or mesothelioma. Patterns of fever may be relevant (p500). *Rigors* are uncontrolled, sometimes violent episodes of shivering which occur with some causes of fever (often acute pyogenic infections ± bacteremia).

Flank pain *Causes:* Pyelonephritis; hydronephrosis; renal calculus; renal tumor; perinephric abscess; pain referred from vertebral column.

Flatulence 400–1300mL of gas are expelled PR per day, and if this, coupled with belching (eructation) and abdominal distension, seems excessive to the patient, he may complain of flatulence. Eructation may occur in those with hiatal hernia—but most patients complaining of flatulence have no GI disease. The most likely cause is air-swallowing (aerophagia).

Frequency (urinary) means ↑frequency of micturition. It is important to differentiate ↑urine production (eg diabetes insipidus p306, diabetes mellitus, polydipsia, diuretics, renal tubular disease, adrenal insufficiency, and alcohol) from frequent passage of small amounts of urine, eg cystitis, urethritis, neurogenic bladder, extrinsic bladder compression (eg pregnancy), bladder tumor, enlarged prostate.

Guarding Reflex contraction of abdominal muscles, eg as you press (gently!) on the abdomen, signifying local or general peritoneal inflammation. It is an imperfect sign of peritonitis, but is one of the best we have; eg if you decide not to operate on someone with right lower quadrant guarding, the risk of missing appendicitis is about 25%. If you *do* operate, the chance of finding appendicitis is 50%.

Gynecomastia p298. **Hematemesis** p204. **Hematuria** p236.

75

Halitosis (bad breath) results from gingivitis (Vincent's angina), metabolic activity of bacteria in plaque, or sulfide-yielding food putrefaction. *Contributory factors:* Smoking, alcohol, drugs (disulfiram; isosorbide); lung disease. Delusional halitosis is quite common. *Treatment:* Try to eliminate anaerobes: • Use the toothbrush more frequently • Dental floss • 0.2% aqueous chlorhexidine gluconate.

The science of halitosis

Locally retained bacteria metabolize sulfur-containing amino acids to yield volatile hydrogen sulfide and methylmercaptane. Not only do these stink, but they also damage surrounding tissue, thereby perpetuating bacterial retention and periodontal disease.

At night and between meals conditions are optimal for odor production—so eating regularly may help. To supplement conventional oral hygienic measures some people advise brushing of the tongue. Oral care products containing metal ions, especially Zn, inhibit odor formation, it is thought, because of affinity of the metal ion to sulfur.

Headache see p320.

Heartburn An intermittent, gripping, retrosternal pain usually worsened by: Stooping/lying, large meals & pregnancy. See **Esophagitis** p197.

Hemiballismus This refers to the uncontrolled unilateral movements of proximal limb joints caused by subthalamic lesions.

Hemoptysis see BOX. Always think of TB ± malignancy; don't confuse with hematemesis: The blood is *coughed up* (eg frothy, alkaline, and bright red, often in a context of known chest disease). NB: Melena occurs if enough blood is swallowed. Hematemesis is acidic and dark ('coffee grounds'). Blood not mixed with sputum suggests infarction or trauma. Consider upper airway source: epistaxis, gum bleeding. Hemoptysis rarely needs treating in its own right, but if massive (eg trauma, TB, hydatid, cancer, AV malformation), call a chest physician/surgeon (the danger is drowning; lobe resection, endobronchial tamponade, or artery embolization may be needed); set up IVF, do CXR, blood gases, CBC, INR/APTT, crossmatch. If distressing, consider *prompt* IV morphine, eg if inoperable malignancy.

Causes of hemoptysis

1 *Respiratory causes of hemoptysis*	
Traumatic	Wounds; post-intubation; foreign body
Infective	Acute bronchitis; pneumonia; lung abscess; bronchiectasis; TB; fungi; paragonimiasis
Neoplastic	Primary or secondary
Vascular	Lung infarction; vasculitis (Wegener's, RA, SLE, Osler–Weber–Rendu); AV fistula; malformations
Parenchymal	Diffuse interstitial fibrosis; sarcoidosis; hemosiderosis; Goodpasture's syndrome; cystic fibrosis
2 *Cardiovascular (pulmonary hypertension)*	Pulmonary edema; mitral stenosis; aortic aneurysm; Eisenmenger's syndrome
3 *Bleeding diatheses*	

Hepatomegaly *Causes: Hepatic congestion:* Right heart failure—may be pulsatile in tricuspid incompetence, hepatic vein thrombosis. *Infection:* Glandular fever, hepatitis viruses, malaria, amoebic abcess, hydatid cyst. *Malignancy:* Metastatic or primary (usually hard ± nodular hepatomegaly), myeloma, leukemia, lymphoma. *Others:* Sickle-cell disease, other hemolytic anemias, porphyria, myeloproliferative disorders (eg myelofibrosis), storage disorders (eg amyloidosis, Gaucher's disease), early cirrhosis, or fatty infiltration.

Hoarseness p54.

Hyperpigmentation See **Skin discoloration** (p81).

Hyperventilation is over-breathing that may be either fast (tachypnea—ie >20breaths/min) or deep (hyperpnea—ie tidal volume ↑). Hyperpnea may not be perceived by the patient (unlike dyspnea), and is usually 'excessive' in that it produces a respiratory alkalosis. This may be appropriate (Kussmaul respiration) or inappropriate—the latter results in palpitations, dizziness, faintness, tinnitus, chest pains, perioral, and peripheral tingling (plasma Ca^{2+}↓). The commonest cause for hyperventilation is anxiety; others include fever and brainstem lesions.

• *Kussmaul respiration* is deep, sighing breathing that is principally seen in metabolic acidoses—diabetic ketoacidosis and uremia.
• *Neurogenic hyperventilation* is produced by pontine lesions.

Insomnia When we are sleeping well this is a trivial and irritating complaint, but if we suffer a few sleepless nights, sleep becomes the most desirable thing imaginable and the ability to bestow sleep the best thing we can do for a patient, second only to relieving pain.

Do not resort to drugs without asking: *What is the cause? Can it be treated?*

Self-limiting causes:	*Psychological:*	*Some typical organic causes:*	
Travel	Jet lag	Depression	Drugs	Nocturia	Alcoholism
Stress	Shift work	Anxiety	Pain/itch	Asthma	Dystonias
Arousal	In hospital	Mania, grief	Tinnitus	Sleep apnea (p189)	

Management: 'Sleep hygiene' • Do not go to bed until you feel sleepy.
• Avoid daytime naps. Establish regular bedtime routines.
• If you can, reserve a room for sleep. Do not eat or watch TV in it.
• Avoid caffeine, nicotine, alcohol—and late-evening hard exercise (sexual activity is the exception: It may produce excellent torpor).
• Consider monitoring with a sleep diary (quantifies sleep pattern and quality), but this could feed insomnia by encouraging obsessions.

Prescribe hypnotics for a few weeks only: They are addictive and cause daytime somnolence ± rebound insomnia on stopping. Warn about driving/machine working. Example: Trazodone 50–100mg at night as less addictive potential.

Internuclear opthalmoplegia This refers to failure of eye adduction (on the affected side) with nystagmus in the other, abducting, eye. It is due to a lesion in the medial longitudinal fasciculus eg caused by MS or stroke.

Itching (pruritus) is common and, if chronic, most unpleasant.

Local causes:	*Systemic:* (Do CBC, ESR, ferritin, LFT, urinalysis, TFT)	
Eczema; atopy; urticaria	Liver disease (bile salts)	Old age; pregnancy
Scabies	Chronic renal failure	Drug reactions
Lichen planus	Lymphomas	Iron deficiency
Dermatitis herpetiformis	Polycythemia	Thyroid disease

Questions: Is there itch with wheals (urticaria); is itching worse at night and are others affected (scabies); what provokes it? After a bath ≈ polycythemia or aquagenic urticaria. Exposure, eg to animals (?atopy) or fiberglass (irritant eczema)? *Look for local causes:* Scabies burrows in the finger webs; lice on hair shafts; knee and elbow blisters (dermatitis herpetiformis). *Systemic:* Splenomegaly, nodes, jaundice, or flushed face or thyroid signs? *Treat* primary diseases; try moisturizing creams, ± emollient bath oils and H1-antihistamines at night, eg hydroxyzine or diphenhydramine.

Jaundice p202.

Jugular venous pulse and pressure p48.

Left iliac fossa pain *Acute:* Gastroenteritis; ureteric colic; UTI; diverticulitis; torted ovarian cyst; salpingitis; ectopic; volvulus; pelvic abscess; cancer in un-descended testis. *Chronic/subacute:* Constipation; irritable bowel syndrome; colon cancer; inflammatory bowel disease; hip pathology.

Left upper quadrant pain *Causes:* Large kidney or spleen; gastric or colonic (splenic flexure) cancer; pneumonia; subphrenic or perinephric abscess; renal colic; pyelonephritis, splenic rupture.

Lid lag is lagging behind of the lid as the eye looks down. **Lid retraction** is the static state of the upper eyelid traversing the eye *above* the iris, rather than over it. *Causes* (both): Thyrotoxicosis and anxiety.

Lymphadenopathy Causes may be divided into:
Reactive: Infective Bacterial (pyogenic, TB, brucella, syphilis); fungal (coccidiomycosis); viral (EBV, CMV, HIV); toxoplasmosis, trypanosomiasis. *Non-infective* Sarcoid; connective tissue disease (rheumatoid); dermatopathic (eczema, psoriasis); drugs (phenytoin); berylliosis.
Infiltrative: Benign Histiocytosis; lipoidoses. *Malignant* Lymphoma, metastases.

Musculoskeletal symptoms Chiefly *pain, deformity, reduced functionPain: Degenerative arthritis* generally produces an aching pain worse with exercise and relieved by rest. Discomfort may be more in certain positions or motions. Cervical or lumbar spine degeneration may also produce subjective changes in sensation not following dermatome distribution. Both inflammatory and degenerative joint disease produce *morning stiffness* in the affected joints but in the former this generally improves during the day, while in the latter the pain is worse at the end of the day. The pain of *bone erosion* due to tumor or aneurysm tends to be deep, boring, and constant. The pain of *fracture* or *infection* of the bone is severe and throbbing and is increased by any motion of the part. *Acute nerve compression* causes a sharp, severe pain radiating along the distribution of the nerve. Joint pain may be referred, eg that from a hip disorder to anterior and lateral aspect of the thigh or to knee; shoulder to the lateral aspect of the humerus; cervical spine to the interscapular area, medial border of scapulae or tips of shoulders + lateral side of arms. (*Back pain*, p366.)
Reduced function: Causes: Pain, bone or joint instability, or restriction of joint movement (eg due to muscle weakness, contractures, bony fusion or mechanical block by intracapsular bony fragments or cartilage).

Nodules *(subcutaneous)* Rheumatoid nodules; PAN; xanthomata; tuberous sclerosis; neurofibromata; sarcoid; granuloma annulare; rheumatic fever.

Oliguria is defined as a urine output of <400mL/24h. This occurs in extreme dehydration, severe cardiac failure, urethral or bilateral ureteral obstruction, acute and chronic renal failure.

Orthopnea See **Dyspnea** above (p73).

Pallor is a non-specific sign and may be racial or familial. Pathology suggested by pallor includes anemia, shock, Stokes–Adams attack, vasovagal faint, myxedema, hypopituitarism, and albinism.

Palmar erythema Causes: Pregnancy; polycythemia; cirrhosis—eg via ↓inactivation of vasoactive endotoxins by the liver.

Palpitations represent to the patient the sensation of feeling his heart beat; to the doctor, the sensation of feeling his heart sink—because the symptom is notoriously elusive. Have the patient tap out the rate and regularity of the palpitations. • Irregular fast palpitations are likely to be paroxysmal AF, or flutter with variable block. • Dropped or missed beats related to rest, recumbency, or eating are likely to be atrial or ventricular ectopics. • Regular pounding is likely to be due to anxiety. • Slow palpitations are likely to be due to drugs such as β-blockers, or to bigeminy. Ask about associated pain, dyspnea, and faints, suggesting hemodynamic compromise. Ask *when* symptoms occur: People often feel their (normal) heart beat in the anxious nocturnal silence of the bedroom.

Often a clinical diagnosis of awareness of normal heart beats may be made, and reassurance is essential. If not, do TSH + transtelephonic event recording (better than 48h ECGs which may miss attacks).

Paraphimosis occurs when a tight foreskin is retracted and then becomes irreplaceable as the glans swells. It can occur when a doctor/nurse fails to replace the patient's foreskin after catheterization. Treat by asking the patient to squeeze the glans for half an hour. Or try soaking a swab in 50% dextrose, and applying it to the edematous area for an hour, and the edema may follow the osmotic gradient.

Pelvic pain *Causes:* UTI; urine retention; bladder stones; menses; labor; pregnancy; endometriosis; salpingitis; endometritis; ovarian cyst. Cancer of: Rectum, colon, ovary, cervix, bladder.

Percussion pain Pain on percussing the abdomen is a sign of peritonitis, and often less painful for the patient than testing Rebound abdominal pain (p430).

Phimosis The foreskin occludes the meatus, obstructing urine. Time (± trials of gentle retraction) usually obviates the need for circumcision.

Polyuria (eg urine >3.5L/24h). Causes: DM; over-enthusiastic IVF treatment; diabetes insipidus (p306); $Ca^{2+}\uparrow$; polydipsia; chronic renal failure.

Postural hypotension is defined as a drop in systolic or diastolic >15mmHg on standing for 3min, compared with lying down. *Causes:* Hypovolemia, Addison's disease (p292), hypopituitarism, autonomic neuropathy (eg diabetes, multisystem atrophy), idiopathic orthostatic hypotension, drugs (eg vasodilators, diuretics).

Prostatism (p476) Symptoms of prostate enlargement are often termed 'prostatism', but it is better to use the terms *cystitis* symptoms or *obstructive* bladder symptoms. Don't assume the cause is prostatic. (1) *Irritative bladder symptoms:* Urgency, dysuria, frequency, nocturia (the last two are also caused by UTI, polydipsia, detrusor instability, hypercalcemia, or uremia); (2) *Obstructive symptoms* (eg reduced size and force of urinary stream, hesitancy and interruption of stream during voiding)—may also be produced by strictures, tumors, urethral valves, or bladder neck contracture. Maximum flow rate of urine is normally ~18–30mL/s.

Pruritus See Itching, p77.

Ptosis is drooping of the upper eyelid. It is best observed with the patient sitting up, his head held by the examiner. The 3rd cranial nerve innervates the main muscle concerned (levator palpebrae), but nerves from the cervical sympathetic chain innervate the superior tarsal muscle, and a lesion of these nerves will cause a mild ptosis which can be overcome on looking up.

Causes: (1) Third nerve lesions usually causing unilateral complete ptosis. Look for other evidence of 3rd nerve lesion (ophthalmoplegia with outward deviation of the eye, pupil dilated and unreactive to light and accommodation). (2) Sympathetic paralysis usually causes unilateral partial ptosis. Look for other evidence of sympathetic lesion (constricted pupil, lack of sweating on same side of the face—Horner's syndrome). (3) Myopathy (dystrophia myotonica, myasthenia gravis). These usually cause bilateral partial ptosis. (4) Congenital (present since birth). May be unilateral or bilateral, is usually partial and is not associated with other neurological signs. (5) Syphilis.

Pulses p48.

Pupillary abnormalities The key questions are: • Are the pupils equal, central, circular, dilated, or constricted? • Do they react to light, directly and consensually? • Do they constrict normally on convergence/accommodation?

79

Irregular pupils are caused by iritis, syphilis, or globe rupture. *Dilated pupils* Causes: 3rd cranial nerve lesions and mydriatic drugs. But always ask: Is this pupil dilated, or is it the other which is constricted? *Constricted pupils* are associated with old age, sympathetic nerve damage (Horner's syndrome, and see **Ptosis** p79), opiates, miotics (eg pilocarpine eye-drops for glaucoma), and pontine damage. *Unequal pupils (anisocoria)* may be due to a unilateral lesion, eye-drops, eye surgery, syphilis, or be a Holmes–Adie pupil (below). Some inequality is normal.

Reaction to light: Test by covering one eye and shining light into the other obliquely. Both pupils should constrict (one by the direct, the other by the consensual or indirect light reflex). Lesion site may be deduced by knowing the pathway: From the retina the message passes up the optic nerve to the superior colliculus (midbrain) and thence to the 3rd nerve nuclei bilaterally. The 3rd nerve causes pupillary constriction. If a light in one eye causes only contralateral constriction, the defect is 'efferent', as the afferent pathways from the retina being stimulated must be intact. Test for a *relative afferent pupillary defect* by moving the light quickly from pupil to pupil. If an eye has severely reduced acuity (eg due to optic atrophy), the affected pupil will paradoxically dilate when the light is moved from the normal eye to the abnormal eye. This is because, in the face of reduced afferent input from the affected eye, the consensual pupillary relaxation response from the normal eye predominates. This phenomenon is also known as the Marcus Gunn sign.

Reaction to accommodation/convergence: If the patient first looks at a distant object and then at the examiner's finger held a few inches away, the eyes will converge and the pupils constrict. The neural pathway involves a projection from the cortex to the nucleus of the 3rd nerve.

Holmes-Adie (myotonic) pupil: This is a benign condition, which occurs usually in women and is unilateral in about 80% of cases. The affected pupil is normally moderately dilated and is poorly reactive to light, if at all. It is slowly reactive to accommodation; wait and watch carefully: It may eventually constrict more than a normal pupil. It is often associated with diminished or absent ankle and knee reflexes, in which case the Holmes–Adie syndrome is present. *Argyll Robertson pupil:* This occurs in neurosyphilis, but a similar phenomenon may occur in diabetes mellitus. The pupil is constricted. It is unreactive to light, but reacts to accommodation. The iris is usually patchily atrophied and depigmented. *Hutchinson pupil:* This is the sequence of events resulting from rapidly rising unilateral intracranial pressure (eg in intracerebral haemorrhage). The pupil on the side of the lesion first constricts then widely dilates. The other pupil then goes through the same sequence.

Rebound abdominal pain is present if, on the sudden removal of pressure from the examiner's hand, the patient feels a *momentary increase* in pain. It signifies local peritoneal inflammation, manifest as pain as the peritoneum rebounds after being gently displaced.

Rectal bleeding Ascertain details about • Pain on defecation? • Is blood mixed with stool, or just on surface? • Is blood just on toilet paper, or also in the toilet bowl? *Causes and classical features:* Diverticulosis (painless, large volumes of blood in bowl); colorectal cancer (blood mixed with stool); hemorrhoids (bright red blood on paper and in bowl); anal fissure (painful, bright red blood on paper and surface of stool); inflammatory bowel disease (blood and mucus mixed with loose stool); trauma; polyps; angiodysplasia; ischemic colitis; iatrogenic (radiation proctitis; post-polypectomy bleeding; aorto-enteric fistula after aortic surgery).

Regurgitation Gastric and esophageal contents are regurgitated effortlessly into the mouth—without contraction of abdominal muscles and diaphragm (so distinguishing it from true vomiting). Regurgitation is rarely preceded by nausea, and when due to gastro-esophageal reflux, it is often associated with heartburn. An esophageal pouch may cause regurgitation. Very high GI obstructions (eg gastric volvulus) cause non-productive retching rather than true regurgitation.

Right iliac fossa pain *Causes:* All causes of left iliac fossa pain (p78) plus appendicitis but usually excluding diverticulitis.

Right upper quadrant pain *Causes:* Gallstones; hepatitis; appendicitis (eg if pregnant); colonic cancer at the hepatic flexure; right kidney pathology (eg renal colic; pyelonephritis); intrathoracic conditions (eg pneumonia); subphrenic or perinephric abscess.

Rigors are uncontrolled, sometimes violent episodes of shivering which occur as a patient's temperature rises quickly from normal. FUO p500.

Skin discoloration Generalized hyperpigmentation due at least in part to melanin, may be genetic, or due to radiation, Addison's (p292), chronic renal failure, pregnancy, oral contraceptive pill, any chronic wasting (eg TB, carcinoma), malabsorption, biliary cirrhosis, hemochromatosis, chlorpromazine, or busulfan. Hyperpigmentation due to other causes occurs in jaundice, carotenemia, and gold therapy.

Splenomegaly Abnormally large spleen. If massive, think of: Leishmaniasis, malaria, myelofibrosis, chronic myeloid leukemia.

Sputum p54

Stridor is an inspiratory sound due to partial obstruction of the upper airways. That obstruction may be due to something within the lumen (eg foreign body, tumor, bilateral vocal cord palsy), within the wall (eg edema from anaphylaxis, laryngospasm, tumor, croup, acute epiglottitis), or extrinsic (eg goiter, lymphadenopathy). It is a medical (or surgical) emergency if the airway is compromised.

Subcutaneous emphysema This is a crackling sensation felt on palpating the skin over the chest or neck, caused by air tracking from the lungs eg due to a pneumothorax. It may rarely occur due to a pneumomediastinum eg following esophageal rupture.

Tactile vocal fremitus p56

Tenesmus This is a sensation felt in the rectum of incomplete emptying following defecation—as if there was something else left behind, which cannot be passed. It is very common in the irritable bowel syndrome, but can be caused by a tumor.

Terminal dribbling Dribbling at the end of urination, often seen in conjunction with incontinence following incomplete urination, is commonly associated with **prostatism** (p79).

Tinnitus p326. **Tiredness** See **Fatigue** p75.

Tremor is rhythmic oscillation of limbs, trunk, head, or tongue. 3 types:

1 *Resting tremor*—worst at rest; feature of parkinsonism, but the tremor is more resistant to treatment than bradykinesia or rigidity. Usually a slow tremor (frequency: 3–5Hz)

2 *Postural tremor*—worst, eg if arms outstretched. Typically a rapid tremor (frequency: 8–12Hz). May be exaggerated physiological tremor (eg anxiety, thyrotoxicosis, alcohol, drugs), metabolic (eg hepatic encephalopathy, CO_2 retention), due to brain damage (eg Wilson's disease, syphilis) or *benign essential tremor* (BET). This is usually a familial (autosomal dominant) tremor of

81

arms and head presenting at any age. It is suppressed by large-ish amounts of alcohol. Rarely progressive. Propranolol (40–80mg/8–12h PO) helps ~30%.

3 *Intention tremor*—worst during movement and occurs in cerebellar disease (eg in MS). No effective drug has been found.

Trousseau's sign This is elicited by inflating a BP cuff on an arm/leg to above systolic pressure. The hands and feet go into spasm (carpopedal spasm) in hypocalcemia. The metacarpophalangeal joints become flexed and the interphalangeal joints are extended. See **Chvostek's sign**, p71.

Urinary changes *Cloudy urine* suggests pus (infection, UTI) but is often normal phosphate precipitation in an alkaline urine. *Pneumaturia* (bubbles in urine as it is passed) occurs with UTI due to gas-forming organisms or may signal an enterovesical (bowel-bladder) fistula from diverticulitis or neoplastic diseases of the gut. *Nocturia* is seen in 'prostatism', diabetes mellitus, UTI, and reversed diurnal rhythm as occurs with renal and cardiac failure. *Hematuria* (RBC in urine) is due to neoplasia or glomerulonephritis until proven otherwise.

- **Visual loss** Get ophthalmic help. *If sudden, ask:* Is the eye painful/red (*glaucoma; iritis*)? *Optic neuritis* may be painful.
- What is each eye's acuity? Is there a contact lens problem (eg *infection*)?
- History of trauma, migraine, TIA, MS, or *diabetes*; what is the blood sugar?
- Any flashes/floaters (*TIA, migraine, retinal artery occlusion; detachment*)?
- Is the cornea cloudy: *Corneal ulcer; glaucoma*?
- Is there a visual field problem/hemianopsia (*stroke, space-occupying lesion, glaucoma*)? Formal field testing requires ophthalmic help.
- Any heart disease/bruits? (*emboli*); hyperlipidemia (xanthoma)?
- Is the BP raised or lowered? Measure it lying and standing.
- Are there focal CNS signs? Is there an afferent pupillary defect (p79)?
- Tender temporal arteries ± ESR ↑ ≈ *giant cell arteritis*: Urgent steroids, p379.
- Any distant signs: *HIV* (causes retinitis), *SLE, sarcoid, Behçet's disease*, etc.?

Voice and disturbance of speech (p64) may be noted by the patient or the doctor. Assess if difficulty is with articulation (*dysarthria*, eg from muscle problems), or of word command (*dysphasia*—always central).

Vomiting Causes of nausea/vomiting include:

Gastrointestinal	*CNS*	*Metabolic/endocrine*
Gastroenteritis	Meningitis/encephalitis	Uremia
Peptic ulceration	Migraine	Hypercalcemia
Pyloric stenosis	↑Intracranial pressure	Hyponatremia
Intestinal obstruction	Brainstem lesions	Pregnancy
Paralytic ileus	Motion sickness	Diabetic ketoacidosis
Acute cholecystitis	Ménière's disease	Addison's disease
Acute pancreatitis	Labyrinthitis	Drugs:
	Psychiatric disorder:	• alcohol
Other	• self-induced	• antibiotics
Myocardial infarction	• psychogenic	• cytotoxics
Autonomic neuropathy	• bulimia nervosa	• digoxin
UTI		• opiates

The history is very important: Ask about timing, relationship to meals, amount, and content (liquid, solid, bile, blood, 'coffee grounds'). Associated symptoms and previous medical history often indicate the cause. *Signs:* Look for signs of dehydration. Examine the abdomen for distension, tenderness, an abdominal mass, a succussion splash (pyloric stenosis), or tinkling bowel sounds (intestinal obstruction).

Non-gastrointestinal causes of vomiting

Never forget these, as they can be a sign of serious disease. The following mnemonic covers the most important non-gastrointestinal causes of vomiting: **ABCDEFGHI**

- **A**cute renal failure/**A**ddison's disease
- **B**rain (eg ↑ICP, p722)
- **C**ardiac (myocardial infarct)
- **D**iabetic ketoacidosis
- **E**ars (eg labyrinthitis, Ménière's disease)
- **F**oreign substances (alcohol, drugs eg opiates)
- **G**ravidity (eg hyperemesis gravidarum)
- **H**ypercalcemia/**H**yponatremia
- **I**nfection (eg UTI, meningitis)

Walking difficulty: In the elderly, this is a common and non-specific presentation: The reason may be *local* (typically osteo- or rheumatoid arthritis, but remember fractured neck of femur), *systemic* (eg pneumonia, UTI, anemia, drugs, hypothyroidism, renal failure, hypothermia), or even a manifestation of depression or bereavement. *It is only rarely a manipulative strategy.*

More specific causes to consider are Parkinson's disease (p348), polymyalgia rheumatica (very treatable, p379), and various neuropathies/myopathies. One of the key questions is 'Is there pain?'—another issue to address is whether there is muscle wasting and, if so, is it symmetrical?

If there is also ataxia, the cause is not always alcohol: Other chemicals may be involved (cannabis, arsenic, thallium, mercury—or prescribed sedatives), or there may be a metastatic or non-metastatic manifestation of malignancy—or a CNS primary or vascular lesion.

Remember also treatable conditions, such as pellagra (p230), B₁₂↓, and beriberi, and infections such as encephalitis, myelitis, Lyme disease, brucellosis, or rarities such as botulism (p53).

Bilateral weak legs in an otherwise fit person suggests a cord lesion p531. If there is associated incontinence ± saddle anesthesia, prompt treatment for cord compression may be needed.

Waterbrash refers to the excessive secretion of saliva, which suddenly fills the mouth. It typically occurs after meals, and may denote G-E reflux disease. It is suggested that this is an exaggeration of the esophago-salivary reflex. It should not be confused with **regurgitation** (p197).

Weight loss is a feature of chronic disease and depression—also of malnutrition, chronic infections, and infestations (eg TB, HIV/enteropathic AIDS), malignancy, diabetes mellitus, and hyperthyroidism (typically in the presence of increased appetite). Severe generalized muscle wasting is also seen as part of a number of degenerative neurological and muscle diseases and in cardiac failure (cardiac cachexia), although in the latter, right heart failure may not make weight loss a major complaint. Do not forget anorexia nervosa as a possible underlying cause of weight loss.

Focus on treatable causes, eg diabetes is easy to diagnose—TB can be very hard. For example, the CXR may look like cancer, so you may forget to send bronchoscopy samples for AFB stain and TB culture (to the detriment not just of the patient, but to the entire ward).

Wheeze p56

Whispered pectoriloquy This refers to the increased transmission of a patient's whispers heard when auscultating over consolidated lung. It is a manifestation of ↑vocal resonance. **NB:** *Vocal resonance* is sound vibration of the patient's spoken or whispered voice transmitted to the stethoscope. *Tactile* *fremitus* is the sound vibration of the spoken or whispered voice transmitted via the lung fields and detected by palpation over the back.

Xanthomata These are localized deposits of fat under the skin surface, commonly occurring over joints, tendons, hands, and feet. They are a sign of hyperlipidemia (p106). *Xanthelasma palpebra* is a xanthoma on the eyelid.

84

Unexplained signs and symptoms: How to refer a patient for an opinion

▶*When you don't know: Ask.*

▶*If you find yourself wondering if you should ask: Ask.*

Frequently, the skills needed will require the help of a consultant. If so, during ward rounds, agree who should be asked for an opinion. You will be left with the job of making the arrangements. This can be a daunting task, if you are very junior and have been asked to contact an intimidating consultant. Don't be intimidated: Perhaps this may be an opportunity to learn something new. A few simple points can help the process go smoothly.

• Have the patient's notes, observations, and drug charts at hand.
• Be familiar with the history: You may be interrogated.
• Ask if it is a convenient time to talk.
• At the outset, state if you are just looking for advice or if you are asking if the patient could be seen. Make it clear exactly what the question is that you want addressed, 'We wonder why Mr Smith's legs have become weak today...' This helps the listener to focus their thoughts while you describe the story and will save you wasting time if the switchboard has put you through to the wrong specialist.
• Give the patient's age and occupation, to give a snapshot of the person.
• Run through a brief history. Do not present the case as if you are in formal rounds—it will take ages to get to the point and the listener will get more and more irritated.
• If you would like the patient to be seen, give warning if you know that they will be going off the ward for a test at a particular time.
• If you are on the ward when the consultant arrives, offer to introduce him/her to the patient.

We thank Martin Zeidler for providing the first draft of this page.

Cardiovascular medicine

Stuart Russell, M.D.

Contents

Cardiovascular health

Ischemic heart disease (IHD), even though ↓ in incidence, is still the most common cause of death worldwide. Encouraging cardiovascular health is not *only* about preventing IHD. The activities that are associated with improving cardiovascular health have many beneficial side effects as well. Exercise will improve cardiovascular health (BP↓, HDL↑) but can also prevent osteoporosis and improve glucose tolerance. People who improve *and maintain* their fitness live longer: *Age-adjusted mortality from all causes is reduced by >40%.* Avoiding obesity helps too, but there is no evidence that losing weight will lengthen life. However, the risk of diabetes *will* diminish if weight loss can be achieved.

Smoking is the major modifiable risk factor for cardiovascular mortality. You *can* help people quit, and quitting *does* undo much of the harm of smoking. *Simple advice works.* Most smokers want to give up. Just because smoking advice does not *always* work, do not stop giving it. Ask about smoking during every visit—especially those concerned with smoking-related diseases.
- Ensure advice is congruent with the patient's beliefs about smoking.
- Concentrate on the benefits of giving up.
- Invite the patient to choose a date (when there will be few stressors) on which he or she will become a non-smoker. You may suggest the birth-day of a loved one or an anniversary so that they stop as a 'gift'.
- Suggest throwing away all accessories (cigarettes, pipes, ashtrays, lighters, matches) in advance; inform friends of the new change; practice saying 'no' to their offers of 'just one cigarette'.
- *Nicotine gum*, chewed intermittently to limit nicotine release: ≥10 × 2mg sticks may be needed/day. *Transdermal nicotine patches* may be easier. Written advice offers no added benefit to advice from nurses. Always offer follow-up.
- *Bupropion* may improve the success rate in those who want to quit to 30% at 1yr vs. 16% with patches and 15.6% for placebo (patches+ bupropion: 35.5%): Consider if the above fails. *Dose:* 150mg PO qD (while still smoking; quit within 2wks); dose may be twice daily from day 7; stop after 7wks. *Warn of SEs:* Seizures (risk <1:1000), insomnia, headache. *CI:* Epilepsy; cirrhosis; pregnancy/lactation; bipolar depression; eating disorders; CNS tumors; on antimalarials etc; alcohol or benzodiazepine withdrawal.

Lipids and BP (p106, p130) are the other major modifiable risk factors (few can change their sex or genes).

Apply preventive measures such as healthy eating (see p192) *early* in life to maximize impact, when there are most years to save, and before bad habits get ingrained.

For more on risk factors and their impact see the American Heart Association *Heart Disease and Stroke Statistics* 2005 update.

Cardiovascular symptoms

Chest pain Cardiac-sounding chest pain may have no serious cause, but always think 'Could this be a MI, dissecting aortic aneurysm, pericarditis, or pulmonary embolism?'.

Nature of pain: Constricting suggests angina, esophageal spasm, or anxiety; a *sharp* pain may be from the pleura or pericardium, especially if exacerbated by inspiration. A prolonged (>½h), dull, central crushing pain or pressure suggests MI. Stabbing, short lasting (<30s), or pain in continually varying location is less likely to be cardiac.

Radiation: To shoulder, either or both arms, or neck/jaw suggests cardiac ischemia. The pain of aortic dissection is classically instantaneous, tearing, and interscapular, but may be retrosternal. Epigastric pain may be cardiac.

Precipitants: Pain associated with cold, exercise, palpitations, or emotion suggest cardiac pain or anxiety; if brought on by food, lying flat, hot drinks, or alcohol, consider esophageal spasm (but meals *can* cause angina).

Relieving factors: If pain is relieved *within minutes* by rest or nitroglycerin, suspect angina. Nitroglycerin can relieve esophageal spasm, but usually more slowly. If antacids help, suspect GI causes. Pericarditis pain improves on leaning forward.

Associations: Dyspnea occurs with cardiac pain, pulmonary embolism, pleurisy, or anxiety. MI may cause nausea, vomiting, or sweating. In addition to coronary artery disease, angina may be caused by aortic stenosis (AS), hypertrophic obstructive cardiomyopathy (HOCM), paroxysmal supraventricular tachycardia (SVT) and be exacerbated by anemia. Chest pain with *tenderness* suggests self-limiting costochondritis (Tietze's syndrome).

Differential diagnosis of chest pain: Pleuritic pain (ie exacerbated by inspiration) implies inflammation of the pleura 2° to pulmonary infection, inflammation, or infarction. The patient may 'catch their breath'. *Musculoskeletal pain:* Exacerbated by pressure on the affected area. *Fractured rib:* Pain on respiration, exacerbated by gentle pressure on the sternum. *Subdiaphragmatic pathology* may also mimic cardiac pain.

Acutely ill patients: • Admit to hospital • Check pulse, BP in both arms, JVP, heart sounds, and examine the legs for DVT • Give O_2 by face mask • Insert an IV line • Relieve pain (eg morphine 5–10mg IV slowly + an antiemetic) • Place on cardiac monitor; do 12-lead ECG • CXR • Arterial blood gas (ABG).

Famous traps: Aortic dissection (a tearing or ripping sensation, often midscapular). Make sure you check all pulses and bilateral BP; Herpes zoster (p510); ruptured esophagus; cardiac tamponade (shock with JVP↑); opiation addiction.

Dyspnea may be from LVF, pulmonary embolism, any respiratory cause, or anxiety. *Severity:* Emergency presentations. Ask about shortness of breath at rest or on exertion, orthopnea, PND, exercise tolerance, and coping with daily tasks. *Associations:* Specific symptoms associated with heart failure are orthopnea (ask about number of pillows used at night or if sitting in a recliner), paroxysmal nocturnal dyspnoea (waking up at night gasping for breath), and peripheral edema. Pulmonary embolism is associated with acute onset of dyspnea and pleuritic chest pain; ask about risk factors for DVT.

Palpitation(s) may be due to premature ventricular contractions, AF, SVT and ventricular tachycardia (VT), thyrotoxicosis, anxiety, and rarely pheochromocytoma. *History:* Ask about previous episodes, precipitating/relieving factors, duration of symptoms, associated chest pain, dyspnea, or dizziness. *Did the patient check their pulse?*

Syncope may reflect cardiac or CNS events. Vasovagal 'faints' are common (pulse↓, pupils dilated). The history from an observer is invaluable in diagnosis. *Prodromal symptoms:* Chest pain, palpitations, or dyspnea point to a cardiac cause, eg arrhythmia. Aura, headache, dysarthria, limb weakness indicate CNS causes. *During the episode:* Was there a pulse? Was there limb jerking, tongue biting, or urinary incontinence? **NB:** Hypoxia from lack of cerebral perfusion may cause seizures. *Recovery:* Was this rapid (arrhythmia) or prolonged and associated with post-ictal drowsiness (seizure)?

How patients communicate ischemic cardiac sensations

In emergency departments we are always hearing questions such as 'Is your pain sharp or dull?' followed by an equivocal answer. The doctor goes on 'Sharp like a knife—or dull and crushing?' The doctor is getting irritated because the patient must know the answer, but is not saying it. Instead of asking the questions that we relate to cardiac chest pain (chest heaviness associated with dyspnea and radiation to the jaw and left arm) allow the patient to tell their story. Patients often avoid using the word 'pain' to describe ischemia: 'Heaviness', 'tightening', 'pressure', 'burning', or 'a lump in the throat' (angina means to choke) may be used. They may say 'sharp' to communicate severity, and not character. So be as vague in your questioning as your patient is in their answers. 'Tell me some more about what you are feeling (long pause)… as if someone was doing *what* to you?' 'Sitting on me', or 'like a hotness' might be the response (suggesting cardiac ischemia). Do not ask 'Does it go into your left arm'. Try 'Is there anything else about it?' (pause)… 'Does it go anywhere?' Note your patient's exact words.

Note also non-verbal clues: The clenched fist placed over the sternum is a telling feature of cardiac pain (Levine sign positive).

A good history, taking account of these features, is the best way to stratify patients likely to have cardiac pain. If the history is non-specific, and there are no risk factors for cardiovascular diseases, and ECG and plasma troponin T (p110) are normal (<0.2mcg/L) 6–12h after the onset of pain, discharge will probably be OK. But when in doubt, get help.

Features making cardiac pain unlikely:
- Stabbing, shooting pain
- Pain lasting <30s, however intense
- Well-localized, left sub-mammary pain ('In my heart, doctor')
- Pains of continually varying location
- Youth.

Do not feel that you must diagnose every pain. *Chest pain with no cause* is common. Extensive testing, including cardiac catheterization and ruling out depression may not find the cause. Do not reject these patients: Explain your findings to them. Some have a 'chronic pain syndrome' which responds to a tricyclic, eg imipramine 50mg at night[1] (this dose does not imply any depression). It is similar to post-herpetic neuralgia.

1 Cannon RO, Quyyumi AA, Mincemoyer R, *et al.* 1994 *NEJM* **330** 1411–7.

ECG—a methodical approach

First confirm the patient's name and age, and the ECG date. Then:

- *Rate:* At usual speed (25mm/s) each 'big square' is 0.2s; each 'small square' is 0.04s. To calculate the rate, divide 300 by the number of big squares per R–R interval (p91).

- *Rhythm:* If the cycles are not clearly regular, use the 'card method': Lay a card along ECG, marking positions of 3 successive R waves. Slide the card to and fro to check that all intervals are equal. If not, note if different rates are multiples of each other (ie varying block), or is it 100% irregular (atrial fibrillation [AF] or ventricular fibrillation, [VF])? *Sinus rhythm* is characterized by a P wave (upright in II, III, & aVF; inverted in aVR) followed by a QRS complex. AF has no discernible P waves and the QRS complexes are irregularly irregular. *Atrial flutter* has a 'sawtooth' baseline of atrial depolarization (~300/min) and regular QRS complexes. *Nodal rhythm* has a normal QRS complex but P waves are absent or occur just before or within the QRS complex. *Ventricular rhythm* has QRS complexes >0.12s with P waves following them.

- *Axis:* The mean frontal axis is the sum of all the ventricular forces during ventricular depolarization. The axis lies at 90° to the isoelectric complex (ie the one in which positive and negative deflections are equal). *Normal axis* is between −30° and +90°. As a simple rule of thumb, if the complexes in leads I and II are both 'positive', the axis is normal. *Left axis deviation* (LAD) is −30° to −90°. Causes: Left anterior hemiblock, inferior MI, VT from LV focus, Wolff–Parkinson–White (WPW) syndrome (some types). *Right axis deviation* (RAD) is +90° to +180°. Causes: RVH, PE, anterolateral MI, left posterior hemiblock (rare), WPW syndrome (some types).

- *P wave:* Normally precedes each QRS complex. *Absent P wave:* AF, sinoatrial block, junctional (AV nodal) rhythm. Dissociation between P waves and QRS complexes indicates complete heart block. *P mitrale:* Bifid P wave in lead II and biphasic P wave in lead V_1, indicates left atrial hypertrophy. *P pulmonale:* Peaked P wave (>2.5mm in lead II), indicates right atrial hypertrophy. Pseudo-P-pulmonale seen if $K^+\downarrow$.

- *P–R interval:* Measure from start of P wave to start of QRS. *Normal range:* 0.12–0.2s (3–5 small squares). A *prolonged P-R interval* implies delayed AV conduction (1st degree heart block). A *short P-R interval* implies unusually fast AV conduction down an accessory pathway, eg WPW (ECG p121). In 2nd degree block some P waves aren't followed by a QRS. If the PR interval ↑ with each cycle until there is a P wave not followed by a QRS, this is Möbitz type I (Wenckebach) AV block. If the PR interval is constant and a P wave is not followed by a QRS, this is Möbitz type II AV block. In 3rd degree block the P waves and QRS waves are independent of each other.

- *QRS complex:* Normal duration: <0.12s. If ≥0.12s suggests ventricular conduction defects, eg a bundle branch block (p93). Large QRS complexes suggest *ventricular hypertrophy* (p93). Normal Q wave <0.04s wide and <2mm deep. *Pathological Q waves* may occur within a few hours of an acute MI.

- *QT interval:* Measure from start of QRS to end of T wave. It varies with rate. Calculate *corrected QT interval (QT^c)* by dividing the measured QT interval by the square root of the cycle length, ie $QT^c = (QT)/(\sqrt{R-R})$. Normal QT^c: 0.38–0.43s. *Prolonged QT interval:* Acute myocardial ischemia, myocarditis, bradycardia (eg AV block), head injury, hypothermia, electrolyte imbalance ($K^+\downarrow$, $Ca^{2+}\downarrow$, $Mg^{2+}\downarrow$), congenital (Romano–Ward & Jervell–Lange–Nielson syndromes); sotalol, quinidine, antihistamines, macrolides (eg erythromycin), amiodarone, phenothiazines, tricyclics.

- *ST segment:* Usually isoelectric. Planar elevation (>1mm) or depression (>0.5mm) usually implies infarction (p111) or ischemia (p99), respectively.

- *T wave:* Abnormal if inverted in I, II, and V_4–V_6. It is peaked in hyperkalemia (ECG 13, p621) and flattened in hypokalemia.

- *U WAVE:* May be prominent in hypokalemia but can also be normal.

- *J WAVE:* Associated with hypothermia.

ECG nomenclature (ventricular activation time, VAT)

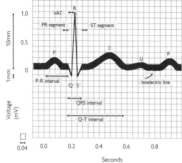

Calculating the R-R interval To calculate the rate, divide 300 by the number of big squares per R-R interval—if the standard ECG speed of 25mm/s is used (elsewhere, 50mm/s may be used: Don't be confused!)

R-R duration(s)	Big squares	Rate (per min)
0.2	1	300
0.4	2	150
0.6	3	100
0.8	4	75
1.0	5	60
1.2	6	50
1.4	7	43

Determining the ECG axis
• The axis lies at 90° to the isoelectric complex (the one in which positive and negative deflections are equal in size).
• If the complexes in I and II are both predominantly positive, the axis is normal.

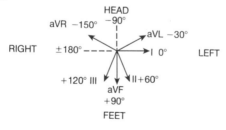

Causes of LAD	*Causes of RAD*
Left anterior hemiblock	RVH
Inferior MI	Pulmonary embolism
VT from LV focus	Anterolateral MI
WPW syndrome (some) p121	Left posterior hemiblock (rare)
Left ventricular hypertrophy	WPW syndrome (some)

ECG—abnormalities

Sinus tachycardia: Rate >100. Anxiety, exercise, pain, fever, sepsis, hypovolemia, heart failure, pulmonary embolism, pregnancy, thyrotoxicosis, beri beri, CO_2 retention, autonomic neuropathy, sympathomimetics, eg caffeine, adrenaline, and nicotine (may produce abrupt changes in sinus rate, and other arrhythmias).

Sinus bradycardia: Rate <60. Physical fitness, vasovagal attacks, sick sinus syndrome, acute MI (esp. inferior), drugs (beta blockers, digoxin, amiodarone, verapamil), hypothyroidism, hypothermia, ↑intracranial pressure, cholestasis.

AF: (ECG p117) Common causes: IHD thyrotoxicosis, hypertension.

1st and 2nd degree heart block: Normal variant, athletes, sick sinus syndrome, IHD, acute carditis, drugs (digoxin, beta blockers).

Complete heart block: Idiopathic (fibrosis), congenital, IHD, aortic valve calcification, cardiac surgery/trauma, digoxin toxicity, infiltration (abscesses, granulomas, tumors, parasites).

ST elevation: Normal variant (high take-off), acute MI, Prinzmetal's angina, acute pericarditis (saddle-shaped), left ventricular aneurysm.

ST depression: Normal variant (upward sloping), digoxin (downward sloping), ischemic (horizontal): Angina, acute posterior MI.

T inversion: In V_1–V_3: Normal (black people and children), right bundle branch block (RBBB), pulmonary embolism. In V_2–V_5: Subendocardial MI, HOCM, subarachnoid hemorrhage, lithium. In V_4–V_6 and aVL: Ischemia, LVH, associated with left bundle branch block (LBBB).

92 **NB:** ST and T wave changes are often non-specific, and must be interpreted in the light of the clinical context.

MI: (ECG p111.)
- Within hours, the T wave may become peaked, and the ST segment may begin to rise.
- Within 24h, the T wave inverts, as ST segment elevation begins to resolve. ST elevation rarely persists, unless a left ventricular aneurysm develops. T wave inversion may or may not persist.
- Within a few days, pathological Q waves begin to form. Q waves usually persist, but may resolve in 10%.

The leads affected reflect the site of the infarct: Inferior (II, III, aVF), anteroseptal (V_{1-4}), anterolateral (V_{4-6}, I, aVL), posterior (tall R and ST↓ in V_{1-2}).

'Non-Q wave infarcts' (formerly called subendocardial infarcts) have ST and T changes without Q waves.

Pulmonary embolism: Sinus tachycardia is commonest. There may be RAD, RBBB (p93), right ventricular strain pattern V_{1-3} or AF. Rarely, the classic '$S_IQ_{III}T_{III}$' pattern occurs: Deep S waves in I, pathological Q waves in III, inverted T waves in III.

Metabolic abnormalities: Digoxin effect: ST depression and inverted T wave in V_{5-6}. In *digoxin toxicity*, any arrhythmia may occur (ventricular ectopy & nodal bradycardia are common). *Hyperkalemia:* Tall, tented T wave, widened QRS, absent P waves, 'sine wave' appearance (ECG 13, p621). *Hypokalemia:* Small T waves, prominent U waves. *Hypercalcemia:* Short QT interval. *Hypocalcemia:* Long QT interval, small T waves.

ECG—additional points

Where to place the chest leads

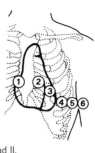

V_1: Right sternal edge, 4th intercostal space

V_2: Left sternal edge, 4th intercostal space

V_3: Half-way between V_2 and V_4

V_4: The patient's apex beat

All subsequent leads are in the same horizontal plane as V_4

V_5: Anterior axillary line

V_6: Mid-axillary line (V_7: Posterior axillary line)

Finish 12-lead ECGs with a long rhythm strip in lead II.

Disorders of ventricular conduction

Bundle branch block (p94, see ECGs 1 and 2) Delayed conduction is evidenced by prolongation of QRS >0.12s. Abnormal conduction patterns lasting <0.12s are incomplete blocks. The area that would have been reached by the blocked bundle depolarizes slowly and late. Taking V_1 as an example, right ventricular depolarization is normally +ve and left ventricular depolarization is normally –ve.

In RBBB, the following pattern is seen: QRS >0.12s, 'RSR' pattern in V_1, dominant R in V_1, inverted T waves in V_1–V_3 or V_4, deep wide S wave in V_6. Causes: Normal variant (isolated RBBB), pulmonary embolism, cor pulmonale.

In LBBB, the following pattern is seen: QRS >0.12s, 'M' pattern in V_5, no septal Q waves, inverted T waves in I, aVL, V_5–V_6. Causes: IHD, hypertension, cardiomyopathy, idiopathic fibrosis. **NB:** If there is LBBB, no comment can be made on the ST segment or T wave.

Bifascicular block is the combination of RBBB and left bundle hemiblock, manifest as an axis deviation, eg LAD in the case of left anterior hemiblock.

Trifascicular block is the combination of bifascicular block and 1st degree heart block.

Ventricular hypertrophy There is no single marker of ventricular hypertrophy: Electrical axis, voltage, and ST wave changes should all be taken into consideration. Relying on a single marker such as voltage may be unreliable as a thin chest wall may result in large voltage whereas a thick chest wall may mask it.

Suspect *left ventricular hypertrophy* (LVH) if the R wave in V_6 >25mm or the sum of the S wave in V_1 and the R wave in V_6 is >35mm (ECG 8 p133).

Suspect *right ventricular hypertrophy* (RVH) if dominant R wave in V_1, T wave inversion in V_1–V_3 or V_4, deep S wave in V_6, RAD.

Other causes of *dominant R wave in V_1*: RBBB, posterior MI, some types of WPW syndrome (p118).

Causes of low voltage QRS complex: (QRS <5mm in all limb leads.) Hypothyroidism, chronic obstructive pulmonary disease (COPD), ↑hematocrit (intra-cardiac blood resistivity is related to hematocrit), changes in chest wall impedance (eg in renal failure, subcutaneous emphysema but *not* obesity), pulmonary embolism, bundle branch block, carcinoid heart disease, myocarditis, cardiac amyloid, adriamycin cardiotoxicity, and other heart muscle diseases, pericardial effusion, pericarditis.

93

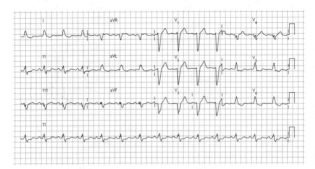

ECG 1—left bundle branch block: Note the W pattern in V_1 and the M pattern in V_6.

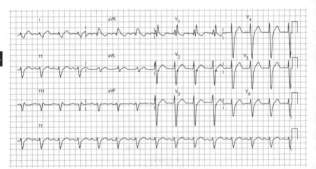

ECG 2—right bundle branch block—note the M pattern in V_1 and the W pattern in V_5.

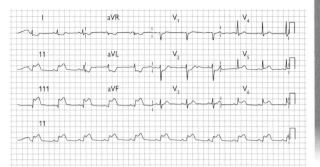

ECG 3—acute infero-lateral myocardial infarction: Note the marked ST elevation in the inferior leads (II, III, aVF), but also in V_5 and V_6, indicating lateral involvement as well. There is also 'reciprocal change' ie ST-segment depression in leads I and aVL. The latter is often seen with a large myocardial infarction.

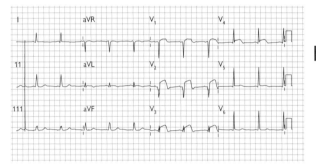

ECG 4—acute anterior myocardial infarction—note the marked ST segment elevation and evolving Q waves in leads V_1–V_4.

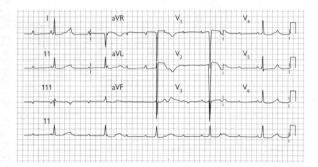

ECG 5—complete heart block. Note the dissociation between the P waves and the QRS complexes. QRS complexes are relatively narrow, indicating that there is a ventricular rhythm originating from the conducting pathway.

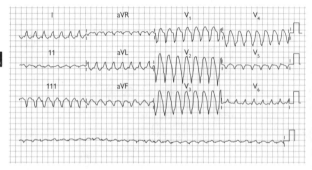

ECG 6—ventricular tachycardia—note the broad complexes.

ECG 7—dual chamber pacemaker. Note the pacing spikes which occur before some of the P waves, and the QRS complexes.

Exercise ECG testing

The patient undergoes a graduated, treadmill exercise test, with continuous 12-lead ECG and BP monitoring. There are numerous treadmill protocols; the 'Bruce protocol' is the most widely used.

Indications:
- To help confirm a suspected diagnosis of IHD.
- Assessment of cardiac function and exercise tolerance.
- Prognosis following MI. Often done pre-discharge (if +ve, worse outcome).
- Evaluation of response to treatment (drugs, angioplasty, coronary artery bypass grafting [CABG]).
- Assessment of exercise-induced arrhythmias.

Contraindications:
- Unstable angina.
- Recent Q wave MI (<5d).
- Severe AS.
- Uncontrolled arrhythmia, hypertension (systemic or pulmonary), or heart failure.

Be cautious about arranging tests that will be hard to perform or interpret. These patients should have some type of imaging in addition to a stress test:
- Complete heart block, LBBB.
- Pacemaker patients.
- Osteoarthritis, COPD, stroke, or other limitations to exercise.

Stop the test if:
- Chest pain or dyspnea occurs. You want to make sure that the patient has a maximal test and would consider not stopping for minor chest pain without EKG changes.
- The patient feels faint, exhausted, or is in danger of falling.
- ST segment elevation/depression >2mm (with or without chest pain).
- Atrial or ventricular arrhythmia (not just ectopy).
- Fall in BP or excessive rise in BP (systolic >230mmHg).
- Development of AV block or LBBB.
- Maximal or 90% maximal heart rate for age is achieved.

Interpreting the test: A +ve test only allows one to assess the *probability* that the patient has IHD. 75% with significant coronary artery disease have a +ve test, but so do 5% of people with normal arteries (the false positive rate is even higher in middle-aged women, eg 20%). The more +ve the result, the higher the predictive accuracy. Down-sloping ST depression is much more significant than up-sloping, eg 1mm J-point depression with down-sloping ST segment is 99% predictive of 2–3 vessel disease.

Morbidity: 24 in 100,000. *Mortality:* 10 in 100,000.

Ambulatory ECG monitoring

Continuous ECG monitoring for 24h may be used to evaluate for paroxysmal arrhythmias. However, >70% of patients will not have symptoms during the period of monitoring. ~20% will have a normal ECG during symptoms and only up to 10% will have an arrhythmia coinciding with symptoms. Give these patients an event recorder they can activate themselves during a symptomatic episode. These episodes can then be transmitted via a telephone for evaluation. Recorders may also be programmed to detect ST segment depression, either symptomatic (to prove angina), or to reveal 'silent' ischemia (predictive of re-infarction or death soon after MI).

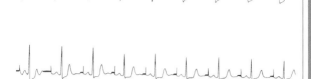

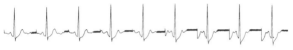

Each complex is taken from sample ECGs (lead V₅) recorded at 1-min intervals during exercise (top line) and recovery (bottom line). At maximum ST depression, the ST segment is almost horizontal. This is a positive exercise test.

This is an exercise ECG in the same format. It is negative because although the J point is depressed, the ensuing ST segment is steeply up sloping.

Cardiac catheterization

This involves the insertion of a catheter into the heart via the femoral (or radial/brachial) artery or vein. The catheter is manipulated within the heart and great vessels to measure pressures. Catheterization can also be used to:
• Sample blood to assess oxygen saturation.
• Inject radiopaque contrast medium to image the anatomy of the heart and flow in blood vessels.
• Perform angioplasty (± stenting), valvuloplasty, and cardiac biopsies.
• Perform intravascular ultrasound to quantify arterial narrowing.

During the procedure, ECG and arterial pressures are monitored continuously.

Indications:
• *Coronary artery disease:* Diagnostic (assessment of coronary vessels and graft patency); therapeutic (angioplasty, stent insertion).
• *Valve disease:* Diagnostic (to assess severity); therapeutic valvuloplasty.
• *Congenital heart disease:* Diagnostic (assessment of severity of lesions); therapeutic (balloon dilatation or septostomy).
• *Other:* Cardiomyopathy; pericardial disease; endomyocardial biopsy.

Pre-procedure checks:
• Brief history/examination; **NB:** Peripheral pulses, bruits, aneurysms.
• Investigations: Electrolytes, BUN/creatinine, CBC, PT/PTT, type & screen, ECG.
• Consent for angiogram ± angioplasty ± stent depending on the indication of the procedure. Explain reason for procedure and possible complications (below).
• IV access, ideally in the left hand.
• Patient should be nothing by mouth (NPO) for at least 6h before the procedure.
• Patients should take all their morning drugs (& pre-medication if needed). Withhold oral hypoglycemics and only give ½ dose of insulin.

Post-procedure checks:
• Pulse, blood pressure, arterial puncture site (for bruising or swelling? false aneurysm), peripheral pulses.
• Investigations: CBC and PT/PTT (if suspected blood loss), ECG.

Complications:
• *Hemorrhage.* Apply firm pressure over puncture site. If you suspect a false aneurysm, diagnostic ultrasound is required. Some require ultrasound guided or surgical repair.
• *Contrast reaction.* This is usually mild with modern contrast agents.
• *Loss of peripheral pulse.* May be due to dissection, thrombosis, or arterial spasm. Occurs in <1% of brachial catheterizations. Rare with femoral catheterization.
• *Angina.* May occur during or after cardiac catheterization. Usually responds to sublingual NTG; if not give analgesia and IV nitrates.
• *Arrhythmias.* Usually transient. Manage along standard lines and remove all catheters from the heart.
• *Pericardial tamponade.* Rare, but should be suspected if the patient becomes hypotensive and/or anuric.
• *Infection.* Post-catheter fever is usually due to a contrast reaction. If it persists for >24h, take blood cultures before giving antibiotics.

Mortality: <1 in 1000 patients, in most centers.

Intra-cardiac electrophysiology This catheter technique can determine types and origins of arrhythmias, and locate (and ablate) aberrant pathways (eg causing atrial flutter or VT). Arrhythmias may be induced, and the effectiveness of control by drugs assessed.

Normal values for intracardiac pressures and saturations

Location	Pressure (mmHg) Mean	Range	Saturation (%)
Inferior vena cava			76
Superior vena cava			70
Right atrium	4	0–8	74
Right ventricle			74
Systolic	25	15–30	
End-diastolic	4	0–8	
Pulmonary artery			74
Systolic	25	15–30	
Diastolic	10	5–15	
Mean	15	10–20	
Pulmonary artery	a	3–12	74
Wedge pressure	v	3–15	
Left ventricle			
Systolic	110	80–140	98
End-diastolic	8	5–12	
Aorta			
Systolic	110	80–140	98
Diastolic	70	60–90	
Mean	85	70–105	
Brachial			
Systolic	120	90–140	98
Diastolic	72	60–90	
Mean	83	70–105	

Gradients across stenotic valves

Valve	Normal gradient (mmHg)	Stenotic gradient (mmHg) Mild	Moderate	Severe
Aortic	0	<30	30–50	>50
Mitral	0	<5	5–15	>15
Prosthetic	5–10			

Diagram of coronary circulation

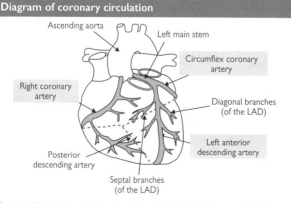

Reproduced from Myerson, SG, Choudhury, RP, and Mitchell ARJ (eds). Emergencies in Cardiology. OUP, 2006. By permission of Oxford University Press.

Echocardiography

This non-invasive technique uses the differing ability of various structures within the heart to reflect ultrasound waves. It not only demonstrates anatomy but also provides a continuous display of the functioning heart throughout its cycle. There are various types of scans:

M-mode (motion mode): Scans are displayed to produce a permanent single dimension (time) image.

2-dimensional (real time): A 2-D, fan-shaped image of a segment of the heart is produced on the screen, which may be 'frozen' and hard-copied. Several views are possible and the 4 commonest are: Long axis, short axis, 4-chamber, and subcostal. 2-D echocardiography is good for visualizing ventricular function, congenital heart disease, LV aneurysm, mural thrombus, LA myxoma, septal defects.

Doppler and color-flow echocardiography: Different colored jets illustrate flow and gradients across valves and septal defects (p148).

Trans-esophageal echocardiography (TEE) can be more sensitive than transthoracic echocardiography (TTE) because the transducer is nearer to the heart and the images are not limited by lung or fat interference. Indications: Diagnosis aortic dissections; assessing prosthetic valves; finding cardiac source of emboli, and endocarditis. Don't do if esophageal disease or cervical spine instability.

Stress echocardiography: Used to evaluate ventricular function, ejection fraction, myocardial thickening, and regional wall motion pre- and post-exercise. Dobutamine or dipyridamole may be used if the patient cannot exercise. Inexpensive and as sensitive/specific as a thallium scan (p104).

Uses of echocardiography

Quantification of global RV and LV function: Echo is useful for detecting focal and global wall motion abnormalities, LV aneurysm, mural thrombus, and LVH (echo is 5–10 times more sensitive than the ECG in detecting this). The size of the ventricle can also be assessed.

Estimating right heart hemodynamics: Doppler studies of pulmonary artery flow allow evaluation of RV function and pressures.

Valve disease: Measurement of pressure gradients and valve orifice areas in stenotic lesions. Detecting valvular regurgitation. Evaluating function of prosthetic valves is another role.

Congenital heart disease: Establishing the presence of lesions and determining their functional significance.

Endocarditis: Vegetations may not be seen if <2mm in size. TTE with color doppler is best for aortic regurgitation (AR). TTE is useful for visualizing mitral valve vegetations, leaflet perforation, or looking for an aortic root abscess.

Pericardial effusion is best diagnosed by echo. Fluid may first accumulate between the posterior pericardium and the left ventricle, then anterior to both ventricles and anterior and lateral to the right atrium. There may be paradoxical septal motion.

HOCM (p144): Echo features include asymmetrical septal hypertrophy, small LV cavity, dilated left atrium, and systolic anterior motion of the mitral valve.

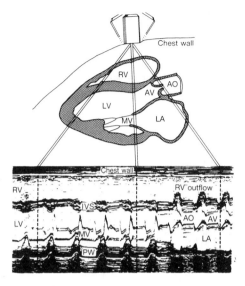

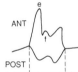

e
ANT
f
POST
1. Normal mitral valve
CLOSED | OPEN | CLOSED

2. Mitral stenosis
 • reduced e–f slope

3. Aortic regurgitation
 • fluttering of ant.
   leaflet

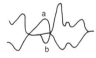

4. (a) Systolic anterior
       leaflet movement
       (SAM) in HOCM
   (b) Mitral valve prolapse
       (late systole)

Normal M-mode echocardiogram (RV=right ventricle; LV=left ventricle; AO=aorta; AV=aortic valve; LA=left atrium; MV=mitral valve; PW=posterior wall of LV; IVS=interventricular septum). After Hall R *Med International* **17** 774.

Nuclear cardiology and other cardiac scans

Myocardial perfusion imaging

A non-invasive method of assessing regional myocardial blood flow and the cellular integrity of myocytes. The technique uses radionuclide tracers, which cross the myocyte membrane and are trapped intracellularly.

Thallium-201, a K$^+$ analog, is the most widely used agent. It is distributed via regional myocardial blood flow and requires cellular integrity for uptake. Newer *technetium-99* based agents are similar to thallium-201 but have improved imaging characteristics, and can also be used to assess myocardial perfusion and LV performance in the same study.

Myocardial territories supplied by unobstructed coronary vessels have normal perfusion whereas regions supplied by stenosed coronary vessels have poorer relative perfusion, a difference which is accentuated by exercise. For this reason, exercise tests are used in conjunction with radionuclide imaging to identify areas at risk of ischemia/infarction. Exercise scans are compared with resting views: *Reperfusion* (ischemia) or *fixed defects* (infarct) can be seen and the coronary artery involved is reliably predicted. Drugs (eg adenosine and dipyridamole) can also be used to induce perfusion differences between normal and underperfused tissues in patients that can't exercise.

Myocardial perfusion imaging has also been used in patients presenting with acute MI (to determine the amount of myocardium salvaged by thrombolysis) and in diagnosing acute chest pain in those without classical ECG changes (to define the presence of significant perfusion defects).

Positron emission tomography (PET)

Severely underperfused tissues, such as those supplied by a critically stenotic coronary artery, switch from fatty acid metabolism to glycolytic metabolism. Such altered cellular biochemistry may be imaged by PET using ^{18}F-labelled deoxyglucose (FDG), which identifies glycolytically active tissue that is viable. This phenomenon called hibernating myocardium occurs in up to 40% of fixed defects seen on thallium-201 scans.

Computer tomography (CT) allows only limited assessment of cardiac structures. It can help evaluate cardiac disease (eg constrictive pericarditis). CT is also part of first line assessment for abnormalities of the ascending and descending aorta, especially in aortic dissection, and for detecting pulmonary emboli. Ultra fast CT can reliably evaluate the proximal parts of coronary arteries and assist with evaluating congenital anomalies.

Magnetic resonance imaging (MRI) MRI is used in assessing congenital heart disease, intra-cardiac structures, and the great vessels. Its advantages over CT are: The lack of exposure to radiation; the wide field of view and high-image resolution; the ability to orient images in multiple planes, and the ability to gate or trigger the MRI scanner, according to the cardiac cycle, allowing stop-frame imaging of the heart and great vessels. Spin-echo MRI has a high sensitivity for detecting false lumina and intra-mural flaps in aortic dissection compared with CT. Its main limitation, compared with TEE (p102) and CT, is its inability to image significantly unstable patients. Additionally, significant artifact occurs in patients who have implantable devices and some patients devices will be altered by the magnet.

New uses of MRI include myocardial phosphorus-31 NMR spectroscopy (^{31}P-NMR) which may demonstrate ischemia in the not-uncommon problem of women with chest pain but normal coronary angiograms. ('syndrome X' denotes this type of uncertain chest pain.) ^{31}P-NMR may suggest abnormal dilator responses of the microvasculature to stress.

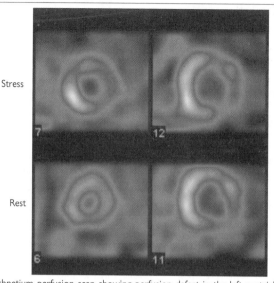

Stress

Rest

Technetium perfusion scan showing perfusion defect in the left ventricle anterior and lateral walls at stress which is reversible (difference between stress and rest images).

Hyperlipidemia

Cholesterol is a major risk factor for coronary heart disease (CHD) and due to the efficacy of the current medications is very treatable. The decision to treat hypercholesterolemia should be based on multiple factors. The Adult Treatment Panel III (ATP III) has established clinical guidelines for cholesterol testing and management. (http://www.nhlbi.nih.gov/guidelines/cholesterol/atp3_rpt.htm). First, determine if the patient has CHD or its equivalent (diabetes, symptomatic carotid artery disease, peripheral vascular disease, or an abdominal aortic aneurysm). Second, determine if the patient has other risk factors for CHD (smoking, BP↑, family history, HDL<40mg/dL, or age: Male >45, female >55). Third, decide to treat based on LDL level and their risk for CHD using the Framingham risk calculator (http://hin.nhlbi.nih.gov/atpiii/calculator.asp?usertype=prof).

Trial evidence that treating hypercholesterolemia is worthwhile
- '4S' study. 2° prevention trial (patients with IHD) using simvastatin ≥20mg/d PO in 4444 men aged 35–70 (cholesterol 212–309mg/dL). Number needed to treat (NNT) to prevent 1 fatal MI was 25 (over 6yrs), and 14 for non-fatal events.
- WOSCOPS. 1° prevention trial in Scotland with over 6500 men (cholesterol >155mg/dL), pravastatin 40mg/24h PO. NNT to prevent 1 fatal MI was 142 (over 5yrs), and for all cardiac events was 55.
- CARE study. 2° prevention trial with pravastatin 40mg/24h PO in 4159 people, post-MI, with 'normal' cholesterol (average 209mg/dL). NNT for fatalities was 91 (over 5yrs), and for non-fatal MI was 38.
- HEART PROTECTION STUDY. 2° prevention trial with 40mg simvastatin to patients irrespective of cholesterol. NNT for death = 55. No evidence of 'threshold of cholesterol' for benefit. 33% of the patients had an LDL <113mg/dL and still demonstrated reduction in mortality and cardiovascular events.

Who to screen
- CHD or risk↑, eg DM, BP↑.
- Family history of hyperlipidemia, or CHD before 65yrs old.
- Xanthoma or xanthelasma.
- Corneal arcus before 50yrs old.

Management
- Exclude familial or 2° hyperlipidemias. Treat as appropriate.
- Lifestyle advice. Aim for BMI of 20–25. Diet with <10% of calories from saturated fats and plenty of fiber. Exercise.
- Treat those with known CHD.
- If 0 or 1 risk factors, treat at LDL >160. If 2 or more risk factors and MI risk <20%, treat at LDL >130mg/dL. If CHD or >20% MI risk, treat at LDL >100mg/dL.
- 'Statins' are first choice; they ↓cholesterol synthesis in the liver (eg simvastatin 10–40mg PO at night). CI: Porphyria, LFT↑. SE: Myositis (stop if CK↑ by ≥10-fold. If any muscle aches, check CK; risk is 1/100,000 treatment yrs); abdominal pain; LFT↑ (stop if AST ≥100U/L).
- 2nd-line therapy: Fibrates, eg bezafibrate (useful in familial mixed hyperlipidemias); cholesterol absorption inhibitors of ezetimibe (useful in combination with a statin to enhance cholesterol reduction); anion exchange resins, eg cholestyramine; & nicotinic acid (HDL↑; LDL↓; SE: Severe flushes—aspirin 325mg ½h pre-dose helps this).
- Hypertriglyceridemia responds best to fibrates, nicotinic acid, or fish oil.

Familial or 1° hyperlipidemias
Risk of CHD↑↑. Lipids travel in blood packaged with proteins as lipoproteins. There are 4 classes: Chylomicrons (mainly triglyceride); LDL (mainly cholesterol, the lipid correlating most strongly with CHD); VLDL (mainly triglyceride); HDL (mainly phospholipid, correlating inversely with CHD). See table opposite.

2° hyperlipidemias A result of diabetes mellitus; alcohol abuse; T4↓; renal failure, nephrosis, and cholestasis.

Xanthomata These yellowish lipid deposits may be: Eruptive (itchy nodules in crops in hypertriglyceridemia); tuberous (yellow plaques on elbows and knees); planar—also called palmar (orange-colored streaks in palmar creases), virtually diagnostic of remnant hyperlipidemia; or deposits in tendons, eyelids (xanthelasmata), or cornea (arcus).

Primary hyperlipidemias			
Familial hyperchylomi-cronemia (lipoprotein lipase deficiency or apoCII deficiency)[I]	Chol <250 Trig 900–1300 Chylomicrons ↑		Eruptive xanthomata; lipemia retinalis; hepatosplenomegaly (HSM)
Familial hypercholesterolemia[II] (LDL receptor defects)	Chol 300–600 Trig <200	LDL↑	Tendon xanthoma; corneal arcus; xanthelasma
Familial defective apoprotein B-100[IIa]	Chol 300–600 Trig <200	LDL↑	Tendon xanthoma; arcus; xanthelasma
Polygenic hyper-cholesterolemia[IIa]	Chol >300 Trig <200	LDL↑	The commonest 1° lipidemia xanthelasma; corneal arcus
Familial combined hyperlipidemia[IIb, IV or V]	Chol 250–400 Trig 200–1000	LDL↑VLDL↑ HDL↓	Next commonest 1°lipidemia xanthe-lasma; arcus
Dysbetalipoproteine-mia (remnant particle disease)[III]	Chol 350–550 Trig 800–1200	IDL↑ HDL↓ LDL↓	Palmar striae; tubero-eruptive xanthoma
Familial hypertri-glyceridemia[IV]	Chol 290–450 Trig 250–550	VLDL↑	
Type V hyperlipopro-teinemia	Trig 850–2500; chylomicrons		Eruptive xanthoma; lipemia retinalis; HSM

Chol = plasma cholesterol (mg/dL)

Trig = plasma triglyceride (mg/dL); **colored numerals** = **WHO** phenotype

1° HDL abnormalities

Hyperalphalipoproteinemia: ↑HDL chol >80

Hypoalphalipoproteinemia (Tangier disease): ↓HDL chol <35

1° Primary LDL abnormalities

Abetalipoproteinemia: Trig <30, Chol <50, missing LDL, VLDL and chylomicrons, and fat malabsorption, retinopathy, and acanthocytosis

Hypobetalipoproteinemia: Chol <60 LDL↓, HDL ↓. ↑ longevity

Atherosclerosis and 'statins'

Think of atheroma as the slow accumulation of snow on a mountain. Nothing much happens until one day an avalanche devastates the community below. The snow is lipid and lipid-laden macrophages; the mountain is an arterial wall; the avalanche is plaque rupture; and the community below is, all too often, myocardium or CNS neurons. The devastation is infarction. In assessing risk of thrombi, remember Rudolph Virchow's (1821–1902) triad of *changes in the vessel wall, changes in blood flow,* and *changes to the blood constituents.*

Plaque biology Atheroma is the result of cycles of vascular wall injury and repair, leading to the accumulation of T lymphocytes, which produce growth factors, cytokines, and chemoattractants. LDL gains access by a process called transcytosis, where it undergoes modification by macrophage-derived oxidative free radicals—a process enhanced by smoking tobacco and hypertension. Rupture of atheromatous plaque triggers most acute coronary events. These plaques have a core of lipid-laden macrophages and a fibrous cap. Many factors predispose to plaque formation, eg genetics, sex (♂), BP, smoking, and diabetes mellitus. Plaques are not static, dead things. They can regress or accumulate, or become inflamed (eg in unstable angina). The balance between LDL efflux and influx is alterable, eg by diet or anti-lipid drugs. Neither is the vessel wall a non-participatory audience to these great events. A sclerotic arterial wall comprises areas of chronic inflammation, with monocytes, macrophages, and T lymphocytes—with smooth muscle proliferation, and elaboration of extracellular matrix. These macrophages make cholesterol, and also produce enzymes (eg interstitial collagenase, gelatinase, and stromelysin), which have been implicated in digesting the plaque cap. The thinner the cap, and the fewer smooth muscle cells involved, the more unstable the plaque and the more likely it is to rupture. Endothelial cells also release a number of anti- and pro-atherogenic molecules including nitric oxide and endothelin-1. Normal endothelial function is lost early in the process of atherosclerosis with a shift to the production of pro-atherogenic molecules.

After plaque rupture, what happens to fibrinogen and passing platelets partly determines the extent of the impending catastrophe. Hypercholesterolemia (if present) is associated with hypercoagulable blood and enhanced platelet reactivity at sites of vascular damage.

Disease prevention What can we do about plaques? First, try to prevent them: Eat a healthy diet (p192), encourage *some* exercise, discourage smoking; treat high BP and diabetes. Once a plaque is there, it can be bypassed, ablated (physically removed or compressed), or stented (with a metal stent). Angioplasty splits the plaque, causing an injury response: Elastic recoil→thrombus formation→inflammation→smooth muscle proliferation→arterial remodeling. An alternative to this drastic change is to give a statin, even if the cholesterol is 'normal' since the whole process described above is favorably influenced by statins. Statins inhibit the enzyme HMG-COA reductase, which is responsible for the *de novo* synthesis of cholesterol in the liver. This leads to an ↑ in LDL receptor expression by hepatocytes and ultimately reduced circulating LDL cholesterol. In the past reducing LDL to <100 was the goal but recent data suggests that even lower levels may be beneficial. Besides this, statins have other favorable effects:

• Thrombotic state↓.
• Suppress inflammation (CRP↓).
• Plaque stabilization.
• Restoration of normal endothelial function.
• Reduction in cholesterol synthesis by within-vessel macrophages.
• Reduction of within-vessel macrophage proliferation and migration.

Other cardiovascular drugs

Antiplatelet drugs Aspirin irreversibly acetylates cyclo-oxygenase, preventing production of thromboxane A_2, thereby inhibiting platelet aggregation. It is commonly used in low dose (eg 81mg) for 2° prevention following MI, TIA/stroke, and for patients with angina or peripheral vascular disease. May have a role in 1° prevention. ADP receptor antagonists (eg clopidogrel) also block platelet aggregation, but may cause less gastric irritation. They have a role if intolerant of aspirin, and post-coronary stent insertion.

β-blockers Block beta-adrenoceptors, thus antagonizing the sympathetic nervous system. Blocking β_1-receptors is negatively inotropic and chronotropic and delays AV conduction, and blocking β_2-receptors induce peripheral vasoconstriction and bronchoconstriction. Drugs vary in their β_1/β_2 selectivity (eg propranolol is non-selective, and bisoprolol relatively β_1 selective), but this does not seem to alter their clinical efficacy. *Uses:* Angina, hypertension, antidysrhythmic, post MI (↓mortality), heart failure (with caution). *CI:* Asthma/COPD, heart block. *Caution:* Peripheral vascular disease, heart failure, diabetes. *SE:* Lethargy, impotence, *depression*, nightmares, headache.

Diuretics Loop diuretics (eg *furosemide*) used in heart failure and hypertension inhibit the Na/K/2Cl co-transporter. Thiazides used in hypertension inhibit Na/Cl co-transporter. *SE: Loop* dehydration, ↓K^+, ↓Ca^{2+}, ototoxic; *thiazides:* ↓K^+, ↑Ca^{2+}, ↓Mg^{2+}, ↑urate (± gout), impotence.

Vasodilators used in heart failure, IHD, and hypertension. Nitrates preferentially dilate veins & the large arteries, ↓ filling pressure (pre-load), while hydralazine primarily dilates the resistance vessels thus ↓ BP (after-load). Prazosin (an α-blocker) dilates arteries and veins.

Calcium antagonists These ↓cell entry of Ca^{2+} via voltage-sensitive channels on smooth muscle cells, thereby promoting coronary and peripheral vasodilatation and reducing myocardial oxygen consumption.

Pharmacology: Effects of specific Ca^{2+} antagonists vary because they have different effects on the L-Ca^{2+}-type channels. The *dihydropyridines* eg nifedipine and amlodipine, are mainly peripheral vasodilators (they also dilate coronary arteries) and can cause a reflex tachycardia, so are often used with a β-blocker. They are used mainly in hypertension and angina. Verapamil and diltiazem (*non-dihydropyridines*) also slow conduction at the atrioventricular and sinoatrial nodes and may be used to treat hypertension, angina, and dysrhythmias. Don't give verapamil with β-blockers (risk of bradycardia ± LVF). *SE:* Flushes, headache, edema (diuretic unresponsive), LV function↓, gingival hypertrophy. *CI:* Heart block.

Digoxin Blocks the Na^+/K^+ pump. It is used to slow the pulse in fast AF (p120; aim for <100). As it is a weak +ve inotrope, its role in heart failure in sinus rhythm may be best reserved if symptomatic despite optimal ACE-i and beta blocker therapy; here there is little benefit with mortality (but admissions for worsening CHF are ↓by ~25%). Old people and people with renal insufficiency are at ↑risk of toxicity: Use lower doses. Check plasma levels >6h post-dose. Typical dose: 0.25mg a day, 0.125mg (or ↓ renal function). Toxicity risk↑ if: K^+↓, Mg^{2+}↓, or Ca^{2+}↑. t½ ≈ 36h. If on digoxin, use less energy in cardioversion (start with 5J). *SE:* Any arrhythmia (supraventricular tachycardia SVT with AV block is suggestive), nausea, appetite↓, yellow vision, confusion, gynecomastia. In toxicity, stop digoxin; check K^+; treat arrhythmias; consider Digibind® by IVI (p736). *CI:* HOCM; WPW syndrome (p121).

ACE-inhibitors p129; **nitrates** p115; **antihypertensives** see p132.

Acute coronary syndromes (ACS)

Definitions ACS includes unstable angina and evolving MI, which share a common underlying pathology—plaque rupture, thrombosis, and inflammation. However, ACS may rarely be due to emboli or coronary spasm in normal coronary arteries, or vasculitis (p378). Usually divided into *ACS with ST-segment elevation* or new onset LBBB—what most of us mean by acute MI; and *ACS without ST-segment elevation*—the ECG may show ST-depression, T-wave inversion, non-specific changes, or be normal (includes non-Q wave or subendocardial MI). The degree of irreversible myocyte death varies, and significant necrosis can occur without ST-elevation. Cardiac troponins (T and I) are the most sensitive and specific markers of myocardial necrosis, and have become the test of choice in patients with ACS (see below).

Risk factors *Non-modifiable:* Age, ♂ sex, family history of IHD (MI in first degree relative <55yrs). *Modifiable:* Smoking, hypertension, DM, hyperlipidemia, obesity, sedentary lifestyle. *Controversial* risk factors include: Stress, type A personality, LVH, apoprotein A↑, fibrinogen↑, hyperinsulinemia, homocysteine levels↑, ACE genotype, and cocaine use.

Diagnosis is based on the presence of at least 2 out of 3 of: Typical history, ECG changes, and cardiac enzyme rise (WHO criteria).

Symptoms Acute central chest pain, lasting >20min, often associated with nausea, diaphoresis, dyspnea, palpitations. May present without chest pain ('silent' infarct) or with atypical chest pain. eg in elderly or diabetics. In such patients, presentations may include: Syncope, pulmonary edema, epigastric pain and vomiting, post-operative hypotension or oliguria, acute confusional state, stroke, diabetic hyperglycemic states.

Signs Distress, anxiety, pallor, sweatiness, pulse↑ or ↓, BP↑ or ↓, 4ᵗʰ heart sound. There may be signs of heart failure (↑ JVP, 3ʳᵈ heart sound and bibasilar crackles) or a pansystolic murmur (papillary muscle dysfunction/rupture, VSD). A low-grade fever may be present. Later, a pericardial friction rub or peripheral edema may develop.

Tests *ECG:* Classically, hyperacute (tall) T waves, ST elevation or new LBBB occur within hours of acute Q wave (transmural infarction). T wave inversion and the development of pathological Q waves follow over hours to days (p92). In other ACS: ST-depression, T-wave inversion, non-specific changes, or normal. *In 20% of MIs, the ECG may be normal initially.*

CXR: Look for cardiomegaly, pulmonary edema, or a widened mediastinum (?aortic dissection). Don't routinely delay ℞ while waiting for a CXR.

Blood: CBC, electrolytes, renal function, glucose↑, lipids↓, cardiac enzymes (CK, troponin)↑. CK is found in myocardial and skeletal muscle. It is raised in: MI; after trauma (falls, seizures); prolonged exercise; myositis; hypothermia; hypothyroidism. Check CK-MB isoenzyme levels if there is doubt as to the source (normal CK-MB/CK ratio <5%). Troponin T better reflects myocardial damage (peaks at 12–24h; elevated for >1wk). If normal ≥6h after onset of pain, and ECG normal, risk of missing MI is tiny (0.3%). Peak post-MI levels also help risk stratification.

Differential diagnosis (p88) Angina, pericarditis, myocarditis, aortic dissection, pulmonary embolism, and esophageal reflux/spasm.

Management See *emergencies* (p690). The management of ACS with and without ST-segment elevation varies. Likewise, if there is no ST-elevation, and symptoms settle without a rise in cardiac troponin, then no myocardial damage has occurred, the prognosis is good, and patients can be discharged. Therefore, the two key questions are: Is there ST-segment elevation; and is there a rise in troponin?

Mortality 50% of deaths occur within 2h of onset of symptom.

Enzyme changes following acute MI

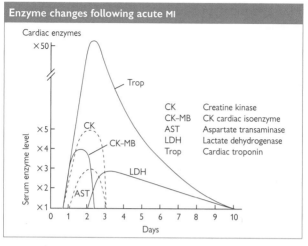

Cardiac enzymes

Serum enzyme level

CK   Creatine kinase
CK–MB CK cardiac isoenzyme
AST   Aspartate transaminase
LDH   Lactate dehydrogenase
Trop   Cardiac troponin

Days

Sequential ECG changes following acute MI

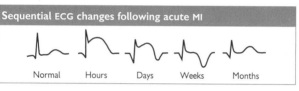

Normal   Hours   Days   Weeks   Months

Management of ACS

Pre-hospital Arrange emergency ambulance. Aspirin 325mg chewed (if no *absolute* CI) and NTG sublingual. Analgesia, eg morphine 5–10mg IV (not IM because of risk of bleeding with thrombolysis). Ask if the patient took a PDE 5 inhibitor (sildenafil, vardenafil, tadalafil) since nitrates are contraindicated in that situation.

In hospital O_2, morphine, aspirin p690.

Then the key question for subsequent management of ACS is whether there is ST-segment elevation (includes new onset LBBB or a true posterior MI).

ST-segment elevation
- *Thrombolysis*, if no contraindication, or 1° angioplasty.
- *β-blocker*, eg atenolol 5mg IV unless contraindicated.
- *ACE-inhibitor:* Consider starting ACE-i (eg lisinopril 2.5mg) in all normotensive patients within 24h of acute MI, especially if there is clinical evidence of heart failure or echo evidence of LV dysfunction.

ACS without st-segment elevation
- *β-blocker*, eg atenolol 5mg IV unless contraindicated.
- *Low molecular weight heparin* (eg enoxaparin).
- *Nitrates*, unless contraindication (usually given intravenously).
- High-risk patients (persistent or recurrent ischemia, ST-depression, diabetes, ↑ troponin) require infusion of a GPIIb/IIIa antagonist (eg tirofiban), and, ideally, urgent angiography. Clopidogrel may be useful in addition to aspirin.
- Low-risk patients (no further pain, flat or inverted T waves, or normal ECG, **and** negative troponin) can be discharged if a repeat troponin is negative. Treat medically and arrange further investigation eg stress test, angiogram.

112

Subsequent management *Bed rest for 48h;* continuous ECG monitoring.
- Daily examination of heart, lungs, and legs for complications (p114).
- Daily 12-lead ECG, electrolytes and renal function, cardiac enzymes for 2–3d.
- *Prophylaxis against thromboembolism:* Eg heparin 5000U/12h SC until fully mobile. If large anterior MI, consider warfarin anticoagulation for 3 months as prophylaxis against systemic embolism from LV mural thrombus. Continue daily *low-dose aspirin* (eg 81mg) indefinitely. Aspirin reduces vascular events (MI, stroke, or vascular death) by 29%.
- *Start oral β-blocker* (eg metoprolol ~50mg/6h, enough to ↓ the pulse to ≤60; continue for at least 1yr). Long-term β-blockade reduces mortality from all causes by ~25% in patients who have had a previous MI. If contraindicated, consider verapamil or diltiazem as an alternative.
- *Continue ACE-i* in all patients: ACE-i in those with evidence of heart failure ↓2yr mortality by 25–30%.
- *Start a statin:* Cholesterol reduction post-MI has been shown to be of benefit in patients with both elevated and normal cholesterol levels. Some treat all patients, others only if total cholesterol >200mg/dL or LDL >130mg/dL.
- *Address modifiable risk factors:* Discourage smoking (p87). Encourage exercise. Identify and treat diabetes mellitus, hypertension, and hyperlipidemia.
- *Exercise ECG:* May be useful in risk stratification post-MI, and in subjects without ST-segment elevation or a troponin rise. Not necessary in patients who received a cardiac cath and appropriate intervention.
- *General advice.* If uncomplicated, discharge after 5–7d. *Work:* Return to work after 4–12wks. A few occupations should not be restarted post-MI: Airline pilots; air traffic controllers; divers. Drivers of public service or heavy goods vehicles may be permitted to return to work if they meet certain criteria. Patients undertaking heavy manual labor should be advised to seek a lighter job. *Diet:* A diet high in fish, fruit, vegetables, and fiber, and low in saturated fats should be encouraged. *Exercise:* Encourage regular daily exercise. *Sex:* Intercourse is best avoided for 1 month. *Travel:* Avoid air travel for 2 months.

Review at 5wks post-MI to review symptoms: Angina? Dyspnea? Palpitations?
• If angina recurs, treat conventionally, and consider coronary angiography.
Review at 3 months
• Check fasting lipids. Does the dose of statin need to be ↑ to reach goal levels.

Acute postero-lateral MI

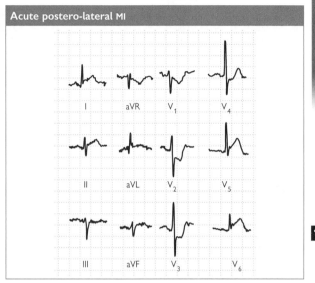

Complications of MI

- *Cardiac arrest* (p675); *cardiogenic shock* (p696).
- *Unstable angina:* Manage along standard lines (p691) and refer to a cardiologist for urgent investigation.
- *Bradycardias or heart block:* Sinus bradycardia: Treat with atropine 0.6–1.2mg IV. Consider temporary cardiac pacing if no response, or poorly tolerated by the patient. 1ˢᵗ degree AV block: Observe closely as approximately 40% develop higher degrees of AV block. Wenckebach (Möbitz type I) block: Does not require pacing unless poorly tolerated. Möbitz type II block: Carries a high risk of developing complete AV block; should be paced. Complete AV block: Insert pacemaker; may not be necessary after inferior MI if narrow QRS and reasonably stable & pulse ≥40–50. Bundle branch block: MI complicated by trifascicular block or non-adjacent bifascicular disease should be paced.
- *Tachyarrhythmias:* **NB:** K⁺↓, hypoxia and acidosis all predispose to arrhythmias and should be corrected. Regular wide complex tachycardia after MI is almost always VT. If hemodynamically stable, give lidocaine or amiodarone. If this fails, can repeat at a lower dose. Would review ACLS protocols. Consider maintenance antidysrhythmic therapy. Early VT (<24h): Give lidocaine by infusion for 12–24h or amiodarone. Late VT (>24h) amiodarone and start oral therapy (amiodarone or sotalol). SVT. AF or flutter: If compromised, DC cardioversion. Otherwise, control rate with digoxin, β-blockers or calcium channel blockers. In atrial flutter or intermittent AF, try amiodarone or sotalol.
- *Left ventricular failure (LVF)* p692.
- *Right ventricular failure (RVF)/infarction:* Presents with low cardiac output and JVP↑. Insert a Swan–Ganz catheter to measure right-sided pressures and guide fluid replacement. If BP remains low after fluid replacement, give inotropes.
- *Pericarditis:* Central chest pain, relieved by sitting forwards. ECG: Saddle-shaped ST elevation. Treatment: NSAIDs. Echo to check for effusion.
- *DVT & PE:* Patients are at risk of developing DVT & PE and should be prophylactically heparinized (5000U/12h SC) until fully mobile.
- *Systemic embolism:* May arise from a LV mural thrombus. After large anterior MIs, consider anticoagulation with warfarin for 3 months.
- *Cardiac tamponade:* (p696) Presents with low cardiac output, pulsus paradoxus, JVP↑, muffled heart sounds. Diagnosis: Echo. Treatment: Pericardial aspiration (provides temporary relief p667), surgery.
- *Mitral regurgitation:* May be mild (minor papillary muscle dysfunction) or severe (chordal or papillary muscle rupture or ischemia). Presentation: Pulmonary edema. Diagnosis: Echo. Treat LVF (p692) and consider valve replacement.
- *Ventricular septal defect:* Presents with pansystolic murmur, JVP↑, cardiac failure. Diagnosis: Echo. Treatment: Surgery. 50% mortality in 1ˢᵗ wk.
- *Late malignant ventricular arrhythmias:* Occur 1–3wks post-MI and are the cardiologist's nightmare. Avoid hypokalemia, the most easily avoidable cause.
- *Dressler's syndrome:* Recurrent pericarditis, pleural effusions, fever, anemia and ESR↑ 1–3wks post-MI. Treatment: NSAIDs; steroids if severe.
- *Left ventricular aneurysm:* This occurs late (4–6wks post-MI), and presents with LVF, angina, recurrent VT, or systemic embolism. ECG: Persistent ST segment elevation. Treatment: Anticoagulate, consider excision.

Angina pectoris

This is due to myocardial ischemia and presents as a central chest tightness or heaviness, which is brought on by exertion and relieved by rest. It may radiate to one or both arms, the neck, jaw or teeth. *Other precipitants:* Emotion, cold weather, and heavy meals. *Associated symptoms:* Dyspnea, nausea, diaphoresis, lightheadedness.

Causes Mostly atheroma. Rarely: Anemia, AS; tachyarrhythmias; HOCM; arteritis/small vessel disease.

Types of angina *Stable angina:* Induced by effort, relieved by rest. *Unstable (crescendo) angina:* Angina of ↑ frequency or severity; occurs on minimal exertion or at rest; associated with ↑↑risk of MI. *Decubitus angina:* Precipitated by lying flat. *Variant (Prinzmetal's) angina:* Caused by coronary artery spasm (rare; may co-exist with fixed stenoses).

Tests ECG: Usually normal, but may show ST depression; flat or inverted T waves; signs of past MI. If resting ECG normal, consider exercise ECG (p98), thallium scan (p104), or coronary angiography.

Management *Alteration of lifestyle:* Stop smoking, encourage exercise, weight loss. *Modify risk factors:* Hypertension, diabetes, etc., p87.
- *Aspirin* (81mg/24h) reduces mortality by 34%.
- *β-blockers:* Eg atenolol 50–100mg/24h PO, unless contra-indications (asthma, COPD, LVF, bradycardia, coronary artery spasm).
- *Nitrates:* For symptoms, give NTG spray or sublingual tabs, up to every ½h. Prophylaxis: Give regular oral nitrate, eg isosorbide mononitrate 10–30mg PO (eg bid; an 8h nitrate-free period to prevent tolerance) or slow-release nitrate (eg Imdur® 60mg/24h). Alternatives: Adhesive nitrate skin patches. SE: Headaches, BP↓.
- *Calcium antagonists:* Amlodipine 5–10mg/24h; diltiazem 90–180mg/12h PO.
- If total cholesterol >200mg/dL give a statin— p108.
- Unstable angina requires admission & urgent treatment: See *emergencies*, p691.

Indications for referral Diagnostic uncertainty; new angina of sudden onset; recurrent angina if past MI or CABG; angina uncontrolled by drugs; unstable angina. Some units routinely do exercise tolerance tests on those <70yrs old, but age alone is a poor way to stratify patients.

Percutaneous transluminal coronary angioplasty (PTCA) involves balloon dilatation of the stenotic vessel(s). *Indications:* Poor response or intolerance to medical therapy; refractory angina in patients not suitable for CABG; previous CABG; post-thrombolysis in patients with severe stenoses, symptoms, or positive stress tests. Comparisons of PTCA vs. drugs alone show that PTCA may control symptoms better but with more frequent cardiac events (eg MI and need for CABG) and little effect on overall mortality. *Complications:* Restenosis (20–30% within 6 months); emergency CABG (<3%); MI (<2%); death (<0.5%). Stenting reduces restenosis rates and the need for bail out CABG. NICE recommends that >70% of angioplasties should be accompanied by stenting. Drug-coated stents reduce restenosis. Antiplatelet agents, eg clopidogrel reduce the risk of stent thrombosis. IV platelet glycoprotein IIb/IIIa-inhibitors (eg eptifibatide) can reduce procedure-related ischemic events.

CABG: Indications: Left main disease, multi-vessel disease; multiple severe stenoses; distal vessel disease; patient unsuitable for angioplasty; failed angioplasty; refractory angina; MI; pre-operatively (valve or vascular surgery). Comparisons of CABG vs. PTCA have found that CABG results in better symptom control and lower re-intervention rate, but longer recovery time and length of inpatient stay.

Arrhythmias

Disturbances of cardiac rhythm or arrhythmias are:
• Common.
• Often benign (but may reflect underlying heart disease).
• Often intermittent, causing diagnostic difficulty.
• Occasionally severe, causing cardiac compromise.

Causes *Cardiac:* MI, coronary artery disease, LV aneurysm, mitral valve disease, cardiomyopathy, pericarditis, myocarditis, aberrant conduction pathways. *Non-cardiac:* Caffeine, smoking, alcohol, pneumonia, drugs (β_2-agonists, digoxin, tricyclics, adriamycin, doxorubicin), metabolic imbalance (K^+, Ca^{2+}, Mg^{2+}, hypoxia, hypercapnia, metabolic acidosis, thyroid disease, pheochromocytoma). Presentation is with palpitation, chest pain, presyncope/syncope, hypotension, or pulmonary edema. Some arrhythmias may be asymptomatic and incidental, eg AF.

History Take a detailed history of palpitations. Ask about precipitating factors, onset, nature (fast or slow, regular or irregular) duration, associated symptoms (chest pain, dyspnea, light headedness). Review drug history. Ask about past medical history or family history of cardiac disease.

Tests CBC, electrolytes, glucose, Ca^{2+}, Mg^{2+}, TSH. ECG: Look for signs of IHD, AF, short P–R interval (WPW syndrome), long QT interval (metabolic imbalance, drugs, congenital), U waves (hypokalemia). 24h ECG monitoring; several recordings may be needed. May need a continuous monitor. Echo: To look for structural heart disease, eg mitral stenosis. Provocation tests: Exercise ECG, cardiac catheterization, and electrophysiological studies may be required.

Treatment If the ECG is normal during palpitations, reassure the patient. Otherwise, treatment depends on the type of arrhythmia.

Bradycardia: (p117) If asymptomatic and rate >40bpm, no treatment is required. Look for a cause (drugs, sick sinus syndrome, hypothyroidism) and stop any drugs that may be contributing (β-blocker, digoxin). If rate <40bpm or patient is symptomatic, give atropine 0.5–1.0mg IV (up to maximum of 3mg). If no response, insert a temporary pacing wire (p668). If necessary, start an isoproterenol infusion or use external cardiac pacing.

Sick sinus syndrome: Sinus node dysfunction causes bradycardia ± arrest, sinoatrial block or SVT alternating with bradycardia/asystole (tachy–brady syndrome). AF and thromboembolism may occur. Pace if symptomatic.

SVT: (p118) Narrow complex tachycardia (rate >100bpm, QRS width <120ms). Acute management: Vagotonic maneuvers followed by IV adenosine or verapamil (if not on β-blocker); DC shock if compromised. Maintenance therapy: β-blockers or verapamil.

AF/flutter: (p120) May be incidental finding. Control ventricular rate with beta blockers, calcium channel blockers, or digoxin: Use flecainide for pre-excited AF. DC shock if compromised (p688).

VT: (p122) Broad complex tachycardia (rate >100bpm, QRS duration >120ms). Acute management: IV lidocaine or amiodarone, if no response or if compromised DC shock. Oral therapy: Amiodarone loading dose (400mg/8h PO for 7d, then 400mg/12h for 7d) followed by maintenance therapy (200–400mg/24h). SE: Corneal deposits, photosensitivity, hepatitis, pneumonitis, lung fibrosis, nightmares, INR↑ (warfarin potentiation), T4↑, T3↓. Monitor LFT and TFT.

Finally, pacing may be used to overdrive tachyarrhythmias, to treat bradyarrhythmias, or prophylactically in conduction disturbances (p124). Implanted automatic defibrillators can save lives and are indicated for patients with an ejection fraction <35% and NYHA class II–III heart failure symptoms.

Diagnosis of bradycardias and AV block

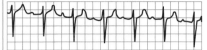

First degree AV block. P–R interval = 0.28s

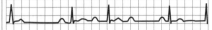

Möbitz type I (Wenckebach) AV block. With each succesive QRS, the P–R interval increases—until there is a non-conducted P wave.

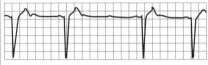

Möbitz type II AV block. Ratio of AV conduction varies from 2:1 to 3:1

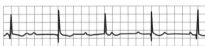

Complete AV block with narrow ventricular complexes. There is no relation between atrial and the slower ventricular activity.

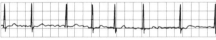

Atrial fibrillation

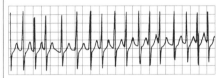

Atrial fibrillation with a rapid ventricular response. Diagnosis is based on the totally irregular ventricular rhythm.

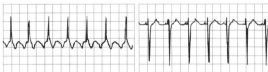

Atrial flutter with 2:1 AV block. Lead aVF (on left) shows the characteristic saw-tooth baseline whereas lead V_1 (on right) shows discrete atrial activity, alternate 'F' waves being superimposed on ventricular T waves.

Narrow complex tachycardia

ECG shows rate of >100bpm and QRS complex duration of <120ms.

Differential diagnosis
- Sinus tachycardia: Normal P wave followed by normal QRS.
- SVT: P wave absent or inverted after QRS.
- AF: Absent P wave, irregular QRS complexes.
- Atrial flutter: Atrial rate usually 300bpm giving 'flutter waves' or 'sawtooth' baseline (p117), ventricular rate often 150bpm (2:1 block).
- Atrial tachycardia: Abnormally shaped P waves, may outnumber QRS.
- Multifocal atrial tachycardia: 3 or more P wave morphologies, irregular QRS complexes.
- Junctional tachycardia: Rate 150–250bpm, P wave either buried in QRS complex or occurring after QRS complex.

Principles of management See algorithm opposite.
- If the patient is compromised, use DC cardioversion (p668).
- Otherwise, identify the underlying rhythm and treat accordingly.
- Vagal maneuvers (carotid sinus massage, Valsalva maneuver) transiently ↑ AV block, and may unmask an underlying atrial rhythm.
- If unsuccessful, give adenosine which causes transient AV block. It has a short half-life (10–15s) and works in 2 ways: By transiently slowing ventricles to show the underlying atrial rhythm; by cardioverting a junctional tachycardia to sinus rhythm.

Give 6mg IV bolus into a large vein; follow by saline flush, while recording a rhythm strip; if unsuccessful, give 12mg, then 12mg again at 2min intervals, unless on dipyridamole or post cardiac transplantation. Warn of SE: Transient chest tightness, dyspnea, headache, flushing. CI: Asthma, 2nd/3rd degree AV block, or sinoatrial disease (unless pacemaker). Drug interactions: Potentiated by dipyridamole, antagonized by theophylline.

Specific management *Sinus tachycardia* Identify and treat the cause.

SVT: If adenosine fails, use verapamil 5–10mg IV over 2min, or over 3min if elderly (not if already on β-blocker). If no response, give further dose of 5mg IV after 5–10min. Alternatives: Atenolol 2.5mg IV at 1mg/min repeated at 5min intervals to a maximum of 10mg or sotalol. If no good, use DC cardioversion.

AF/flutter: Manage along standard lines (p120).

Atrial tachycardia: Rare. If due to digoxin toxicity, stop digoxin; consider digoxin-specific antibody fragments (p736). Maintain K+ at 4–5mmol/L.

Multifocal atrial tachycardia: Most commonly occurs in COPD. Correct hypoxia and hypercapnia. Consider verapamil if rate remains >110bpm.

Junctional tachycardia: There are 3 types of junctional tachycardia: AV nodal re-entry tachycardia (AVNRT), AV re-entry tachycardia (AVRT), and His bundle tachycardia. Where anterograde conduction through the AV node occurs, vagal maneuvers are worth trying. Adenosine will usually cardiovert a junctional rhythm to sinus rhythm. If it recurs, treat with a β-blocker or amiodarone. Radiofrequency ablation is increasingly being used in AVRT and in some patients with AVNRT.

WPW syndrome (ECG p121) Caused by congenital accessory conduction pathway between atria and ventricles. Resting ECG shows short P–R interval and widened QRS complex due to slurred upstroke or 'delta wave'. 2 types: WPW type A (+ve δ wave in V_1), WPW type B (–ve δ wave in V_1). Patients present with SVT which may be due to an AVRT, pre-excited AF, or pre-excited atrial flutter. Refer to cardiologist for electrophysiology and ablation of the accessory pathway.

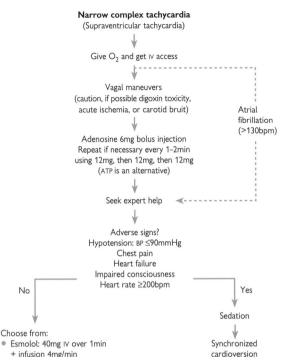

Narrow complex tachycardia
(Supraventricular tachycardia)

↓

Give O₂ and get IV access

↓

Vagal maneuvers
(caution, if possible digoxin toxicity,
acute ischemia, or carotid bruit)

↓

Adenosine 6mg bolus injection
Repeat if necessary every 1–2min
using 12mg, then 12mg, then 12mg
(ATP is an alternative)

↓

Atrial
fibrillation
(>130bpm)

Seek expert help ←- - - - -

↓

Adverse signs?
Hypotension: BP ≤90mmHg
Chest pain
Heart failure
Impaired consciousness
Heart rate ≥200bpm

No ↓   ↓ Yes

No:

Choose from:
- Esmolol: 40mg IV over 1min
  + infusion 4mg/min
  (IV injection can be repeated
  with increments of infusion
  to 12mg/min)
- Digoxin: max IV dose 500mcg
  over 30min ×2
- Verapamil: 5–10mg IV over 2min
- Amiodarone: 300mg over IV
  1hr; may be repeated once
  if necessary via a central
  line if possible
- Overdrive pacing—not AF

Yes:

Sedation

↓

Synchronized
cardioversion
100J: 200J: 360J

↓

Amiodarone 150mg IV
over 10min then 300mg
over 1hr if necessary
preferably by central
line, and repeat
cardioversion

119

Atrial fibrillation (AF) and flutter

AF is a chaotic, irregular atrial rhythm at 300–600bpm. The AV node responds intermittently, hence the irregular ventricular rate. It is common in the elderly (≤9%). The main risk is of embolic stroke, which is preventable by warfarin (reducible to 1%/yr from 4%; higher risk if old, poor LV function, DM, past TIA or stroke, or large left atrium on echocardiogram).

Common causes: Heart failure; hypertension; cardiac ischemia; MI (seen in 22%); mitral valve disease; pneumonia; hyperthyroidism; alcohol.

Rare causes: Cardiomyopathy, constrictive pericarditis, sick sinus syndrome, bronchial carcinoma, atrial myxoma, endocarditis, hemochromatosis, sarcoidosis, or other causes of atrial dilatation. 'Lone' AF means none of the above causes.

Signs & symptoms: It may be asymptomatic (found incidentally) or present with chest pain, palpitations, dyspnea, or presyncope. On examination, the pulse is *irregularly irregular*, the apical pulse rate is greater than the radial rate and the 1ˢᵗ heart sound is of variable intensity. Look for signs of mitral valve disease or hyperthyroidism.

Tests: ECG shows absent P waves, irregular QRS complexes. *Blood tests:* Electrolytes, cardiac enzymes, thyroid function tests. Echo to look for LA enlargement, mitral valve disease, poor LV function, and other structural abnormalities.

Acute AF (eg ≤72h):
- Treat any associated acute illness (eg MI, pneumonia).
- Control ventricular rate with either a β-blocker or a calcium channel blocker—intravenously if necessary. Digoxin can also be used but is not considered a first line agent. If AF does not resolve, consider drug or electrical cardioversion.
- Drug cardioversion: Amiodarone IVI (5mg/kg over 1h then ~900mg over 24h via a central line max 1.2g in 24h) or PO (200mg/8h for 1wk, 200mg/12h for 1wk, 100–200mg/24h maintenance). Alternative (if hemodynamically stable and no known IHD): Flecainide 2mg/kg IV over >25min (max 150mg) with ECG monitoring. 300mg stat PO may also work.
- DC cardioversion is indicated: (1) electively, following a first attack of AF with an identifiable cause; (2) as an emergency, if the patient is compromised. Protocol: 200J→300J→360J (100J may be tried first, but is successful in <20%).
- Anticoagulation is not required if AF is of recent onset (<48h) with a structurally normal heart on echo, but aspirin may be given. Otherwise, anticoagulate with warfarin for at least 3wks before and 4wks after DC cardioversion.

Chronic AF:
- Control rate with β-blockers or calcium channel blockers. If the rate is not controlled on high doses of one consider adding a second agent. Digoxin can be used but will not control the rate during exercise. Alternative: Amiodarone PO.
- Anticoagulate with warfarin if >60 unless contraindication. Aim for an INR of 2.0–3.0. For those aged <60yrs with no other risk factors (eg hypertension, diabetes, LV dysfunction, ↑ LA size, rheumatic valve disease, MI, structural heart disease), or those in whom warfarin is contraindicated, aspirin (325mg PO) can be used.

Paroxysmal AF:
- Many antiarrhythmic agents can be used to try to maintain sinus rhythm. Be cautious to not use an agent contraindicated in a certain patient population (eg flecainide in ischemic heart disease). Anticoagulate with warfarin.

Summary of treatment of AF

- Treat any reversible cause.
- Control ventricular rate.
- Consider cardioversion to sinus rhythm, if onset within last 12 months (do echo first; is heart structurally normal?).
- Prevent emboli: Warfarin (or aspirin).

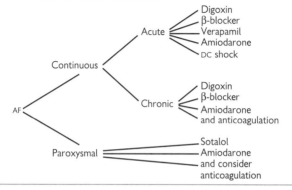

- AF
  - Continuous
    - Acute
      - Digoxin
      - β-blocker
      - Verapamil
      - Amiodarone
      - DC shock
    - Chronic
      - Digoxin
      - β-blocker
      - Amiodarone and anticoagulation
  - Paroxysmal
    - Sotalol
    - Amiodarone and consider anticoagulation

Note on atrial flutter

- ECG: Continuous atrial depolarization (eg ~300/min, but very variable) produces a sawtooth baseline with variable block 2:1 or 3:1 usually.
- Carotid sinus massage or IV adenosine transiently block the AV node and may unmask flutter waves.
- Treatment: Same as AF. Consider cavotricuspid isthmus ablation (this 'flutter isthmus' is low in the right atrium).

Wolff–Parkinson–White syndrome

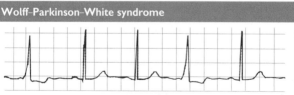

ECG of WPW syndrome (p118) in 1st & 4th beats; compared with the other beats, it can be seen how the delta wave both broadens the ventricular complex, and shortens the PR interval.

Wide complex tachycardia

ECG shows rate of >100 and QRS complexes >120ms (>3 small squares, p90). If no clear QRS complexes, it is VF or asystole, p123.

Principles of management
• Identify the underlying rhythm and treat accordingly.
• If in doubt, treat as VT (the commonest cause).

Differential diagnosis
• VT; includes Torsade de pointes, see below.
• SVT with aberrant conduction, eg AF, atrial flutter.

(**NB:** Premature ventricular beats should not cause confusion when occurring singly; but if >3 together at rate of >120, this constitutes VT.)

Identification of the underlying rhythm (see opposite) may be difficult, seek expert help. Diagnosis is based on the history (IHD ↑ the likelihood of a ventricular arrhythmia), a 12-lead ECG, and the lack of response to IV adenosine (p119). ECG findings in favor of VT:
• +ve QRS concordance in chest leads.
• Marked LAD.
• AV dissociation (occurs in 25%) or 2:1 or 3:1 AV block.
• Fusion beats or capture beats.
• RSR complex in V_1 (with +ve QRS in V_1).
• QS complex in V_6 (with –ve QRS in V_1).

Concordance means QRS complexes are all +ve or –ve. A *fusion beat* is when a 'normal beat' fuses with a VT complex to create an unusual complex, and a *capture beat* is a normal QRS between abnormal beats (see opposite).

122

Management Connect to a cardiac monitor; have a defibrillator to hand.
• Give high-flow oxygen by face mask.
• Obtain IV access and take blood for electrolytes, cardiac enzymes, Ca^{2+}, Mg^{2+}.
• Obtain 12-lead ECG.
• ABG (if evidence of pulmonary edema, reduced conscious level, sepsis).

VT: Hemodynamically stable.
• Correct hypokalemia and hypomagnesemia.
• Amiodarone 150mg IV over 10min, then 1mg/min IV x 6 hours.
• OR lidocaine 1–1.5mg/kg over 2min repeated every 5min to 300mg max.
• If this fails, or cardiac arrest occurs, use DC shock.
• After correction of VT, establish the cause from history/investigations.
• Maintenance antiarrhythmic therapy may be required. If VT occurs <24h after MI, give IV lidocaine or amiodarone IVI for 12–24h. If VT occurs >24h after MI, give IV lidocaine or amiodarone infusion and start oral antiarrhythmic: Eg amiodarone.
• Prevention of recurrent VT: Surgical isolation of the arrhythmogenic area or implantation of an automatic defibrillator may help.

VF: (ECG, see opposite) Use asynchronized DC shock (p668): See also the *American Heart Association ACLS Guidelines* (p677).

Ventricular extrasystoles (PVCs) are the commonest post-MI arrhythmia but they are also seen in healthy people (≥10/h). Post-MI they suggest electrical instability, and there is a risk of VF if the 'R on T' pattern (ie no gap before the T wave) is seen. If frequent (>10/min), treat with lidocaine 100mg IV as above. Otherwise, just observe patient and replace electrolytes.

Torsade de pointes: Looks like VF but is VT with varying axis (ECG, see opposite). It is due to ↑QT interval (congenital, drug-induced, or biochemical) and also occurs post MI. R: Mg sulfate ± overdrive pacing.

Fusion and capture beats

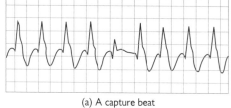

(a) A capture beat

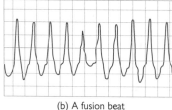

(b) A fusion beat

Specimen rhythm strips

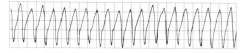

VT with a rate of 235/min.

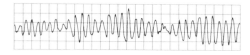

VF.

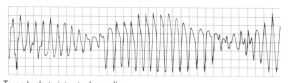

Torsade de pointes tachycardia.

Pacemakers

Pacemakers supply electrical initiation to myocardial contraction. The pacemaker lies subcutaneously where it may be programed through the skin as necessary. Pacemakers usually last 7–15yrs.

Indications for temporary cardiac pacing
- Symptomatic bradycardia, unresponsive to atropine.
- Acute conduction disturbances following MI:
  - After acute *anterior* MI, prophylactic pacing is required in:
    - Complete AV block
    - Möbitz type II AV block
    - Non-adjacent bifascicular or trifascicular block (p93).
  - After *inferior* MI, pacing may not be needed in complete AV block if reasonably stable, and rate is >40–50, and QRS complexes are narrow.
- Suppression of drug-resistant tachyarrhythmias, eg SVT, VT.
- Special situations: During general anesthesia; during cardiac surgery; during electrophysiological studies; drug overdose (eg digoxin, β-blockers, verapamil).

Indications for a permanent pacemaker
- Complete AV block (Stokes–Adams attacks, asymptomatic, congenital) or Möbitz type II AV block p117 with symptoms or HR <40 or >3s asystole.
- Persistent AV block after anterior MI.
- Symptomatic bradycardias (eg sick sinus syndrome, p116).
- Drug-resistant tachyarrhythmias.

Some say persistent bifascicular block after MI requires a permanent system: This remains controversial.

Pre-operative assessment: CBC, PT/PTT. Insert IV cannula. Consent for procedure under local anesthetic. Consider pre-medication. Give antibiotic coverage 20min before, and 1 and 6h after.

Post-procedure assessment: Prior to discharge, check wound for bleeding or hematoma; check position on CXR; check pacemaker function. During 1st week, inspect for wound hematoma, dehiscence, or muscle twitching. Count apical rate (p70): If this is ≥6bpm less than the rate quoted for the pacemaker, suspect malfunction. Other problems: Lead fracture; pacemaker interference (eg from patient's muscles).

Types of pacemakers: 3-letter pacemaker codes enable the identification of the pacemaker: The 1st letter indicates the chamber paced (A = atria, V = ventricles, D = dual chamber); the 2nd letter identifies the chamber sensed (A = atria, V = ventricles, D = dual chamber, 0 = none), and the 3rd letter indicates the pacemaker response (T = triggered, I = inhibited, D = dual, R = reverse). DDD pacemakers are the only pacemakers that sense and pace both chambers. The 4th letter (if present) is for rate responsiveness while exercising.

ECG of paced rhythm: (ECG 7, p97, and opposite for rhythm strip) If the system is on 'demand' of 60bpm, a pacing spike will only be seen if the intrinsic heart rate is <60bpm. If it is cutting in at a higher rate, its sensing mode is malfunctioning. If it is failing to cut in at slower rates, its pacing mode is malfunctioning, ie the lead may be dislodged, the pacing threshold is too high, or the lead (or insulation) is faulty. If you see spikes but no capture (ie no systole), suspect dislodgment.

Some confusing pacemaker terms

Fusion beat: Union of native depolarization and pacemaker impulse.

Pseudofusion: The pacemaker impulse occurs just after cardiac depolarization, so it is ineffective, but it distorts the QRS morphology.

Pseudopseudofusion beat: If a DVI pacemaker gives an atrial spike within a native QRS complex, the atrial output is non-contributory.

Pacemaker syndrome: In single-chamber pacing, retrograde conduction to the atria, which then contract during ventricular systole. This leads to retrograde flow in pulmonary veins, and ↓cardiac output.

Pacemaker tachycardia: In dual-chamber pacing, a short-circuit loop goes between the electrodes, causing an artificial WPW-like syndrome. Solution: Single-chamber pacing.

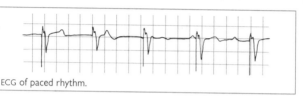

ECG of paced rhythm.

Heart failure—basic concepts

Definition Heart failure occurs when the heart fails to maintain the cardiac output and BP to meet the body's requirements. Prognosis is poor with >50% of patients dying within 5yrs of diagnosis.

Classification LVF and RVF may occur independently, or together as *congestive heart failure (CHF). Low-output cardiac failure:* The heart's output is inadequate (eg ejection fraction <0.35), or is only adequate with high filling pressures. Causes: Usually ischemia, hypertension, valve disorders, or ↑alcohol use.

- *Pump failure due to:*
  - *Heart muscle disease:* IHD; cardiomyopathy (p144).
  - *Restricted filling:* Constrictive pericarditis, tamponade, restrictive cardiomyopathy. This may be the mechanism of action of fluid overload: An expanding right heart impinges on the LV, so filling is restricted by the ungiving pericardium.
  - *Inadequate heart rate:* β-blockers, heart block, post MI.
  - *Negative inotropic drugs:* Eg most antiarrhythmic agents.
- *Excessive preload:* Eg mitral regurgitation or fluid overload (eg NSAID causing fluid retention). Fluid overload may cause LVF in a normal heart if renal excretion is impaired or big volumes are involved (eg IVI running too fast). More common if there is simultaneous compromise of cardiac function and in the elderly.
- *Chronic excessive afterload:* Eg AS, hypertension.

NB: High-output failure is rare. Here, output is normal or ↑ in the face of much ↑ needs. Failure occurs when cardiac output fails to meet needs. It will occur with a normal heart, but even earlier if there is heart disease. *Causes:* Heart disease with anemia or pregnancy, hyperthyroidism, Paget's disease, arteriovenous malformation or fistulas, beri beri. *Consequences:* Initially features of RVF; later LVF becomes evident.

Symptoms depend on which ventricle is more affected. LVF: Dyspnea, poor exercise tolerance, fatigue, orthopnea, paroxysmal nocturnal dyspnea (PND), nocturnal cough (±pink frothy sputum), wheeze (cardiac 'asthma'), nocturia, cool peripheries, weight loss, muscle wasting. RVF: Peripheral edema (up to thighs, sacrum, abdominal wall), abdominal distension (ascites), nausea, anorexia, facial engorgement, pulsation in neck and face (tricuspid regurgitation), epistaxis. In addition, patients may be depressed or complain of drug-related side effects.

Signs The patient may look ill and exhausted, with cool peripheries, and peripheral cyanosis. Pulse: Resting tachycardia, pulsus alternans. Systolic BP↓, narrow pulse pressure, Raised JVP. Precordium: Displaced apex (LV dilatation), RV heave (pulmonary hypertension), Auscultation: S₃ gallop (p50), murmurs of mitral or aortic valve disease. Chest: Tachypnea, bibasal end-inspiratory crackles, wheeze ('cardiac asthma'), pleural effusions. Abdomen: Hepatomegaly (pulsatile in tricuspid regurgitation), ascites, peripheral edema.

Investigations

Blood tests: CBC; electrolytes; BNP; TSH; iron studies. *CXR:* Cardiomegaly (cardiothoracic ratio >50%), prominent upper lobe veins (upper lobe diversion), peribronchial cuffing, diffuse interstitial or alveolar shadowing, classical perihilar 'bat's wing' shadowing, fluid in the fissures, pleural effusions, Kerley B lines (variously attributed to interstitial edema and engorged peripheral lymphatics). *ECG* may indicate cause (look for evidence of ischemia, MI, or ventricular hypertrophy). It is rare to get a completely normal ECG in chronic heart failure. *Echocardiography* is the key investigation. It may indicate the cause (MI, valvular heart disease) and can confirm the presence or absence of LV dysfunction. *Endomyocardial biopsy* is rarely needed.

New York classification of heart failure: Summary

I Heart disease present, but no dyspnea with ordinary activity.
II Comfortable at rest; dyspnea with ordinary activities.
III Dyspnea present with mild activity.
IV Dyspnea present at rest or with minimal activity.

The CXR in left ventricular failure (see also x-ray Plate 2)

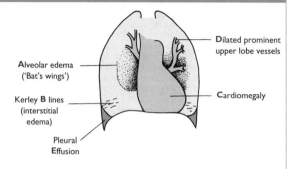

Alveolar edema ('Bat's wings')

Kerley **B** lines (interstitial edema)

Pleural **E**ffusion

Dilated prominent upper lobe vessels

Cardiomegaly

These features can be remembered as **A, B, C, D, E**.

Heart failure—management

Acute heart failure is a medical emergency (p692).

Chronic heart failure Treat the cause (eg if arrhythmias; valve disease).
- Treat exacerbating factors (anemia, thyroid disease, infection, ↑BP).
- Avoid exacerbating factors, eg NSAIDs (cause fluid retention and ↓ the effectiveness of ACE inhibitors).
- Stop smoking. Eat less salt. Maintain optimal weight and nutrition.
- Drugs: The following are used:

  1 *Diuretics:* Loop diuretics routinely used to relieve symptoms eg furosemide; ↑ dose and frequency as necessary. SE:Mg, K^+↓, renal impairment. Monitor electrolytes and add K^+ sparing diuretic (eg *spironolactone*) if K^+ <3.2mEq/L, predisposition to arrhythmias, concurrent digoxin therapy (K^+↓ ↑ risk of digoxin toxicity), or pre-existing K^+-losing conditions. If refractory fluid, consider adding *metolazone* 5mg/24h PO prior to the furosemide dose.

  2 *ACE-inhibitor:* Consider in all patients with left ventricular systolic dysfunction; improves symptoms and prolongs life (see opposite). If cough is a problem an angiotensin receptor antagonist may be substituted (eg losartan 25mg/d; max 100mg PO).

  3 *β-blockers* (eg carvedilol, metropolol XL) Recent randomized trials show that β-blockers ↓mortality in heart failure. These benefits appear to be additive to those of ACE-i in patients with heart failure due to LV dysfunction. Should be initiated after diuretic and ACE-I only if the patient is euvolemic. Use with caution: 'Start low and go slow'; if in doubt seek specialist advice first.

  4 *Spironolactone:* The RALES trial showed that spironolactone (25mg/24h PO) ↓mortality by 30% when added to conventional therapy. It should be initiated in NYHA III-IV patients. It improves endothelial dysfunction (↑nitric oxide bio-activity) and inhibits vascular angiotensin I/angiotensin II conversion. Spironolactone is K^+-sparing and hyperkalemia should be monitored closely in the elderly or those with renal insufficiency.

  5 *Digoxin* improves symptoms even in those with sinus rhythm (data from the RADIANCE and other trials). Use it if diuretics, ACE-i, and β-blocker do not control symptoms, or in patients with AF. Dose: 0.125–0.25mg/24h PO. Monitor K^+ and maintain at 4–5mEq/L. Other inotropes are unhelpful in terms of outcome.

  6 *Vasodilators:* Long-acting nitrates ↓preload by causing venodilatation, eg isosorbide mononitrate 60mg/24h PO. 2nd line agents include arterial vasodilators, which reduce afterload (eg hydralazine, SE: Drug-induced lupus) or α-blockers, which are combined arterial and venous vasodilators, eg prazosin. Vasodilators improve arterial hemodynamics and ↓mortality (so especially valuable if ACE-i is contraindicated).

Intractable heart failure Reassess the cause. Is the patient taking their drugs? At maximum dose? Are they compliant with diet? Admit to hospital for:
- Bed rest.
- IV furosemide ± metolazone.
- IV opiates and nitrates may relieve symptoms—rarely used.
- Daily weight & frequent electrolytes (K^+↓).
- DVT prophylaxis: Heparin 5000U/12h SC and TED stockings.
- *In extremis,* IV inotropes (p696) may be needed but will not prolong life (it may be difficult to wean patients off them).
- *Consider 'tailoring therapy' with a right heart catheterization.*
- Finally, consider a heart transplant or left ventricular assist device.

How to start ACE-inhibitors

Check that there are no contraindications/cautions:
- Renal failure (serum creatinine >2.5mg/dL; but not an absolute CI)
- Hyperkalemia: K⁺ >5.0mEq/L
- Hyponatremia: Caution if <130mEq/L (relates to a poorer prognosis)
- Hypovolemia
- Hypotension (systolic BP <90mmHg)
- AS or LV outflow tract obstruction
- Pregnancy or lactation
- Severe COPD or cor pulmonale (not an absolute CI)
- Renal artery stenosis[1]. (Suspect if arteriopathic, eg cerebrovascular disease, IHD, peripheral vascular disease. ACE-inhibitors reduce GFR and may precipitate acute renal failure.)

Warn the patient about possible side effects:
- Hypotension, especially with 1st dose (so lie down after swallowing)
- Dry cough (1:10)
- Taste disturbance
- Hyperkalemia
- Renal impairment
- Urticaria and angioedema (<1:1000)
- Rarely: Proteinuria, leukopenia, fatigue

Starting ace-inhibitors:

Hypertensive patients can be safely started on ACE-inhibitors as outpatients. Warn them about postural hypotension and advise them to take the 1st dose on going to bed. Use a long-acting ACE-inhibitor at low doses.

Patients with CHF are best started on ACE-inhibitors under close medical supervision. Start with small dose and ↑ every 2wks until at target dose (equivalent of 40mg lisinopril a day) or side effects supervene (↓BP, ↑creatinine). Review in ~1wk for assessment; monitor CHEM 7 regularly. Patients on high doses of diuretics (>80mg furosemide a day) may need a reduction in their diuretic dose first—seek expert help.

129

1 If renovascular disease precludes the use of ACE-i and frusemide (=furosemide) is providing no answer, consider maximal vasodilatation with nitrates and hydralazine: seek expert advice.

Hypertension

Hypertension is a major risk factor for stroke and MI. It is usually asymptomatic, so screening is vital.

Defining hypertension BP has a skewed normal distribution within the population, and risk is continuously related to BP. Therefore, it is impossible to define 'hypertension'. We choose to select a value above which risk is significantly ↑, and the benefit of treatment is clear cut, see below. BP should be assessed over a period of time (don't rely on a single reading). The 'observation' period depends on the BP and the presence of other risk factors or end-organ damage.

Who to treat All patients with malignant hypertension or a sustained pressure ≥140/90mmHg should be treated (p131). For those ≤140/90, the decision depends on the risk of coronary events, presence of diabetes or end-organ damage; see the *Joint National Committee Guidelines*, *(JNC VII)* (see opposite).

Systolic or diastolic pressure? For many years diastolic pressure was considered to be more important than systolic pressure. However, evidence from the Framingham and the MrFIT studies indicates that systolic pressure is the most important determinant of cardiovascular risk in the over 50s.

Systolic hypertension in the elderly: The age-related rise in systolic BP was considered part of the 'normal' aging process, and isolated systolic hypertension (ISH) in the elderly was largely ignored. But evidence from major studies indicates, beyond doubt, that benefits of treating are even greater than treating moderate hypertension in middle-aged patients.

'Malignant' hypertension: This refers to severe hypertension (eg systolic >200, diastolic >130mmHg) in conjunction with bilateral retinal hemorrhages and exudates; papilledema may or may not be present. Symptoms are common, eg headache ± visual disturbance. Alone it requires urgent treatment. However, it may precipitate acute renal failure, heart failure, or encephalopathy, which are hypertensive emergencies. Untreated, 90% die in 1yr; treated, 70% survive 5yrs. Pathological hallmark is fibrinoid necrosis. It is more common in younger patients and in black people. Look hard for any underlying cause.

Causes

Essential hypertension (primary, cause unknown). ~95% of cases.

2° hypertension. ~5% of cases. Causes include:
- *Renal disease:* The most common 2° cause. 75% are from *intrinsic renal disease:* Glomerulonephritis, polyarteritis nodosa (PAN), systemic sclerosis, chronic pyelonephritis, or polycystic kidneys. 25% are due to *renovascular disease,* most frequently atheromatous (elderly ♂ cigarette smokers, associated peripheral vascular disease) or rarely fibromuscular dysplasia (young ♀), p260.
- *Endocrine disease:* Cushing's (p290) and Conn's syndromes (p294), pheochromocytoma (p295), acromegaly, hyperparathyroidism.
- *Others:* Coarctation, pregnancy, steroids, MAOI.

Signs & symptoms Usually asymptomatic (except malignant hypertension above). Always examine the CVS system fully and check for retinopathy. Are there features of an underlying cause (pheochromocytoma, p295), signs of renal disease, radiofemoral delay, or weak femoral pulses (coarctation), renal bruits, palpable kidneys, or Cushing's syndrome? Look for end-organ damage LVH, retinopathy & proteinuria—indicates severity and duration of hypertension and associated with a poorer prognosis.

Investigations *Basic:* Electrolytes, creatinine, cholesterol, glucose, ECG, urine analysis (for protein, blood). *Specific* (exclude a secondary cause): Renal ultrasound, renal arteriography, 24-h urinary VMA and metanephrines, urinary free cortisol, renin, and aldosterone. ECHO and 24-h ambulatory BP monitoring may be helpful in some cases eg white coat or borderline hypertension

Hypertensive retinopathy

Grade
I   Tortuous arteries with thick shiny walls (silver or copper wiring)
II   A–V nicking (narrowing where arteries cross veins)
III Flame hemorrhages and cotton wool spots
IV   Papilledema.

Seventh Report of the Joint National Committee on Prevention, Detection, Evaluation, and Treatment of High Blood Pressure (JNC 7)[1]

ALGORITHM FOR TREATMENT OF HYPERTENSION

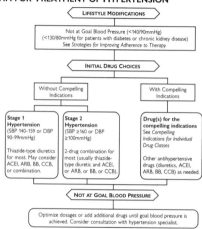

| LIFESTYLE MODIFICATIONS |

Not at Goal Blood Pressure (<140/90mmHg)
(<130/80mmHg for patients with diabetes or chronic kidney disease)
See *Strategies for Improving Adherence to Therapy*

| INITIAL DRUG CHOICES |

Without Compelling Indications

Stage 1 Hypertension
(SBP 140–159 or DBP 90–99mmHg)

Thiazide-type diuretics for most. May consider ACEI, ARB, BB, CCB, or combination.

Stage 2 Hypertension
(SBP ≥160 or DBP ≥100mmHg)

2-drug combination for most (usually thiazide-type diuretic and ACEI, or ARB, or BB, or CCB).

With Compelling Indications

Drug(s) for the compelling indications
See *Compelling Indications for Individual Drug Classes*

Other antihypertensive drugs (diuretics, ACEI, ARB, BB, CCB) as needed.

| NOT AT GOAL BLOOD PRESSURE |

Optimize dosages or add additional drugs until goal blood pressure is achieved. Consider consultation with hypertension specialist.

131

Classification of Blood Pressure (BP)

Category	SBP mmHg		DBP mmHg
Normal	<120	and	<80
Prehypertension	120–139	or	80–89
Hypertension, Stage 1	140–159	or	90–99
Hypertension, Stage 2	≥160	or	≥100

Key: SBP = systolic blood pressure DBP = diastolic blood pressure

Compelling indications for Individual Drug Classes

Compelling Indication	Initial Therapy Options
• Heart failure	THIAZ, BB, ACEI, ARB, ALDO ANT
• Post myocardial infarction	BB, ACEI, ALDO ANT
• High CVD risk	THIAZ, BB, ACEI, CCB
• Diabetes	THIAZ, BB, ACEI, ARB, CCB
• Chronic kidney disease	ACEI, ARB
• Recurrent stroke prevention	THIAZ, ACEI

Key: THIAZ = thiazide diuretic, ACEI= angiotensin converting enzyme inhibitor, ARB = angiotensin receptor blocker, BB = beta blocker, CCB = calcium channel blocker, ALDO ANT = aldosterone antagonist

www.nhlbi.nih.gov/guidelines/hypertension/phycard.pdf

Hypertension—management

Look for and treat underlying causes (eg renal disease, acute pain).

Treatment goal For most patients aim for BP <140/90, but 130/80 in patients with diabetes and renal disease. Reduce blood pressure gradually; a rapid reduction can be fatal, especially in the context of stroke.

Lifestyle changes ↓Concomitant risk factors: Stop smoking; low-fat diet. Reduce alcohol and salt intake; ↑ exercise; reduce weight if obese. (See DASH diet; http://www.nhlbi.nih.gov/health/public/heart/hbp/dash/new_dash.pdf.)

Drugs Explain the need for long-term treatment. Essential hypertension is not 'curable'. The recent ALLHAT study suggests that adequate BP reduction is more important than the specific drug used. However, ACE-i may provide additional renal benefit if co-existing diabetes.

- *Thiazide diuretics:* Are 1st choice, ↑ the dose brings no benefit, and produces more SEs: Hypokalemia, hyponatremia, postural hypotension, impotence.
- *β-blockers:* Eg atenolol 50mg/24h PO. Higher doses provide little additional benefit. SE: Bronchospasm, heart failure, lethargy, impotence. CI: Asthma; caution in heart failure.
- *ACE-i:* Eg lisinopril 2.5–20mg/24h PO (max 40mg/d) or enalapril. ACE-i may be 1st choice if co-existing LVF, or in diabetics with microalbuminuria or proteinuria. SE: Cough, K$^+$↑, renal failure, angioedema. CI renal artery stenosis, AS.
- *Ca^{2+}-channel antagonist:* Eg nifedipine SR 30–90mg/24h PO. SE: Flushing, fatigue, gum hyperplasia, ankle edema. Avoid short-acting drugs.
- *Others:* Angiotensin receptor antagonists (eg losartan), methyldopa (used in pregnancy), and doxazosin (an α-blocker). For refractory cases: Clonidine, minoxidil, or hydralazine (causes a reflex tachycardia unless given with a β-blocker and may cause an SLE-like syndrome).

The 4 main classes of agent happen to start with ABCD. There is some evidence that in monotherapy A&B are more effective in younger people and C&D in older individuals (and black people). This may guide initial therapy and if one drug fails, switch between groups. When adding drugs, it makes sense to combine A or B with C or D eg a thiazide and ACE-i, or β-blocker and Ca^{2+}—channel antagonist—the 'ABCD rule'. Remember that most drugs take 4–8wks to produce their maximum effect, and don't assess efficacy on the basis of a single clinic BP measurement.

Malignant hypertension Most patients can be managed with oral therapy except for those with encephalopathy. The aim is for a controlled reduction in BP over days, not hours. Avoid sudden drops in BP as cerebral autoregulation is poor (so stroke risk↑).

- Bed rest; start a loop diuretic, eg furosemide (40–80mg daily ± a thiazide). There is no ideal antihypertensive therapy, but labetalol, atenolol, or long-acting calcium blockers may be used orally.
- Encephalopathy (headache, focal CNS signs, seizures, coma): Aim to reduce BP to ~110mmHg diastolic over 4h. Admit to monitored area. Insert intra-arterial line for pressure monitoring. Furosemide 40–80mg IV; then either IV labetalol (eg 50mg IV over 1min, repeated every 5min, max 200mg), or sodium nitroprusside infusion (0.5mcg/kg/min IV titrated up to 8mcg/kg/min eg 50mg in 1L dextrose 5%; expect to give 100–200mL/h for a few hours only, to avoid cyanide risk). Labetalol or hydralazine can also be used intravenously. Avoid hydralazine if CAD.

Never use sublingual (SL) nifedipine to reduce BP (it can cause an uncontrollable drop in BP and stroke).

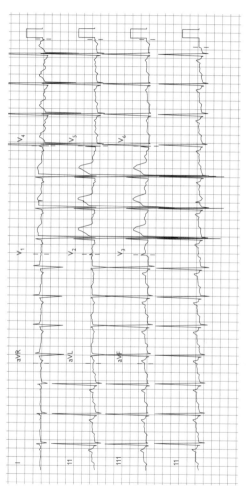

ECG 8—left ventricular hypertrophy—this is from a patient with malignant hypertension—note the sum of the S-wave in V_2 and R-wave in V_6 is >35mm.

Rheumatic fever

This systemic infection is still common in the Third World, although increasingly rare in the West. Peak incidence: 5–15yrs. Tends to recur unless prevented. Pharyngeal infection with Lancefield Group A β-hemolytic streptococci triggers rheumatic fever 2–4wks later, in the susceptible 2% of the population. An antibody to the carbohydrate cell wall of the streptococcus cross-reacts with valve tissue (antigenic mimicry) and may cause permanent damage to the heart valves.

Diagnosis Use the *revised Jones criteria*. There must be evidence of recent strep infection plus 2 major criteria, or 1 major + 2 minor.

Evidence of streptococcal infection:
- Recent streptococcal infection.
- History of scarlet fever.
- +ve throat swab.
- ↑ in antistreptolysin O titer ASOT >200U/mL.
- ↑ in DNase B titer.

Major criteria:
- *Carditis:* Tachycardia, murmurs (mitral or AR, Carey Coombs' murmur, p52), pericardial rub, CCF, cardiomegaly, conduction defects (45–70%). An apical systolic murmur may be the only sign.
- *Arthritis:* A migratory arthritis; usually affects the larger joints (75%).
- *Subcutaneous nodules:* Small, mobile painless nodules on extensor surfaces of joints and spine (2–20%).
- *Erythema marginatum:* Geographical-type rash with red, raised edges and clear center; occurs mainly on trunk, thighs, arms in 2–10%.
- *Sydenham's chorea (St Vitus' dance):* Occurs late in 10%. Unilateral or bilateral involuntary semi-purposeful movements. May be preceded by emotional lability and uncharacteristic behavior.

Minor criteria:
- Fever.
- Raised ESR or CRP.
- Arthralgia (but not if arthritis is one of the major criteria).
- Prolonged P–R interval (but not if carditis is major criterion).
- Previous rheumatic fever.

Management
- Penicillin G 0.6–1.2 million units IM stat then penicillin V 250mg/6h PO.
- Analgesia for carditis/arthritis: Aspirin 100mg/kg/d PO in divided doses (maximum 8g/d) for 2d, then 70mg/kg/d for 6wks. Monitor salicylate level. Toxicity causes tinnitus, hyperventilation, metabolic acidosis. Alternative: NSAIDs.
- Steroids are thought not to have a major impact on sequelae, but they may improve symptoms.
- Immobilize joints in severe arthritis.
- Diazepam for the chorea.

Prognosis 60% with carditis develop chronic rheumatic heart disease. This correlates with the severity of the carditis. Acute attacks last an average of 3 months. Recurrence may be precipitated by further streptococcal infections, pregnancy, or use of oral contraceptives. Cardiac sequelae affect mitral (70%), aortic (40%), tricuspid (10%), and pulmonary (2%) valves. Incompetent lesions develop during the attack, stenoses years later.

Secondary prophylaxis Penicillin V 250mg/12h PO until no longer at risk (>30yrs). Thereafter, give antibiotic prophylaxis for dental or other surgery (p142). Erythromycin can be used if penicillin allergic.

Mitral valve disease

Mitral stenosis *Causes:* Rheumatic; congenital, mucopolysaccharidoses, endocardial fibroelastosis, malignant carcinoid, prosthetic valve.

Presentation: Dyspnea; fatigue; palpitations; chest pain; systemic emboli; hemoptysis; chronic bronchitis-like picture ± complications (below).

Signs: Malar (ie cheek) flush; low-volume pulse; AF common; tapping, undisplaced, apex beat (palpable S_1). On auscultation: Loud S_1; opening snap (pliable valve); rumbling mid-diastolic murmur (heard best in expiration, as the patient lies on their left side). Graham Steell murmur (p52) may occur. *Severity:* The more severe the stenosis, the longer the diastolic murmur, and the closer the opening snap is to S_2.

Tests: ECG: AF; P-mitrale if in sinus rhythm; RVH; progressive RAD. *CXR:* Left atrial enlargement; pulmonary edema; mitral valve calcification. *Echocardiography* is diagnostic. Significant stenosis exists if the valve orifice is $<1cm^2/m^2$ body surface area. Indications for *cardiac catheterization:* Previous valvotomy; signs of other valve disease; angina; severe pulmonary hypertension; calcified mitral valve.

Management: If in AF, *rate control is crucial;* (add a β-blocker or calcium channel blocker if needed to keep the pulse rate <90); anticoagulate with warfarin. Diuretics ↓preload and pulmonary venous congestion. If this fails to control symptoms, balloon valvuloplasty (if pliable, non-calcified valve), open mitral valvotomy or valve replacement. SBE/IE prophylaxis for dental or surgical procedures (p142). Oral penicillin as prophylaxis against recurrent rheumatic fever if <30yrs old.

Complications: Pulmonary hypertension; emboli, pressure from large LA on local structures, eg hoarseness (recurrent laryngeal nerve), dysphagia (esophagus), bronchial obstruction; infective endocarditis (rare).

Mitral regurgitation *Causes:* Functional (LV dilatation); annular calcification (elderly); rheumatic fever, infective endocarditis, mitral valve prolapse, ruptured chordae tendinae; papillary muscle dysfunction/rupture; connective tissue disorders (Ehlers–Danlos, Marfan's); cardiomyopathy; congenital (may be associated with other defects, eg ASD, AV canal); appetite suppressants (eg fenfluramine, phentermine).

Symptoms: Dyspnea; fatigue; palpitations; infective endocarditis. *Signs:* AF; displaced, hyperdynamic apex; RV heave; soft S_1; split S_2; loud P_2 (pulmonary hypertension) pansystolic murmur at apex radiating to axilla. *Severity:* The more severe, the larger the left ventricle.

Tests: ECG: AF ± P-mitrale if in sinus rhythm (may mean left atrial size↑); LVH. *CXR:* Big LA & LV; mitral valve calcification; pulmonary edema.

Echocardiogram to assess LV function (trans-esophageal to assess severity and suitability for repair rather than replacement). *Doppler echo* to assess size and site of regurgitant jet. *Cardiac catheterization* to confirm diagnosis, exclude other valve disease, assess coronary artery disease.

Management: Digoxin for fast AF. Anticoagulate if: AF; history of embolism; prosthetic valve; additional mitral stenosis. Diuretics improve symptoms. Surgery for deteriorating symptoms; aim to repair or replace the valve before LV irreversibly impaired. Antibiotics to prevent endocarditis.

Mitral valve prolapse *Prevalence:* ~5%. Occurs alone or with: ASD, patent ductus arteriosus, cardiomyopathy, Turner syndrome, Marfan syndrome, osteogenesis imperfecta, pseudoxanthoma elasticum, WPW (p118). *Symptoms:* Asymptomatic—or atypical chest pain and palpitations. *Signs:* Mid-systolic click and/or a late systolic murmur. *Complications:* Mitral regurgitation, cerebral emboli, arrhythmias, sudden death. *Tests: Echocardiography* is diagnostic. ECG may show inferior T wave inversion. *Treatment:* β-blockers may help palpitations and chest pain. Give endocarditis prophylaxis (p142), if co-existing mitral regurgitation.

Aortic valve disease

Aortic stenosis (AS) *Causes:* Senile calcification is the commonest. Also congenital bicuspid valve.

Presentation: Angina; dyspnea; dizziness; syncope; systemic emboli if infective endocarditis; CCF; sudden death. *Signs:* Slow rising pulse with narrow pulse pressure (feel for diminished and delayed carotid upstroke—'parvus et tardus'); heaving, undisplaced apex beat; LV heave; aortic thrill; ejection systolic murmur (heard at the base, left sternal edge and the aortic area, radiates to the carotids). As stenosis worsens, A_2 is increasingly delayed, giving first a single S_2 and then reversed splitting. But this sign is rare. More common is a quiet A_2. In severe AS, A_2 may be inaudible (calcified valve). There may be an ejection click (pliable valve) or an audible S_4 (said to occur more commonly with bicuspid valves, but not in all populations).

Tests: ECG: P-mitrale, LVH with strain pattern; LAD (left anterior hemiblock); poor R wave progression; LBBB or complete AV block (calcified ring). *CXR:* LVH; calcified aortic valve; post-stenotic dilatation of ascending aorta. *Echo* is diagnostic (p102). *Doppler echo* can estimate the gradient across valves: Severe stenosis if gradient ≥50mmHg and valve area <0.5cm^2. If the aortic jet velocity is >4m/s (or is ↑ by >0.3m/s per year) risk of complications is ↑. *Cardiac catheter* can assess: Valve gradient; LV function; coronary artery disease; the aortic root.

Differential diagnosis: Hypertrophic obstructive cardiomyopathy (HOCM).

Management: Symptomatic patients have a poor prognosis: 2–3yr survival if angina/syncope; 1–2yr survival with cardiac failure. Prompt valve replacement (p138) is recommended. In asymptomatic patients with severe AS and a deteriorating ECG, valve replacement is also recommended. If the patient is not medically fit for surgery, percutaneous valvuloplasty may be attempted. Endocarditis prophylaxis (p142).

Aortic sclerosis is senile degeneration of the valve. There is an ejection systolic murmur, no carotid radiation, and a normal pulse and S_2.

Aortic regurgitation (AR) *Causes: Congenital. Valve disease:* Rheumatic fever; infective endocarditis, rheumatoid arthritis; SLE; pseudoxanthoma elasticum; appetite suppressants (eg fenfluramine, phentermine). *Aortic root disease:* Hypertension; trauma; aortic dissection; seronegative spondyloarthritis (ankylosing spondylitis; reactive arthritis; psoriatic arthritis); Marfan syndrome; osteogenesis imperfecta; syphilitic aortitis.

Symptoms: Dyspnea; palpitations; cardiac failure. *Signs:* Collapsing (water-hammer) pulse; wide pulse pressure; displaced, hyperdynamic apex beat; high-pitched early diastolic murmur (heard best in expiration, with patient sitting forward). Associated signs: Corrigan's sign (carotid pulsation); Quincke's sign (capillary pulsations in nail beds); Duroziez's sign (femoral diastolic murmur as blood flows backwards in diastole); Traube's sign ('pistol shot' sound over femoral arteries). In severe AR, an Austin Flint murmur may be heard (p52).

Investigations: ECG: LVH. *CXR:* Cardiomegaly; dilated ascending aorta; pulmonary edema. *Echocardiography* is diagnostic. *Cardiac catheterization* to assess: Severity of lesion; anatomy of aortic root; LV function; coronary artery disease; other valve disease.

Management: Indications for surgery: ↑ symptoms; enlarging heart on CXR/echo; ECG deterioration (T wave inversion in lateral leads); infective endocarditis refractory to medical therapy. Aim to replace the valve before significant LV dysfunction occurs. Endocarditis prophylaxis (p142).

Right heart valve disease

Tricuspid regurgitation *Causes:* Pulmonary hypertension; rheumatic fever; infective endocarditis (IV drug abusers); carcinoid syndrome; congenital (eg ASD, AV canal, Ebstein's anomaly).

Symptoms: Fatigue; hepatic pain on exertion; ascites; edema. *Signs:* Giant v waves and prominent y descent in JVP (p48); RV heave; pansystolic murmur, heard best at lower sternal edge in inspiration; pulsatile hepatomegaly; jaundice; ascites. *Management:* Treat underlying cause. Drugs: Diuretics, digoxin, ACE-inhibitors. Valve replacement (20% operative mortality).

Tricuspid stenosis *Cause:* Rheumatic fever; almost always occurs with mitral or aortic valve disease. *Symptoms:* Fatigue, ascites, edema. *Signs:* Giant a wave and slow y descent in JVP (p48); opening snap, early diastolic murmur heard at the left sternal edge in inspiration. *Diagnosis:* Doppler echo. *Treatment:* Diuretics; surgical repair.

Pulmonary stenosis *Causes:* Usually congenital (Turner's syndrome, Noonan's syndrome, William's syndrome, Fallot's tetralogy, rubella). Acquired causes: Rheumatic fever, carcinoid syndrome. *Symptoms:* Dyspnea; fatigue; edema; ascites. *Signs:* Dysmorphic facies (congenital causes); prominent a wave in JVP; RV heave. In mild stenosis, there is an ejection click, ejection systolic murmur (which radiates to the left shoulder); widely split S_2. In severe stenosis, the murmur becomes longer and obscures A_2. P_2 becomes softer and may be inaudible. *Tests:* ECG: RAD, P-pulmonale, RVH, RBBB. CXR: Post-stenotic dilatation of pulmonary artery; RV hypertrophy; right atrial hypertrophy. Cardiac catheterization is diagnostic. *Treatment:* Pulmonary valvuloplasty or valvotomy.

Pulmonary regurgitation is caused by any cause of pulmonary hypertension (p188). A decrescendo murmur is heard in early diastole at the left sternal edge (the Graham Steell murmur).

Cardiac surgery

Valvuloplasty can be used in mitral or pulmonary stenosis (pliable, noncalcified valve, no regurgitation). A balloon catheter is inserted across the valve and inflated.

Valvotomy Closed valvotomy is rarely performed now. Open valvotomy is performed under cardiopulmonary bypass through a median sternotomy.

Valve replacements *Mechanical valves* may be of the ball-cage (Starr–Edwards), tilting disc (Bjork–Shiley), or double tilting disc (St. Jude) type. These valves are very durable but the risk of thromboembolism is high; patients require lifelong anticoagulation. *Xenografts* are made from porcine valves or pericardium. These valves are less durable and may require replacement at 8–10yrs. Anticoagulation is not required unless there is AF. *Homografts* are cadaveric valves. They are particularly useful in young patients and in the replacement of infected valves. *Complications of prosthetic valves:* Systemic embolism, infective endocarditis, hemolysis, structural valve failure, arrhythmias.

CABG see opposite.

Cardiac transplantation Consider this when cardiac disease is *severely* curtailing quality of life, and survival is not expected beyond 6–12 months. Refer to a specialty center. Main contraindications: Malignancy, age >70, significant peripheral or cerebrovascular disease, diabetes with end organ dysfunction, non-compliance.

Coronary artery bypass grafts

Indications for CABG: To improve survival
- Left main disease
- Triple vessel disease involving proximal part of the left anterior descending, especially with LV dysfunction

To relieve symptoms
- Angina unresponsive to drugs
- Unstable angina (sometimes)
- If angioplasty is unsuccessful

Procedure: Surgery is planned based on the result of angiograms. Not all stenoses are bypassable. The heart is stopped and blood is oxygenated and pumped artificially by a machine outside the body (cardiac bypass).

The patient's own saphenous vein or internal mammary artery is used as the graft. Several grafts may be placed.

>50% of vein grafts close in 10yrs (low-dose aspirin helps prevent this). Internal mammary artery grafts last longer (but may cause chest-wall numbness).

After CABG: If angina persists or recurs (from poor run-off from the graft, distal disease, new atheroma, or graft occlusion) restart anti-anginal drugs, and consider angioplasty (repeat surgery is dangerous). Mood, sex, and intellectual problems are common early. Rehabilitation helps:
- Exercise: Walk→cycle→swim→jog
- Drive at 1 month: No need to tell DMV
- Get back to work eg at 3 months
- Address smoking cessation; BP; lipids
- Aspirin, statin for life.

Infective endocarditis

Fever + new murmur = endocarditis until proven otherwise.

Classification
- 50% of all endocarditis occurs on *normal valves.* It follows an *acute course,* and presents with acute heart failure.
- Endocarditis on *abnormal valves* tends to run a *subacute course.* Predisposing cardiac lesions: Aortic or mitral valve disease; tricuspid valves in IV drug users; coarctation; patent ductus arteriosus; VSD; prosthetic valves. Endocarditis on prosthetic valves may be 'early' (acquired at the time of surgery, poor prognosis) or 'late' (acquired hematogenously).

Causes *Bacteria:* Any cause of bacteremia exposes valves to the risk of bacterial colonization (eg dental work; UTI; urinary catheterization; cystoscopy; respiratory infection; endoscopy (controversial); colonic carcinoma; gall bladder disease; skin disease; IV cannulation; surgery; abortion; fractures). Quite often, no cause is found. *Streptococcus viridans* is the commonest (35–50%). Others: Enterococci; *Staphylococcus aureus/epidermidis;* diphtheroids and microaerophilic streptococci. Rarely: HACEK group of Gram –ve bacteria (*Haemophilus–Actinobacillus–Cardiobacterium–Eikenella–Kingella*); *Coxiella burnetii; Chlamydia. Fungi:* These include *Candida, Aspergillus,* and *Histoplasma. Other causes:* SLE (Libman–Sacks endocarditis); malignancy.

Clinical features The patient may present with any of the following: *Signs of infection:* Fever, rigors, night sweats, malaise, weight loss, anemia, splenomegaly, and clubbing. *Cardiac lesions:* Any new murmur, or a change in the nature of a pre-existing murmur, should raise the suspicion of endocarditis. Vegetations may cause valve destruction, and severe regurgitation, or valve obstruction. An aortic root abscess causes prolongation of the P–R interval, and may lead to complete AV block. LVF is a common cause of death. *Immune complex deposition:* Vasculitis (p378) may affect any vessel. Microscopic hematuria is common; glomerulonephritis and acute renal failure may occur. Roth spots (boat-shaped retinal hemorrhage with pale center); splinter hemorrhages (on finger or toe nails); Osler's nodes (painful pulp infarcts in fingers or toes) and Janeway lesions (painless palmar or plantar macules) are pathognomonic. *Embolic phenomena:* Emboli may cause abscesses in the relevant organ, eg brain, heart, kidney, spleen, GI tract. In right-sided endocarditis, pulmonary abscesses may occur.

Diagnosis The *Duke* criteria for definitive diagnosis of endocarditis are given opposite. *Blood cultures:* Take 3 sets at different times and from different sites at peak fever. 85–90% are diagnosed from the first 2 sets; 10% are culture-negative. *Blood tests:* Normochromic, normocytic anemia, neutrophil leukocytosis, high ESR/CRP. Also check electrolytes, Mg^{2+}, LFTs. *Urinalysis* for microscopic hematuria. *CXR* (cardiomegaly) and *ECG* (prolonged P–R interval) at regular intervals. *Echocardiography* TTE may show vegetations, but only if >2mm. TEE is more sensitive, and better for visualizing mitral lesions and possible development of aortic root abscess.

Management Consultation with Infectious Disease and Cardiology should be considered.
- Antibiotics: see opposite.
- Consider surgery if: Heart failure, progressive heart block, valvular obstruction; repeated emboli; fungal endocarditis; persistent bacteremia; myocardial abscess; unstable infected prosthetic valve.

Prognosis 30% mortality with staphylococci; 14% with bowel organisms; 6% with sensitive streptococci.

Duke criteria for infective endocarditis

Major criteria:
- Positive blood culture:
  - typical organism in 2 separate cultures or
  - persistently +ve blood cultures, eg 3, >12h apart (or majority if ≥4)
- Endocardium involved:
  - +ve echocardiogram (vegetation, abscess, dehiscence of prosthetic valve) or
  - new valvular regurgitation (change in murmur not sufficient).

Minor criteria:
- Predisposition (cardiac lesion; IV drug abuse)
- Fever >38°C
- Vascular/immunological signs
- +ve blood culture that do not meet major criteria
- +ve echocardiogram that does not meet major criteria.

How to diagnose: Definite infective endocarditis: 2 major **or** 1 major and 3 minor **or** all 5 minor criteria (if no major criterion is met).

Antibiotic therapy for infective endocarditis

- Consult Infectious Disease for the appropriate regimen based on bacterial sensitivities in your hospital. The following are guidelines only:
- *Empirical therapy:* Nafcillin or oxacillin 2g/4h IV + gentamicin or tobramycin 1mg/kg q12h IV.
- *Streptococci:* PCN G 20–30 million U/d IV for 4–6wks; then amoxicillin 1g/8h PO for 2wks. Monitor minimum inhibitory concentration (MIC) and add gentamicin 1mg/kg q8-12h IV for the first 2wks. Monitor gentamicin levels.
- *Enterococci:* Ampicillin[1] 1g/6h IV + gentamicin 1mg/kg q 8-12h IV for 4wks. Monitor gentamicin levels.
- *Staphylococci:* Oxacillin or nafcillin 2g/4h IV + gentamicin 1mg/kg q12h IV. Treat for 6–8wks; stop gentamicin after 1wk.
- *Coxiella:* Doxycycline 100mg/12h PO indefinitely + co-trimoxazole, rifampin, or ciprofloxacin.
- *Fungi:* Flucytosine 3g/6h IVI over 30mins followed by fluconazole 50mg/24h PO (a higher dose may be needed). Amphotericin if flucytosine resistance or *Aspergillus*. Miconazole if renal function is poor.

---

[1] For penicillin allergy, use vancomycin 1g/12h IV.

Prevention of endocarditis

Anyone with congenital heart disease, acquired valve disease, or prosthetic valves is at risk of infective endocarditis and should take prophylactic antibiotics before procedures which may result in bacteremia. The recommendations of the American Heart Association are:

Which conditions?

Prophylaxis recommended
- Prosthetic valve(s)
- Previous endocarditis
- Septal defects
- Mitral prolapse with regurgitation
- Acquired valve disease
- Surgical shunts

Prophylaxis not recommended
- Mitral prolapse (no regurgitation)
- Functional/innocent murmur

Which procedures?

Prophylaxis recommended
- Dental procedures
- Upper respiratory tract surgery
- Esophageal dilatation
- Sclerotherapy of varices
- Surgery/instrumentation of lower bowel, gall bladder, or GU tract

Prophylaxis not recommended
- Flexible bronchoscopy
- Diagnostic upper GI endoscopy
- TEE (p102)
- Cesarean or normal delivery
- Cardiac catheterization (unless high-risk patient)

Which regimen?

- *Dental procedures*
  - *Local or no anesthetic:* Amoxicillin 2g PO, 1h before the procedure. Alternative (if penicillin allergy or >1 dose of penicillin in previous month): Clindamycin 600mg PO or cephalexin 2g PO or azithromycin/clarithromycin 500mg 1h pre procedure.
  - *Intolerant of oral meds:* Ampicillin 2g IV 30min pre procedure.
- *Upper respiratory tract procedures*
  - As for dental procedures.
- *Gastrointestinal and genitourinary procedures*
  - High risk (prosthetic valve, prior endocarditis, surgical shunt): Ampicillin 2g IM/IV + gentamicin 1.5mg/kg IV/IM 30min pre procedure. Vancomycin 1g IV + gentamicin if penicillin allergy.
  - Moderate risk: Amoxicillin 2g PO 1h pre-procedure. Vancomycin 1g IV if penicillin allergy.

Diseases of heart muscle

Acute myocarditis *Causes:* Inflamed myocardium from viruses (coxsackie, polio, HIV, Lassa fever); bacteria (Clostridia, diphtheria, Meningococcus, Mycoplasma, psittacosis); spirochetes (Leptospirosis, syphilis, Lyme disease); protozoa (Chagas' disease); drugs; toxins; vasculitis, (p378).

Signs & symptoms: Fatigue, dyspnea, chest pain, palpitations, tachycardia, soft S_1, S_4 gallop.

Tests: ECG: ST segment elevation/depression, T wave inversion, atrial arrhythmias, transient AV block. Serology may be helpful.

Management: Treat the underlying cause. Supportive measures. Patients may recover or get intractable heart failure (p128).

Dilated cardiomyopathy A dilated, poorly contractile heart of unknown cause. Associations: Alcohol, ↑BP, hemochromatosis, viral infection, autoimmune, peri- or postpartum, thyrotoxicosis, congenital (X-linked). *Prevalence:* 0.2%.

Presentation: Fatigue, dyspnea, pulmonary edema, RVF, emboli, AF, VT. *Signs:* ↑Pulse, ↓BP, ↑JVP, displaced, diffuse apex, S_3 gallop, mitral or tricuspid regurgitation (MR/TR), pleural effusion, edema, jaundice, hepatomegaly, ascites.

Tests: CXR: Cardiomegaly, pulmonary edema. *ECG:* Tachycardia, non-specific T wave changes, poor R wave progression. *Echo:* Globally dilated hypokinetic heart with low ejection fraction. Look for MR, TR, LV mural thrombus.

Management: Bed rest, diuretics, digoxin, ACE-inhibitor, beta blockers, anticoagulation. Consider cardiac transplantation. *Mortality:* Variable depending on severity of symptoms.

Hypertrophic cardiomyopathy *HOCM* ≈ LV outflow tract (LVOT) obstruction from asymmetric septal hypertrophy.

Prevalence: 0.2%. Autosomal dominant inheritance, but 50% are sporadic. 70% have mutations in genes encoding β-myosin, α-tropomyosin, and troponin T. May present at any age. Ask about family history or sudden death.

The patient: Angina; dyspnea; palpitation; syncope; sudden death (VF is amenable to implantable defibrillators). Pulse with rapid upstroke; *a* wave in JVP; double apex beat; systolic thrill at lower left sternal edge; harsh ejection systolic murmur.

Tests: ECG: LVH; progressive T wave inversion; deep Q waves (inferior + lateral leads); AF; WPW syndrome (p118); ventricular ectopy; VT. *Echo:* Asymmetrical septal hypertrophy; small LV cavity with hypercontractile posterior wall; midsystolic closure of aortic valve; systolic anterior movement of mitral valve. *Cardiac catheterization* may provoke VT. It helps assess: Severity of gradient; coronary artery disease or mitral regurgitation. Electrophysiological studies may be needed (WPW). Exercise test ± Holter monitor to risk stratify.

Management: β-blockers or verapamil for symptoms (p109). Amiodarone 100–200mg/d for arrhythmias (AF, VT). Anticoagulate for paroxysmal AF or systemic emboli. Septal myectomy (surgical, or chemical, with alcohol, to ↓LV outflow tract gradient) is reserved for those with severe symptoms. Consider implantable defibrillator.

Mortality: 5.9%/yr if <14yrs; 2.5%/yr if >14yrs. *Poor prognostic factors:* Age <14yrs or syncope at presentation; family history of HOCM/sudden death.

Restrictive cardiomyopathy *Causes:* Amyloidosis; hemochromatosis; sarcoidosis; scleroderma; Löffler's eosinophilic endocarditis, endomyocardial fibrosis. *Presentation* is like constrictive pericarditis (p146). Features of RVF predominate: ↑JVP, with prominent x and y descents; hepatomegaly; edema; ascites. *Diagnosis:* Cardiac catheterization.

Cardiac myxoma Rare benign cardiac tumor. Prevalence ≤5/10,000, ♀:♂ ≈ 2:1. Usually sporadic, may be familial (autosomal dominant). It may mimic infective endocarditis (fever, weight loss, clubbing, ↑ESR), or mitral stenosis (left atrial obstruction, systemic emboli, AF). A 'tumor plop' may be heard, and signs may vary according to posture. *Tests:* Echocardiography. *Treatment:* Excision.

The heart in various, mostly rare, systemic diseases

This list reminds us to look at the heart *and* the whole patient, not just in exams (where those with odd syndromes congregate), but always.

Acromegaly: (p304) BP↑; LVH; hypertrophic cardiomyopathy; high output cardiac failure; coronary artery disease.

Amyloidosis: (p587) Restrictive cardiomyopathy.

Ankylosing spondylitis: (p372) Conduction defects; AV block; AR.

Behçet's disease: (p378) AR; arterial ± venous thrombi.

Cushing's syndrome: (p290) Hypertension.

Down's syndrome: ASD; VSD; mitral regurgitation.

Ehlers–Danlos syndrome: Mitral valve prolapse + hyperelastic skin ± aneurysms and GI bleeds. Joints are loose and hypermobile; mutations exist, eg in genes for procollagen (COL3A1); there are 6 types.

Friedreich's ataxia: Hypertrophic cardiomyopathy.

Hemochromatosis: (p216) AF; cardiomyopathy.

Holt-Oram syndrome: ASD or VSD with upper limb defects.

Human immunodeficiency virus: (p518) Myocarditis; dilated cardiomyopathy; effusion; ventricular arrhythmias; SBE/IE; non-infective thrombotic (murantic) endocarditis; RVF (pulmonary hypertension); metastatic Kaposi's sarcoma.

Hypothyroidism: (p282) Sinus bradycardia; low pulse pressure; pericardial effusion; coronary artery disease; low voltage ECG.

Kawasaki disease: Coronary arteritis similar to PAN; commoner than *rheumatic fever* as a cause of acquired heart disease.

Klinefelter's syndrome:♂ ASD. Psychopathy; learning difficulties; libido↓; gynecomastia; sparse facial hair and small firm testes. XXY.

Marfan's syndrome: Mitral valve prolapse; AR; aortic dissection. Look for long fingers and a high-arched palate.

Noonan's syndrome: ASD; pulmonary stenosis ± low-set ears.

PAN: (p378) Small and medium vessel vasculitis + angina; MI; arrhythmias; CHF; pericarditis and conduction defects.

Rheumatoid nodules: Conduction defects; pericarditis; LV dysfunction; AR; coronary arteritis. Look for arthritis signs, (p368).

Sarcoidosis: (p182) Infiltrating granulomas may cause complete AV block; ventricular or supraventricular tachycardia; myocarditis; CHF; restrictive cardiomyopathy. ECG may show Q waves.

Syphilis: (p538) Myocarditis; ascending aortic aneurysm.

Systemic lupus erythematosus: (p374) Pericarditis/effusion; myocarditis; Libman–Sacks endocarditis; mitral valve prolapse; coronary arteritis.

Systemic sclerosis: (p374) Pericarditis; pericardial effusion; myocardial fibrosis; myocardial ischemia; conduction defects; cardiomyopathy.

Thyrotoxicosis: (p280) Pulse↑; AF ± emboli; wide pulse pressure; hyperdynamic apex; loud heart sounds; ejection systolic murmur; pleuropericardial rub; angina; high output cardiac failure.

Turner's syndrome:♀ Coarctation of aorta. Look for webbed neck. XO.

William's syndrome: Supravalvular aortic stenosis (visuo-spatial IQ↓).

Pericardial diseases

Acute pericarditis Inflammation of the pericardium which may be 1° or 2° to systemic disease.

Causes: • Viruses (coxsackie, flu, Epstein–Barr, mumps, varicella, HIV) • Bacteria (pneumonia, rheumatic fever, TB) • Fungi • Myocardial infarct • Dressler's • Uremia • Rheumatoid arthritis • SLE • Myxedema • Trauma • Surgery • Malignancy • Radiotherapy • Procainamide; hydralazine.

Clinical features: Central chest pain worse on inspiration or lying flat ± relief by sitting forward. A pericardial friction rub may be heard. Look for evidence of a pericardial effusion or cardiac tamponade (see below).

Tests: ECG classically shows concave (saddle-shaped) ST segment elevation, but may be normal or non-specific (10%). Can also see PR depression. *Blood tests:* CBC, ESR, electrolytes, cardiac enzymes, viral serology, blood cultures, and, if indicated, autoantibodies, fungal cultures, thyroid function tests. Cardiomegaly on CXR may indicate a pericardial effusion. *Echo* to evaluate cardiac function and evaluate for effusions.

Treatment: Analgesia, eg ibuprofen 400mg/8h PO with food. Treat the cause. Consider colchicine before steroids/immunosuppressants if relapse or continuing symptoms occur. 15–40% do recur.

Pericardial effusion Accumulation of fluid in the pericardial space.

Causes: Any cause of pericarditis (see above).

Clinical features: Dyspnea, raised JVP (with prominent x descent, p48), bronchial breathing at left base (Ewart's sign: Large effusion compressing left lower lobe). Look for signs of cardiac tamponade (see below).

Diagnosis: CXR shows an enlarged, globular heart. ECG shows low voltage QRS complexes and alternating QRS morphologies (electrical alternans). *Echocardiography* shows an echo-free zone surrounding the heart.

Management: Treat the cause. Pericardiocentesis may be *diagnostic* (suspected bacterial pericarditis) or *therapeutic* (cardiac tamponade). Send pericardial fluid for culture, TB culture, and cytology.

Constrictive pericarditis The heart is encased in a rigid pericardium.

Causes: Often unknown; also TB, or after *any* pericarditis.

Clinical features: These are mainly of right heart failure with ↑JVP (with prominent x and y descents, p48); Kussmaul's sign (JVP rising paradoxically with inspiration); soft, diffuse apex beat; quiet heart sounds; S₃; diastolic pericardial knock, hepatosplenomegaly, ascites, and edema.

Tests: CXR: Small heart ± pericardial calcification (if none, CT/MRI helps distinguish from other cardiomyopathies). *Echo*; cardiac catheterization.

Management: Surgical excision.

Cardiac tamponade Accumulation of pericardial fluid raises intrapericardial pressure, hence poor ventricular filling and fall in cardiac output.

Causes: Any pericarditis (above); aortic dissection; hemodialysis; warfarin; trans-septal puncture at cardiac catheterization; post cardiac biopsy.

Signs: Pulse↑, BP↓, pulsus paradoxus, JVP↑, Kussmaul's sign, muffled S_1 & S_2.

Diagnosis: Beck's triad: Falling BP; rising JVP; small, quiet heart. CXR: Big globular heart (if >250mL fluid). ECG: Low voltage QRS ± electrical alternans. *Echo* is diagnostic: Echo-free zone (>2cm, or >1cm if acute) around the heart ± diastolic collapse of right atrium and right ventricle.

Management: Seek expert help. The pericardial effusion needs urgent drainage. Send fluid for culture, ZN stain/TB culture & cytology.

Pericarditis

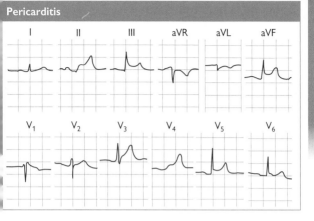

Congenital heart disease

The spectrum of congenital heart disease in adults is considerably different from that in infants and children; adults are unlikely to have complex lesions. The commonest lesions, in descending order of frequency, are:

Bicuspid aortic valve These function well at birth and go undetected. Most eventually develop AS (requiring valve replacement) and/or AR (predisposing to IE/SBE). (p140).

Atrial septal defect (ASD) A hole connects the atria. *Ostium secundum* defects (high in the septum) are commonest; *ostium primum* defects (opposing the endocardial cushions) are associated with AV valve anomalies. Primum ASDs present early. Secundum ASDs are often asymptomatic until adulthood, as the L→R shunt depends on compliance of the right and left ventricles. The latter ↓ with age (esp. if BP↑). This augments L→R shunting causing dyspnea and heart failure, eg at age 40–60. There may be pulmonary hypertension, cyanosis, arrhythmia, hemoptysis, and chest pain.

Signs: AF; ↑JVP; wide, fixed split S2; pulmonary ejection systolic murmur. Pulmonary hypertension may cause pulmonary or tricuspid regurgitation.

Complications: Paradoxical embolism (rare). Reversal of left to right shunt (**Eisenmenger complex**); Eisenmenger complex is a congenital heart defect at first associated with a left to right shunt, which may lead to pulmonary hypertension and shunt reversal. If so, cyanosis develops (± heart failure and respiratory infections), and Eisenmenger's syndrome is present.

Tests: ECG: RBBB with LAD and prolonged P–R interval (primum defect) or RAD (secundum defect). CXR: Small aortic knuckle, pulmonary plethora, progressive atrial enlargement. Echocardiography is diagnostic. Cardiac catheterization shows step up in O2 saturation in the right atrium.

Treatment: In children, surgical closure is recommended before age 10yrs. In adults, closure is recommended if symptomatic, or if asymptomatic but having pulmonary to systemic blood flow ratios of ≥1.5:1.

Ventricular septal defect (VSD) A hole connecting the 2 ventricles.

Causes: Congenital (prevalence 2:1000 births); acquired (post-MI).

Symptoms: May present with severe heart failure in infancy, or remain asymptomatic and be detected incidentally in later life.

Signs: These depend upon the size and site of the VSD: Smaller holes, which are hemodynamically less significant, give louder murmurs. Classically, a harsh pansystolic murmur is heard at the left sternal edge, accompanied by a systolic thrill, ± left parasternal heave. Larger holes are associated with signs of pulmonary hypertension.

Complications: AR, infundibular stenosis, infective endocarditis, pulmonary hypertension, Eisenmenger complex (see opposite).

Tests: ECG: Normal (small VSD), LAD + LVH (moderate VSD) or LVH + RVH (large VSD). CXR: Normal heart size ± mild pulmonary plethora (small VSD) or cardiomegaly, large pulmonary arteries and marked pulmonary plethora (large VSD). Cardiac catheter: Step up in O2 saturation in right ventricle.

Treatment: This is medical, at first, as many VSDs close spontaneously. Indications for surgical closure: Failed medical therapy, symptomatic VSD, shunt >3:1, SBE/IE. Give SBE/IE prophylaxis for untreated defects (p141).

Coarctation of the aorta Congenital narrowing of the descending aorta; usually occurs just distal to the origin of the left subclavian artery. More common in boys. *Associations:* Bicuspid aortic valve, Turner's syndrome. *Signs:* Radio-femoral delay, weak femoral pulse, BP↑, scapular bruit, systolic murmur (best heard over the left scapula). *Complications:* Heart failure, infective endocarditis. *Tests:* CXR shows rib notching. *Treatment:* Surgery.

Pulmonary stenosis may occur alone or with other lesions (p137).

Driving and the heart

The rules on driving with heart conditions vary from state to state and you should become familiar with the laws in your state before discussing driving with your patients. In general, it is the responsibility of the driver but you should guide your patients appropriately.

Pulmonary medicine

Albert J. Polito, M.D.

Contents

Investigations

Diseases and conditions

Chest x-ray

Films are usually taken with the patient standing in front of the film with the x-ray source behind (PA film). Emergency films may be done in the opposite direction (AP), which magnifies heart size. There are 4 radiographic densities: Air, fat, water/soft tissue, bone. A border is only seen at an interface of 2 densities, eg heart (water) and lung (air); this 'silhouette' is lost if air in the lung is replaced by consolidation (water). This is the silhouette sign and helps localize pathology (eg middle lobe pneumonia or collapse causing loss of distinction of the right heart border).

Trachea should be central.

Heart is normally <½ the width of the thorax. It may appear tall and narrow if the chest is hyperinflated (COPD) or larger, if an AP film is taken.

Mediastinum may be widened in many disorders: Retrosternal thyroid, lymph node enlargement (sarcoidosis, lymphoma, metastases, TB), tumor (thymoma, teratoma, neurogenic tumors), aortic aneurysm, cysts (bronchogenic cyst, pericardial cyst), paravertebral mass (TB), esophageal dilatation (achalasia, hiatus hernia).

Hila The left hilum is higher than the right. Hila may be pulled up or down by fibrosis or collapse. (1) *Enlarged hila:* Nodes; pulmonary arterial hypertension; bronchial ca. (2) *Calcification:* Past TB; silicosis; histoplasmosis.

The diaphragm (Right side is usually slightly higher). *Causes of a raised hemidiaphragm:* Lung volume loss, stroke, phrenic nerve palsy (from: Trauma, MND, cancer), hepatomegaly, subphrenic abscess; subpulmonic effusion and diaphragm rupture cause apparent elevation. **NB:** Bilateral palsies (polio, muscular dystrophy) cause hypoxia.

Lung fields Shadowing may be described as nodular, reticular (network of fine lines, interstitial), or alveolar (fluffy).

Nodular shadows:
• Neoplasia (metastases, lung carcinoma, adenoma, hamartoma)
• Infections (varicella pneumonia, hydatid, septic emboli)
• Granulomas (miliary TB, sarcoidosis, histoplasmosis, Wegener's)
• Pneumoconioses (except asbestosis), Caplan's syndrome

Reticular shadows: Usually acute interstitial changes (cardiac or non-cardiac pulmonary interstitial edema, atypical pneumonia, eg viral). Also:
• Chronic infections (TB; histoplasmosis)
• Neoplasia (lymphangitic carcinomatosis)
• Sarcoidosis; silicosis; asbestosis
• Idiopathic pulmonary fibrosis; rheumatoid.
• Extrinsic allergic alveolitis (EAA) • Wegener's; SLE; PAN; CREST

Alveolar shadows: Usually pulmonary edema from LVF (p692). Also:
• Pneumonia   • Renal or liver failure
• Hemorrhage   • ARDS (p174); DIC (p577)
• Drugs (heroin, cytotoxics)   • Head injury, or after neurosurgery
• Smoke inhalation (p741)   • Alveolar proteinosis
• O_2 toxicity   • Near-drowning
• Fat emboli, ~7d post-fracture • Heat stroke (p686).

'Ring' shadows: Either airways seen end-on (pulmonary edema, bronchiectasis), or cavitating lesions, eg abscess (bacterial, fungal, amoebic), tumor, or pulmonary infarct (triangular with a pleural base).

Linear opacities: Septal lines (Kerley's B lines, ie interlobular lymphatics seen with fluid, tumor, or dusts). Atelectasis.

Apparently normal CXR Check for apical pneumothorax, tracheal compression, absent breast shadow (mastectomy), rib pathology (fractures, metastases, or notching), air under diaphragm (perforated viscus), double left heart border (left lower lobe collapse), fluid level behind the heart (hiatus hernia, achalasia), and paravertebral abscess (TB).

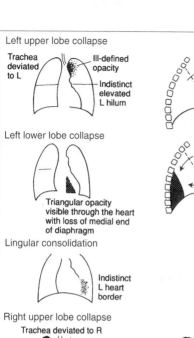
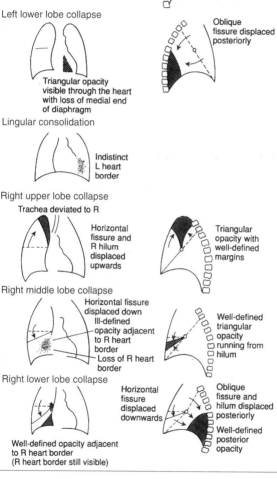

Left upper lobe collapse

Trachea deviated to L — Ill-defined opacity — Indistinct elevated L hilum

Sharply defined posterior border due to anterior displacement of oblique fissure

Left lower lobe collapse

Triangular opacity visible through the heart with loss of medial end of diaphragm

Oblique fissure displaced posteriorly

Lingular consolidation

Indistinct L heart border

Right upper lobe collapse

Trachea deviated to R

Horizontal fissure and R hilum displaced upwards

Triangular opacity with well-defined margins

Right middle lobe collapse

Horizontal fissure displaced down
Ill-defined opacity adjacent to R heart border
Loss of R heart border

Well-defined triangular opacity running from hilum

Right lower lobe collapse

Horizontal fissure displaced downwards

Oblique fissure and hilum displaced posteriorly

Well-defined posterior opacity

Well-defined opacity adjacent to R heart border (R heart border still visible)

Bedside tests in chest medicine

Sputum examination Collect a good sample; if necessary ask a respiratory therapist to help. Note the appearance: Clear and colorless (chronic bronchitis), yellow/green (pulmonary infection), red (hemoptysis), black (smoke, coal), or frothy white/pink (pulmonary edema). Send the sample to the laboratory for microscopy (stain for bacteria, fungi and mycobacteria, if indicated), culture, and cytology.

Peak expiratory flow (PEF) is measured by a maximal forced expiration through a peak flow meter. It correlates well with the forced expiratory volume in 1 second (FEV_1) and is used as an estimate of airway caliber. Peak flow rates should be measured regularly in asthmatics to monitor response to therapy and disease control.

Pulse oximetry allows non-invasive assessment of peripheral O_2 saturation. It provides a useful tool for monitoring those who are acutely ill or at risk of deterioration. On most pulse oximeters, the alarm is set at 90%. An oxygen saturation of ≤80% is clearly abnormal and action is required (unless this is normal for the patient, eg in COPD. Here, check arterial blood gases (ABG) as P_aCO_2 may be rising despite a normal P_aO_2). Erroneous readings may be caused by: Poor perfusion, motion, excess light, skin pigmentation, nail varnish, dyshemoglobinemias, and carbon monoxide poisoning. As with any bedside test, be skeptical, and check ABG, whenever indicated (p177).

Arterial blood gas (ABG) analysis Heparinized blood is taken from the radial, brachial, or femoral artery, and pH, P_aO_2, and P_aCO_2 are measured using an automated analyzer. Remember to note the FiO_2 (fraction or percentage of inspired oxygen).

- *Acid–base balance:* Normal pH is 7.35–7.45. A pH <7.35 indicates *acidosis* and a pH >7.45 indicates *alkalosis*.
- *Oxygenation:* Normal P_aO_2 is 80–100mmHg. Hypoxia is caused by one or more of the following reasons: Ventilation/perfusion ($\dot{V}/\dot{Q}$) mismatch, hypoventilation, abnormal diffusion, right to left cardiac shunts. Of these, $\dot{V}/\dot{Q}$ mismatch is the commonest cause. Severe hypoxia is defined as a P_aO_2 <60mmHg.
- *Ventilatory efficiency:* Normal P_aCO_2 is 35–45mmHg. P_aCO_2 is directly related to alveolar ventilation. A P_aCO_2 <35mmHg indicates *hyperventilation* and a P_aCO_2 >45mmHg indicates *hypoventilation*. Type I respiratory failure is defined as P_aO_2 <60mmHg and P_aCO_2 <45mmHg, whereas Type II respiratory failure is defined as P_aO_2 <60mmHg and P_aCO_2 >45mmHg.

Alveolar–arterial O_2 concentration gradient may be calculated from the FiO_2, P_aO_2, and P_aCO_2: See OPPOSITE.

Spirometry measures functional lung volumes. FEV_1 and forced vital capacity (FVC) are measured from a full forced expiration into spirometer; exhalation continues until no more breath can be exhaled. FEV_1 is less effort-dependent than PEF. The FEV_1/FVC ratio gives a good estimate of severity of airflow obstruction; normal ratio is 75–80%.

- *Obstructive defect* (eg asthma, COPD) FEV_1 is reduced more than the FVC and the FEV_1/FVC ratio is <70%.
- *Restrictive defect* (eg lung fibrosis) FVC is reduced and the FEV_1/FVC ratio is normal or raised. Other causes: Sarcoidosis; pneumoconiosis, interstitial pneumonias; connective tissue diseases; pleural effusion; obesity; kyphoscoliosis; neuromuscular problems.

(Aa)PO₂: The Alveolar-arterial (Aa) oxygen gradient

This is the difference in the O_2 partial pressures between the alveolar and arterial sides. In type II respiratory failure it helps tell if hypoventilation is from lung disease or poor respiratory effort.

(Aa)PO₂ = $P_AO_2 - P_aO_2$. How do we find P_AO_2, the partial pressure of oxygen in the alveoli? Respiratory physiology teaches that this depends on **R**, the respiratory quotient (≈0.8, nearer to 1 if eating all carbohydrates); barometric pressure (**P_B** ≈ 760mmHg at sea level); and **P_{H₂O}**, the water saturation of airway gas ($P_{H₂O}$ ≈ 47mmHg as inspired air is usually fully saturated by the time it gets to the carina). P_AO_2 clearly depends on F_iO_2, the fractional concentration of O_2 in inspired air eg F_iO_2 is 0.5 if breathing 50% O_2, and 0.21 if breathing room air). So...

$$P_AO_2 = (P_B - P_{H₂O}) \times F_iO_2 - P_aCO_2/R$$
$$= (760 - 47) \times F_iO_2 - P_aCO_2/0.8 \text{ (at sea level)}$$
$$= 713 \times F_iO_2 - 1.25 \times P_aCO_2$$

Breathing air and having a P_aCO_2 of 60mmHg
In this case, P_AO_2 = 713 × 0.21 − (1.25 × 60) = 75mmHg. *Aa normal ranges breathing air*: 2–12mmHg at 25yrs old; ↑ with age to 12–25 at 75yrs.
Examples of expected Aa gradients: 50 at an F_iO_2 of 0.5 ($P_AO_2 - P_aO_2$ = 335 − 285 = 50) and 120 for an F_iO_2 of 1.0 ($P_AO_2 - P_aO_2$ = 668 − 548 = 120).

Normal peak expiratory flow (PEF)

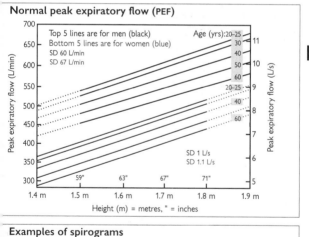

Examples of spirograms

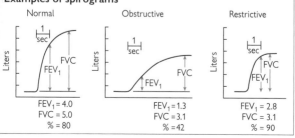

Normal	Obstructive	Restrictive
FEV₁ = 4.0	FEV₁ = 1.3	FEV₁ = 2.8
FVC = 5.0	FVC = 3.1	FVC = 3.1
% = 80	% = 42	% = 90

Further investigations in chest medicine

Lung function tests PEF, FEV$_1$, FVC (p154). *Total lung capacity* (TLC) and *residual volume* (RV) are useful in distinguishing obstructive and restrictive diseases. TLC and RV are ↑ in obstructive airways disease and reduced in restrictive lung diseases and musculoskeletal abnormalities. The *diffusing capacity* (DLCO) across alveoli is calculated by measuring carbon monoxide uptake from a single inspiration in a standard time (usually 10s). Low in emphysema and interstitial lung disease, high in alveolar hemorrhage. DLCO can be corrected for alveolar volume in appropriate circumstances[1]. *Flow volume loop* measures flow at various lung volumes. Characteristic patterns are seen with intrathoracic airways obstruction (asthma, emphysema) and extrathoracic airways obstruction (vocal cord paralysis).

Radiology *Chest x-ray* (p152). *Ultrasound* is used in the diagnosis and drainage of pleural effusions (particularly loculated effusions) and empyema. *Radionuclide scans Ventilation/perfusion* ($\dot{V}/\dot{Q}$) *scans* are used to diagnose pulmonary embolism (PE) (unmatched perfusion defects are seen). *Bone scans* are used to diagnose bone metastases. *Computer tomography* (CT) of the thorax is used for diagnosing and staging lung ca, imaging the hila, mediastinum and pleura, and guiding biopsies. Thin (1–1.5mm) section high resolution CT (HRCT) is used in the diagnosis of interstitial lung disease and bronchiectasis. *Spiral CT pulmonary angiography* (CTPA) is used increasingly in the diagnosis of PE. *Pulmonary angiography* is also used for diagnosing PE and pulmonary hypertension.

Fiberoptic bronchoscopy is performed under local anesthetic via the nose or mouth. *Diagnostic indications:* Suspected lung malignancy, slowly resolving pneumonia, pneumonia in the immunosuppressed, interstitial lung disease. Bronchial lavage fluid may be sent to the lab for microscopy, culture, and cytology. Mucosal abnormalities may be brushed (cytology) and biopsied (histopathology). *Therapeutic indications:* Aspiration of mucus plugs causing lobar collapse or removal of foreign bodies. *Pre-procedure investigations:* CBC, CXR, spirometry, pulse oximetry and arterial blood gases (if indicated). Check clotting if recent anticoagulation and a biopsy may be performed. *Complications:* Respiratory depression, bleeding, pneumothorax (X-RAY PLATE 6).

Bronchoalveolar lavage (BAL) is performed at the time of bronchoscopy by instilling and aspirating a known volume of warmed, buffered 0.9% saline into the distal airway. *Diagnostic indications:* Suspected malignancy, pneumonia in the immunosuppressed (especially HIV), suspected TB (if sputum negative), interstitial lung diseases (eg sarcoidosis, extrinsic allergic alveolitis, histocytosis X). *Therapeutic indications:* Alveolar proteinosis. *Complications:* Hypoxia (give supplemental O$_2$), transient fever, transient CXR shadow, infection (rare).

Lung biopsy may be performed in several ways. *Percutaneous needle biopsy* is performed under radiological guidance and is useful for peripheral lung and pleural lesions. *Transbronchial biopsy* performed at bronchoscopy may help in diagnosing diffuse lung diseases, eg sarcoidosis. If these are unsuccessful, an *open lung biopsy* may be performed under general anesthetic.

Surgical procedures are performed under general anesthetic. *Rigid bronchoscopy* provides a wide lumen, enables larger mucosal biopsies, controlling bleeding, and removal of foreign bodies. *Mediastinoscopy and mediastinotomy* enable examination and biopsy of the mediastinal lymph nodes/lesions. *Thoracoscopy* allows examination and biopsy of pleural lesions, drainage of pleural effusions, and talc pleurodesis.

1 D Johnson 2000 *Respir Med* **94** 28–37.

Lung volumes: Physiological and pathological

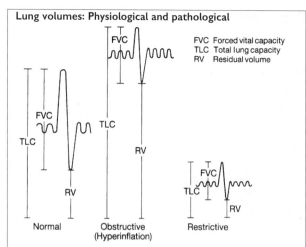

FVC   Forced vital capacity
TLC   Total lung capacity
RV   Residual volume

Normal

Obstructive
(Hyperinflation)

Restrictive

Flow volume loops

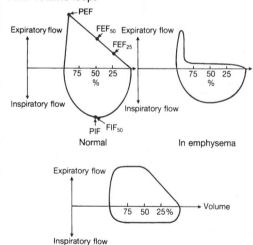

PEF = peak expiratory flow; FEF$_{50}$ = forced expiratory flow at 50% TLC; FEF$_{25}$ = forced expiratory flow at 25% TLC; PIF = peak inspiratory flow; FIF$_{50}$ = forced inspiratory flow at 50% TLC.

Pneumonia

An acute lower respiratory tract illness associated with fever, symptoms and signs in the chest, and abnormalities on the chest x-ray. Incidence: 1–3/1000 population. Mortality: 10% (patients admitted to the hospital).

Classification and causes

1 *Community-acquired* pneumonia (CAP) may be 1° or 2° to underlying disease. *Streptococcus pneumoniae* is the commonest cause, followed by *Haemophilus influenzae* and *Mycoplasma pneumoniae*. *Staphylococcus aureus, Legionella species, Moraxella catarrhalis,* and *Chlamydia* account for most of the remainder. Gram negative bacilli, *Coxiella burnetii* and anaerobes are rare. Viruses account for up to 15%.

2 *Hospital acquired (Nosocomial)* (>48h after hospital admission). Most commonly Gram negative enterobacteria or *Staph. aureus*. Also *Pseudomonas, Klebsiella, Bacteroides,* and *Clostridia.*

3 *Aspiration* Those with stroke, myasthenia, bulbar palsies, ↓consciousness (eg post-ictal or drunk), esophageal disease (achalasia, reflux), or with poor dental hygiene, risk aspirating oropharyngeal anaerobes.

4 *Immunocompromised patient* Strep. pneumoniae, H. influenzae, Staph. aureus, M. catarrhalis, M. pneumoniae, Gram –ve bacilli and *Pneumocystis jiroveci*. Other fungi, viruses (CMV, HSV), and mycobacteria.

Clinical features *Symptoms:* Fever, rigors, malaise, anorexia, dyspnea, cough, purulent sputum, hemoptysis, and pleuritic chest pain. *Signs:* Fever, cyanosis, confusion (may be the only sign in the elderly), tachypnea, tachycardia, hypotension, signs of consolidation (diminished expansion, dull percussion note, ↑ tactile vocal fremitus/vocal resonance, bronchial breathing), and a pleural rub.

Tests aim to establish diagnosis, identify pathogen, and assess severity (see below). *CXR* (X-RAY PLATES 5 & 8): Lobar or multilobar infiltrates, cavitation or pleural effusion. *Assess oxygenation:* Oxygen saturation (ABGs if S_aO_2 <92% or severe pneumonia). *Blood tests:* CBC, electrolytes, LFT, CRP, blood cultures. *Sputum* for microscopy and culture. In severe cases, check for Legionella (sputum culture, urine antigen), atypical organism/viral serology (complement fixation tests acutely and paired serology) and some centers may check for pneumococcal antigen in urine, sputum, or blood. *Pleural fluid* may be aspirated for culture. Consider *bronchoscopy* and bronchoalveolar lavage if patient is immunocompromised or in the ICU.

Management (p708) *Antibiotics* (p159), orally if not severe and not vomiting. *Oxygen* keep P_aO_2 >60 and/or saturation ≥92%. *IV fluids* (anorexia, dehydration, shock). *Analgesia* if pleurisy—eg acetaminophen 1g/6h. If severe pneumonia should have IV antibiotics and consider ICU if failure to improve quickly, shock, hypercapnia, or uncorrected hypoxia.

Complications (p161) Pleural effusion, empyema, lung abscess, respiratory failure, septicemia, brain abscess, pericarditis, myocarditis, cholestatic jaundice. Repeat CRP and CXR in patients not progressing satisfactorily.

Preventing pneumococcal infection Offer pneumococcal vaccine (23-valent Pneumovax II® 0.5mL SC) to those with: • Chronic heart or lung conditions • Cirrhosis • Nephrosis • Diabetes mellitus • Immunosuppression (eg splenectomy, AIDS, or on chemotherapy). CI: Pregnancy, lactation, fever. If high risk of fatal pneumococcal infection (asplenia, sickle-cell disease, nephrosis, post-transplant), revaccinate after 5yrs (3–5yrs in children >2yrs old), unless they had a severe vaccine reaction.

Empirical treatment of pneumonia

Clinical setting	Organisms	Antibiotic
Community acquired		
Mild not previously ℞	*Streptococcus pneumoniae* *Haemophilus influenzae*	Amoxicillin 500mg–1.0g/8h or erythromycin[1] 500mg/6h PO
Mild	*Streptococcus pneumoniae* *Haemophilus influenzae* *Mycoplasma pneumoniae*	Amoxicillin 500mg–1.0g/8h PO + erythromycin[1] 500mg/6h PO or fluoroquinolone if IV required: ampicillin 500mg/6h + erythromycin[1] 500mg/6h IV
Severe	As above	Cephalosporin IV (eg cefotaxime 2g/6h IV) AND erythromycin[1] 1g/6h IV
Atypical	*Legionella pneumophilia*	Clarithromycin 500mg/12h PO/IV ± rifampin
	Chlamydia species	Tetracycline
	Pneumocystis jiroveci	High-dose co-trimoxazole (p521)
Hospital acquired		
	Gram negative bacilli Pseudomonas Anaerobes	Aminoglycoside IV + antipseudomonal penicillin IV or 3rd gen. cephalosporin IV (p494)
Aspiration		
	Streptococcus pneumoniae Anaerobes	3rd gen. cephalosporin IV + clindamycin 600mg/6h IV
Neutropenic patients		
	Gram positive cocci Gram negative bacilli	Aminoglycoside IV + antipseudomonal penicillin IV or 3rd gen. cephalosporin IV
	Fungi (p164)	Consider antifungals after 48h

3rd gen = 3rd generation, eg cefotaxime, p494; gentamicin is an example of an aminoglycoside (p496).

159

[1] Clarithromycin 500mg bid PO/IV or azithromycin 500mg qd PO/IV may be used in place of erythromycin throughout these recommendations.

Specific pneumonias

Pneumococcal pneumonia is the commonest bacterial pneumonia. It affects all ages, but is commoner in the elderly, alcoholics, post-splenectomy, immuno-suppressed, and patients with chronic heart failure or pre-existing lung disease. Clinical features: Fever, pleurisy, herpes labialis. CXR shows lobar consolidation. Treatment: Amoxicillin or cephalosporin.

Staphylococcal pneumonia may complicate influenza infection or occur in the young, elderly, IV drug users, or patients with underlying disease (eg leukemia, lymphoma, cystic fibrosis (CF)). It causes a bilateral cavitating bronchopneu-monia. Treatment: Oxacillin (vancomycin if methicillin-resistant strain).

Klebsiella pneumonia occurs in the elderly and causes a cavitating pneumonia, particularly of the upper lobes. Treatment: Cefuroxime.

Pseudomonas is a common pathogen in bronchiectasis and CF. It also causes hospital acquired infections, particularly in the ICU or after surgery. Treat-ment: Anti-pseudomonal penicillin, ceftazidime, meropenem, or ciprofloxacin.

Mycoplasma pneumoniae occurs in epidemics about every 4yrs. It presents insidiously with flu-like symptoms (headache, myalgia, arthralgia) followed by a dry cough. CXR shows bilateral patchy consolidation. Diagnosis: Myco-plasma serology. Cold agglutinins may cause an autoimmune hemolytic anemia. Complications: Skin rash (erythema multiforme (PLATE 17), Stevens–Johnson syndrome), meningoencephalitis or myelitis; Guillain–Barré syn-drome. Treatment: Macrolide or tetracycline.

Legionella pneumophilia colonizes water tanks kept at <60°C (eg hotel air-conditioning and hot water systems) causing outbreaks of Legionnaire's disease. Flu-like symptoms (fever, malaise, myalgia) precede a dry cough and dyspnea. Extra-pulmonary features include anorexia, diarrhea, vomiting, hepatitis, renal failure, confusion, and coma. CXR shows bi-basal consolida-tion. Blood tests may show lymphopenia, hyponatremia, and deranged LFTs. Urinalysis may show hematuria. Diagnosis: Legionella serology/urine antigen. Treatment: Macrolide ± rifampin, or fluoroquinolone. 10% mortality.

Chlamydia pneumoniae is the commonest chlamydial infection. Person-to-person spread occurs, causing a biphasic illness: Pharyngitis, hoarseness, otitis, followed by pneumonia. Diagnosis: *Chlamydia* serology (non-specific). Treatment: Tetracycline.

Chlamydia psittaci causes psittacosis, an ornithosis acquired from infected birds (typically parrots). Symptoms include headache, fever, dry cough, leth-argy, arthralgia, anorexia, and diarrhea. Extra-pulmonary features are legion but rare, eg meningoencephalitis, infective endocarditis, hepatitis, nephritis, rash, splenomegaly. CXR shows patchy consolidation. Diagnosis: *Chlamydia* serology. Treatment: Tetracycline.

Viral pneumonia The commonest cause is influenza. Other viruses that can affect the lung are: Measles, CMV, and varicella zoster.

Pneumocystis jiroveci pneumonia This causes pneumonia in the immunosup-pressed (eg HIV). It presents with a dry cough, exertional dyspnea, fever, bilateral crepitations. CXR may be normal or show bilateral perihilar intersti-tial shadowing. Diagnosis: Visualization of the organism in induced sputum, bronchoalveolar lavage, or in a lung biopsy specimen. Treatment: High-dose co-trimoxazole, or pentamidine by slow IVI for 2–3wks (p521). Steroids are beneficial if severe hypoxemia. Prophylaxis is indicated if the CD4 count is <200 × 10^6/L or after the 1st attack.

Complications of pneumonia

Respiratory failure (p176) Type I respiratory failure (P_aO_2 <60mmHg) is relatively common. Treatment is with high-flow (60%) oxygen. *Transfer the patient to ICU if hypoxia does not improve with O_2 therapy or P_aCO_2 rises to >45mmHg.* Careful O_2 administration is required in COPD patients; check arterial blood gases frequently and consider elective mechanical ventilation if rising P_aCO_2 or worsening acidosis. Aim to keep SaO_2 at 90–94%.

Hypotension may be due to a combination of dehydration and vasodilatation due to sepsis. If systolic BP is <90mmHg, give an IV fluid challenge of 250mL colloid/crystalloid over 15min. If BP does not rise, insert a central line and give IV fluids to maintain the systolic BP >90mmHg. If systolic BP remains <90mmHg despite fluid therapy, request ICU assessment for inotropic support (phenylephrine, norepinephrine) .

Atrial fibrillation (p120) is quite common, particularly in the elderly. It usually resolves with treatment of the pneumonia. Digoxin may be required to slow the ventricular response rate in the short term.

Pleural effusion Inflammation of the pleura by adjacent pneumonia may cause fluid exudation into the pleural space. If this accumulates in the pleural space faster than it is reabsorbed, a pleural effusion develops. If this is small it may be of no consequence. If it becomes large and symptomatic, or infected (empyema), drainage is required (p180, p661).

Empyema is pus in the pleural space. It should be suspected if a patient with a resolving pneumonia develops a recurrent fever. Clinical features and the CXR indicate a pleural effusion. The aspirated pleural fluid is typically yellow and turbid with a pH <7.2, glucose↓, and LDH↑. The empyema should be drained using a chest drain, preferably inserted under radiological guidance. Although intrapleural streptokinase (250,000U in 50mL 0.9% saline/12h for 3d) has been used to break down the adhesions the latest data indicate no benefit.

Lung abscess is a cavitating area of localized, suppurative infection within the lung.

Causes: • Inadequately treated pneumonia • Aspiration (eg alcoholism, esophageal obstruction, bulbar palsy) • Bronchial obstruction (tumor, foreign body) • Pulmonary infarction • Septic emboli (septicemia, right heart endocarditis, IV drug use) • Subphrenic or hepatic abscess.

Clinical features: Swinging fever; cough; purulent, foul-smelling sputum; pleuritic chest pain; hemoptysis; malaise; weight loss. Look for: Finger clubbing; anemia; crepitations. Empyema develops in 20–30%.

Tests: Blood: CBC (anemia, neutrophilia), ESR, CRP, blood cultures. *Sputum:* Microscopy, culture, and cytology. *CXR:* Walled cavity, often with a fluid level. Consider CT scan to exclude obstruction, and bronchoscopy to obtain diagnostic specimens.

Treatment: Antibiotics as indicated by sensitivities; continue until healed (4–6 wks). Postural drainage. Repeated aspiration, antibiotic instillation, or surgical excision may be required.

Septicemia may occur as a result of bacterial spread from the lung parenchyma into the bloodstream. This may cause metastatic infection, eg infective endocarditis, meningitis. Treatment is with IV antibiotic according to sensitivities.

Pericarditis and myocarditis may also complicate pneumonia.

Jaundice This is usually cholestatic, and may be due to sepsis or 2° to antibiotic therapy (particularly penicillin derivatives).

Cystic fibrosis (CF)

One of the commonest life-threatening autosomal recessive conditions (1:2000 live births) affecting Caucasians. Other races also are affected. Caused by mutations in the CF transmembrane conductance regulator (CFTR) gene on chromosome 7 (>800 mutations have now been identified). This leads to a combination of defective chloride secretion and ↑ sodium absorption across airway epithelium. The changes in the composition of airway surface liquid predisposes the lung to chronic pulmonary infections and bronchiectasis.

Clinical features *Neonate:* Failure to thrive; meconium ileus; rectal prolapse. *Children and young adults: Respiratory:* Cough; wheeze; recurrent infections; bronchiectasis; pneumothorax; hemoptysis; respiratory failure; cor pulmonale. *Gastrointestinal:* Pancreatic insufficiency (diabetes mellitus, steatorrhea); distal intestinal obstruction syndrome (meconium ileus equivalent); gallstones; cirrhosis. *Other:* Male infertility; osteoporosis; arthritis; vasculitis; nasal polyps; sinusitis; and hypertrophic pulmonary osteoarthropathy (HPOA). *Signs:* Cyanosis; finger clubbing; bilateral coarse crackles.

Diagnosis *Sweat test:* Sweat sodium and chloride >60mmol/L; chloride usually >sodium. *Genetics:* Screening for known common CF mutations should be considered. *Fecal elastase* is a simple and useful screening test for exocrine pancreatic dysfunction.

Tests *Blood:* CBC, electrolytes, LFTs; clotting; vitamin A, D, E levels; annual glucose tolerance test. *Bacteriology:* Cough swab, sputum culture. *Radiology: CXR:* Hyperinflation; bronchiectasis. *Abdominal ultrasound:* Fatty liver; cirrhosis; chronic pancreatitis; *Spirometry:* Obstructive defect. *Aspergillus serology/ skin test* (20% develop ABPA, p164). *Biochemistry:* Fecal fat analysis.

Management

Patients with CF are best managed by a multidisciplinary team including physician, physiotherapist, specialist nurse, and dietitian with attention to psychosocial as well as physical well-being. Gene therapy (transfer of CFTR gene using liposome or adenovirus vectors) is not yet possible.

Chest Physiotherapy regularly (postural drainage, active cycle techniques, or forced expiratory techniques); Antibiotics are given for acute infective exacerbations (PO for *Staph. aureus*, IV for *P. aeruginosa*) and prophylactically PO (flucloxacillin) or nebulized (colistin or tobramycin); mucolytics may be useful (eg DNase 2.5mg daily nebulized); bronchodilators.

Gastrointestinal Pancreatic enzyme replacement; fat soluble vitamin supplements (A, D, E, K); ursodeoxycholic acid for impaired liver function; cirrhosis may require liver transplantation.

Other Treatment of CF-related diabetes; screening for and treatment of osteoporosis; treatment of arthritis, sinusitis, and vasculitis; fertility and genetic counseling.

Advanced lung disease Oxygen, diuretics (cor pulmonale); non-invasive ventilation; lung or heart/lung transplantation.

Prognosis Median survival is now over 30yrs.

Bronchiectasis

Pathology Chronic infection of the bronchi and bronchioles leading to permanent dilatation of these airways. Main organisms: *H. influenzae*; *Strep. pneumoniae*; *Staph. aureus*; *Pseudomonas aeruginosa*.

Causes *Congenital:* CF; Young's syndrome; primary ciliary dyskinesia; Kartagener's syndrome. *Post-infection:* Measles; pertussis; bronchiolitis; pneumonia; TB; HIV. *Other:* Bronchial obstruction (tumor, foreign body); allergic bronchopulmonary aspergillosis (ABPA p164); hypogammaglobulinemia; rheumatoid arthritis; ulcerative colitis; idiopathic.

Clinical features *Symptoms:* Persistent cough; copious purulent sputum; intermittent hemoptysis. *Signs:* Finger clubbing; coarse inspiratory crepitations, wheeze (asthma, COPD, ABPA). *Complications:* Pneumonia, pleural effusion; pneumothorax; hemoptysis; cerebral abscess; amyloidosis.

Investigations *Sputum* culture. *CXR:* Cystic shadows, thickened bronchial walls (tram-tracking and ring shadows). *HRCT chest:* To assess extent and distribution of disease. *Spirometry* often shows an obstructive pattern; reversibility should be assessed. *Bronchoscopy* to locate site of hemoptysis or exclude obstruction. *Other tests:* Serum immunoglobulins; CF sweat chloride test; *Aspergillus* precipitins or skin-prick test.

Management *Postural drainage* should be performed twice daily. Chest physiotherapy may aid sputum expectoration and mucous drainage. *Antibiotics* should be prescribed according to bacterial sensitivities. Patients known to culture *Pseudomonas* will require either oral ciprofloxacin or IV antibiotics. *Bronchodilators* (eg nebulized albuterol) may be useful in patients with asthma, COPD, CF, ABPA. *Corticosteroids* (eg prednisone) for ABPA. *Surgery* may be indicated in localized disease or to control severe hemoptysis.

Fungi and the lung

Aspergillus This group of fungi affects the lung in 5 ways:

1 *Asthma:* Type I hypersensitivity (atopic) reaction to fungal spores, p168.

2 *Allergic bronchopulmonary aspergillosis (ABPA):* This results from a Type I and III hypersensitivity reaction to *Aspergillus fumigatus*. Early on, the allergic response causes bronchoconstriction, but as the inflammation persists, permanent damage occurs, causing bronchiectasis. *Symptoms:* Wheeze, cough, sputum (plugs of mucus containing fungal hyphae), dyspnea, and 'recurrent pneumonia'. *Investigations:* CXR (transient segmental collapse or consolidation, bronchiectasis); *Aspergillus* in sputum; positive aspergillus skin test and/or aspergillus-specific IgE RAST; positive serum precipitins; eosinophilia; raised serum IgE. *Treatment:* Prednisone 30–40mg/24h PO for acute attacks; maintenance dose 5–10mg/d. Sometimes itraconazole is used in combination with corticosteroids. Bronchodilators for asthma. Sometimes bronchoscopic aspiration of mucous plugs is needed.

3 *Aspergilloma (mycetoma):* A fungus ball within a pre-existing cavity (often caused by TB, sarcoidosis). It is usually asymptomatic but may cause cough, hemoptysis, lethargy ± weight loss. *Investigations:* CXR (round opacity within a cavity, usually apical); sputum culture; strongly positive serum precipitins; *Aspergillus* skin test (30% +ve). *Treatment* (only if symptomatic): Consider surgical excision for solitary symptomatic lesions or severe hemoptysis. Oral itraconazole and other antifungals have been tried with limited success. Local instillation of amphotericin paste under CT-guidance yields partial success in carefully selected patients, eg in massive hemoptysis.

4 *Invasive aspergillosis: Risk factors:* Immunocompromised, eg HIV, leukemia, burns, Wegener's, and SLE, or after broad-spectrum antibiotic therapy. *Investigations:* Sputum culture; serum precipitins; CXR (consolidation, abscess). Early chest CT and serial serum measurements of galactogamman (an *Aspergillus* antigen) can be very helpful. Diagnosis may only be made at lung biopsy or autopsy. *Treatment:* IV amphotericin B (see below). Alternatives: IV voriconazole or itraconazole. *Prognosis:* Very poor.

5 *Extrinsic allergic alveolitis (EAA)* is caused by sensitivity to *Aspergillus clavatus* ('malt worker's lung'). Clinical features and treatment are as for other causes of EAA (p184). Diagnosis is based on a history of exposure and the presence of serum precipitins to *A. clavatus*. Pulmonary fibrosis may occur if untreated.

Using amphotericin B test dose: 1mg in 20mL 5% dextrose IV over 20–30min. There are many different preparations. Consult your pharmacist. *Do not give any other drug in the same IVI.* SE: Anaphylaxis; fever; rash; anorexia; nausea; diarrhea; headache; myalgia; arthralgia; anemia; ↓K⁺; ↓Mg²⁺; nephrotoxicity; hepatotoxicity; arrhythmias; hearing loss; diplopia; seizures; peripheral neuropathy; phlebitis. *Monitor* electrolytes *daily*. Ambisome® (liposomal amphotericin) has fewer SEs, but is expensive; it is indicated in systemic or deep mycoses where nephrotoxicity precludes conventional amphotericin; IV initial test dose: 1mg over 10min, then 1mg/kg/d, as a single IVI dose; gradually ↑ if needed to 3–5mg/kg/d. Alternatives: Abelcet® & Amphotec®.

Other fungal infections *Candida* and *Cryptococcus* may cause pneumonia in the immunosuppressed (p548).

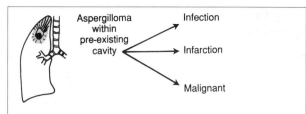

Aspergilloma within pre-existing cavity

Infection

Infarction

Malignant

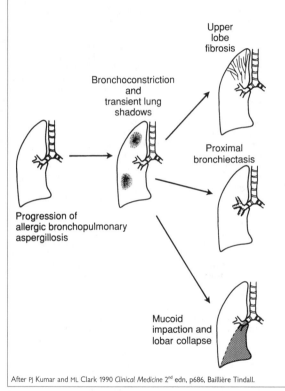

Bronchoconstriction and transient lung shadows

Upper lobe fibrosis

Proximal bronchiectasis

Progression of allergic bronchopulmonary aspergillosis

Mucoid impaction and lobar collapse

After PJ Kumar and ML Clark 1990 *Clinical Medicine* 2nd edn, p686, Baillière Tindall.

Lung tumors

Carcinoma of the bronchus Accounts for ≈19% of all cancers and 27% of cancer deaths (≈170,000 new cases/yr in the US). Incidence is ↑ in women.

Risk factors: Cigarette smoking is the major risk factor. Others: Asbestos, chromium, arsenic, iron oxides, and radiation (radon gas).

Histology: Squamous (30%); adenocarcinoma (30%); small (oat) cell (25%); large cell (15%); alveolar cell carcinoma (rare, <1%).

Symptoms: Cough (80%); hemoptysis (70%); dyspnea (60%); chest pain (40%); recurrent or slowly resolving pneumonia; anorexia; weight loss.

Signs: Cachexia; anemia; clubbing; HPOA (hypertrophic pulmonary osteoarthropathy, causing wrist pain); supraclavicular or axillary lymphadenopathy. *Chest signs:* May be none; consolidation; collapse; pleural effusion. *Metastases:* Bone tenderness; hepatomegaly; confusion; seizures; myopathy; peripheral neuropathy.

Complications: Local: Recurrent laryngeal nerve palsy; phrenic nerve palsy; SVC obstruction; Horner's syndrome (Pancoast's tumor); rib erosion; pericarditis; AF. *Metastatic:* Brain; bone (bone pain, anemia, ↑Ca^{2+}); liver (hepatomegaly); adrenals (Addison's). *Endocrine:* Ectopic hormone secretion, eg SIADH (↓Na^+ and ↑ADH) and ACTH (Cushing's) by small cell tumors; PTH (↑Ca^{2+}) by squamous cell tumors. *Non-metastatic neurological:* Confusion; seizures; cerebellar syndrome; proximal myopathy; peripheral neuropathy; polymyositis; Eaton–Lambert syndrome (p356). *Other:* Finger clubbing; HPOA; dermatomyositis; acanthosis nigricans; thrombophlebitis migrans.

Tests: Cytology: Sputum & pleural fluid. *CXR:* Peripheral circular opacity; hilar enlargement; consolidation; lung collapse (X-RAY PLATE 4); pleural effusion; bony metastases. Peripheral lesions and superficial lymph nodes may be amenable to *percutaneous fine needle aspiration/biopsy. Bronchoscopy:* To give histological diagnosis and assess operability. *CT:* To stage the tumor (OPPOSITE). *Radionuclide bone scan:* For suspected metastases. *Lung function tests.*

Treatment: Non-small cell tumors: Excision is the treatment of choice for peripheral tumors, with no metastatic spread (~25%). *Curative radiotherapy* is an alternative in patients with inadequate respiratory reserve. *Small cell tumors* are almost always disseminated at presentation. They may respond to *chemotherapy* with a combination of cyclophosphamide, doxorubicin, vincristine, etoposide, or cisplatin. *Palliation:* Radiotherapy is used for bronchial obstruction, SVC obstruction, hemoptysis, bone pain, and cerebral metastases. SVC stent + radiotherapy/dexamethasone for SVC obstruction. *Endobronchial therapy* includes tracheal stenting, cryotherapy, laser therapy, and brachytherapy (a radioactive source is placed close to the tumor). *Pleural drainage/pleurodesis* for symptomatic pleural effusions. *Drug therapy:* Analgesia; corticosteroids; antiemetics; codeine; bronchodilators; antidepressants.

Prognosis: Non-small cell: 50% 2yr survival without spread; 10% with spread. *Small cell:* Median survival is 3 months if untreated; 1–1½yrs if treated.

Prevention: Actively discourage smoking. Prevent occupational exposure to carcinogens.

Other lung tumors *Bronchial adenoma:* Rare, slow-growing tumor. 90% are carcinoid tumors; 10% are cylindromas. Treatment: Surgery. *Hamartoma:* Rare, benign tumor. CT scan: Lobulated mass with flecks of calcification. Often excised to exclude malignancy. *Mesothelioma* (p186).

Coin lesions of the lung

- Malignancy (1° or 2°)
- Abscess
- Granuloma
- Carcinoid tumor
- Pulmonary hamartoma
- Arteriovenous malformation
- Encysted effusion (fluid, blood, pus)
- Cyst
- Foreign body
- Skin tumor (eg seborrheic wart)

TNM staging for lung cancer

Primary tumor (T)	TX	Malignant cells in bronchial secretions, no other evidence of tumor	
	Tis	Carcinoma *in situ*	
	T0	None evident	
	T1	≤3cm, in lobar or more distal airway	
	T2	>3cm and >2cm distal to carina *or* any size if pleural involvement *or* obstructive pneumonitis extending to hilum, but not all the lung	
	T3	Involves the chest wall, diaphragm, mediastinal pleura, pericardium, or <2cm from, but not at, carina	
	T4	Involves the mediastinum, heart, great vessels, trachea, esophagus, vertebral body, carina, *or* a malignant effusion is present	
Regional nodes (N)	N0	None involved (after mediastinoscopy)	
	N1	Peribronchial and/or ipsilateral hilum	
	N2	Ipsilateral mediastinum or subcarinal	
	N3	Contralateral mediastinum or hilum, scalene, or supraclavicular	
Distant metastasis (M)	M0	None	
	M1	Distant metastases present	

Stage	*Tumor*	*Lymph nodes*	*Metastasis*
Occult	TX	N0	M0
I	Tis, T1, or T2	N0	M0
II	T1 or T2	N1	M0
	T3	N0	M0
IIIa	T3	N1	M0
	T1–T3	N2	M0
IIIb	T1–T4	N3	M0
	T4	N0–N2	M0
IV	T1–T4	N0–N3	M1

Asthma

Asthma affects 5–8% of the population. It is characterized by recurrent episodes of dyspnea, cough, and wheeze caused by reversible airways obstruction. Three factors contribute to airway narrowing: *Bronchial muscle contraction*, triggered by a variety of stimuli; *mucosal swelling/inflammation*, caused by mast cell and basophil degranulation resulting in the release of inflammatory mediators; ↑ *mucus production*.

Symptoms Intermittent dyspnea, wheeze, cough (often nocturnal) and sputum. Ask specifically about:
- *Precipitants:* Cold air, exercise, emotion, allergens (house dust mite, pollen, animal fur), infection, drugs (eg aspirin, NSAIDs, β-blockers).
- *Diurnal variation* in symptoms or peak flow. Marked morning dipping of peak flow is common and can tip the patient over into a serious attack, despite having normal peak flow at other times.
- *Exercise:* Quantify the exercise tolerance.
- *Disturbed sleep:* Quantify as nights per week (a sign of serious asthma).
- *Acid reflux:* This has a known association with asthma.
- *Other atopic disease:* Eczema, hay fever, allergy, or family history?
- *The home (especially the bedroom):* Pets? Carpet? Feather pillows or duvet? Floor cushions and other 'soft furnishings'?
- *Occupation:* If symptoms remit at weekends or holidays, something at work may be a trigger. Ask the patient to measure their peak flow at work and at home (at the same time of day) to confirm this.
- *Days per week off work or school.*

Signs Tachypnea; audible wheeze; hyper-inflated chest; hyper-resonant percussion note; diminished air entry; widespread, polyphonic wheeze. *Severe attack:* Inability to complete sentences; pulse >110bpm; respiratory rate >25/min; PEF 33–50% of predicted. *Life-threatening attack:* Silent chest; cyanosis; bradycardia; exhaustion; PEF <33% of predicted; confusion; feeble respiratory effort.

Tests *Chronic asthma:* PEF monitoring (p154): A diurnal variation of >20% on ≥3d a wk for 2wks. Spirometry: Obstructive defect (↓FEV_1/FVC, ↑RV); usually ≥15% improvement in FEV_1 following β₂ agonists or steroid trial. CXR: Hyperinflation. Skin-prick tests may help to identify allergens. Histamine or methacholine challenge. *Aspergillus* serology. *Acute attack:* PEF, sputum culture, CBC, electrolytes, CRP, blood cultures. ABG analysis usually shows a normal or slightly reduced P_aO_2 and low P_aCO_2 (hyperventilation). If P_aO_2 normal but the patient is hyperventilating, watch carefully and repeat the ABG a little later. *If P_aCO_2 is raised, transfer to a step-down unit or ICU for mechanical ventilation.* CXR (to exclude infection or pneumothorax).

Treatment Chronic asthma (p170). Emergency treatment (p702).

Differential diagnosis Pulmonary edema ('cardiac asthma'); COPD (often co-exists); large airway obstruction (eg foreign body, tumor); SVC obstruction (wheeze/dyspnea not episodic); pneumothorax; PE; bronchiectasis; obliterative bronchiolitis (suspect in elderly).

Associated diseases Acid reflux; polyarteritis nodosa (PAN); Churg–Strauss syndrome; ABPA.

Natural history Most childhood asthmatics either grow out of asthma in adolescence, or suffer much less as adults. A significant number of people develop chronic asthma late in life.

Mortality Death certificates give a figure of ≈4000/yr (US). 50% are >65yrs old.

Management of chronic asthma

Lifestyle education Stop smoking and avoid precipitants. Check inhaler technique. Teach patients to use a peak flow meter to monitor PEF twice a day. Educate patients to manage their disease by altering their medication in response to changes in symptoms or PEF. Give specific advice about what to do in an emergency; provide a written action plan.

National Asthma Education and Prevention Program (NAEPP) guidelines Start at the step most appropriate to severity. Review treatment every 1–6 months. A gradual stepwise reduction in treatment may be possible; alternatively, consider step up if control is not maintained. A short course of prednisone may be used to gain control as quickly as possible.

Step 1 **Mild intermittent asthma** Occasional short-acting inhaled β_2-agonist as required for symptom relief. If daytime symptoms occur more than 2 days per week (but not every day), or if nocturnal symptoms occur more than 2 nights per month, go to Step 2.

Step 2 **Mild persistent asthma** Add low-dose inhaled steroid: beclomethasone 40–120mcg/12h, budesonide 100–200mcg/12h, or fluticasone 44–132mcg/12h. If symptoms occur daily or more than 1 night per week, go to Step 3.

Step 3 **Moderate persistent asthma** Add long-acting β_2-agonist (eg salmeterol 50mcg/12h or formoterol 12mcg/12h). If benefit—but still inadequate control—continue and ↑dose of inhaled steroid to medium-dose (beclomethasone 120–240mcg/12h, budesonide 200–600mcg/12h, or fluticasone 132–330mcg/12h). If symptoms are continual or occur frequently at night, go to Step 4.

Step 4 **Severe persistent asthma** Continue long-acting β_2-agonist and ↑dose of inhaled steroid to high-dose (beclomethasone up to 320mcg/12h, budesonide up to 800mcg/12h, or fluticasone up to 440mcg/12h).

Drugs *β_2-adrenoreceptor agonists* relax bronchial smooth muscle, acting within minutes. Albuterol is best given by inhalation (aerosol, powder, nebulizer), but may also be given PO. SE: Tachyarrhythmias, ↓K^+, tremor, anxiety. Long-acting inhaled β_2-agonist (eg salmeterol, formoterol) can help nocturnal symptoms and reduce morning dips. They should never be used as mono-therapy for asthma and should only be added when symptoms are inadequately controlled on inhaled corticosteroids. SE: Same as albuterol, tolerance, arrhythmias, paradoxical bronchospasm (salmeterol), ? ↑risk of death.

Corticosteroids are best inhaled, eg beclomethasone via spacer (or powder), but may be given PO or IV. They act over days to ↓bronchial mucosal inflammation. Rinse mouth after inhaled steroids to prevent oral candidiasis. Oral steroids are used acutely (high-dose, short courses, eg prednisone 30–40mg/24h PO for 7d) and longer term in lower dose (eg 5–10mg/24h) if control is not optimal on inhalers. Warn about SEs.

Aminophylline (metabolized to theophylline) may act by inhibiting phosphodiesterase, thus ↓bronchoconstriction by ↑CAMP levels. Stick with one brand name (bioavailability variable). It may be useful as 'add-on' treatment if inhaled therapy is inadequate. In acute severe asthma, it may be given IVI. It has a narrow therapeutic ratio, causing arrhythmias, GI upset, and seizures in the toxic range. Check theophylline levels, and do ECG monitoring and check plasma levels after 24h if IV therapy is used.

Anticholinergics (eg ipratropium) may ↓muscle spasm synergistically with β_2-agonists. They may be of more benefit in COPD than in asthma. Try each alone, and then together; assess with spirometry.

Cromolyn May be used as prophylaxis in mild and exercise-induced asthma (always inhaled), especially in children. It may precipitate asthma.

Leukotriene receptor antagonists (eg montelukast, zafirlukast) block the effects of cysteinyl leukotrienes in the airways. May be used as 'add-on' therapy to recommended inhaler regimens.

Doses of some inhaled drugs used in bronchoconstriction

	Inhaled aerosol	Inhaled powder	Nebulized *(supervised)*
Albuterol			
Dose example:	90–180mcg/4–6h		2.5–5mg/6h
(the same for **CFC** and **CFC**-free devices Proventil HFA® is an example of a **CFC**-free inhaler)			
Salmeterol			
Dose/puff	—	50mcg	—
Recommended regimen	—	50mcg/12h	—
Ipratropium bromide			
Dose/puff	17mcg	—	500mcg/mL
Recommended regimen	20–80mcg/6h	—	500mcg/6h
Steroids			
(Flovent HFA®= fluticasone; Qvar®= beclomethasone; Pulmicort®= budesonide)			
Fluticasone (Flovent HFA®)			
Doses available/ puff (CFC-free)	44, 110, & 220mcg	—	—
Recommended regimen	88–440mcg/12h	—	—
Beclomethasone (Qvar®)			
Doses available/ puff (CFC-free)	40 & 80mcg	—	—
Recommended regimen	40–320mcg/12h		
Budesonide (Pulmicort®)			
Doses available/ puff (CFC-free)	—	200mcg	—
Recommended regimen	—	200–800mcg/12h	—

Any puff/dose ≥250mcg≈significant steroid absorption: Carry a steroid card.

Changing to a CFC-free device: Soon *all* inhalers will be **CFC**-free. Tell patients their inhaler may taste different and that **CFCs** will not have harmed them. They may not like the new taste: Anticipate this point, and reassure.

Chronic obstructive pulmonary disease (COPD)

Definitions COPD is a common progressive disorder of airway obstruction (↓FEV$_1$, ↓FEV$_1$/FVC, p154) with little or no reversibility. COPD includes chronic bronchitis and emphysema (COPD is the preferred term). Usually patients have *either* COPD *or* asthma, not both: COPD is favored by: • Age of onset >35yrs • Smoking related • Chronic dyspnea • Sputum production • No marked diurnal or day-to-day FEV$_1$ variation. *Chronic bronchitis* is defined *clinically* as cough, sputum production on most days for 3 months of 2 successive years. There is no ↑ in mortality if lung function is normal. Symptoms improve in 90% if they stop smoking. *Emphysema* is defined *histologically* as enlargement of the air spaces distal to the terminal bronchioles, with destruction of the alveolar walls.

Prevalence ~14 million in the US COPD mortality: 115,000 deaths/yr in the US.

Pink puffers and blue bloaters (two ends of a spectrum) *Pink puffers* have ↑alveolar ventilation, a near normal P$_a$O$_2$ and a normal or low P$_a$CO$_2$. They are breathless but not cyanotic. They may progress to type I respiratory failure (p176). *Blue bloaters* have ↓alveolar ventilation, with a low P$_a$O$_2$ and high P$_a$CO$_2$. They can be cyanotic but usually not breathless and may go on to develop cor pulmonale. Their respiratory centers are relatively insensitive to CO$_2$ and they rely on their hypoxic drive to maintain respiratory effort—*supplemental oxygen should be given with care.*

Clinical features *Symptoms:* Cough, sputum, dyspnea, and wheeze. *Signs:* Tachypnea; use of accessory muscles of respiration; hyper-inflation; ↓crico-sternal distance (<3cm); ↓expansion; resonant or hyper-resonant percussion note; quiet breath sounds (eg over bullae); wheeze; cyanosis; cor pulmonale. *Complications:* Acute exacerbations ± infection; polycythemia; respiratory failure; cor pulmonale (edema; JVP↑); pneumothorax (ruptured bullae); lung ca.

Tests *CBC:* PCV↑. *CXR:* Hyperinflation (>6 anterior ribs seen above diaphragm in mid-clavicular line); flat hemidiaphragms; large central pulmonary arteries; ↓peripheral vascular markings; bullae. *ECG:* Right atrial and ventricular hypertrophy (cor pulmonale). *ABG:* P$_a$O$_2$↓ ± hypercapnia. *Lung function (p154):* Obstructive + air trapping (FEV$_1$ <80% of predicted—see below, FEV$_1$/FVC ratio <70%, TLC↑, RV↑, DLCO↓ in emphysema). Learn how to do FEV$_1$ and FVC from an experienced spirometrist: Ensure *maximal* expiration of the full breath (it takes ≥6s; it's *not* a quick puff out).

Treatment *Chronic stable:* See BOX; *Emergency R$_x$* p704. Offer *smoking cessation* advice with firm concern. BMI is often low: *Diet advice ± supplements* may help. *Mucolytics* may help chronic productive cough. Disabilities may cause serious, treatable *depression;* screen for this. *Respiratory failure* p176. *Flu and pneumococcal vaccinations.*

Long term O$_2$ therapy (LTOT): A MRC trial showed that if P$_a$O$_2$ was maintained ≥60mmHg for 15h a day, 3yr survival improved by 50%. LTOT should be given for: (1) clinically stable non-smokers with P$_a$O$_2$ <55mmHg—despite maximal R$_x$. These values should be stable on two occasions >3 wks apart. (2) If P$_a$O$_2$ 55–60 *and* pulmonary hypertension (eg RVH; loud S$_2$) + cor pulmonale. O$_2$ can also be prescribed for terminally ill patients.

Predicted FEV$_1$ *(Caucasian males; liters, ↓level in other races)* [1]										*(Caucasian females)*									
Height cm	150	155	160	165	170	175	180	185	190	195	145	150	155	160	165	170	175	180	185	190
♂**Age(yr)** 10	2.5	2.8	3.0	3.2	3.5	3.7	3.9	4.1	4.4	4.6	2.1	2.2	2.3	2.5	2.6	2.7	2.9	3.0	3.1	3.3
25	2.9	3.2	3.4	3.7	4.0	4.2	4.3	4.7	5.0	5.3	2.6	2.7	2.9	3.0	3.1	3.3	3.4	3.5	3.7	3.8
30	2.8	3.1	3.3	3.6	3.8	4.1	4.3	4.6	4.9	5.1	2.5	2.6	2.8	2.9	3.0	3.2	3.3	3.4	3.6	3.7
40	2.7	3.0	3.3	3.6	3.8	4.1	4.3	4.6	4.6	4.9	2.3	2.4	2.5	2.7	2.8	3.0	3.0	3.2	3.3	3.5
50	2.2	2.5	2.8	3.0	3.3	3.5	3.8	4.0	4.3	4.6	2.1	2.2	2.3	2.5	2.6	2.7	2.9	3.0	3.1	3.3
60	2.2	2.5	2.8	3.0	3.3	3.5	3.8	4.0	4.3		1.7	2.0	2.1	2.3	2.4	2.5	2.7	2.8	2.9	3.1
70	1.7	2.0	2.2	2.5	2.7	3.0	3.3	3.5	3.8	4.0	1.6	1.8	1.9	2.1	2.2	2.3	2.5	2.6	2.7	2.9
80	1.4	1.7	2.0	2.2	2.5	2.7	3.0	3.3	3.5	3.8	1.4	1.6	1.7	1.9	2.0	2.1	2.2	2.4	2.5	2.7

1 African FEV$_1$ is 10–15% lower; Chinese: 20% lower; Indian: 10% lower; note: PEF varies little between groups.

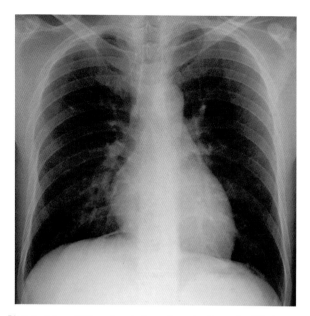

Plate 1. A few millilitres of gas in the peritoneal cavity can be difficult to see. The best way is with a CXR after remaining erect for 10 min. This may be a small pneumoperitoneum at the right cardiophrenic angle. Check with another view or a CT if necessary. If you strongly suspected a perforated ulcer and the CXR and AXR showed no signs of pneumoperitoneum, could you exclude the diagnosis? No. Only 75% of perforations have evidence of pneumoperitoneum.

The authors and publishers would like to thank Peter Scally for permission to use these plates taken from Scally, P. (1999) *Medical imaging: an Oxford core text*. Oxford University Press, Oxford

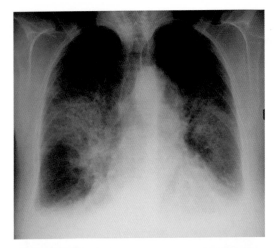

(a)

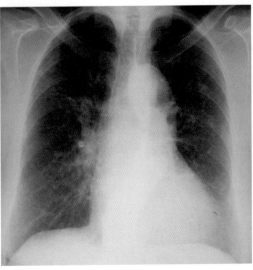

(b)

Plate 2. (a) (b) Two radiographs, 4 days apart. *Lungs*: The major abnormality in the initial film is in the lungs; perihilar opacities that are poorly defined. This is consolidation. But what is the cause? Pulmonary oedema, infection, or blood? The lungs are filled with fluid and unable to expand fully. *Pleura*: The hemidiaphragms are not visible because of pleural effusions, seen curving up the side walls. *Mediastinum*: The heart is enlarged. *Hila, bones, soft tissues*: normal. These are the changes of severe left heart failure. The pulmonary venous pressure has been so high that fluid has flowed from the capillaries, into the interstitium, and then into the alveoli. Look at how the lungs have expanded and the heart borders and hemidiaphragms have sharpened up after treatment.

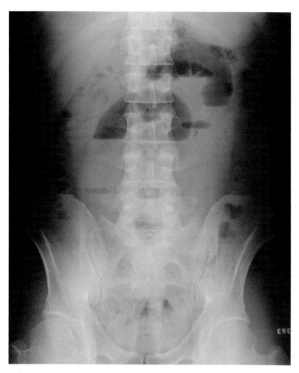

Plate 3. Erect. The fluid levels are immediately obvious in the erect film, but let's approach it in a systematic way. *Gas* can be seen in the colon from the rectum back to the caecum. The stomach bubble is barely visible. That leaves several loops with fluid levels to be explained. They must be small intestine, being centrally placed and with a few valvulae conniventes. The loops are dilated, 3 cm wide, and are probably ileum as the valvulae conniventes are less pronounced here than in the jejunum. By comparison, if the large bowel was obstructed it would show as a few peripheral loops, often over 5 cm in diameter, containing faeces and showing a haustral (scalloped) pattern. Folds in the mucosa of the colon do not extend completely across the lumen. No sign of *calcification in the biliary tree or urinary tract.* The *bones* and *soft tissues* are normal. We would be looking for evidence of a cause of small bowel obstruction: a hernia, surgical clips, or any other signs of surgery.

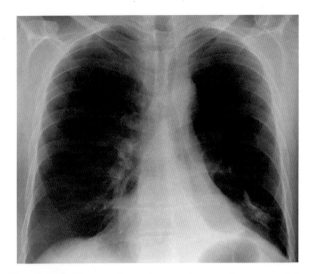

Plate 4. *Lungs*: These are of normal volume. Fewer markings are seen in the left lung except at the base. *Pleura*: Following the pleura reveals loss of the clarity of the left hemidiaphragm. *Mediastinum*: In the mediastinum the left main bronchus is pulled down and there is a triangular opacity behind the heart on the left. This is a collapsed left lower lobe. It also depresses the left *hilum*. *Bones*: Check the bones for metastatic disease because the left lower lobe bronchus may be obstructed by a neoplasm. *Soft tissues*: appear unremarkable.

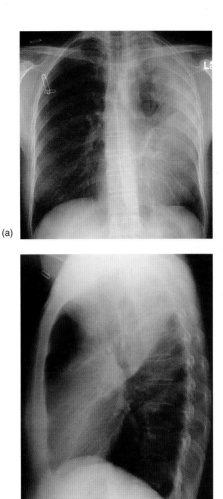

(a)

(b)

Plate 5. (a) (b) *Lungs*: Normal lung volumes. A poorly defined opacity in the left lung obliterates the left heart border and therefore is in the upper lobe. The air-bronchogram indicates consolidation. *Pleura*: The pleura in the right hemithorax seem normal. *Mediastinum*: This is central but the oblique fissure on the lateral film is bowed inferiorly because of a slight increase in volume. *Hila*: The left hilum is not visible. *Bones, soft tissues*: normal. Left upper lobe pneumonia (lobar pneumonia). Pneumonia is an infection of the lung, classified as lobar, broncho, and atypical. Usually the pathology progresses through four stages: congestion, red hepatization, grey hepatization, and resolution. This would be one of the stages of hepatization.

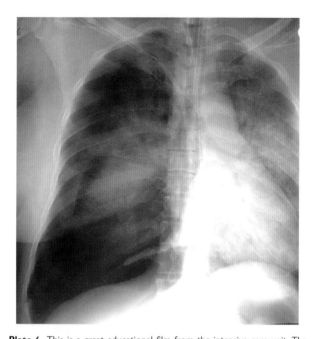

Plate 6. This is a great educational film from the intensive care unit. The inexperienced doctor could be distracted by the poor quality, badly centred film. The technicians do the best they can under difficult conditions. To ask for another in this instance would be a mistake. There is adequate information to make a life-saving decision. After checking the name of the patient, see that the tubes and lines are well positioned—the endotracheal and nasogastric tubes and the right subclavian central venous line. *Lungs*: The left lung shows consolidation. The right hemithorax is too black and hyperexpanded. Right hemidiaphragm is depressed. *Pleura*: The pleural recess is seen at the right base. *Mediastinum*: This is shifted to the left, obstructing venous return and decreasing cardiac output, a threat to life. Is it being pushed or pulled? *Hila, bones*, and *soft tissues*: Check these structures. Is the endotracheal tube down the right main bronchus, inflating the right lung and collapsing the left? No. Is the right lung collapsed? Yes. Right tension pneumothorax. Beware of the half-toning of the hemidiaphragm in a supine film. In the supine position, a pneumothorax will be anterior and the lung will fall posteriorly. A chest tube is needed immediately. The consolidation in the left lung could be a result of any of the causes of the acute respiratory distress syndrome (ARDS). Consolidation/collapse often occurs in intubated patients at the left base. Suction catheters to clear the lungs pass down the ETT and preferentially into the right main bronchus.

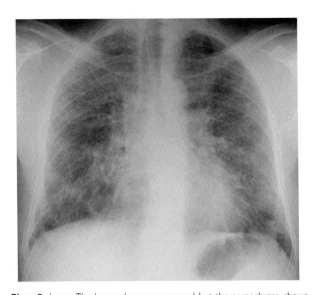

Plate 7. *Lungs*: The lung volumes are normal but the parenchyma shows increased markings that extend out to the chest wall. Normally vessels (arteries and veins) are only seen for 80% of the distance from hilum to pleura. The bronchi should barely be visible. *Pleura*: Following the pleura demonstrates that the heart borders are poorly defined, reflecting interstitial disease in the lung adjacent to the heart. *Mediastinum*: The mediastinal structures themselves are normal. *Hila*: The hila are difficult to interpret. So what? It is not unusual to be missing a piece of information when making a clinical decision. No need for wringing of hands and gnashing of teeth. Either go ahead without it or, if it is essential, find it. In this case, further information is available by comparison with old films or by requesting a CT. *Bone* and *soft tissues*: No abnormality. This is interstitial lung disease. It has a similar appearance to the interstitial oedema of moderate left heart failure but without a big heart. Check the previous film to see if it is acute. It was not. The diagnosis in this example is fibrosing alveolitis.

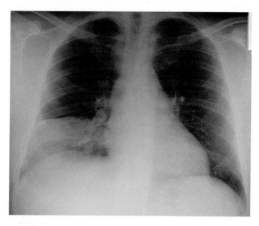

(a)

(b)

Plate 8. (a) (b) *Lungs*: An opacity can be seen at the base of the right lung. *Pleura*: The silhouette of the pleura over the right hemidiaphragm is lost because of adjacent lung disease. The right heart border is also unclear. *Mediastinum, hila, bones, soft tissues*: normal. The middle lobe has two segments. The consolidation of lobar pneumonia here involves principally the lateral segment. The medial segment is affected to a lesser extent, shown by the loss of clarity of the right heart border. Also well seen on the lateral projection, but the PA view has adequate information.

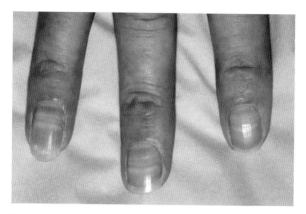

Plate 9. Beau's lines.

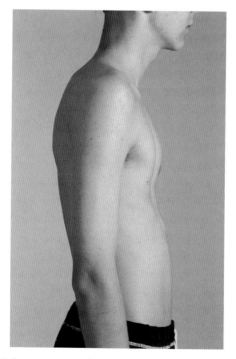

Plate 10. Pectus excavatum. The medical term for funnel or sunken chest. Associations: scoliosis; restrictive spirometry; Marfan's syndrome; Ehlers–Danlos syndrome (plate 24).

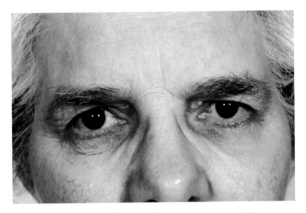

Plate 11. Xanthelasma. *Xanthos* is Greek for yellow, and *elasma* means plate. Xanthelasma are lipid-laden yellow plaques congregating around the lids. They are typically a few mm wide, and signify hyperlipidaemia.

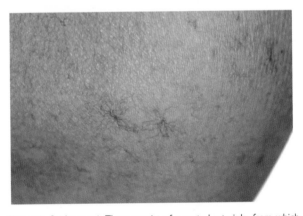

Plate 12. Spider naevi. These consist of a central arteriole, from which numerous vessels radiate (like the legs of a spider). These fill from the centre. They occur most commonly in skin drained by the superior vena cava. Up to 5 are said to be normal (they are common in young females). Causes include liver failure, contraceptive steroids, and pregnancy (ie changes in oestrogen metabolism).

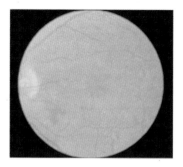

Plate 13. Diabetes, background retinopathy. There are scattered blot haemorrhages and sparse hard exudates but vision is normal.

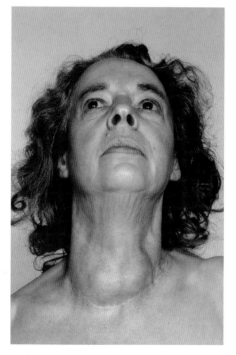

Plate 14. Nodular goitre.

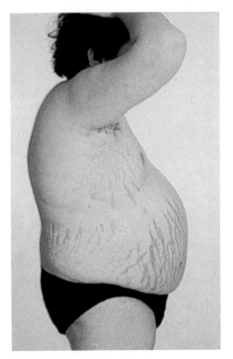

Plate 15. Cushing's disease. Signs of Cushings include purple abdominal striae and wasting, eg in the thighs.

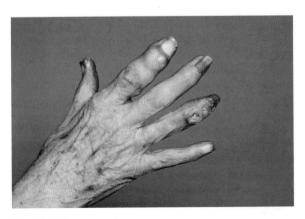

Plate 16. Tophaceous gout.

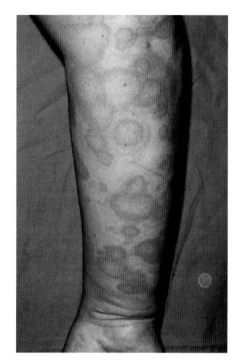

Plate 17. Erythema multiforme. Target lesions eg caused by drugs, herpes or mycoplasma.

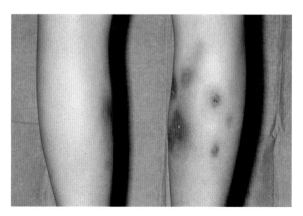

Plate 18. Erythema nodosum. Causes include sarcoidosis, drugs, streps, TB, and UC/Crohn's disease.

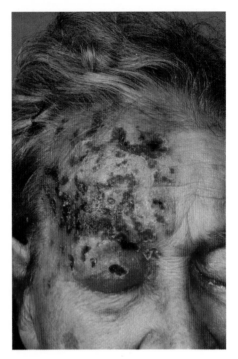

Plate 19. Shingles (herpes zoster) involving the ophthalmic (Vi) division of the trigeminal nerve.

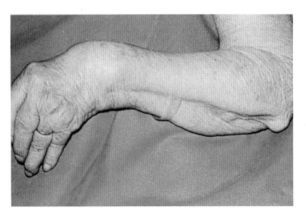

Plate 20. Rheumatoid arthritis. Note ulnar deviation of fingers.

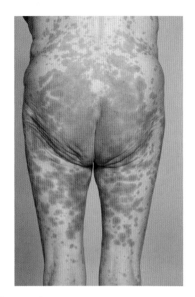

Plate 21. Drug reaction.

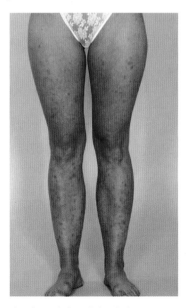

Plate 22. Vascultic skin rash from Behcet's disease.

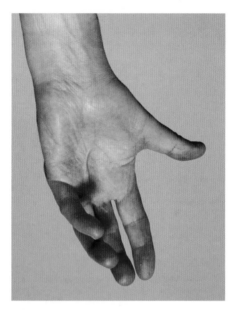

Plate 23. Dupuytren's contracture.

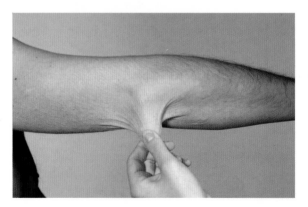

Plate 24. Ehlers–Danlos syndrome. Note the hyperelasticity of the skin. Associations: aneurysms; GI bleeds/perforations; hypermobile joints; flat feet. It is a disorder of collagen.

Global Initiative for Chronic Obstructive Lung Disease (GOLD) 2003 guidelines

Assessment of COPD	Spirometry (FEV_1/FVC <70%)
	Bronchodilator response
	Trial of oral steroids is a poor predictor of response to inhaled steroids.
	CXR ?Bullae ?Other pathology
	ABG ?Hypoxia ?Hypercapnia
Severity of COPD (Stage)	At risk (0) Normal spirometry
	Mild (I) FEV_1 ≥80% predicted
	Moderate (II) FEV_1 50–79% predicted
	Severe (III) FEV_1 30–49% predicted
	Very severe (IV) FEV_1 <30% predicted

Treating stable COPD

NB: Patients who fly should be able to maintain an in-flight P_iO_2 ≥50mmHg.

Non-pharmacological	Stop smoking, encourage exercise, treat poor nutrition or obesity, influenza and pneumococcal vaccination, pulmonary rehabilitation/palliative care.
Pharmacological: Mild	Add PRN short-acting bronchodilator (inhaled ipratropium, albuterol, or combination of two)
Moderate	Add long-acting inhaled β_2 agonist (salmeterol or formoterol) or inhaled anticholinergic (tiotropium).
Severe	Add inhaled steroids if repeated exacerbations. (Advair® combines salmeterol and fluticasone.)

173

More advanced COPD
- Consider pulmonary rehabilitation in patients with moderate or worse COPD.
- Consider LTOT if P_aO_2 <55mmHg (see OPPOSITE).
- Indications for surgery: Recurrent pneumothoraces; isolated bullous disease; lung volume reduction surgery or lung transplantation in selected patients.
- Assess home set-up and support needed. Treat depression.

Indications for specialist referral
- Uncertain diagnosis.
- Suspected severe COPD or a rapid decline in FEV_1.
- Onset of cor pulmonale.
- Assessment for oral corticosteroids, nebulizer therapy, or LTOT.
- Bullous lung disease (to assess for surgery).
- <10 pack-years smoking (=PYS = the number of packs/day × number of years of smoking). Smokers have an excess loss of FEV_1 of 7.4–12.6mL per pack year for men and 4.4–7.2mL per pack year for women.
- Symptoms disproportionate to pulmonary function tests.
- Frequent infections (to exclude bronchiectasis).
- COPD in patient <40yrs (eg is the cause α_1-antitrypsin deficiency?).

Acute respiratory distress syndrome (ARDS)

ARDS, or acute lung injury, may be caused by direct lung injury or occur secondary to severe systemic illness. Lung damage and release of inflammatory mediators cause ↑ capillary permeability and non-cardiogenic pulmonary edema, often accompanied by multiorgan failure.

Causes *Pulmonary:* Pneumonia; gastric aspiration; inhalation; injury; vasculitis; contusion. *Other:* Shock; septicemia; hemorrhage; multiple transfusions; DIC (p577); pancreatitis; acute liver failure; trauma; head injury; malaria; fat embolism; burns; obstetric events (eclampsia; amniotic fluid embolus); drugs/toxins (aspirin, heroin, paraquat).

Clinical features Cyanosis; tachypnea; tachycardia; peripheral vasodilatation; bilateral fine inspiratory crackles.

Investigations CBC, electrolytes, LFT, amylase, clotting, CRP, blood cultures, ABG. CXR shows bilateral pulmonary infiltrates. Pulmonary artery catheter to measure pulmonary capillary wedge pressure (PCWP).

Diagnostic criteria One consensus requires these 4 to exist: **(1)** Acute onset. **(2)** CXR: Bilateral infiltrates. **(3)** PCWP <19mmHg or a lack of clinical congestive heart failure. **(4)** Refractory hypoxemia with P_aO_2 : FiO_2 <200 for ARDS. Others include total thoracic compliance <30mL/cm H_2O.

Management Admit to ICU, give supportive therapy, and treat the underlying cause.
- *Respiratory support* In early ARDS continuous positive airway pressure (CPAP) with 40–60% oxygen may be adequate to maintain oxygenation, but most patients need mechanical ventilation. Indications for ventilation: P_aO_2: <60mmHg despite 60% O_2; P_aCO_2: >45mmHg. The large tidal volumes (10–15mL/kg) produced by conventional ventilation plus reduced lung compliance in ARDS may lead to high peak airway pressures ± pneumothorax. Positive end-expiratory pressure (PEEP) ↑ oxygenation but at the expense of venous return, cardiac output, and perfusion of the kidneys and liver. Other approaches include inverse ratio ventilation (inspiration > expiration), permissive hypercapnia, high-frequency jet ventilation, and other low-tidal-volume techniques.
- *Circulatory support* Invasive hemodynamic monitoring with an arterial line and Swan–Ganz catheter aids the diagnosis and may be helpful in monitoring PCWP and cardiac output. Maintain cardiac output and O_2 delivery with inotropes (eg dobutamine 2.5–10mcg/kg/min IV), vasodilators, and blood transfusion. Consider treating pulmonary hypertension with low-dose (20–120 parts per million) nitric oxide, a selective pulmonary vasodilator. Hemofiltration may be needed in renal failure and to achieve a negative fluid balance.
- *Sepsis* Identify organism(s) and treat accordingly. If clinically septic, but no organisms cultured, use empirical broad-spectrum antibiotics (p159). Avoid nephrotoxic antibiotics.
- *Other:* Nutritional support: Enteral is best. Steroids don't ↓mortality in the acute phase, but may help later on (>7d), particularly if eosinophilia in blood or in fluid from broncho-alveolar lavage.

Prognosis Overall mortality is 50–75%. Prognosis varies with age of patient, cause of ARDS (pneumonia 86%, trauma 38%), and number of organs involved (3 organs involved for >1wk is 'invariably' fatal).

Risk factors for ARDS

- Sepsis
- Hypovolemic shock
- Trauma
- Pneumonia
- Diabetic ketoacidosis
- Gastric aspiration
- Pregnancy
- Eclampsia
- Amniotic fluid embolus
- Drugs/toxins
- Paraquat, heroin, aspirin
- Pulmonary contusion

- Massive transfusion
- Burns
- Smoke inhalation
- Near drowning
- Acute pancreatitis
- DIC
- Head injury
- ICP↑
- Fat embolus
- Heart/lung bypass
- Tumor lysis syndrome
- Malaria

Respiratory failure

Respiratory failure occurs when gas exchange is inadequate, resulting in hypoxia. It is defined as a P_aO_2 <60mmHg and subdivided into 2 types according to P_aCO_2 level.

Type I respiratory failure is defined as hypoxia (P_aO_2 <60mmHg) with a normal or low P_aCO_2. It is caused primarily by ventilation/perfusion ($\dot{V}/\dot{Q}$) mismatch. Causes include:

- Pneumonia
- Pulmonary edema
- PE
- Asthma
- Emphysema
- Pulmonary fibrosis
- ARDS (p174).

Type II respiratory failure is defined as hypoxia (P_aO_2 <60mmHg) with hypercapnia (P_aCO_2 is >45mmHg). This is caused by alveolar hypoventilation, with or without $\dot{V}/\dot{Q}$ mismatch. Causes include:

- *Pulmonary disease:* Asthma, COPD, pneumonia, pulmonary fibrosis, obstructive sleep apnea (OSA, p189).
- *Reduced respiratory drive:* Sedative drugs, CNS tumor, or trauma.
- *Neuromuscular disease:* Cervical cord lesion, diaphragmatic paralysis, poliomyelitis, myasthenia gravis, Guillain–Barré syndrome.
- *Thoracic wall disease:* Flail chest, kyphoscoliosis.

Clinical features are those of the underlying cause together with symptoms and signs of hypoxia, with or without hypercapnia.

Hypoxia: Dyspnea; restlessness; agitation; confusion; central cyanosis. If long-standing hypoxia: Polycythemia; pulmonary hypertension; cor pulmonale.

Hypercapnia: Headache; peripheral vasodilatation; tachycardia; bounding pulse; tremor/flap; papilledema; confusion; drowsiness; coma.

Investigations are aimed at determining the underlying cause:
- Blood tests: CBC, electrolytes, CRP, ABG
- Radiology: CXR
- Microbiology: Sputum and blood cultures (if febrile)
- Spirometry (COPD, neuromuscular disease, Guillain–Barré syndrome).

Management depends on the cause:

Type I respiratory failure
- Treat underlying cause.
- Give oxygen (35–60%) by face mask to correct hypoxia.
- Assisted ventilation if P_aO_2 <60mmHg despite 60% O_2.

Type II respiratory failure The respiratory center may be relatively insensitive to CO_2 and respiration could be driven by hypoxia. *Oxygen therapy should be given with care.* Nevertheless, don't leave the hypoxia untreated.
- Treat underlying cause.
- Controlled oxygen therapy: Start at 24% O_2.
- Recheck ABG after 20min. If P_aCO_2 is steady or lower, ↑ O_2 concentration to 28%, If P_aCO_2 has risen >12mmHg and the patient is still hypoxic, consider assisted ventilation, ie non-invasive positive pressure ventilation).
- If this fails, consider intubation and ventilation, if appropriate.

When to consider arterial blood gas (ABG) measurement

In these clinical scenarios:

Any unexpected deterioration in an ill patient.

Anyone with an acute exacerbation of a chronic chest condition.

Anyone with impaired consciousness.

Anyone with impaired respiratory effort.

Or if any of these signs or symptoms are present:

Bounding pulse, drowsiness, tremor (flapping), headache, pink palms, papilledema (signs of CO_2 retention).

Cyanosis, confusion, visual hallucinations (signs of hypoxia).

Or to monitor the progress of a critically ill patient:

Monitoring the treatment of known respiratory failure.

Anyone ventilated in the ICU.

After major surgery.

After major trauma.

To validate measurements from transcutaneous pulse oximetry:

Pulse oximetry (p154) *sometimes* suffices when it is not critical to know P_aCO_2. Even so, it is wise to do periodic blood gas checks.

Learn arterial puncture from an expert (local anesthesia *does* ↓pain).

Pulmonary embolism (PE)

Causes PEs usually arise from a venous thrombosis in the pelvis or legs. Clots break off and pass through the venous system and the right side of the heart before lodging in the pulmonary circulation. Rare causes include: Right ventricular thrombus (post-MI); septic emboli (right-sided endocarditis); fat, air, or amniotic fluid embolism; neoplastic cells; parasites. *Risk factors:* Any cause of immobility or hypercoagulability:

- Recent surgery
- Thrombophilia/antiphospholipid syn. (p590)
- Recent stroke or MI
- Prolonged bed rest
- Disseminated malignancy
- Pregnancy; postpartum; oral contraceptives/HRT
- Prolonged travel without stopping

Clinical features These depend on the number, size, and distribution of the emboli; small emboli may be asymptomatic whereas large emboli are often fatal. *Symptoms:* Acute breathlessness, pleuritic chest pain, hemoptysis; dizziness; syncope. Ask about risk factors (above), past history or family history of thromboembolism. *Signs:* Pyrexia; cyanosis; tachypnea; tachycardia; hypotension; raised JVP, pleural rub; pleural effusion. Look for signs of a cause, eg deep vein thrombosis; scar from recent surgery.

Tests
- *CXR* may be normal, or may show dilated pulmonary artery, linear atelectasis, small pleural effusion, wedge-shaped opacities or cavitation (rare).
- *ECG* may be normal, or show tachycardia, right bundle branch block, right ventricular strain (inverted T in V_1 to V_4), The classical $S_IQ_{III}T_{III}$ pattern is rare.
- *ABG* may show a low P_aO_2 and a low P_aCO_2.

Treatment (p710) Anticoagulate with low molecular weight heparin (eg enoxaparin 1mg/kg/12h SC) and start oral warfarin 10mg (p574). Stop heparin when INR is >2 and continue warfarin for a minimum of 3 months; aim for an INR of 2–3. Consider placement of a *vena caval filter* in patients who develop emboli despite adequate anticoagulation (NB ↑ risk if placed without concomitant anticoagulation).

Prevention Give heparin (7500U/12h or 5000U/8h) to all immobile patients. Prescribe TED stockings and encourage early mobilization. Women should stop HRT and oral contraceptives pre-op (if reliable with another form of contraception). Patients with a past or family history of thromboembolism should be investigated for thrombophilia.

Pneumothorax

Management p706 & X-RAY PLATE 6

Causes Often spontaneous (especially in young thin men) due to rupture of a subpleural bulla. Other causes: Asthma; COPD; TB; pneumonia; lung abscess; carcinoma; cystic fibrosis; lung fibrosis; sarcoidosis; connective tissue disorders (Marfan's syndrome, Ehlers–Danlos syndrome), trauma; iatrogenic (subclavian CVP line insertion, pleural aspiration or biopsy, percutaneous liver biopsy, positive pressure ventilation).

Clinical features *Symptoms:* There may be no symptoms (especially in fit young people with small pneumothoraces) or there may be sudden onset of dyspnea and/or pleuritic chest pain. Patients with asthma or COPD may present with a sudden deterioration. Mechanically ventilated patients may present with hypoxia or an ↑ in ventilation pressures. *Signs:* Reduced expansion, hyper-resonance to percussion and diminished breath sounds on the affected side. *With a tension pneumothorax, the trachea will be deviated away from the affected side.*

Management and tension pneumothorax see p706

Placing a chest drain p662.

Investigation of suspected PE

- First assess the likely probability of a PE
- Numerous scoring systems are available
- One simple system is the presence of clinical features of a PE (SOB and tachypnea, with or without pleuritic chest pain and hemoptysis) and either *a)* the absence of another reasonable explanation, or *b)* the presence of a major risk factor. If *a* and *b* co-exist, the probability is high; if only one exists, intermediate; if neither exist, low.
- *D-dimers* Only perform in those patients **without** a high probability of a PE. A negative D-dimer test only excludes a PE in those with a low clinical probability, and imaging is NOT required. However, a positive test does not prove a diagnosis of a PE, and imaging is required.
- *Imaging* The conventional 1st-line, if the CXR is normal, is a V̇/Q̇ scan (p156; look for perfusion defects with no corresponding ventilation defects). If 'normal', a PE is reliably excluded. If non-diagnostic, further imaging is required, but may give some false positives. The recommended 1st-line imaging modality now is a spiral CT scan, which can show clots down to 5th-order pulmonary arteries (after the 4th branching). This may also be useful for subjects with indeterminate isotope scans. Bilateral leg ultrasound (or rarely venograms) may also be sufficient to CONFIRM, but not exclude, a PE in patients with a co-existing clinical DVT.

Major risk factors for PE
- Surgery
  - Major abdominal/pelvic
  - Hip/knee replacement
- Obstetrics
  - Late pregnancy; post-partum
  - Cesarean section
- Lower limb problems
  - Fracture
  - Varicose veins
- Malignancy
- Reduced mobility
- Previous PE

Pleural effusion

Definitions A pleural effusion is fluid in the pleural space. Effusions can be divided by their protein and LDH concentrations into *transudates* and *exudates*, see OPPOSITE. Blood in the pleural space is a *hemothorax*; pus in the pleural space is an *empyema*, and chyle (lymph with fat) is a *chylothorax*. Both blood and air in the pleural space is called a *hemopneumothorax*.

Causes *Transudates* may be due to ↑venous pressure (cardiac failure, constrictive pericarditis, fluid overload), or hypoproteinemia (cirrhosis, nephrotic syndrome, malabsorption). Also occur in hypothyroidism and Meigs' syndrome (right pleural effusion and ovarian fibroma). *Exudates* are mostly due to ↑ leakiness of pleural capillaries secondary to infection, inflammation, or malignancy. Causes: Pneumonia; TB; pulmonary infarction; rheumatoid arthritis; SLE; bronchogenic carcinoma; malignant metastases; lymphoma; mesothelioma; lymphangitic carcinomatosis.

Symptoms Asymptomatic—or dyspnea, pleuritic chest pain.

Signs ↓ *expansion; dull percussion note; diminished breath sounds* occur on the affected side. Tactile vocal fremitus and vocal resonance are ↓ (inconstant and unreliable). Above the effusion, where lung is compressed, there may be *bronchial breathing* and *egophony* (bleating vocal resonance). With large effusions there may be *tracheal deviation* away from the effusion. Look for aspiration marks and signs of associated disease: Malignancy (cachexia, clubbing, lymphadenopathy, radiation marks, mastectomy scar); stigmata of chronic liver disease; cardiac failure; hypothyroidism; rheumatoid arthritis; butterfly rash of SLE.

Tests *CXR* Small effusions blunt the costophrenic angles, larger ones are seen as water-dense shadows with concave upper borders. A completely horizontal upper border implies that there is also a pneumothorax.

Ultrasound is useful in identifying the presence of pleural fluid and in guiding diagnostic or therapeutic aspiration.

Diagnostic aspiration: Percuss the upper border of the pleural effusion and choose a site 1 or 2 intercostal spaces below it. Infiltrate down to the pleura with 5–10mL of 1% lidocaine. Attach a 21G needle to a syringe and insert it just above the upper border of an appropriate rib (avoids neurovascular bundle). Draw off 10–30mL of pleural fluid and send it to the lab for *clinical chemistry* (protein, glucose, pH, LDH, amylase); *bacteriology* (gram and AFB staining, bacterial and TB culture) and *cytology*.

Pleural biopsy: If pleural fluid analysis is inconclusive, consider parietal pleural biopsy. Thoracoscopic or CT-guided pleural biopsy ↑ diagnostic yield (by enabling direct visualization of the pleural cavity and biopsy of suspicious areas).

Management is of the underlying cause.
- *Drainage* If the effusion is symptomatic, drain it, repeatedly if necessary. Fluid is best removed slowly (≤2L/24h). It may be aspirated in the same way as a diagnostic tap, or using an intercostal drain (p661).
- *Pleurodesis* with tetracycline, bleomycin, or talc may be helpful for recurrent effusions. Thoracoscopic talc pleurodesis is most effective for malignant effusions. Empyemas (p161) are best drained using a chest drain, inserted under ultrasound or CT guidance.
- *Intrapleural streptokinase* Probably no benefit.
- *Surgery* Persistent collections and ↑ pleural thickness (on ultrasound) require surgery.

Pleural fluid analysis

Gross appearance	*Cause*
Clear, straw-coloured	Transudate, exudate
Turbid, yellow	Empyema, parapneumonic effusion
Hemorrhagic	Trauma, malignancy, pulmonary infarction

Cytology	
Neutrophils ++	Parapneumonic effusion, PE
Lymphocytes ++	Malignancy, TB, RA, SLE, sarcoidosis
Mesothelial cells ++	Pulmonary infarction
Abnormal mesothelial cells	Mesothelioma
Multinucleated giant cells	RA
Lupus erythematosus cells	SLE

Clinical chemistry	
Pleural fluid/serum protein <0.5 AND	If all 3 criteria are met, effusion is a transudate. Otherwise, it is an exudate
Pleural fluid/serum LDH <0.6 AND	
Pleural fluid LDH <2/3 top normal serum LDH	
Glucose <60mg/dL	Empyema, malignancy, TB, RA, SLE
pH <7.2	Empyema, malignancy, TB, RA, SLE
LDH↑ (pleural:serum >0.6)	Empyema, malignancy, TB, RA, SLE
Amylase↑	Pancreatitis, carcinoma, bacterial pneumonia, esophageal rupture

Sarcoidosis

A multisystem granulomatous disorder of unknown cause. Prevalence in US: $5/10^5$ population among Caucasians, $40/10^5$ among African Americans. Commonly affects adults aged 20–40yrs. African Americans are affected more severely than Caucasians, particularly by extrathoracic disease.

Clinical features *Asymptomatic* In 20–40%, the disease is discovered incidentally, after a routine CXR. *Acute sarcoidosis* often presents with erythema nodosum (PLATE 18) ± polyarthralgia. It usually resolves spontaneously.

Pulmonary disease 90% have abnormal CXRs with bilateral hilar lymphadenopathy (**BHL**) ± pulmonary infiltrates or fibrosis. *Symptoms:* Dry cough, progressive dyspnea, ↓exercise tolerance and chest pain. In 10–20% symptoms progress, with concurrent deterioration in lung function.

Non-pulmonary manifestations are legion: Lymphadenopathy; hepatomegaly; splenomegaly; uveitis; conjunctivitis; keratoconjunctivitis sicca; glaucoma; terminal phalangeal bone cysts; enlargement of lacrimal and parotid glands; Bell's palsy; neuropathy; meningitis; brainstem and spinal syndromes; space-occupying lesion; erythema nodosum (PLATE 18); lupus pernio; subcutaneous nodules; cardiomyopathy; arrhythmias; hypercalcemia; hypercalciuria; renal stones; pituitary dysfunction.

Investigations *Blood tests:* ↑ESR, lymphopenia, abnormal LFTs, ↑serum ACE, ↑immunoglobulins. *24h urine:* Ca^{2+}↑; hypercalciuria. *Tuberculin skin test* is –ve in two-thirds;. *CXR* is abnormal 90%. *Stage 0:* Normal. *Stage 1:* BHL. *Stage 2:* BHL + peripheral pulmonary infiltrates. *Stage 3:* Peripheral pulmonary infiltrates alone. *Stage 4:* Progressive pulmonary fibrosis; bulla formation (honeycombing); pleural involvement.

ECG may show arrhythmias or bundle branch block. *Lung function tests* may be normal or show reduced lung volumes, impaired gas transfer, and a restrictive ventilatory defect. *Tissue biopsy* (lung, liver, lymph nodes, skin nodules. or lacrimal glands) is diagnostic and shows non-caseating granulomata.

Bronchoalveolar lavage (BAL) shows ↑lymphocytes in active disease; ↑neutrophils with pulmonary fibrosis.

Ultrasound may show nephrocalcinosis or hepatosplenomegaly.

Bone x-rays show 'punched out' lesions in terminal phalanges.

CT/MRI may be useful in assessing severity of pulmonary disease or diagnosing neurosarcoidosis. *Ophthalmology assessment* (slit lamp examination, fluorescein angiography) is indicated in ocular disease. *Kveim tests* are obsolete.

Management Patients with BHL alone do not require treatment since the majority recover spontaneously. *Acute sarcoidosis:* Bed rest, NSAIDs, *Indications for corticosteroid therapy:*
• Parenchymal lung disease (symptomatic, static, or progressive)
• Uveitis
• Hypercalcemia
• Neurological or cardiac involvement.

Prednisone (40mg/24h) PO for 4–6wks, then ↓dose over 1yr according to clinical status. A few patients relapse and may need a further course or long-term therapy. In severe illness, IV methylprednisolone or immunosuppressants (methotrexate, cyclosporin, azathioprine, cyclophosphamide) may be needed.

Prognosis 60% of patients with thoracic sarcoidosis show spontaneous resolution within 2yrs. 20% of patients respond to steroid therapy. In the remainder, improvement is unlikely despite therapy.

Causes of bilateral hilar lymphadenopathy (BHL)

Infection	TB
	Mycoplasma
Malignancy	Lymphoma
	Carcinoma
	Mediastinal tumors
Industrial dust disease	Silicosis
	Berylliosis
Extrinsic allergic alveolitis	

Differential diagnosis of granulomatous diseases

Infections	Bacteria	TB
		Leprosy
		Syphilis
		Cat scratch fever
	Fungi	*Cryptococcus neoformans*
		Histoplasma capsulatum
		Coccidioides immitis
	Protozoa	Schistosomiasis
Autoimmune	Primary biliary cirrhosis	
	Granulomatous orchitis	
Vasculitis	Giant cell arteritis	
	Polyarteritis nodosa	
	Takayasu's arteritis	
	Wegener's granulomatosis	
Industrial dust disease	Silicosis	
	Berylliosis	
Idiopathic	Crohn's disease	
	de Quervain's thyroiditis	
	Sarcoidosis	
Extrinsic allergic alveolitis		
Histiocytosis X		

Extrinsic allergic alveolitis (EAA)

In sensitized individuals, inhalation of allergens (fungal spores or avian proteins) provokes a hypersensitivity reaction. In the acute phase, the alveoli are infiltrated with acute inflammatory cells. With chronic exposure, granuloma formation and obliterative bronchiolitis occur.

Causes (representative examples among numerous described in the literature)
• Bird fancier's and pigeon fancier's lung (proteins in bird droppings).
• Farmer's and mushroom worker's lung (*Micropolyspora faeni, Thermoactinomyces vulgaris*).
• Malt worker's lung (*Aspergillus clavatus*).
• Bagassosis (*Thermoactinomyces sacchari*).

Clinical features *4-6h post-exposure:* Fever, rigors, myalgia, dry cough, dyspnea, crackles (no wheeze). *Chronic:* ↑ dyspnea, weight↓, exertional dyspnea, Type I respiratory failure, cor pulmonale.

Tests *Acute: Blood:* CBC (neutrophilia); ESR↑; ABGs; positive serum precipitins (indicate exposure only). *CXR:* Mid-zone mottling/consolidation; hilar lymphadenopathy (rare). *Lung function tests:* Reversible restrictive defect; reduced gas transfer during acute attacks.

Chronic: Blood: Positive serum precipitins. *CXR:* Upper-zone fibrosis; honeycomb lung. *Lung function tests:* Persistent changes (see above). Bronchoalveolar lavage *(BAL)* fluid shows ↑ lymphocytes and mast cells.

Management *Acute attack:* Remove allergen and give O_2 (35–60%), then:
• Hydrocortisone 200mg IV.
• Oral prednisone (40mg/24h PO), followed by reducing dose.

Chronic: Avoid exposure to allergens, or wear a face mask or +ve pressure helmet. Long-term steroids often achieve CXR and physiological improvement.

Idiopathic pulmonary fibrosis (X-RAY PLATE 7)

A disease of unknown cause, characterized by an inflammatory cell infiltrate and pulmonary fibrosis.

Symptoms Dry cough; exertional dyspnea; malaise; weight↓; arthralgia.

Signs Cyanosis; finger clubbing; fine end-inspiratory crepitations.

Complications Type I respiratory failure; ↑ risk of lung cancer.

Tests *Blood:* ABG (P_aO_2↓; P_aCO_2↑); CRP↑; immunoglobulins↑; ANA (30% +ve), rheumatoid factor (10% +ve). *CXR:* (X-RAY PLATE 7) Lung volume↓; bilateral lower zone reticulo-nodular shadows; honeycomb lung (advanced disease). *Spirometry:* Restrictive (p154); ↓DLCO. *BAL* may indicate activity of alveolitis: Lymphocytes↑ (good response/prognosis) or neutrophils and eosinophils↑ (poor response/prognosis). *Lung biopsy* may be needed for diagnosis.

Management A large proportion of patients have chronic irreversible disease which is unresponsive to treatment. Prednisone 60mg/24h PO for 6wks, followed by a reducing dose. Alternative: Cyclophosphamide 100–150mg/24h PO + prednisone 20mg/24h PO. Monitor response with symptom inquiry, CXR, and lung function tests. The patient may be suitable for lung transplantation.

Prognosis 50% overall 5yr survival rate.

Industrial dust diseases

Coal worker's pneumoconiosis (CWP) results from inhalation of coal dust particles (1–3mcm in diameter) over 15–20yrs. These are ingested by macrophages which die, releasing their enzymes and causing fibrosis.

Clinical features: Asymptomatic, but co-existing chronic bronchitis is common. CXR: Many round opacities (1–10mm), especially upper zone.

Management: Avoid exposure to coal dust; treat co-existing chronic bronchitis.

Progressive massive fibrosis (PMF) is due to progression of CWP, which causes progressive dyspnea, fibrosis, and eventually, cor pulmonale. CXR: Upper-zone fibrotic masses (1–10cm).

Management: Avoid exposure to coal dust.

Caplan's syndrome is the association between rheumatoid arthritis, pneumoconiosis, and pulmonary rheumatoid nodules.

Silicosis is caused by inhalation of silica particles, which are very fibrogenic. A number of jobs may be associated with exposure, eg metal mining, stone quarrying, sandblasting, and pottery/ceramic manufacture.

Clinical features: Progressive dyspnea, ↑incidence of TB, CXR shows diffuse miliary or nodular pattern in upper and mid-zones and egg-shell calcification of hilar nodes. PMF may occur. Spirometry: Restrictive ventilatory defect.

Management: Avoid exposure to silica.

Asbestosis is caused by inhalation of asbestos fibers. Chrysotile (white asbestos) is the least fibrogenic—crocidolite (blue asbestos) is the most fibrogenic. Amosite (brown asbestos) is the least common and has intermediate fibrogenicity. Asbestos was commonly used in the construction industry for fire proofing, pipe lagging, electrical wire insulation, and roofing felt. Degree of asbestos exposure is related to degree of pulmonary fibrosis.

Clinical features: Similar to other fibrotic lung diseases with progressive dyspnea, clubbing, and fine end-inspiratory crackles. Also causes pleural plaques, ↑risk of bronchial adenocarcinoma and mesothelioma.

Management: Symptomatic. Patients are often eligible for workers compensation.

Malignant mesothelioma is a tumor of mesothelial cells which usually occurs in the pleura, and rarely in the peritoneum or other organs. It is associated with occupational exposure to asbestos, but the relationship is complex. 90% report previous exposure to asbestos, but only 20% of patients have pulmonary asbestosis. The latent period between exposure and development of the tumor may be up to 45yrs.

Clinical features include chest pain, dyspnea, weight loss, finger clubbing, recurrent pleural effusions. If the tumor has metastasized there may be lymphadenopathy, hepatomegaly, bone pain/tenderness, abdominal pain/obstruction (peritoneal malignant mesothelioma).

Tests: CXR/CT: Pleural thickening/effusion. Bloody pleural fluid.

Diagnosis is made on histology, following a pleural biopsy or thoracoscopy. Often the diagnosis is only made post-mortem.

Management: Symptomatic.

Prognosis is very poor (<2yrs, ≈2400 deaths/yr in the US).

Causes of interstitial lung disease

Granulomatous diseases	Tuberculosis
	Sarcoidosis
Drugs	Amiodarone
	Bleomycin
	Busulfan
	Nitrofurantoin
	Sulfasalazine
Connective tissue diseases	Ankylosing spondylitis
	Rheumatoid arthritis
	Systemic lupus erythematosus
	Systemic sclerosis
Extrinsic allergic alveolitis (EAA) (p184)	Bird fancier's lung
	Farmer's lung
	Malt worker's lung
	Mushroom picker's lung
	Pigeon fancier's lung
Industrial dust diseases	Asbestosis
	Berylliosis
	Pneumoconiosis
	Silicosis
Radiation	
Chronic pulmonary edema (mitral stenosis)	
Bronchiolitis obliterans organizing pneumonia	
Idiopathic pulmonary fibrosis	

Cor pulmonale

Cor pulmonale is right heart failure caused by chronic pulmonary hypertension. Causes include chronic lung disease, pulmonary vascular disorders, and neuromuscular and skeletal diseases (see BOX).

Clinical features Symptoms include dyspnea, fatigue, or syncope. Signs: Cyanosis; tachycardia; raised JVP with prominent *a* and *v* waves; RV heave; loud P$_2$, pansystolic murmur (tricuspid regurgitation); early diastolic Graham Steell murmur; hepatomegaly and edema.

Investigations *CBC:* Hb and hematocrit↑ (secondary polycythemia). *ABG:* Hypoxia, with or without hypercapnia. *CXR:* Enlarged right atrium and ventricle, prominent pulmonary arteries. *ECG:* Pulmonale; right axis deviation; right ventricular hypertrophy/strain.

Management
- *Treat underlying cause*—eg COPD and pulmonary infections.
- *Treat respiratory failure*—in the acute situation give 24% oxygen if P_aO_2 <60mmHg. Monitor ABG and gradually ↑ oxygen concentration if P_aCO_2 is stable. In COPD patients, long-term oxygen therapy (LTOT) for 15h/d ↑ survival. Patients with chronic hypoxia when clinically stable should be assessed for LTOT.
- *Treat cardiac failure* with diuretics such as furosemide (eg 40–160mg/24h PO). Monitor electrolytes and give amiloride or potassium supplements if necessary. Alternative: Spironolactone.
- Consider *phlebotomy* if the hematocrit is >55%.
- Consider *heart-lung transplantation* in young patients.

Prognosis Poor. 50% die within 5yrs.

Causes of cor pulmonale

- *Lung disease*
  Asthma (severe, chronic)
  COPD
  Bronchiectasis
  Pulmonary fibrosis
  Lung resection
- *Pulmonary vascular disease*
  Pulmonary emboli
  Pulmonary vasculitis
  Primary pulmonary hypertension
  ARDS
  Sickle-cell disease
  Parasite infestation
- *Thoracic cage abnormality*
  Kyphosis
  Scoliosis
  Thoracoplasty
- *Neuromuscular disease*
  Myasthenia gravis
  Poliomyelitis
  Motor neuron disease
- *Hypoventilation*
  Sleep apnea
  Enlarged adenoids in children
  Cerebrovascular disease

Obstructive sleep apnea syndrome

This disorder is characterized by intermittent closure/collapse of the pharyngeal airway which causes apneic episodes during sleep. These are terminated by partial arousal.

Clinical features The typical patient is an overweight, middle-aged man (or a postmenopausal woman) who presents because of snoring or daytime somnolence. His partner often describes apneic episodes during sleep.
• Snores loudly in sleep • Daytime somnolence • Poor sleep quality
• Morning headache • ↓ libido • Cognitive performance↓

Complications Pulmonary hypertension; Type II respiratory failure (p176). Sleep apnea is also reported as an independent risk factor for hypertension.

Investigations Simple studies (eg pulse oximetry, video recordings) may be all that are required for diagnosis. Polysomnography (which monitors oxygen saturation, airflow at the nose and mouth, ECG, EMG chest and abdominal wall movement during sleep) is diagnostic. The occurrence of 15 or more episodes of apnea or hypopnea during 1h of sleep indicates significant sleep apnea.

Management
• Weight reduction
• Avoidance of tobacco and alcohol
• CPAP via a nasal mask during sleep is effective
• Surgical procedures to relieve pharyngeal obstruction (tonsillectomy, uvulopalatopharyngoplasty, or tracheostomy) are occasionally needed, but only after seeing a specialist in sleep disorders.

Gastroenterology

Jonathan Buscaglia, M.D., and Sanjay Jagannath, M.D.

Contents

Oral manifestations of GI diseases

The oropharynx can provide diagnostic clues to a variety of GI diseases. Some examples are noted below.

Leukoplakia: A potentially pre-malignant white thickening of the tongue or oral mucosa. When in doubt, refer all intra-oral white lesions. *Causes:* Poor dental hygiene; smoking; sepsis; aphthous stomatitis; squamous papilloma; verucca vulgaris; 2° syphilis. Oral hairy leukoplakia is a painless, shaggy whitish streaky patch on the side of the tongue due to EBV which is often seen in patients with AIDS.

Necrotizing stomatitis: Severe periodontal disease charcterized by inflammation and necrosis of gingiva to adjacent soft tissue and nonalveolar bone. Often seen in patients with AIDS.

Aphthous ulcers: Minute, painful shallow white ulcers distributed along mucous membranes. Affects 20% of the population. *Causes:* Associated conditions include inflammatory bowel disease, Behçet's disease, trauma, celiac sprue, erythema multiforme (PLATE 17), lichen planus, pemphigus, pemphigoid, infections (Herpes simplex, syphilis). Can be seen in otherwise healthy individuals. *Treatment* can be difficult: Steroid creams, treatment of underlying condition.

Candidiasis (thrush): White patches or erythema of the buccal mucosa. Patches may be hard to remove and bleed if scraped. *Risk factors:* Extremes of age; DM; antibiotics; immunosuppression (long-term corticosteroids, including inhalers; cytotoxics; malignancy; HIV). Oropharyngeal candidiasis in an apparently healthy patient suggests underlying HIV infection *Treatment:* Nystatin swish and swallow suspension, fluconazole.

Angular cheilitis: Fissuring at the angles of the mouth. Commonly associated with vitamin B deficiencies (riboflavin, niacin, pyridoxine). Infectious causes include *Staphylococcus* and *Candida*.

Gingivitis: Gum inflammation ± hypertrophy occurs with poor oral hygiene, drugs (phenytoin, cyclosporin, nifedipine), pregnancy, vitamin C deficiency (scurvy), acute myeloid leukemia (p579), or Vincent's angina.

Microstomia: The mouth is too small due to thickening and tightening of the perioral skin after burns or in epidermolysis bullosa (destructive skin and mucous membrane blisters ± ankyloglossia) or systemic sclerosis (p374) (look for facial telangiectasia; sclerodactyly; Raynaud's; calcinosis).

Oral pigmentation: Perioral melanin spots characterize Peutz–Jeghers' syndrome. Multiple telangiectasias of the buccal cavity suggest Osler–Weber–Rendu syndrome. Blue rubber bleb nevi syndrome can present with a mound-like venous anomaly on mucous membranes. Can be a cause of clinically overt or occult GI bleeding

Teeth: A blue line at the gum–tooth margin suggests lead poisoning. Prenatal or childhood tetracycline exposure causes yellowish-brown discoloration.

Tongue: *Ulcerated tongue:* May be seen in patients with graft-versus-host disease. Associated with tetrad of painful oral mucositis, enteritis, dermatitis, and hepatic dysfunction.

Glossitis: A smooth, red, sore tongue often caused by iron, folate, or B_{12} deficiency. If *local* loss of papillae leads to ulcer-like lesions that change in color and size, use the term *geographic tongue* (harmless migratory glossitis).

Macroglossia: Diffusely enlarged tongue. Look for evidence of repeated tongue biting. *Causes:* Myxedema; acromegaly; amyloid.

Healthy, enjoyable eating

There are no good or bad *foods*, and no universally good or bad *diets*. We must not consider diet out of context with a desired lifestyle, and nor should we assume that everyone wants to be thin, healthy, and live forever. If we are walking to the South Pole, we need a diet full of fat; taking any other food would be a waste of space (fat is energy-rich). But if we live a sedentary life, the converse is not necessarily (or even probably) true.[1]

Current recommendations must take into account 3 facts:
- Obesity is an escalating epidemic costing health services as much as smoking.
- Diabetes mellitus is burgeoning: In some places prevalence is >7% (p270).
- Past advice has not changed eating habits in large sections of the population.

Advice is likely to focus on the following:
1 *Body mass index:* *Weight in kilogram/(height in meters)*; aim for 20–25; ie *eat less.* Controlling quantity may be more important than quality. In hypertension, eating the 'right' things lowered BP by 0.6mmHg, but controlling weight caused a 3.7mmHg reduction in 6 months in 1 randomized trial.

2 *Fish oil:* (Rich in omega-3 fatty acid, eg mackerel, herring, salmon). This helps those with hyperlipidemia. If canned fish, avoid those in unspecified oils. Nuts are also valuable: Walnuts lower total cholesterol and have one of the highest ratios of polyunsaturates to saturates (7:1). Soya protein lowers cholesterol, low-density lipoproteins, and triglycerides.

3 *Refined sugar:* (see BOX for its deleterious effects) Use fruit to add sweetness. Have low-sugar drinks. Don't add sugar to drinks or cereals.

4 *Eat enough fruit and fiber*—see BOX. Reduce salt.

Avoid this diet if: • <5yrs old • Need for low residue (Crohn's, UC, p224) or special diet (celiac, p232) • If weight *loss* expected (eg HIV +ve). *Emphasis may be different in:* Dyslipidemia (p106); DM; obesity; constipation; liver failure; chronic pancreatitis; renal failure (less protein); BP↑.[2]

192

---

1 Randomized trials (not without problems) show how an *Atkins-type diet* low in carbohydrate (∴ ↑fat & ↑protein) can *improve* lipid profiles and insulin resistance. Possibe SEs: renal problems; excessive calcium excretion. Foster G 2003 *NEJM* **348** 2082 & Samaha F 2003 *NEJM* **348** 2074.
2 Dietary approaches to stop hypertension *DASH diet* emphasizing fruits, vegetables, & ↓↓fat dairy items lowers BP and can make losartan more effective. Conlin P 2003 *Am J Hypertens* **16** 337.

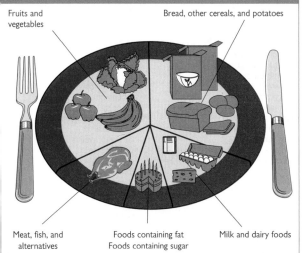

Traditional low-fat nutritional advice: The balance of good health

Fruits and vegetables

Bread, other cereals, and potatoes

Meat, fish, and alternatives

Foods containing fat
Foods containing sugar

Milk and dairy foods

This shows rough proportions of food types that make up the putatively ideal meal. It is a model against which other diets are compared

Starchy foods: Bread, rice, pasta, potatoes, etc. form the main energy source (especially wholemeal). ↑Fluid intake with a diet high in non-starch polysaccharide (NSP)—eg 8 cups (1–2½ pints) daily. Warn about bulky stools. NSP ↓calcium and iron absorption, so restrict main intake to 1 meal a day.

Fruit, vegetables: Eg >6 different pieces of fruit (ideally with skins) or portions of pulses, beans, or lightly cooked greens per day. This may ↓cardiovascular and cancer mortality.

Meat and alternatives: Meat should be cooked without additional fat. Lower fat alternatives, such as white meat (poultry, without skin), white fish, and vegetable protein sources (eg pulses, soya) are encouraged.

Dairy foods: Low-fat skim milk/yogurt; cottage cheese.

Fat and sugary foods: Avoiding extra fat in cooking is advised ('grill, boil, steam, or bake, but don't fry'). Fatty spreads (eg butter) are kept to a minimum and snack foods (crisps, sweets, biscuits, or cake) are avoided.

Avoiding obesity: Excess sugar causes caries, diabetes, and obesity (this contributes to osteoarthritis, cancer, and hypertension, and ↑oxidative stress—so raising cardiovascular mortality).

Drugs for obesity? Orlistat lowers fat absorption (hence SE of oily fecal incontinence).

Dysphagia or Odynophagia

Dysphagia is difficulty in swallowing and odynophagia is pain with swallowing. Progressive or new-onset dysphagia lasting >3wks deserves detailed investigation.

Causes may be classified as oropharyngeal or esophageal:

Mechanical block
Malignant stricture
Esophageal cancer
Metastatic cancer
Benign strictures
Esophageal web or ring
Peptic stricture
Extrinsic pressure
Lung cancer
Mediastinal lymph nodes
Retrosternal goiter
Aortic aneurysm
Left atrial enlargement
Pharyngeal pouch.

Motility disorders
Achalasia
Diffuse esophageal spasm
Systemic sclerosis
Myasthenia gravis
Bulbar palsy
Pseudobulbar palsy
Syringobulbia
Bulbar poliomyelitis
Chagas' disease.

Others
Esophagitis
Infection (*Candida*, HSV)
Reflux esophagitis
Globus hystericus.

Clinical features: A careful history can establish whether dysphagia or odynophagia is oropharyngeal or esophageal in location, and whether it is neuromuscular or structural in origin. Some discerning questions to ask include the following:

1 Does dysphagia occur within one second of swallowing? This implicates the oropharyngeal location.
2 Is the dysphagia localized to the retrosternal or subxiphoid region? Often implicates an esophageal source.
3 Was there difficulty in swallowing liquids and solids from the onset? An affirmative answer implies a motility disorder (achalasia, neurological dysfunction), whereas a negative answer implies a structural abnormality (stricture, ring or web).
4 Is it painful to swallow? Implicates mucosal disease (eg esophageal ulcerations due to malignancy, infections, or esophagitis).
5 Is the dysphagia intermittent, or progressive? Intermittent implies esophageal spasm.
6 Does the neck bulge or gurgle on drinking? Suspect a pharyngeal pouch (eg Zenker's diverticulum).

Investigations: The first question is whether to obtain a barium swallow study prior to upper endoscopy? Patients with suspected oropharyngeal dysphagia should have a cine-esophagram performed first. A structural abnormality is often adequately treated with upper endoscopy. Findings suggestive of esophageal dysmotility or spasm should be further evaluated with esophageal manometry ± pH probe. Treatment is based on diagnosis.

Specific conditions: *Diffuse esophageal spasm (DES)* is a disease characterized by rapid, nonperistaltic wave progression through the esophagus. Symptoms include intermittent dysphagia (30–60%) ± chest pain (80–90%). Barium swallow: Abnormal, non-peristaltic contractions eg corkscrew esophagus. Medical therapy, which has limited success, includes smooth muscle relaxants or tricyclic antidepressants. *Achalasia* is the most common motor disorder of the esophagus, and is characterized by incomplete relaxation of the lower esophageal sphincter (LES) (due to degeneration of the myenteric plexus). Secondary achalasia can result from Chagas' disease and pseudoachalasia. Symptoms include dysphagia, regurgitation, substernal cramps, and weight loss. Barium swallow: Dilated tapering esophagus (bird's beak), and usually without peristalsis. Diagnosis is made with manometry revealing non-propagating low amplitude peristalsis of the esophagus and incomplete LES relaxation. Treatment: Medications (smooth muscle relaxants), local injection (Botulinum toxin), endoscopic and acid supression dilatation or Heller's myotomy—then proton pump inhibitors (PPIs). *Benign esophageal stricture:* Caused by gastroesophageal reflux disease (GERD) (p197), corrosives, surgery, or radiotherapy. Treatment is with endoscopic balloon dilatation. *Esophageal cancer:* Associations: GERD, tobacco, alcohol, Barrett's esophagus, achalasia. *Paterson-Brown-Kelly (Plummer-Vinson) syndrome* Post-cricoid web + iron-deficiency anemia.

Nausea and vomiting

Nausea is the subjective sensation of an impending urge to vomit, and vomiting is the forceful evacuation of gastric contents via the mouth. Causes of nausea and vomiting are protean and may originate from different body systems. Gross classifications include medications, CNS disorders, GI and peritoneal disorders, endocrine and metabolic abnormalities, infectious and miscellaneous causes.

Tests: *Blood tests* including comprehensive metabolic panel. A metabolic alkalosis (pH >7.45, HCO_3↑) suggests severe vomiting. A plain upright AXR may suggest a suspected bowel obstruction. Consider upper GI *endoscopy* if vomiting persists. Identify and *treat the underlying cause.*

Treatment: *Fluids* Give IV fluids for rehydration. *Drugs* Various anti-emetics may be chosen, and administered IV or per rectum, if not tolerated orally. Avoid those anti-emetics with prokinetic properties until bowel obstruction is ruled out. Metoclopramide 10mg IV for GI causes (except intestinal obstruction). Avoid drugs in pregnancy.

Dyspepsia and peptic ulceration

Dyspepsia (indigestion) is a non-specific group of symptoms (abdominal pain, bloating, nausea) related to the upper GI tract. Causes of dyspeptic symptoms may include: Peptic ulcer disease (duodenal and gastric ulcers), gastritis, esophagitis, gastro-esophageal reflux disease, malignancy, or non-ulcer dyspepsia (diagnosis of exclusion).

Symptoms & signs: Physical examination, often normal, may reveal epigastric tenderness, tympanic percussion due to bloating, etc. These physical examination signs are non-specific.

Management of dyspepsia: The initial management of patients with uninvestigated dyspepsia remains controversial. Clinical suspicion and economics often dictate when to test and perform invasive procedures on patients. A reasonable approach is to prescribe an empiric trial of a proton-pump inhibitor for 4–8wks in patients <50yrs old with intermittent symptoms and without alarm signs. For patients at least 50yrs old, long standing symptoms, or with alarm signs, upper endoscopy is indicated.

Peptic ulcer disease (PUD)

Abdominal pain occurs in 94% of patients with PUD. Typically described as burning, non-radiating epigastric pain, that is often relieved with food or antacids. The pain may awaken patients in the middle of the night. Two-thirds of duodenal ulcer patients and one-third of gastric ulcer patients present with symptoms. Symptomatic pain is non-specific, however, since one-third of patients with non-ulcer dyspepsia also have similar pain. **Warning signs** of complicated PUD include signs of perforation, penetration, or hemorrhage. Ask for acute exacerbations in frequency, location, or severity of symptoms. Question patients for melena (90% of melena is due to upper GI hemorrhage), hemetemesis, and radiating pain.

Duodenal ulcers (DU) are 4× more common than GU. *Risk factors:* H. pylori (~90%); drugs (aspirin; NSAIDs; steroids). Diseases associated with DU include: Zollinger–Ellison syndrome, systemic mastocytosis, Multiple endocrine neoplasia type I, chronic pulmonary disease, chronic renal failure, cirrhosis, nephrolithiasis, and alpha-1-antitrypsin deficiency.

Diagnosis: Upper GI endoscopy. Test for H. pylori (see BOX). Gastrin concentrations should be measured if Zollinger–Ellison syndrome is suspected.

Gastric ulcers (GU) occur primarily in the elderly, on the lesser curve of the stomach. Ulcers elsewhere are more likely to be malignant. *Risk factors:* H. pylori (~70%); smoking; NSAID; stress-related ulcers (Cushing's or Curling's ulcers). *Diagnosis:* Upper GI endoscopy must be performed to exclude malignancy; take multiple biopsies from the rim and base of the ulcer (histology, H. pylori) and brushings (cytology).

Treatment of peptic ulcers *Lifestyle:* Avoid food that worsens symptoms. Stop smoking (slows healing in GU; ↑relapse rates in DU). Medical therapy includes antacids, H₂ receptor antagonists, proton-pump inhibitors, and cytoprotective agents (sucralfate, misoprostol). Misoprostol is contraindicated in women of child-bearing age and dose-related diarrhea is often the limiting factor in patient compliance. *H. pylori eradication:* Triple[1] or quadruple therapy. *NSAID-associated ulcers:* Stop NSAID if possible (if not, use H₂-receptor antagonist, PPI, or misoprostol for prevention). If symptoms persist, re-endoscope, recheck for H. pylori, and reconsider the differential diagnosis. *Surgery:* (p460) May be indicated for complications of PUD.

---

1 Triple therapy for 7–14d: (1) PPI (eg lansprazole 30mg twice daily). (2) Amoxicillin 1gm twice daily. (3) Clarithromycin 500mg twice daily.

Gastroesophageal reflux disease (GERD)

The development of signs, symptoms, or complications related to the retrograde passage of gastric contents into the esophagus is termed gastro-esophageal reflux disease (GERD). GERD is extremely common with equal prevalence among genders, however, there is a male predominance for complications. Factors associated with GERD include the potency of the refluxate, anti-reflux barriers, luminal acid clearance mechanisms, esophageal tissue resistance, and gastric emptying. Dysfunction of the lower esophageal sphincter predisposes to the gastroesophageal reflux of acid. If reflux is prolonged or excessive, it may cause inflammation of the esophagus (esophagitis), benign esophageal stricture, Barrett's esophagus and esophageal adenocarcinoma.

Associations: Smoking, alcohol, hiatal hernia, pregnancy, obesity, large meals, surgery in achalasia, drugs (tricyclics, anticholinergics, nitrates); systemic sclerosis. GERD can also contribute to asthma and other extraintestinal manifestations.

Symptoms Heartburn (burning, retrosternal discomfort related to meals, lying down, and straining, relieved by antacids); belching; acid brash (acid or bile regurgitation); waterbrash (excessive salivation); odynophagia (painful swallowing, eg from esophagitis or stricture); nocturnal asthma (cough/wheeze with apparently minimal inhalation of gastric contents).

Complications: Esophagitis, ulcers, iron deficiency anemia, benign strictures, Barrett's esophagus, and esophageal adenocarcinoma.

Tests Isolated symptoms do not require investigation. *Indications for upper GI endoscopy:* Age >50yrs; symptoms >4wks; dysphagia; persistent symptoms despite treatment; relapsing symptoms; weight loss or other alarm signs/symptoms. Barium swallow may show hiatus hernia. 24h esophageal pH monitoring ± esophageal manometry may be needed to distinguish GERD from other causes.

The Los Angeles (LA) classification: Minor diffuse changes (erythema, edema; friability) are not included, and the term *mucosal break* is used to encompass the old terms erosion and ulceration. There are 4 grades.

1 One or more mucosal breaks <5mm long, not extending beyond 2 mucosal fold tops. A mucosal break is a well-demarcated area of slough/erythema.
2 Mucosal break >5mm long limited to the space between 2 mucosal fold tops.
3 Mucosal break continuous between the tops of 2 or more mucosal folds but which involves less than 75% of the esophageal circumference.
4 Mucosal break involving ≥75% of the esophageal circumference.

Treatment

1 *Lifestyle: Encourage:* Weight loss; raise bed head; small, regular meals. *Avoid:* Hot drinks, alcohol, and eating <3h before bed. Avoid drugs affecting esophageal motility (nitrates, anticholinergics, tricyclic antidepressants) or that damage the mucosa (NSAID, K^+ salts, alendronate).
2 *Drugs: Antacids* to relieve symptoms. If symptoms persist for >4wks (or weight↓; dysphagia; excessive vomiting; GI bleeding), *refer for GI endoscopy*. If esophagitis confirmed, try a PPI (the most effective option). *Prokinetic drugs:* These help gastric emptying (eg metoclopramide; dystonias can be a serious side-effect).
3 *Endoscopy/surgery:* Endoscopic options are emerging. Nissen fundoplication, is not indicated unless symptoms are bad *and* there is radiological or pH-monitoring evidence of *severe* reflux. Laparoscopic repairs are favorable. **NB:** Surgery is better than drugs at improving asthma (less acid spill-over into the lung).[1]

---

1 In one randomized study (*n* = 62), surgery produced a 43% improvement in asthma symptom scores, compared with <10% in medical and control patients. There was a worsening of asthma in 12% of the surgical group, 36% of medical patients, and 48% of the control group. *Am J Gastroenterol* 2003 **98** 987.

Diarrhea

The normal daily stool weight is 100–200g, and in the US, a daily stool weight >200g is abnormal. *Diarrhea* means ↑ stool water (hence ↑ stool volume, eg >200mL daily), and this ↑ stool frequency and the passage of liquid stool. If it is the stool's fat content that is ↑, the diarrhea is termed *steatorrhea*. Distinguish both from *fecal urgency* (may be caused by cancers or UC, p224).

Conditions that cause diarrhea are broadly classified into **osmotic diarrhea** (stool output diminishes with reduced oral intake), **secretory diarrhea** (stool output persists despite reduction in oral intake), and **mucosal injury** categories. In reality, high-output diarrhea is usually a combination of these mechanisms. Normal-output diarrhea (stool volume <200g/d) is typically related to anorectal dysfunction. Foul-smelling, greasy stools are characteristic of steatorrhea.

Common causes	Uncommon	Rare
Gastroenteritis	Microscopic colitis[1]	Autonomic neuropathy
– viral	Celiac disease	Addison's disease
– bacterial	Chronic pancreatitis	Ischemic colitis
– parasites/protozoa	Thyrotoxicosis	Amyloidosis
Irritable bowel	Laxative abuse; food allergy	Tropical enteropathy
Drugs (below)	Lactose intolerance	Gastrinoma, VIPoma[2]
Colorectal cancer	Ileal/gastric resection	Carcinoid syndrome
Ulcerative colitis (UC)	Bacterial overgrowth	Medullary thyroid ca
Crohn's disease	Pseudomembranous colitis	Pellagra

Clinical features It is important to take a detailed and accurate history:

Is it acute (<3wks duration) or chronic (>3wks duration)? Acute: Usually infectious, or drug-induced. Ask about recent travel, sexual practices, ingestion of well water or inadequately cooked food and shellfish. Question for exposure to ill contacts

Chronic: Usually requires extensive history and further testing. Ask about prior bowel surgery and a family history. Additional testing should include: Stool studies for lactoferrin (fecal leukocytes), ova and parasites, cultures, and c. dificile toxin. Check for signs of labs of malabsorbption, including vitamins, and evaluate stool for steatorrhea (sudan stain). Often, radiographic and endoscopic evaluation with biopsies is required if above testing is normal.

- *Is the large or small bowel the source?* Large bowel symptoms: Watery stool ± blood or mucus; pelvic pain relieved by defecation; tenesmus; urgency. Small bowel symptoms: Periumbilical (or RIF) RLQ pain, not relieved by defecation; watery stool or steatorrhea.
- *Is there blood, mucus, or pus?* Bloody diarrhea: *Campylobacter, Shigella, Salmonella, E. coli*, amebiasis, Inflammatory bowel disease, malignancy, pseudomembranous colitis, ischemic colitis. *Mucus* occurs in IBS, colonic adenocarcinoma, polyps. *Pus* suggests inflammatory bowel disease or diverticulitis.
- *Could there be a non-GI cause?* Think of drugs (antibiotics; PPIs; cimetidine; propranolol; cytotoxics; NSAIDs; digoxin; alcohol; laxative abuse) and medical conditions (thyrotoxicosis, autonomic neuropathy, Addison's disease).

Examination *Look for:* weight↓, anemia, dehydration, oral ulcers, clubbing, rashes, and abdominal scars. *Feel for:* Enlarged thyroid or an abdominal mass. *Do a rectal examination:* Any rectal mass (rectal carcinoma), or impacted feces (overflow diarrhea)? Test stools for fecal occult blood.

---

1 Think of microscopic colitis in any chronic diarrhoea; do biopsy (may be +ve on normal looking colon mucosa—reported as 'lymphocytic' or 'collagenous' colitis). Prognosis: good. Bismuth subsalicylate may help (eg Pepto-Bismol®). L Schiller 2000 *Lancet* **355** 1198 & *Gastrointest Dis* 2000 **10** 145.
2 Vasoactive intestinal polypeptide-secreting tumor—suspect if hypokalaemic acidosis; Ca^{2+}↑; Mg^{2+}↓.

ests *Bloods:* In addition to above tests, look for evidence of iron deficiency r celiac sprue.

tool for pathogens & *C. dificile* toxin (pseudomembranous colitis). Fecal fat xcretion or ^{13}C-hiolein breath test if symptoms of chronic pancreatitis, nalabsorption, or steatorrhea are present.

Colonoscopy/Barium enema: In colitis, and to exclude malignancy. If normal, onsider small bowel radiology (Crohn's) ± endoscopic ultrasound or endo-copic retrograde cholangiopancreatography (ERCP) (p208, eg chronic pancreatitis).

Management Treat causes. Oral rehydration is preferable to IV rehydration. If severely dehydrated, give 0.9% saline + 20mmol K$^+$/L IVI. Codeine phos-hate 30mg/6h PO reduces stool frequency. Avoid antibiotics unless the atient has infective diarrhea and is systemically unwell.

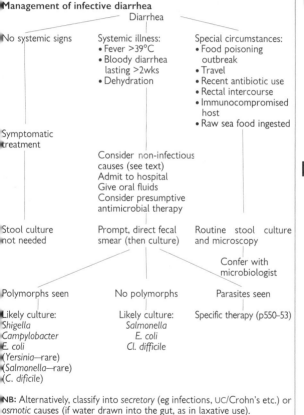

Management of infective diarrhea

Diarrhea

No systemic signs

Systemic illness:
• Fever >39°C
• Bloody diarrhea lasting >2wks
• Dehydration

Special circumstances:
• Food poisoning outbreak
• Travel
• Recent antibiotic use
• Rectal intercourse
• Immunocompromised host
• Raw sea food ingested

Symptomatic treatment

Consider non-infectious causes (see text)
Admit to hospital
Give oral fluids
Consider presumptive antimicrobial therapy

Stool culture not needed

Prompt, direct fecal smear (then culture)

Routine stool culture and microscopy

Confer with microbiologist

Polymorphs seen

Likely culture:
Shigella
Campylobacter
E. coli
(*Yersinia*—rare)
(*Salmonella*—rare)
(*C. dificile*)

No polymorphs

Likely culture:
Salmonella
E. coli
Cl. difficile

Parasites seen

Specific therapy (p550–53)

NB: Alternatively, classify into *secretory* (eg infections, UC/Crohn's etc.) or *osmotic* causes (if water drawn into the gut, as in laxative use).

199

Constipation

Constipation is defined as the symptomatic ↓ in stool frequency to ≤3 bowel movements per week, or difficulty in defecation, with straining or discomfort.

Causes of constipation are numerous and relate either to colonic transit impairment or to structure or functional obstruction to fecal evacuation (see BOX).

Clinical features Ask about frequency, nature, and consistency of the stool and in comparison to their past habits. Is there blood or mucus in/on the stools? Is there diarrhea alternating with constipation? Has there been a recent change in bowel habit? Ask about diet and drugs. Rectal examination is essential.

Tests Most constipation does not need investigation, especially young, mildly affected patients. Indications for investigation: Age >40yrs; recent change in bowel habit; associated symptoms (weight loss, rectal bleeding, mucous discharge, or tenesmus). *Blood tests:* TSH. *Colonoscopy* and biopsy of abnormal mucosa if testing is abnormal. Special investigations (eg transit studies anorectal physiology) are rarely indicated.

Treatment Treat the cause (see BOX). Advise exercise and adequate fluid intake (a high-fiber diet is often advised, but this may cause bloating without helping the constipation). Consider drugs only if these measures fail, and try to use them for short periods only. Often, a stimulant such as senna ± a bulking agent is more effective and cheaper than agents such as polyethylene glycol solutions.

Bulking agents ↑Fecal mass and thus stimulate peristalsis. CI: Difficulty in swallowing; intestinal obstruction; colonic atony; fecal impaction. *Stimulant laxatives* ↑ intestinal motility and should be avoided in intestinal obstruction. Prolonged use may cause colonic atony and hypokalemia. Pure stimulant laxatives include *bisacodyl* tablets (5–10mg at night) or suppositories (10mg in the mornings) and *senna* (2–4 tablets at night). *Glycerol suppositories* act as a rectal stimulant.

Stool softeners: Docusate sodium acts as a stool softener. *Liquid paraffin* should not be used for a prolonged period (SE: Anal seepage, lipoid pneumonia malabsorption of fat-soluble vitamins).

Osmotic laxatives retain fluid in the bowel. *Lactulose*, a semisynthetic disaccharide, produces an osmotic diarrhea of low fecal pH that discourages growth of ammonia-producing organisms. It is useful in hepatic encephalopathy, and used frequently for constipation. A major side effect is bloating that can often worsen the abdominal pain in constipated patients. A better alternative is polyethylene glycol (Miralax®) which is an osmotic laxative. *Magnesium salts* (eg magnesium hydroxide and magnesium sulfate) are useful when rapid bowel evacuation is required. *Sodium salts* (eg Microlette® and Micralax® enemas) should be avoided as they may cause sodium and water retention. *Phosphate enemas* are useful for rapid bowel evacuation prior to procedures.

What if laxatives don't help? A multi-disciplinary approach with behavior therapy, psychological support, habit training ± sphincter-action biofeedback may help. 5HT4 agonists are available with clinical trials underway.

Causes of constipation

Poor diet
Inadequate fluid intake or dehydration
Immobility (or lack of exercise)
Irritable bowel syndrome
Elderly
Post-operative pain

Anorectal disease
Anal fissure
Anal stricture
Rectal prolapse

Intestinal obstruction
Colorectal carcinoma
Strictures (eg Crohn's disease)
Pelvic mass (eg fibroids)
Diverticular disease (stricture formation)
Congenital abnormalities
Pseudo-obstruction

Metabolic/endocrine
Hypothyroidism
Hypercalcemia
Hypokalemia
Porphyria
Lead poisoning

Drugs
Opiate analgesics (eg morphine, codeine)
Anticholinergics (tricyclics, phenothiazines)
Iron

Neuromuscular (slow transit with ↓propulsive activity)
Spinal or pelvic nerve injury
Aganglionosis (Chagas' disease, Hirschsprung's disease)
Systemic sclerosis
Diabetic neuropathy

Other causes
Chronic laxative abuse (rare—diarrhea is more common)
Idiopathic slow transit
Idiopathic megarectum/colon
Psychological (eg associated with depression or abuse as a child).

Jaundice

Jaundice (icterus) refers to a yellow pigmentation of skin, sclera, and mucos due to an elevated plasma bilirubin level (visible at >3mg/dL). Jaundice may be classified by the type of circulating bilirubin (conjugated or unconjugated) or by the site of the problem (pre-hepatic, hepatocellular, or choles tatic/obstructive). *Bilirubin metabolism:* Bilirubin is formed from the break down of hemoglobin. It is conjugated with glucuronic acid by hepatocytes making it water soluble. Conjugated bilirubin is secreted into bile and passe into the duodenum. In the small intestine, bile is converted to urobilinogen by the gut flora. Most (>90%) of the urobilinogen is actively reabsorbed in the ileum and transported via the portal circulation to the liver. Some of the portal urobilinogen is re-taken by the hepatocytes and re-secreted into the bile (**enterohepatic circulation**). A portion of the bile bypasses the live and is excreted by the kidneys into the urine. The remainder of urobilinogen that is not reabsorbed in the ileum is converted to stercobilin in the dista small intestine or proximal colon, giving feces its characteristic brown color.

Pre-hepatic jaundice If there is excess bilirubin production (hemolysis inadequate liver uptake, or deficient hepatic conjugation), unconjugated bilirubin enters the blood. Because unconjugated bilirubin is water insoluble it is not excreted in urine, resulting in an *unconjugated (indirect) hyper bilirubinemia. Causes:* Physiological (neonatal); hemolysis; ineffective erythro poiesis; glucuronyl transferase deficiency (eg Gilbert's syndrome; Crigler-Najjar syndrome).

Hepatocellular jaundice There is hepatocyte damage ± cholestasis. *Causes Viruses:* Hepatitis (p516, eg, A, B, C, etc.), CMV, EBV (p511); drugs (see BOX) alcoholic hepatitis; cirrhosis; liver metastases/abscess; hemochromatosis; auto immune hepatitis (AIH); sepsis; leptospirosis; alpha-1-antitrypsin deficiency Budd–Chiari syndrome; Wilson's disease (p218); failure to excrete conjugated bilirubin (Dubin-Johnson and Rotor syndromes); right heart failure, causing sinusoidal congestion; toxins, eg carbon tetrachloride; fungi (*Amanita phal loides*).

Cholestatic (obstructive) jaundice Blockage or obstruction of the com mon bile duct results in *conjugated hyperbilirubinemia.* Conjugated bilirubin i water soluble and thus easily excreted into the urine. Jaundiced patient complain of dark, tea-colored urine. The lack of conjugated bilirubin reaching the gut (due to bile duct obstruction) prevents adequate urobilinogen forma tion. This causes the feces to become clay-colored. *Causes:* Choledocholithi asis; pancreatic cancer; lymph nodes at the porta hepatis; drugs (see BOX) cholangiocarcinoma; sclerosing cholangitis; primary biliary cirrhosis (PBC) choledochal cyst; biliary atresia.

Clinical features Ask about clues to a possible viral hepatitis such as bloo transfusions before 1990, IV drug use, body piercing, tattoos, sexual activity travel abroad, jaundiced contacts, etc. Also, query family history, alcoho consumption, and *all* medications (eg old drug charts and records). *Examine* for signs of chronic liver disease, hepatic encephalopathy, lymphadenopathy hepatomegaly, splenomegaly, palpable gall bladder, and ascites. Pale stools & dark urine ≈ obstructive jaundice.

Tests *Urine:* Bilirubin is absent in pre-hepatic causes; urobilinogen is absent in obstructive jaundice. *Hematology:* Signs of hemolysis (anemia, elevated LDH, low haptoglobin, elevated reticulocyte count, positive Coombs' test). *Biochemistry* LFT (bilirubin—direct and indirect, ALT, AST, alk phos, total protein, albumin) *Virology:* EBV, CMV, HAV, HBV, & HCV serologies. *Other specific tests,* eg for hemo chromatosis (elevated ferritin and iron:TIBC ratio, causing a high serum % iro saturation (>55–60%); alpha-1-antitrypsin deficiency (serum for genetic analysis) Wilson's disease (eg low serum and high urine copper levels, low serum ceruloplasmin (p218): PBC (high anti-mitochondrial antibody titres, AMA), and

AIH (high anti-nuclear and anti-smooth muscle antibodies). *Ultrasound:* Are the bile ducts dilated (obstruction)? Are there gallstones, hepatic metastases or pancreatic masses? Request *MRCP* (p209) OR *ERCP* if bile ducts are dilated. Consider performing a *liver biopsy* (p208) if the bile ducts are normal. Consider abdominal *CT or MRI scan*.

Drug-induced jaundice

Hepatitis	Phenytoin, carbamazepine, valproic acid
	Anti-TB meds (isoniazid, rifampin, pyrazinamide); nitrofurantoin; antifungals (ketoconazole, fluconazole, itraconazole); antivirals (DDI, AZT)
	Statins
	ACE-inhibitors, methyldopa, calcium channel blockers
	MAOI's, amitriptyline, imipramine
	Halothane (general anesthetic); NAIDs (ibuprofen, sulindac, diclofenac, indomethacin)
Cholestasis	Antibiotics (erythromycin, nitrofurantoin, rifampin)
	Anabolic steroids
	Oral contraceptives
	Chlorpromazine
	Prochlorperazine,
	Sulfonylureas, chlorpropamide
	Gold salts, cyclosporin

Causes of jaundice in a previously stable patient with cirrhosis

- Sepsis
- Alcohol
- Drugs
- Malignancy (eg hepatocellular carcinoma)
- GI bleeding

Upper gastrointestinal bleeding 1

Hematemesis is vomiting of blood. It may be bright or resemble coffee grounds. *Melena* is black, tarry-like stool (signifies altered blood) with a characteristic odor. Both indicate upper GI bleeding.

Causes

Common	Rare
Peptic ulcers	Bleeding disorders
Gastritis/gastric erosions	Portal hypertensive gastropathy
Mallory–Weiss tear	Aorto–enteric fistula; angiodysplasia
Duodenitis	Hemobilia (bleeding from biliary tree)
Esophageal varices	Dieulafoy lesion (rupture of a submu-
Esophagitis	cosal arteriole)
Malignancy	Meckel's diverticulum
Drugs (NSAIDs, steroids	Peutz–Jeghers' syndrome
thrombolytics, anticoagulants)	Osler–Weber–Rendu syndrome

Assessment Brief history and examination to assess severity.

History: Elicit a focused history evaluating for risk factors or conditions that are associated with severe GI bleeding. Assess for: Prior history of GI bleeding, history of PUD, known bleeding diathesis, underlying cirrhosis and portal hypertension, dysphagia, vomiting, weight loss, NSAID use, alcohol consumption. *Examination:* Look for stigmata of chronic liver disease and perform a digital rectal examination to check for melena. Assess for signs of vascular shock:
• Peripheral vasoconstriction (cool and clammy).
• Tachycardic (pulse >100bpm, and JVP not elevated).
• Hypotensive (systolic BP <100mmHg).
• Postural drop in BP (Orthostatic)
• Poor urine output, eg <30mL/h.

Calculating the *Rockall risk score* (see BOX) may help to risk-stratify the patient.

Acute management (p712) Critical to management is fluid resuscitation of a bleeding patient. In summary:
• Protect airway and give high-flow oxygen.
• Insert 2 large-bore (14–16G) IV cannula and draw blood for hemoglobin levels, clotting assessment, and type and cross for 4–6U PRBCs (1U per g/dL <14g/dL).
• Give IV colloid while waiting for blood to be cross-matched. In an emergency, give group O Rh-ve blood.
• Transfuse until hemodynamically stable.
• Correct clotting abnormalities (vitamin K, FFP, platelets).
• Monitor pulse, BP, and CVP at least hourly until stable.
• Insert a urinary catheter and monitor hrly urine output.
• Consider a CVP line to monitor CVP and guide fluid replacement.
• Obtain a CXR, ECG, and ABG in high-risk patients.
• Arrange an urgent endoscopy (p208).
• Notify surgeons of all severe bleeds on admission.

Further management
• Re-examine after 4h and give FFP if >4U transfused.
• Monitor pulse, BP, CVP, and urine output hourly; ↓frequency to 4h if hemodynamically stable.
• Check CBC, CMP, LFT, and clotting daily.
• Transfuse to keep Hb >10g/dL; always keep 2U of blood in reserve.
• Keep 'NPO' for 24h. Allow clear fluids after 24h and light diet after 48h, if no evidence of re-bleeding. Discuss with consulting gastroenterologist, if needed.
• IV or oral proton pump inhibitor.

Rockall risk-scoring system for GI bleeds

Score	0	1	2	3
Age	<60yrs	60–79yrs	80yrs	
Shock: Systolic BP pulse rate	BP >100mmHg <100/min	BP >100mmHg Pulse >100/min	BP <100mmHg	
Co-morbidity	No major	Cardiac failure Ischemic heart disease	Renal failure Liver failure	Metastases
Diagnosis	Mallory–Weiss tear; no lesion; no sign of recent bleeding	All other diagnoses	Upper GI malignancy	
Signs of recent haemorrhage on endoscopy	None, or dark-red spot		Blood in upper GI tract; Adherent clot; Visible vessel	

Rockall scores help predict risk of rebleeding and death after upper GI bleeding. A score >6 is said to be an indication for surgery—but decisions relating to surgery are rarely taken on the basis of Rockall scores alone.

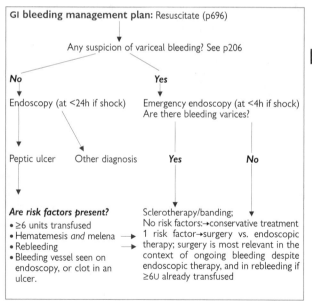

GI bleeding management plan: Resuscitate (p696)

Any suspicion of variceal bleeding? See p206

No

Endoscopy (at <24h if shock)

Peptic ulcer   Other diagnosis

Are risk factors present?
• ≥6 units transfused
• Hematemesis *and* melena
• Rebleeding
• Bleeding vessel seen on endoscopy, or clot in an ulcer.

Yes

Emergency endoscopy (at <4h if shock) Are there bleeding varices?

Yes   **No**

Sclerotherapy/banding;
No risk factors:→conservative treatment
1 risk factor→surgery vs. endoscopic therapy; surgery is most relevant in the context of ongoing bleeding despite endoscopic therapy, and in rebleeding if ≥6U already transfused

Endoscopy should be arranged after resuscitation, within 4h if variceal hemorrhage is suspected, or bleeding is ongoing—and otherwise within 12–24h of admission. It can identify the site of bleeding, be used to estimate the risk of rebleeding, and to administer endoscopic treatment. Stigmata of high risk rebleeding lesions for PUD include: Actively bleeding vessel (60%), adherent clot (40%), visible vessel (20%), flat spot (10%), clean base (5%).

Rebleeding Since rebleeders have ↑ mortality, identify these patients and monitor them closely for signs of rebleeding.

Guidelines for considering surgery
- Severe bleeding or bleeding despite transfusing 6U if >60yrs (8U if <60yrs)
- Rebleeding
- Active bleeding at endoscopy that cannot be controlled
- Rockall score >6 (p205).

Varices Portal hypertension causes dilated collateral veins (varices) at sites of porto-systemic anastomosis. Varices are most prevalently in the distal esophagus, but may also be found in the stomach (gastric varices), around the umbilicus (caput medusae—rare) and in the rectum (rectal varices) and duodenum (duodenal varices). Varices develop in patients with cirrhosis once portal pressure (measured by hepatic venous pressure gradient) is >10mmHg; if >12mmHg, variceal bleeding may develop—associated with a mortality of 30–50% per episode.

Causes of portal hypertension can be divided into: *Pre-hepatic:* Portal vein thrombosis; splenic vein thrombosis, Arterioportal fistula, splenomegaly. *Intrahepatic:* Cirrhosis; fulminant hepatitis, veno-occlusive disease, Budd-Chiari syndrome, schistosomiasis (common worldwide); sarcoidosis; myeloproliferative diseases; congenital hepatic fibrosis, metastatic malignnacy. *Post-hepatic:* Budd–Chiari syndrome; right heart failure; constrictive pericarditis; Inferior vena cava web.

Risk factors for variceal hemorrhage: ↑Portal pressure; variceal size, endoscopic features of the variceal wall, eg fresh clot, red wale sign, etc. and Child–Pugh score ≥8 (see BOX).

Suspect varices as a cause of GI bleeding if there is alcohol abuse or cirrhosis. Look for signs of chronic liver disease, encephalopathy, splenomegaly ± ascites.

Prophylaxis—primary: Without treatment, ~30% of cirrhotic patients with varices bleed. This is reduced to 15% by: (1) Non-selective β-blockers (propranolol) ± nitrates (isosorbide mononitrate). (2) Endoscopic ligation (banding) is be indicated for large varices. This ↓ risk of 1st bleeding when compared with propranolol. **NB:** Endoscopic sclerotherapy is not used as complications may outweigh benefits. *Secondary:* After an initial variceal bleed, risk of further bleeding is high. Options are (1) and (2) as above, + transjugular intrahepatic porto–systemic shunting **(TIPS)**[1] or surgical shunts. Endoscopic banding is better than sclerotherapy (lower bleeding rates & fewer complications). TIPS is also used in uncontrolled variceal hemorrhage. Consider surgical shunts if TIPS is impossible for technical reasons.

Acute variceal bleeding: Get expert help at the bedside from your experts.
- Resuscitate until hemodynamically stable (do not give 0.9% saline).
- Correct clotting abnormalities with vitamin K and FFP.
- Start IVI of octreotide (for 5d).
- Endoscopic therapy: **B**and ligation Y ± sclerotherapy—only if vasoactive drugs fail **NB:** Banding may be impossible (∵ limited visualization).
- If bleeding uncontrolled, a **M**innesota tube or **S**engstaken–**B**lakemore tube should be placed by someone with experience—or TIPS as above.

NB intensive sclerotherapy regimens ↓risk of rebleeding but may not ↑ survival.

1 TIPS works by shunting blood away from the portal circulation.

Balloon tamponade with a Sengstaken–Blakemore tube

In life-threatening variceal bleeding, this can buy time to arrange transfer to a specialist liver center or surgical decompression.

It uses balloons to compress gastric and esophageal varices.

Before insertion, inflate balloons with a measured volume (120–300mL) of air giving pressures of 60mmHg (check with a sphygmomanometer).

- Deflate, and clamp exits.
- Pass the lubricated tube (try to avoid sedation) and inflate the gastric balloon with the predetermined volume of air. **NB:** The tube is easier to pass when it is cold, which is why it is kept in the refrigerator.
- Inflate the esophageal balloon. Check pressures (should be 20–30mmHg greater than on the trial run). This phase of the procedure is dangerous: Do not over inflate the balloon (risk of esophageal necrosis or rupture). Often, hemodynamic stability can be achieved with inflation of the gastric balloon alone.
- Tape to patient's forehead to ensure the gastric balloon impacts gently on the gastroesophageal junction.
- Place the esophageal aspiration channel on continuous low suction and arrange for the gastric channel to drain freely.
- Leave *in situ* until bleeding stops. Remove after <24h.

Various other techniques of insertion may be used, and tubes vary in structure. *Do not try to pass one yourself if you have no or little experience:* Ask an expert; if unavailable, transfer urgently to a specialist liver center.

Endoscopy and biopsy

Upper GI endoscopy *Diagnostic indications*
- Dyspepsia, especially if >50yrs old
- Gastric biopsy (suspected malignancy)
- Duodenal biopsy (eg celiac disease)
- Hematemesis
- Persistent vomiting
- Iron-deficiency anemia.

Therapeutic: Primarily injection/coagulating of bleeding lesions. Also:
- Sclerotherapy or banding of esophageal varices
- Dilatation of strictures (esophageal, pyloric)
- Palliation of esophageal cancer (stent insertion, laser therapy, photodynamic therapy).
- Palliation of malignant obstruction (stent insertion).

Pre-procedure: NPO after midnight except for medications. Obtain informed written consent. Advise the patient not to drive for 24h if sedation is being given. Arrange follow-up.

Procedure: Sedation may be given (eg midazolam 2mg IV; monitor O_2 saturation with a pulse oximeter). The pharynx may be sprayed with local anesthetic and a flexible endoscope is swallowed. Continuous suction must be available to prevent aspiration. *Complications:* Transient sore throat; amnesia following sedation; perforation (<0.1%); cardiorespiratory arrest (<0.1%).

Duodenal biopsy is the gold standard for diagnosing celiac disease. Endoscopy with biopsy is also useful in investigating unusual causes of malabsorption, eg giardiasis, lymphoma, Whipple's disease, amyloid, eosinophilic gastroenteritis, or microscopic colitis.

Colonoscopy *Diagnostic indications:* Lower GI bleeding; iron deficiency; persistent diarrhea; biopsy of a known lesion or polyp; to assess for Crohn's or UC; colorectal cancer surveillance; *Strep. bovis* endocarditis.

Therapeutic indications: Polypectomy; Lower GI bleeding treatment; treating malignant obstruction, pseudo-obstruction or volvulus.

Preparation: Various prep solutions exist. Most commonly used is polyethylene glycol solution (1 gallon). Obtain written consent.

Procedure: Sedation and analgesia are given before a flexible colonoscope is passed per rectum around the colon.

Complications: Abdominal discomfort; incomplete examination; perforation (0.2%); hemorrhage after biopsy or polypectomy.

Percutaneous liver biopsy *Indications:* Abnormal LFT, chronic viral hepatitis; alcoholic hepatitis; auto-immune hepatitis (AIH); suspected cirrhosis; suspected carcinoma; biopsy of hepatic lesions; investigation of FUO.

Pre-procedure: NPO after midnight. Check clotting (INR <1.3) and platelet count (>100 × 10^9/L). Obtain written consent. Prescribe analgesia.

Procedure: Sedation (eg diazepam 5mg IV) may be given, but usually not required. The liver borders are percussed and local anesthethic (2% lidocaine) is injected to the region of maximal dullness in the midaxillary line during expiration. Breathing is rehearsed and a needle biopsy is taken with the breath held in expiration. Afterwards the patient lies on the right side for 2h, then in bed for 6h while regular pulse and BP observations are taken.

Complications: Local pain; pneumothorax/hemothorax; bleeding (<0.5%); death (<0.1%); biopsy of adjacent organ (eg gallbladder, kidney).

Radiological GI procedures

Abdominal ultrasound is used for the investigation of abdominal pain, abnormal LFT, jaundice, hepatomegaly or abdominal masses. Patients should be NPO by mouth for 4h before the scan in order to allow visualization of the gallbladder.

Pelvic ultrasound requires the bladder to be full. Ultrasound may also be used to guide diagnostic biopsy or therapeutic aspiration.

Endoscopic retrograde cholangiopancreatography (ERCP) *Diagnostic indications:* With the advent of MRCP (below), diagnostic ERCP is less commonly performed. Indications to perform ERCP prior to MRCP are for therapeutic intervention or when clinical suspicion is high for therapeutic intervention. Indications for ERCP include: Cholangitis; jaundice with dilated intrahepatic ducts; recurrent pancreatitis, symptomatic choledocholithiasis, biliary obstruction, biliary strictures. *Pre-pro-cedure:* Check clotting and platelet count. NPO after midnight. Informed consent. Sedation is accomplished similarly to other endoscopic procedures. *Procedure:* A catheter is advanced from a side-viewing duodenoscope via the ampulla into the common bile duct and/or pancreatic duct. Contrast medium is injected and x-rays taken to show lesions in the biliary tree and pancreatic ducts. *Complications:* Pancreatitis; bleeding; cholangitis; perforation. *Mortality:* <0.2% overall; 0.4% if stone removal.

Small bowel follow through After bowel preparation, barium is ingested and serial x-ray films are taken every 30min until barium reaches the caecum. Enhanced films are taken of areas of interest, eg terminal ileum.

Small bowel enema After bowel preparation, barium is introduced via duodenal intubation. Although technically more demanding than a barium follow-through, this method results in better mucosal definition.

Barium enema Always do a rectal exam first ± rigid sigmoidoscopy & biopsy. Preparation is per colonoscopy (p208). For double contrast barium enema, barium and air are introduced per rectum. Special views may be needed to visualize the areas of interest. Gastrografin may be used instead of barium in suspected colonic obstruction. It may show diverticular disease, or cancers (eg an irregular 'apple-core' narrowing of the lumen). In Crohn's disease, look for 'cobblestoning', 'rose thorn' ulcers, colonic strictures with rectal sparing. *Disadvantages:* Significant radiation dose; no biopsy possible.

Computer tomography (CT) is indicated if ultrasound is technically difficult or non-diagnostic. It allows better visualization of retroperitoneal structures but requires skilled interpretation. Oral or IV contrast may be given to enhance definition. The main disadvantage is the high radiation dose.

Magnetic resonance imaging (MRI) provides superior soft tissue imaging and enables the distinction of benign and malignant lesions. The other advantage over CT is the lack of radiation. Disadvantages are that patients with pacemakers and certain metal implants cannot be scanned, and that the scanner itself can induce claustrophobia. *Magnetic resonance cholangiopancreatography (MRCP)* MRCP enables in vivo anatomic exploration of the main pancreatic duct. Horizontal sections provide helpful radio-anatomic information. The technique nevertheless remains limited by poor spatial resolution. MRCP had a sensitivity of 83% and a specificity of 99% for diagnosing common bile duct stones, and according to some authorities, is the investigation of choice—partly, no doubt, due to lack of side-effects.

Endoscopic ultrasound: An ultrasound transducer is placed at the tip of an endoscope, allowing for unprecedented visualization of the GI tract and its adjacent structures. The layers of the GI tract can be discerned (allows for unprecendented evaluation of submucosal lesions), and adjacent organs (pancreas, mediastinal structures). A fine needle aspiration (FNA) can be accomplished through the endoscope, allowing for tissue acquistion. eus has revolutionized cancer diagnosis and staging of esophageal, pancreaticobiliary, gastric, and colorectal cancers.

Imaging via a wireless enteroscopy capsule This capsule is swallowed and sends images to a recorder worn by the patient. It allows for visualization of the small bowel mucosa, and is indicated for obscure GI bleeding, detection of IBD, etc. Recently, it is approved for evaluation of the esophagus, as well. Robotic biopsy and therapeutic procedures are not yet possible.

Liver failure

Definitions Liver failure may occur suddenly in the previously healthy liver: *Acute hepatic failure*; or more commonly, it may occur as a result of decompensation of chronic liver disease: *Acute-on-chronic hepatic failure*. *Fulminant hepatic failure* refers to severe acute liver injury with synthetic dysfunction and encephalopathy occurring within 8wks of the onset symptoms. *Subfulminant hepatic failure* refers to impaired synthetic function and encephalopathy occurring within 9–26wks (<6 months).

Causes *Infections:* Viral hepatitis, yellow fever, leptospirosis.
Drugs: Acetaminophen overdose, halothane, isoniazid.
Toxins: Amanita phalloides mushrooms, carbon tetrachloride.
Vascular: Budd–Chiari syndrome, veno-occlusive disease.

Clinical features *Hepatic encephalopathy* is graded as follows:
Others: 1° biliary cirrhosis, hemochromatosis, autoimmune hepatitis, alpha-1 antitrypsin deficiency, Wilson's disease, fatty liver of pregnancy, malignancy.
Grade I   Altered mood or behavioral changes, day-night reversal, hyperreflexia
Grade II   ↑ drowsiness or hypersomnia, confusion, slurred speech, asterixis
Grade III Stupor, incoherence, restlessness or severe agitation, clonus
Grade IV Coma, decerebrate posturing

Other features: Jaundice, fetor hepaticus (sweat pungent smell), constructional apraxia (ask the patient to draw a five-pointed star). Signs of chronic liver disease suggest acute-on-chronic hepatic failure.

Investigations

Blood tests: CBC (infection, GI bleed); chemistry (renal failure); LFT (bilirubin, AST, ALT, and alk phos); hepatic synthetic function (albumin, bilirubin, PT/INR); glucose (hypoglycemia), Acetaminophen level, ETOH level, hepatitis serologies, ferritin and iron studies, alpha-1-antitrypsin level, serum ceruloplasmin level.
Microbiology: Blood culture; urine culture; cell count/culture of ascites; ascitic neutrophils >250/mm³ indicates spontaneous bacterial peritonitis (SBP). Total ascitic WBC >500/mm³ also indicates SBP.
Radiology: CXR, abdominal ultrasound; Doppler flow studies of the portal vein and hepatic artery (and hepatic vein, in suspected Budd–Chiari).
Neurophysiological studies: EEG may show diffuse high-voltage slow waveforms.

Management Beware sepsis, hypoglycemia, and encephalopathy:
• Nursing care with a 20–30° head elevation in fulminant hepatic failure to reduce ICP and avoid aspiration. May also protect the airway by inserting an NG tube and removing any blood or other contents from stomach.
• Monitor temperature; pulse; RR; BP; pupils (uncal herniation due to ↑ ICP in fulminant hepatic failure); urine output hourly.
• Check CBC, chemistry, LFTs, and INR daily.
• Give 10% dextrose IV, 1L/12h to avoid hypoglycemia. Give 50mL 50% dextrose IV if blood glucose <60mg/dL (do every 1–4h in acute liver failure).
• Treat the cause, if known (eg acetaminophen poisoning, p738).
• If malnourished, obtain nutrition help (eg diet rich in carbohydrate- and protein-derived calories, preferably orally; in encephalopathy, avoid excessive protein in the diet (branched-chain amino acids may have a role in achieving +ve nitrogen balance). Give thiamine and folate supplements as needed.
• Hemofiltration or hemodialysis, if renal failure develops (see BOX).
• Avoid sedatives or other drugs with hepatic metabolism.
• Communicate early with your nearest liver transplant center regarding the appropriateness of transfer (see BOX).

Prognosis Poor prognostic factors: Grade III or IV encephalopathy, age >40yrs, albumin <3.0g/dL, drug-induced liver failure, subfulminant hepatic failure worse than fulminant failure—only 65% survival post-transplantation.

Treating the complications of acute hepatic failure

Bleeding: Vitamin K 10mg/d IV for 3d; platelets and/or FFP for active bleeding or procedures; PRBCs as needed; Recombinant activated Factor VII for invasive procedures

Infection: Until sensitivities are known, give ceftriaxone 1–2g/24h IV. Avoid gentamicin or other nephrotoxic meds (↑ risk of renal failure).

Ascites: Fluid restriction, low-sodium diet, diuretics; daily weights.

Hypoglycemia: Check blood glucose regularly and give 50mL of 50% glucose IV if levels fall below 60mg/dL. Monitor plasma K⁺.

Encephalopathy: Avoid sedatives; 20–30° head elevation in acute hepatic failure; lactulose to alter the gut flora and thus reduce nitrogen (ammonia) production. Aim for 3 soft stools/d; Be careful with oral neomycin—may worsen renal failure; consider oral rifaximin instead.

Cerebral edema: Give mannitol IV bolus at 0.5–1.0g/kg. Hyperventilation in times of impending herniation. Consider hypertonic saline, barbiturates, corticosteroids, or physician-induced hypothermia.

Hepatorenal syndrome (HRS): HRS occurs in ~18% of cirrhotic patients with ascites; due to intense renal vasoconstriction in the setting of splanchnic vasodilation; reduced GFR without significant proteinuria, and *normal* renal histology. *R:* Albumin IV ± hemodialysis. **NB:** ↑levels of neuropeptide Y (NPY) occur in HRS worsening renal vasoconstriction—terlipressin may help. (NPY is a renal vasoconstrictor peptide released on stimulation of sympathetic nervous system). Other possible therapies include midodrine and octreotide.

King's College Hospital UK criteria for liver transplantation

Acetaminophen related fulminant hepatic failure (FHF)	Arterial pH <7.3 following fluid resuscitation, regardless of the stage of encephalopathy *Or all of the following:* INR >6.5 Creatinine >3.4mg/dL Grade III or IV encephalopathy
Non-acetaminophen related FHF	INR >6.5

Or 3 out of 5 of the following:

1 Drug/toxin-induced liver failure, *or* indeterminate cause	**3** >1wk duration of jaundice prior to onset of encephalopathy
2 Age <10 or >40yrs old	**4** INR > 3.5
	5 Bilirubin >17mg/dL

In some centers, transplantation is either *cadaveric* or from *live donors* (eg. right lobe).

Prescribing in liver failure

Avoid opiates and benzodiazepines if possible. Be careful with diuretics (↑ risk of encephalopathy) and avoid oral hypoglycemic agents. Warfarin effects are enhanced, therefore monitor the INR closely. Avoid IV saline solutions which are hypotonic. Hepatotoxic drugs include: Acetaminophen, methotrexate, phenothiazines, isoniazid, azathioprine, estrogen, 6-mercaptopurine, salicylates, tetracycline, mitomycin, and several other antibiotics, antivirals, antifungals, antidepressants, etc… When in doubt, refer to the specific medication's package insert concerning potential adverse effects when prescribing a new medicine.

Cirrhosis

Cirrhosis implies irreversible liver damage. Histologically, there is loss of normal hepatic architecture with fibrosis and nodular regeneration.

Causes Chronic alcohol abuse, chronic viral hepatitis infections, primary biliary cirrhosis, hereditary hemochromatosis, and others: See BOX.

Presentation varies from asymptomatic with abnormal LFT's, to decompensated end-stage liver disease with all its associated complications. *Chronic liver disease:* Leukonychia—white nails without clear demarcation of the lunulae; Terry's nails—white proximally, but distal 30% reddened with telangiectasias; hypoalbuminemia with ascites; palmar erythema (hyperdynamic circulation); spider nevi or angiomas; Dupuytren's contracture (in alcoholic cirrhosis); gynecomastia; testicular atrophy; parotid gland enlargement; clubbing; hepatomegaly, or shrunken/fibrotic liver in late disease.

Complications *Hepatic failure:* Coagulopathy (low levels of factors II, VII, IX, & X cause elevated INR); encephalopathy—asterixis and confusion, coma; hypoalbuminemia (edema, leukopenia, ascites); sepsis (spontaneous bacterial peritonitis) hypoglycemia; GI bleeding; renal failure.

Portal hypertension: Ascites; splenomegaly; portosystemic shunts including esophageal varices (frequently present as a life-threatening upper GI bleed) and 'caput medusae' (enlarged superficial periumbilical veins). ↑Risk of hepatocellular carcinoma.

Tests *Blood:* LFT: ↔ or ↑bilirubin, ↑AST, ↑ALT, ↑alk phos & ↑GGT. Later, with loss of synthetic function, look for ↓albumin ± ↑PT/INR. Low WBC and platelets indicate hypersplenism. *Find the cause:* Ferritin, iron/total iron-binding capacity (p216); hepatitis serologies; quantitative immunoglobulins (p221); autoantibodies (ANA, AMA, SMA); alpha-fetoprotein (p219) level-AFP-; ceruloplasmin (p218); alpha-1-antitrypsin (p222).

Liver ultrasound may show hepatomegaly, splenomegaly, focal liver lesion(s), hepatic vein thrombi, reversal of flow in the portal vein, or ascites. *MRI:* Caudate lobe size↑, smaller islands of regenerating nodules, and the presence of the right posterior hepatic notch are more frequent in alcoholic cirrhosis than in virus-induced cirrhosis. MRI scoring systems based on spleen volume, liver volume, and the presence of ascites or varices/collaterals can quantify the severity of cirrhosis in a manner that correlates well with Child–Pugh grades (see BOX).

Ascitic tap should always be performed and fluid sent for urgent cell count, C&S: An ascitic neutrophil count of >250/mm³ indicates spontaneous bacterial peritonitis. Also, a total WBC>500/mm³ indicates SBP. *Liver biopsy* confirms the clinical diagnosis. This may be done percutaneously (if the INR=1.5 or less, and the platelet count=50K or greater) or via the transjugular route with FFP or activated recombinant Factor VII.

Management *General:* Good nutrition (avoid protein excess), low-sodium diet (especially if ascites); alcohol abstinence; avoid NSAIDs, sedatives, and opiates; vaccinate against HAV and HBV; Cholestyramine may help pruritus (4g PO bid, 1h after other drugs). Consider ultrasound and AFP level every 3–6 months to screen for HCC, p222.

Specific treatments: Pegylated interferon alpha plus ribaviron improves liver biochemistries and may prevent the development decompensated liver disease and/or hepatocellular cancer (HCC) in HCV-induced cirrhosis. Meta-analyses show some benefit of ursodeoxycholic acid in PBC and PSC. Penicillamine for Wilson's disease (p218), aggressive phlebotomy for hereditary hemochromatosis.

Ascites: Fluid restriction (<1.5L/d), low-sodium diet (40–100mmol/d). Spironolactone (aldactone), start 50–100mg/24h PO (usually given in two divided doses as bid); ↑dose every 48h to 400mg/24h if necessary to control ascites and edema; carefully monitor serum K⁺ levels; chart daily weights, aim for weight loss of ≤½kg/d. If response to aldactone is poor, add furosemide 40–120mg/24h PO (usually given in a ratio of 4:10 with aldactone—eg. furosemide 40mg and aldactone 100mg, or furosemide 80mg and aldactone 200mg); check BUN/creatinine and serum Na⁺ often; Therapeutic paracentesis with concomitant albumin infusion (6–8g/L fluid removed) may be tried—albumin infusion during large volume paracentesis may prevent HRS.

Spontaneous bacterial peritonitis: Treatment: Eg ceftriaxone 1–2g/24h or Zosyn 3.375g q6 (pay special attention to dosing; it depends on degree of liver failure and renal failure); fine tune antibiotic coverage after the sensitivities are known. *Prophylaxis:* Bactrim DS tab PO 3–5x/wk; norfloxacin 400mg PO qd; ciprofloxacin 750mg PO qwk.

Prognosis Overall 5yr survival is ~50%. Poor prognostic indicators: Encephalopathy; serum Na⁺<110mEq/L; serum albumin <2.5g/dL; ↑INR.

Liver transplantation is the only definitive treatment for cirrhosis. This ↑ 5yr survival from ~20% in end-stage disease to ~70%.

Causes of cirrhosis

- Chronic alcohol abuse
- Chronic HBV or HCV infection
- Autoimmune disease: PBC (p220); primary sclerosing cholangitis (PSC) (p221); autoimmune hepatitis.
- Genetic disorders: Alpha-1-antitrypsin deficiency (p219); Wilson's disease (p218); hereditary hemochromatosis (p216).
- Others: Budd–Chiari syndrome (hepatic vein thrombosis).
- Drugs: Eg amiodarone, methyldopa, methotrexate

Child–Pugh grading and risk of variceal bleeding

213

Risk ↑↑ if score ≥8

	1 point	2 points	3 points
Bilirubin (mg/dL)	<2	2–3	>3
Albumin (g/dL)	>3.5	2.8–3.5	<2.8
INR	<1.7	1.7–2.3	>2.3
Ascites	None	Slight	Moderate
Encephalopathy	None	1–2	3–4

Alcoholism

An alcoholic is one whose repeated drinking leads to harm in their work or social life. Denial is a leading feature of alcoholism, so it may be helpful to query relatives. Screening tests: MCV↑; gamma-GT↑.

CAGE questions Screening for alcohol abuse: Ever felt you ought to **C**UT down on your drinking? Have people **a**nnoyed you by criticizing your drinking? Ever felt bad or **g**uilty about your drinking? Ever had an **e**ye-opener to steady nerves in the morning? CAGE is quite good at detecting alcohol abuse and dependence (sensitivity, 43–94%; specificity, 70–97%).

Organs affected by alcohol • *The liver:* (Normal in 50% of alcoholics.)

Fatty liver: Acute and reversible, but may progress to cirrhosis if drinking continues (also seen in obesity, DM, and with certain medications). *Cirrhosis:* 5yr survival is 48% if drinking continues (if not, 77%). *Hepatitis:* TPR↑, anorexia, tender hepatomegaly ± jaundice, bleeding, ascites, WBC↑, INR↓, AST↑, MCV↑, urea↑ (HRS). 80% progress to cirrhosis (hepatic failure in 10%). *Biopsy:* Mallory bodies ± neutrophil infiltrate. ℞: See BOX.

- *CNS:* Poor memory/cognition: Multiple high-potency vitamins IM may reverse it; cortical atrophy; retrobulbar neuropathy; fits; falls; wide-based gait neuropathy; Korsakoff's ± Wernicke's encephalopathy.
- *Gut:* Obesity, diarrhea; gastric erosions; peptic ulcers; varices; pancreatitis (acute and chronic).
- *Blood:* MCV↑; anemia from: Marrow depression, GI bleeds, alcoholism-associated folate deficiency, hemolysis; sideroblastic anemia.
- *Heart:* Arrhythmia; BP↑ cardiomyopathy; sudden death in binge drinkers.

Withdrawal signs Pulse↑; BP↓; tremor; fits; hallucinations (*delirium tremens*) may be visual or tactile, eg of animals crawling under one's skin.

Alcohol contraindications Driving; hepatitis; cirrhosis; peptic ulcer; drugs (eg antihistamines); carcinoid; pregnancy (fetal alcohol syndrome—IQ↓, short palpebral fissure, absent filtrum, and small eyes).

Management *Alcohol withdrawal:* Admit; do BP + TPR/4h. Beware BP↓. For the 1st 3d give generous chlordiazepoxide, eg 10–50mg/6h PO, weaning over 7–14d; alternative exist. Vitamins required.

Treating established alcoholics may be rewarding, particularly if they really want to change. If so, *group therapy* or self-help (eg 'Alcoholics Anonymous') may be useful.

Relapse: 50% will relapse in the months following initiation of treatment: *Anxiety, insomnia, and craving* may be intense, and is mitigated by *acamprosate*; CI: Pregnancy, severe liver failure, creatinine >120mcmol/L; SE: D&V, libido ↑ or ↓; dose example: 666mg/8h PO if >60kg and <65yrs old.

Reducing pleasure that alcohol brings (and ↓craving): Naltrexone 50mg/24h PO can halve relapse rates. SE: Vomiting, drowsiness, dizziness, cramps, arthralgia. CI: Liver failure. It is costly. Confer with experts if drugs are to be used.

Patterns of lab tests in alcoholic and other liver disease

	AST *Aspartate aminotransferase*	ALT *Alanine aminotransferase*	MCV *Mean cell volume*
Alcoholic liver disease	↑↑ *(twice as high as ALT)*	↑	↑↑
Hepatitis C (HCV)	↑ or ↔*	↑↑ *(higher than AST)*	↔
Non-alcoholic fatty liver disease	↑	↑↑	↑ or ↔

*In HCV, AST:ALT ratio is typically <1; ratio may reverse if cirrhosis develops. GGT may be ↑↑ in alcoholic liver disease, but is rather non-specific.

Managing alcoholic hepatitis

- Stop alcohol consumption (for withdrawal symptoms, if chlordiazepoxide by the oral route is impossible, try lorazepam IM).
- High-dose B vitamins IV.
- Optimize nutrition (35–40kcal/kg/d non-protein energy) + 1.5g/kg/d of protein (use ideal body weight for calculations eg if malnourished). This prevents encephalopathy, sepsis, and some deaths.
- Daily weight; LFT; BMP; INR. If creatinine↑, get help with this HRS, ie renal failure where the underlying pathology is hepatic. Na⁺↓ is common, but water restriction may make matters worse.
- Culture ascites fluid—appropriate antibiotics in the light of sensitivities.
- Prednisolone 40mg/d for 5d tapered off over 3wks *may* help.[1] Contraindications includes GI bleeding and infection. Anti-tumor necrosis factor antibodies, pentoxifylline may be helpful for acute alcoholic hepatitis. Liver transplantation is not an option for patients with acute alcoholic hepatitis or without history of documented abstinence.

215

---

1 Perhaps only if encephalopathy is present; see *Drug Ther Bul* 2003 **41** (July) 49.

Hereditary hemochromatosis (HH)

This is an inherited disorder of iron metabolism in which ↑ intestinal iron absorption leads to its deposition in multiple organs (joints, liver, heart, pancreas, and pituitary). Middle-aged males are more frequently and severely affected than women, in whom the disease tends to present ~10yrs later (menstrual blood loss is protective). Disease onset is usually at 40–50yrs in men, and 50–60yrs in women.

Genetics HH is one of the most common inherited diseases in those of Northern European ancestry (carrier rate of ~1 in 10 and a frequency of homozygosity of ~1:200–1:400). The gene responsible for most HH is the HFE gene located on chromosome 6. Two major mutations are termed C282Y and H63D. C282Y accounts for 60–100% of HH, and H63D accounts for 3–7%, with compound heterozygotes accounting for 1–4%. Penetrance is unknown but is clearly <100%.

Clinical features Asymptomatic early on—then fatigue, weakness, lethargy and arthralgias (MCP and large joints) usually develop. Later, look for slate-grey skin pigmentation, diabetes mellitus ('bronze diabetes'), and stigmata of chronic liver disease; hepatomegaly early on; small and shrunken cirrhotic liver later on; heart failure (dilated cardiomyopathy) and conduction disturbances; hypogonadism, (pituitary dysfunction, or via cirrhosis) and associated osteoporosis. Other endocrinopathies include hyporeninemic hypoaldosteronism.

Tests *Blood:* Abnormal LFT; ↑serum ferritin; ↑serum iron:TIBC ratio; transferrin saturation >60%, often >80%. HFE genotyping. Blood glucose to look for diabetes. *Joint x-rays* may show chondrocalcinosis. *Liver biopsy:* Perl's stain quantifies iron loading (hepatic iron index (HII) >1.9mcmol/kg/yr) and assesses disease severity. *MRI* also helps estimate hepatic iron loading. Do EKG & echo if you suspect cardiomyopathy.

216

Management *Phlebotomize* ~1U/wk until mildly iron-deficient. Iron will continue to accumulate, so maintenance phlebotomy (1U every 2–3 months) is needed for life. Maintain hemoglobin at about 10–12g/dL, serum ferritin <50ng/mL, and transferrin saturation <50%. *Other monitoring:* Diabetes. Hb$_{A1c}$ levels may be falsely low as phlebotomy reduces the time available for Hb glycosylation. *Over-the-counter self-medication:* Make sure that vitamin preparations etc. contain no iron. *Screening:* Test serum ferritin, transferring saturation, and genotype in 1st-degree relatives. Prevalence of iron overload in asymptomatic C282Y homozygotes is 4.5 per 1000 persons screened. How many will go on to develop iron overload is unknown.

Prognosis Phlebotomy returns life expectancy to normal if non-cirrhotic and non-diabetic. Arthropathy may not improve or even worsen. Gonadal failure is irreversible. In non-cirrhotic patients, phlebotomy may improve liver histology. Cirrhotic patients have >10% chance of developing HCC. Sources vary on the exact risk: Some authorities quote 30%; others 22%. One cause of variability is varying co-factors: Age over 50yrs ↑risk by 13-fold; being HBsAg positive by 5-fold, and alcohol abuse by 2-fold.

Secondary hemochromatosis may occur in any hematological condition where many transfusions (~80U) have been given. To reduce the need for transfusions, find out if the hematological condition responds to erythropoietin or marrow transplantation before the irreversible effects of iron overload become too great.

Autoimmune hepatitis (AIH)

An inflammatory liver disease of unknown cause characterized by suppressor T-cell defects with autoantibodies directed against hepatocyte surface antigens. This disease is a steroid-responsive hepatitis. Two types are distinguished by the presence of circulating autoantibodies:

Type I   Affects both adults or children
             Anti-nuclear antibodies (ANA) and/or
             Anti-smooth muscle antibodies (ASMA) positive in 80%.
             Other autoantibodies associated with type I include: Anti-soluble liver Ab (ASLA), anti-dsDNA Ab, and P-ANCA.
Type II   Affects children; generally girls and some young women
             Anti-liver/kidney microsomal type 1 (ALKM-1) antibodies.
             Other autoantibodies associated with type II include:
             Anti-liver cytosol antigen (ALC-1)

Clinical features Predominantly affects young and middle-aged women. 25% of patients present with acute hepatitis and features of an autoimmune disease (eg fever, malaise, urticarial rash, polyarthritis, pleurisy, or glomerulonephritis). The remainder present insidiously or are asymptomatic and diagnosed incidentally with signs of chronic liver disease. Amenorrhea is common.

Associations

Pernicious anemia	Autoimmune hemolysis	Ulcerative colitis
Diabetes	Glomerulonephritis	HLA A1, B8, & DR3 haplotype
Autoimmune thyroiditis	PSC	PBC

Tests Abnormal LFT (AST AND ALT↑), hypergammaglobulinemia (especially IgG), positive autoantibodies: ANA, ASMA, ALKM-1, ETC. (see above). Anemia, leukopenia and thrombocytopenia indicate hypersplenism. Liver biopsy shows a mononuclear infiltrate (usually plasma cells) within the portal, and then periportal areas. This may be followed by piecemeal necrosis, bridging fibrosis, or cirrhosis. ERCP helps exclude PSC if the alk phos is disproportionately ↑.

217

Diagnosis depends on excluding other diseases as there is no pathognomonic sign or lab test. There is genuine overlap with PBC. Diagnostic criteria exist but are not fully validated.

Management *Prednisone* 30–40mg/d PO for 1 month; ↓by 5mg a month to a maintenance dose of 5–10mg/d PO. Corticosteroids can sometimes be stopped after a few years, but relapse occurs in 50–86%. *Azathioprine* (50–100mg/d PO) may be used alone as a steroid-sparing agent, or in combination with lower doses of prednisone. Remission is achievable in 80% of patients within 3yrs. *10- and 20yr survival rates:* >80%. The goal is to achieve a sustained remission without the need for further drug therapy; achievable in 10–40% of patients overall.

Non-standard proposed therapies to avoid steroid side-effects: Cyclosporin, budesonide, tacrolimus, mycophenolate mofetil, ursodeoxycholic acid, methotrexate, cyclophosphamide, 6-mercaptopurine, and free radical scavengers.

Liver transplantation is indicated for decompensated cirrhosis, but recurrence may occur. Post-transplant 10yr survival rate is 75%.

Wilson's disease/hepatolenticular degeneration

A rare inherited disorder with toxic accumulation of copper (Cu) in liver and CNS (especially basal ganglia, eg globus pallidus hypodensity ± putamen cavitation). It is treatable, so screen all young patients with evidence of liver disease. *Genetics:* Autosomal recessive (gene on chromosome 13; codes for a copper transporting ATPase, ATP7B). 27 mutations are known; HIS1069GLU is the most common.

Signs Children usually present with *liver disease* (hepatitis, cirrhosis, fulminant hepatic failure); young adults often start with *CNS signs:* Tremor; dysarthria; dysphagia; dyskinesias; dystonias; purposeless stereotyped movements (eg hand clapping); dementia; parkinsonism; micrographia; ataxia/clumsiness. *Affective features:* Depression/mania; labile emotions; ↑ libido; personality changes. *Cognitive/behavioral:* Memory deficits; quick to anger; slow to solve problems; decline in IQ. *Psychosis:* Delusions; mutism. *Kayser-Fleischer rings:* Cu deposits in the cornia around the iris (Descemet's membrane), pathognomonic but not always present; may need slit lamp to detect. *Also:* Hemolysis; blue lunulae (nails); polyarthritis; hypermobile joints; grey skin; hypoparathyroidism.

Tests Serum copper and ceruloplasmin usually low. 24h urinary copper excretion is elevated (>100mcg/24h, normal <40mcg). Liver biopsy: ↑hepatic copper content. Molecular genetic testing can confirm the diagnosis. MRI: Basal ganglia degeneration (± fronto-temporal, cerebellar, and brain stem atrophy).

Management *Chelation:* Lifelong penicillamine (1000–1500mg/24h in 2–4 divided doses for the first 4–6 months; then maintenance dosing at 750–1000mg/24h in 2 divided doses). SE: Nausea, rash, leukopenia, anemia, thrombocytopenia, hematuria, nephrotic range proteinuria, lupus. Watch closely for those patients with a known PCN allergy—will likely have a reaction to penicillamine as well. Monitor CBC & urinary Cu (and protein) excretion. Stop if WBC <2.5×10⁹/L, or platelets falling <100k. *Alternative:* Trientine dihydrochloride 750–1500mg/24h in 2–3 divided doses (SE: Rash; sideroblastic anemia). *Liver transplant* if *severe* liver disease. *Screen siblings* as asymptomatic homozygotes need treatment.

Prognosis Pre-cirrhotic liver disease is reversible. Neurological damage less so. Death occurs from liver failure, variceal hemorrhage, or infection (the typical complications associated with end-stage liver disease).

Alpha-1-antitrypsin deficiency

Alpha-1-antitrypsin is one of a family of serine protease inhibitors controlling inflammatory cascades. It is synthesized in the liver, making up 90% of serum alpha globulin on electrophoresis. Alpha-1-antitrypsin deficiency is the chief genetic cause of liver disease in children. In adults, its deficiency causes emphysema, chronic liver disease, and HCC. *Other associations:* Asthma, pancreatitis, gallstones, Wegener's. ↓ risk of stroke. *Prevalence:* 1:2000–1:7000.

Genetics *Carrier frequency:* 1:10. Genetic variants are typed by their electrophoretic mobility as *medium* (M), *slow* (S), or *very slow* (Z). S and Z types are due to single amino acid substitutions at positions 264 and 342, respectively. These result in diminished production of alpha-1-antitrypsin (S=60%, Z=15%). The normal genotype is PIMM, the homozygote is PIZZ; heterozygotes are PIMZ & PISZ.

Symptomatic patients (eg *cholestatic jaundice*/cirrhosis; *dyspnea* from emphysema) usually have PIZZ genotype. **NB:** Cholestasis often remits in adolescence. In adults, cirrhosis ± HCC affects 25% of all alpha-1-antitrypsin-deficient individuals >50yrs.

Tests *Serum alpha-1-antitrypsin* levels are low. *Liver biopsy:* Periodic acid Schiff (PAS) positive; diastase-resistant globules. *Phenotyping* by isoelectric focusing requires expertise to distinguish SZ and ZZ phenotypes. *Prenatal diagnosis* is possible by DNA analysis of chorionic villus samples obtained at 11–13wks gestation. DNA tests are likely to find greater use in the future.

Management *Supportive* for emphysema and hepatic complications. Smoking cessation; consider *augmentation therapy* with human alpha-1-antitrypsin if FEV1 <80% of predicted (expensive!) ± *liver transplant* in decompensated cirrhosis.

Primary biliary cirrhosis (PBC)

Interlobular, intrahepatic bile ducts are damaged by chronic granulomatous inflammation causing progressive cholestasis, cirrhosis, and portal hypertension. *Cause:* ?autoimmune. *Female:male ratio*≈9:1. *Prevalence:* 19–51 cases per million population. *Peak presentation:* ~50yrs old.

Clinical features 50–60% of patients are asymptomatic and diagnosed only after finding ↑alk phos on routine LFTs. Lethargy and pruritus are the most common symptoms in symptomatic patients, and they may precede jaundice by months to years. Signs: Jaundice; skin pigmentation (due to melanosis) xanthelasma; xanthomata; hepatomegaly; and splenomegaly.

Complications: Osteoporosis is common. Malabsorption of fat-soluble vitamins (A, D, K, E) results in osteomalacia and coagulopathy. Other complications: Portal hypertension; ascites; variceal hemorrhage; hepatic encephalopathy; HCC (p222).

Tests *Blood tests:* ↑Alk phos, ↑GGT and 5'-nucleotidase levels, and mildly ↑AST and ALT; late disease: ↑bilirubin, low albumin, ↑PT/INR. 98% are antimitochondrial antibody (AMA) M$_2$ subtype positive (highly specific). Other autoantibodies, such as ANA, may occur in low titers. Immunoglobulins are ↑ (especially IgM). TSH and cholesterol may be ↑.

Radiology: Ultrasound, & ERCP OR MRCP to exclude extrahepatic cholestasis

Liver biopsy: Granulomas around the intrahepatic bile ducts, progressing to cirrhosis.

Treatment *Symptomatic:* Pruritus: Try cholestyramine 4g PO BID–TID. Diarrhea (usually from steatorrhea): PRN imodium or loperamide; can also use pancreatic enzymes as there is often an associated pancreatic insufficiency as well. Osteoporosis prevention (p286).

Specific: Fat-soluble vitamin prophylaxis: Vitamin A, D, and K. Consider *ursodeoxycholic acid* (UDCA), 13–15mg/kg/d to all patients which may obviate the need for *liver transplantation*, which is the last recourse for patients with end stage disease and/or intractable pruritus. Recurrence in the graft may occur but appears not to influence graft success. Other therapies that have been tried besides UCDA include colchicine and methotrexate.

Prognosis Once jaundice develops, survival is <2yrs. In one study, at 2yr post-transplant, predicted survival without retransplant was 55% and actual survival was 79%. At 7yrs, these figures were 22% and 68%, respectively.

Primary sclerosing cholangitis (PSC)

A disorder of unknown cause characterized by inflammation, fibrosis, and strictures of both the intra- and extra-hepatic bile ducts. Immunological mechanisms are implicated. Associations: Ulcerative colitis, 80% of PSC patients also have UC, but only 5% of UC patients have PSC; also associated with HLA-A1, B8, & DR3.

Clinical features Chronic biliary obstruction and secondary biliary cirrhosis lead to liver failure and death (or transplantation) over ~10–12yrs.

Symptoms: Patients may be asymptomatic and diagnosed incidentally after finding an elevated alk phos on routine LFTs; or patients may experience fluctuating symptoms such as jaundice, pruritus, RUQ abdominal pain, and fatigue. *Signs:* Jaundice; hepatomegaly; portal hypertension.

Complications: Bacterial cholangitis; cholangiocarcinoma (10–15% lifetime risk); ↑risk of colorectal cancer in those patients with concomitant UC; 30% of patients in some series have an overlap syndrome with type 1 AIH (p217).[1]

Tests *Blood:* ↑Alk phos initially followed by ↑bilirubin; hypergammaglobulinemia (often first manifested as an elevated serum total protein level); AMA negative, but ANA, ASMA, & P-ANCA may be +ve. *ERCP OR MRCP* shows multiple strictures of the biliary tree (characteristic 'beaded' appearance). *Liver biopsy* shows a fibrous obliteration of the bile ducts with concentric replacement by connective tissue in an 'onion skin' fashion.

Management *Drugs:* Corticosteroids and other immunosuppressives have shown little benefit in stopping the progression of disease and delaying the need for liver transplantation; Ursodeoxycholic acid (UCDA) in higher doses (20–30mg/kg/d) has been shown to improve liver biochemistries and histology in a few small pilot studies. Larger scale prospective studies assessing its effect on overall mortality and time to transplantation are underway; Cholestyramine 4g PO bid/tid for pruritus; Antibiotics (ciprofloxacin) for bacterial cholangitis, and for prophylaxis before invasive GI procedures.

221

Endoscopic or radiologic stenting helps symptomatic dominant strictures. *Liver transplantation* is indicated in end-stage disease. Recurrence occurs in 20%; 5yr graft survival is >60%.

Disease associations

Primary biliary cirrhosis (PBC)
- Thyroid disease
- Rheumatoid arthritis
- Sjögren's syndrome (70%)
- Keratoconjunctivitis, sicca syndrome
- Progressive systemic sclerosis
- Renal tubular acidosis
- Membranous glomerulonephritis

Primary sclerosing cholangitis (PSC)
- Ulcerative colitis (5% of those with UC have PSC; 80% of those with PSC have UC)
- Crohn's disease (much rarer); HIV infection

---

1 Do anti-mitochondrial, anti-nuclear, anti-smooth muscle, anti-liver kidney microsomal type 1, anti-liver cytosol type 1, perinuclear anti-neutrophil nuclear, & anti-soluble liver antigen antibodies.

Liver tumors

The most common liver tumors are secondary (metastatic) tumors. They frequently arise from primary malignancies in the breast, lung, or gastrointestinal tract. Primary hepatic tumors are much less common and may be benign or malignant.

Symptoms Fever, malaise, anorexia, weight loss, RUQ pain (due to liver capsule stretch). Jaundice is late (except with cholangiocarcinoma). Benign tumors are often asymptomatic; if they are large enough, they may cause symptoms due to shear mass effect. Tumors may rupture causing life-threatening intraperitoneal hemorrhage.

Signs Hepatomegaly (smooth, or hard and irregular, eg metastases, cirrhosis, HCC). Look for signs of chronic liver disease and evidence of decompensation (jaundice, ascites). Feel for an abdominal mass or primary lesion. Listen for an arterial bruit over the liver (HCC).

Tests *Blood:* CBC, PT/INR, LFTs, hepatitis serologies, AFP level (↑ in 80% of HCC), CEA level.

Imaging: Ultrasound or CT to identify lesions and guide diagnostic biopsies. MRI is better for distinguishing benign from malignant lesions. ERCP and biopsy/brushings should be performed for suspected cholangiocarcinoma.

Biopsy under ultrasound or CT guidance may achieve a histological diagnosis; exercise extreme care and caution, as seeding along biopsy tract may occur.

Other investigations for metastases (eg CXR, mammography, endoscopy, colonoscopy, CT, marrow biopsy) are tailored according to the suspected primary.

Liver metastases signify advanced disease for any primary malignancy. Treatment and prognosis vary with the type and extent of primary tumor. Chemotherapy may be effective (eg for lymphomas, germ cell tumors). Small, solitary metastases may be amenable to resection. In most, treatment is palliative. Prognosis: <6–9 months.

Hepatocellular carcinoma (HCC) A malignant tumor of hepatocytes accounting for 90% of primary liver cancers. Rare in the West (2–3% of all cancers), but more common in China and sub-Saharan Africa (40% of cancers).

Causes: Cirrhosis, due to any underlying cause (eg alcohol, chronic viral hepatitis, PBC, hereditary hemochromatosis, etc.); in the US, HCV-associated liver disease is a more common cause than HBV; yet in Asia and Africa, chronic HBV-associated liver disease is the more common underlying etiology; other causes include: Aflatoxin, parasites (*Clonorchis sinensis*), drugs (anabolic & contraceptive steroids).

Management: Older studies that reported on liver transplantation as treatment for HCC had disappointing results. However, with newer selection criteria (eg, 3 or fewer tumor nodules that are no more than 3cm in diameter, or a single nodule less than 5cm and without vascular invasion) better outcomes are being achieved. Some studies show 4-year survival rates as high as 75% after transplant. Surgical resection of solitary tumors <3cm diameter gives a 3yr survival rate of 59% (baseline 3yr survival rate is 13%). Local ablative therapy and intra-arterial chemoembolization are reasonable options with decent 5yr survival rates for those patients who are not surgical candidates. Systemic chemotherapy has yielded disappointing results.

Prognosis: Often <6 months without any intervention—95% 5yr mortality. A subtype of HCC known as fibrolamellar HCC, which occurs in children/young adults, has a better prognosis (60% 5yr survival).

Prevention is the key. Ensure HBV vaccination (see BOX). Do not reuse needles. Reduce exposure to aflatoxins (anti-humidity measures such as sun-drying to ↓spread of this common fungal contaminant in stored maize); this is especially important for those who harbor chronic HBV (risk is highly synergistic).

Cholangiocarcinoma (=Biliary tree malignancy; ~10% of liver primaries.) 1/3 are intrahepatic cholangiocellular cancers, and 2/3 are extrahepatic ductal cholangiocarcinomas.

Causes: PSC—occurring in 8–13% of these patients; congenital biliary cysts; biliary–enteric drainage surgery;

The patient: Fever, abdominal pain (±ascites), malaise, bilirubin↑; alk phos↑↑, jaundice.

Pathology: Usually slow-growing. Most are distal extrahepatic or perihilar. A Klatskin tumor is a nodular cholangiocarcinoma arising at the bifurcation of the common hepatic duct; it is frequently associated with a collapsed gallbladder.

Management: 70% are not surgically resectable. Of those that are resectable, 76% recur. Surgery: Eg major hepatectomy + extrahepatic bile duct excision + caudate lobe resection. Post-op problems: Liver failure (15%), bile leak (17%), GI bleeding (6%); wound infection (6.5%). Palliative stenting and decompression of an obstructed extrahepatic biliary tree—percutaneously or via ERCP—improves quality of life. Prognosis: ~5 months.

Benign tumors Hemangiomas are the most common benign liver tumors. They are often an incidental finding on ultrasound or CT scan and do not require treatment. Biopsy should be avoided! Hepatocellular adenomas are common. Causes: Anabolic steroids, oral contraceptives; pregnancy. Only treat if symptomatic. Other common benign tumors of the liver include focal nodular hyperplasia; like hepatocellular adenomas, they commonly occur in women, but oral contraceptives do not seem to be implicated as an underlying cause.

Primary liver tumors

Malignant	Benign
HCC	Cysts
Cholangiocarcinoma	Hemangioma
Angiosarcoma	Adenoma
Hepatoblastoma (children)	Focal nodular hyperplasia
Fibrosarcoma	Fibroma
Leiomyosarcoma	Leiomyoma

Origin of secondary liver tumors

Common in males	Common in females
Stomach	Breast
Lung	Colon
Colon	Stomach
	Uterus

Preventing of hepatitis B, hepatitis B-associated cirrhosis, chronic hepatitis, and hepatic neoplasia

Use hepatitis B vaccine, 1mL into the deltoid muscle; repeat at 1 and 6 months Indications: Everyone. This strategy is expensive, but not as expensive as trying to rely on the ultimately unsuccessful strategy of vaccinating at-risk groups (eg health care workers, IV drug users, unsafe sexual practices, hemodialysis patients, and the sexual partners of known hepatitis B$_e$ antigen +ve carriers. The immunocompromised and others may need further doses. Serologies help in the timing booster shots, and find poor or nonresponders (correlates with older age, smoking, and male sex).

NB: Protective immunity begins about 6wks after the 1st immunizing dose. If an exposure occurs in an unvaccinated person, give hepatitis B immune globulin (HBIG) within the first 96h, and start the HBV vaccine series. If an exposure occurs in a previously vaccinated person, check the hepatitis B surface AB titer; if >10IU/mL, then no therapy; if <10IU/mL, then give HBIG and a booster shot.

Ulcerative colitis (UC)

UC is a relapsing and remitting inflammatory disorder of the colonic mucosa. It may affect just the rectum (proctitis) or extend proximally to involve part or all of the colon (pancolitis). It 'never' spreads proximally to the ileocaecal valve (except for 'backwash ileitis'). *Pathology:* Hyperemic/hemorrhagic granular colonic mucosa ± 'pseudopolyps' formed by inflammation. Punctate ulcers may extend deep into the lamina propria. *Histology:* See *biopsy, below*. *Cause:* Unknown; there is some genetic susceptibility. *Incidence:* 4–11/100,000 in the developed world. Most present aged 15–30yrs. UC is twice as common in non-smokers (the opposite is true for Crohn's disease).

Symptoms Gradual onset of diarrhea ± blood & mucus. Crampy abdominal discomfort is common; bowel frequency is related to severity of disease (see below). Systemic symptoms are common during attacks, eg fever, malaise, anorexia, weight loss. Urgency and tenesmus occur with rectal disease.

Signs May be none: In acute, severe UC: Fever, tachycardia, and a tender, distended abdomen. *Extra-intestinal signs* Clubbing, aphthous oral ulcers, erythema nodosum (PLATE 18), pyoderma gangrenosum, conjunctivitis, episcleritis, iritis, large joint arthritis, sacroiliitis, ankylosing spondylitis, fatty liver, PSC, cholangiocarcinoma—and, very rarely, renal stones, osteomalacia, nutritional deficiencies, and systemic amyloidosis.

Tests *Blood:* CBC, ESR, CRP, BMP, LFT, and blood cultures. Consider iron studies. *Stool: Fecal leukocytes, ova and parasites, routine culture, C. dificile toxin.* To exclude infectious diarrhea (*Cl. difficile, Salmonella, Shigella, Campylobacter, E. coli*, amebae). *Abdominal x-ray:* No fecal shadows; mucosal thickening/islands; colonic dilatation (toxic dilatation >6cm); perforation. *Sigmoidoscopy:* Inflamed, friable mucosa. *Rectal biopsy:* Inflammatory infiltrate; goblet cell depletion; glandular distortion; mucosal ulcers; crypt abscesses. *Barium enema:* Loss of haustra; granular mucosa; shortened colon. Never do a barium enema during an acute severe attack. *Colonoscopy* shows disease extent, and allows biopsies to be taken.

Complications Perforation and bleeding are two serious complications. Others include:
- 'Toxic megacolon' which is dilatation of colon (mucosal islands, colonic diameter >6cm).
- Colonic cancer: Risk ≈ 15% with pancolitis for 20yrs; ↑ risk after 8+ years of having UC. Yearly colonoscopy surveillance with biopsy for dysplasia and early cancer is recommended. Recent studies show chromoendoscopy to be valuable in improving dysplasia detection rates.

Management: Below is a reasonable treatment algorithm, however, medications and doses need to be individualized for each patient.

Mild UC: If <4 motions/d and the patient is well, give prednisolone (eg 20mg/d PO) + mesalazine, eg Asacol MR® (=400mg tabs; in an acute attack 2tabs/8h; maintenance: 1 tab/8h). This may be combined with twice-daily steroid foams PR, or prednisolone 20mg retention enemas. If symptoms improve, ↓steroids gradually. If no improvement after 2wks, treat as moderate UC.

Moderate UC: If 4–6 motions/d, but otherwise well, give oral prednisolone 40mg/d for 1wk, then 30mg/d for 1wk, then 20mg for 4 more weeks + sulfasalazine 1g/12h PO + and twice-daily steroid enemas. If improving, ↓steroids gradually. If no improvement after 2wks, treat as a severe UC.

Severe UC: If systemically unwell and passing >6 motions daily, admit for:
- Nothing by mouth and IV hydration (eg 1L of 0.9% saline + 2L dextrose-saline/24h, + 20mmol K⁺/L; less if elderly).
- Hydrocortisone 100mg/6h IV, or solumedrol 40mg IV per day.
- Rectal steroids, eg hydrocortisone 100mg in 100mL 0.9% saline/12h PR.
- Monitor T°, pulse, and BP—and record stool frequency/character.

- Twice-daily exam: Document distension, bowel sounds and tenderness.
- Daily CBC, ESR, CRP, BMP, LFTS, ± abdominal x-ray.
- Consider the need for blood transfusion (if Hb <10g/dL) and parenteral nutrition (if severely malnourished). Give IM vitamins.
- If improving in 5d, transfer to oral prednisolone (40mg/24h) with a 5-ASA (below, eg sulfasalazine 1g/12h) to maintain remission. Sulfasalazine is a combination of 5-aminosalicylic acid (5-ASA) and sulfapyridine (which carries the 5-ASA to the colon).
- Lack of improvement mandates surgical consultation.

Topical therapies: Proctitis may respond to *suppositories* (prednisolone 5mg or mesalazine, eg Asacol® 250mg/8h PR or Pentasa® 1g at bedtime).
- Procto-sigmoiditis may respond to *foams* (20mg Predfoam®/12–24h or 5-ASA, eg Asacol® 1g/d PR); disposable applicators aid accurate delivery.
- *Retention enemas* (eg 20mg Predsol®) may be needed in left-sided colitis.

Meta-analyses favour topical 5-ASAs over topical steroids.

Indications for surgery: Typically perforation or massive hemorrhage or:
- 'Toxic megacolon' with dilatation of colon (mucosal islands, colonic diameter >6cm).
- Failure to respond to drugs. 85% of those with stool frequency >8/d (or stool frequency 3–8/d and CRP >45) on day 3 will need colectomy. *Procedures:* Proctocolectomy + terminal ileostomy (it may be possible to retain the ileocecal valve, and hence reduce liquid loss); colectomy with later ileoanal pouch. Total surgical mortality: 2–7%; with perforation, 50%.

Novel therapies: Cyclosporine can benefit patients with steroid refractory UC, although there are reservations about its long-term efficacy. Typical dose: 2–4mg/kg IV. SE: Eg nephrotoxicity; K+↑; BP↑ (do BMP, LFT, cholesterol, and BP often; stop if raised and get expert help). Low cholesterol levels (<120mg/dL) is a relative contraindication to cyclosporine use. A small trial showed *tacrolimus* may be superior to cyclosporine in maintaining remission. A monoclonal anti-TNF antibody, *infliximab* (p227) may give rapid control and tissue healing in some inflammatory bowel diseases. Patients should be evaluated for latent tuberculosis prior to therapy. Common adverse effects are abdominal pain, nausea, and vomiting. Serious side effects include worsening of congestive heart failure, bone marrow suppression, hepatotoxicity, drug-induced lupus erythematosus. Do not administer to patients with ongoing infections.

Maintaining remission All 5-ASAs (sulfasalazine, mesalazine, and olsalazine) ↓relapse rate from 80% to 20% at 1yr. Maintenance is continued for life. *Sulfasalazine* (1g/12h PO) remains 1st-line if a cheap drug is essential. SEs relate to sulfapyridine intolerance—headache, nausea, anorexia, and malaise. Other allergic/toxic SEs: Fever, rash, hemolysis, hepatitis, pancreatitis, paradoxical worsening of colitis, and reversible oligospermia. Monitor CBC. *Newer 5-ASAs* deliver the active ingredient (sulfasalazine) but minimize SEs (dyspepsia, nausea ± headache can occur; olsalazine may cause secretory diarrhea). Rare hypersensitivity reactions: Worsening colitis, pancreatitis, pericarditis, nephritis. Examples: *Mesalazine* (400–500mg/8h PO) or *olsalazine* (500mg/12h PO)—indicated in sulfasalazine intolerance and young men (less effect on sperm).

Azathioprine (2–2.5mg/kg/d PO) is indicated as a steroid-sparing agent in those with steroid side-effects or those who relapse quickly when steroids are reduced. Treatment should be continued for several months, during which CBC and TSH should be monitored every 4–6wks. The enzyme responsible for inactivation of the 6-MP is thiopurine S-methyltransferase (TPMT). Levels of TPMT can vary among ethnic groups (10% of the population is heterozygous for the gene), and TPMT levels correlates inversely with 6-TGN levels (the active form of azathioprine). It is now possible to measure enzymes and intermediate metabolite (6-MMP) to help monitor efficacy, risk of hepatotoxicity, and therapeutic levels of active drug. Dosing no longer empirically weight based.

Crohn's disease

Crohn's disease is a chronic inflammatory GI disease characterized by trans-mural granulomatous inflammation. It may affect any part of the gut, but favors the terminal ileum and proximal colon. Unlike UC, there is unaffected bowel between areas of active disease (skip lesions).

Cause: Unknown. Mutations of the NOD2/CARD15 gene ↑risk. *Prevalence.* 100/100,000. Smoking ↑risk 3–4-fold. *Associations:* High sugar, low-fiber diet; infective agents (anaerobes); mucins; altered cell-mediated immunity.

Symptoms & signs Diarrhea, abdominal pain, and weight loss are common. Fever, malaise, anorexia occur with active disease. Look for: Aphthous ulceration; abdominal tenderness; right iliac fossa mass; perianal abscesses/fistulae/skin tags; anal/rectal strictures.

Extra-intestinal signs: Clubbing, erythema nodosum (PLATE 18), pyoderma gangrenosum, conjunctivitis, episcleritis, iritis, large joint arthritis, sacroiliitis ankylosing spondylitis, fatty liver, primary sclerosing cholangitis, cholangio-carcinoma (rare), renal stones, osteomalacia, malnutrition, amyloidosis.

Complications Small intestinal obstruction; toxic dilatation (colonic diameter >6cm); abscess formation (abdominal, pelvic, or ischiorectal); fistulae, eg colo-vesical (bladder), colo-vaginal, perianal, entero-cutaneous; perforation; rectal hemorrhage; colonic carcinoma.

Tests *Blood:* CBC, ESR, CRP, BMP, LFT, blood culture. Serum iron, B_{12}, and red cell folate if anemia. *Markers of activity:* Hb↓; ↑ESR; ↑CRP; ↑WBC; ↓albumin.

Stool microscopy/culture and Clostridium difficile toxin (CDT) to exclude infec-tious diarrhea (*C. difficile, Salmonella, Shigella, Campylobacter, E. coli*).

Colonoscopy and biopsy should be performed even when the mucosa is mac-roscopically normal (20% have microscopic granulomas).

Small bowel enema: To detect ileal disease (strictures, proximal dilatation, inflammatory mass or fistula). *Barium enema:* This may show 'cobblestoning', 'rose thorn' ulcers, colonic strictures with rectal sparing.

Management: Below is a reasonable treatment algorithm, however, medica-tions and doses need to be individualized for each patient. Severity is harder to assess than in UC. Severe symptoms (fever; pulse↑; ↑ESR; ↑CRP; ↑WCC; ↓albumin) merit admission. Endoscopic findings do not reflect overall sever-ity of a Crohn's flare.

Mild attacks: Patients are symptomatic but systemically well. Prednisolone 30mg/d PO for 1wk, then 20mg/d for 1 month. See in clinic every 2–4wks. If symptoms resolve, reduce steroids by 5mg every 2–4wks. Stop steroids only when all parameters have returned to normal.

Severe attacks: Admit for IV steroids, nothing by mouth, and IV hydration (eg 1L 0.9% saline + 2L dextrose-saline/24h, + 20mmol K⁺/L, less if elderly). Then:
- Hydrocortisone 100mg/6h IV or Solumedrol 60mg IV qd.
- Treat rectal disease, if present, with rectal steroids twice daily (hydrocorti-sone 100mg in 100mL 0.9% saline/12h PR).
- Metronidazole 400mg/8h PO, or 500mg/8h IV, helps, especially in perianal disease or super-infection. SE: Alcohol intolerance; irreversible neuropathy.
- Monitor T°, pulse, BP, and record stool frequency/character.
- Physical examination twice daily.
- Daily CBC, ESR, CRP, BMP, and plain abdominal x-ray.
- Consider need for transfusion (if Hb <10g/dL) and parenteral nutrition.
- If improving after 5d, transfer on to oral prednisolone (40mg/24h).
- If no response (or deterioration) during IV therapy, seek surgical advice.

Additional therapies in Crohn's disease

Azathioprine (2–2.5mg/kg/d PO) is a steroid-sparing agent, eg for those with steroid side-effects or if relapsing rapidly after dose reduction. It takes 6–10wks to work.

Sulfasalazine: 1g/12h PO and other 5-ASAs (p225) are minimally helpful in active Crohn's. They may be reserved for maintenance, eg in preventing the common problem of relapse after resection (Asacol® 2 × 400mg/8h PO has prevented some recurrence, particularly if this dose produces high mucosal levels of 5-ASA).

Elemental diets: Are as good as steroids in active disease, but are unpalatable and relapse is more common.

Methotrexate: A Cochrane review finds good evidence from a single large randomized trial on which to recommend 25mg IM weekly for induction of remission and complete withdrawal from steroids in patients with refractory Crohn's disease. NNT ≈ 5. There is no evidence on lower doses. Monitor LFTS for methotrexate-induced hepatotoxicity.

Surgery: 50–80% of patients need ≥1 operation in their life. *Indications for surgery:* Usually failure to respond to drugs—or:
• Intestinal obstruction from strictures
• Intestinal perforation
• Local complications (fistulae, abscesses).

Surgery is never curative: The aim is limited resection of the worst areas. Bypass and pouch surgery is *not* done in Crohn's (∴ ↑risk of recurrence).

Infliximab: This is an anti-tumor necrosis factor monoclonal antibody. It can ↓ Crohn's disease activity. A single dose of infliximab is given by IVI over 2h in an infusion center. NNT ≈ 3–4 (p34). Response may be short-lived. It may be repeated at 8wks. *CI:* Sepsis, LFT↑ >3-fold above top end of normal, concurrent cyclosporine or tacrolimus. *SE:* Rash; ?↑ risk of malignancy.

Irritable bowel syndrome (IBS)

IBS is used to describe a heterogeneous group of abdominal symptoms for which no organic cause can be found. Most are probably due to disorders of intestinal motility.

Clinical features Patients are usually 20–40yrs old and ♀ are more frequently affected than ♂. *Symptoms:* Central or lower abdominal pain (relieved by defecation); abdominal bloating; altered bowel habit (constipation alternating with diarrhea); tenesmus; mucus PR. Less commonly: Nausea, dyspareunia; pain in the back, thigh, or chest; urinary frequency; depression. Symptoms are chronic (>3 months over 12 month-period), and may be exacerbated by stress, menstruation, or gastroenteritis. *Signs:* Examination is often unremarkable although generalized abdominal tenderness is common. Insufflation of air during endoscopy may reproduce the pain.

Markers of organic disease: (ie it may well not be IBS) Age >40yrs; history <6 months; anorexia; weight↓; waking at night with pain/diarrhea; mouth ulcers; rectal bleeding; abnormal investigations. Management: See BOX.

Carcinoma of the pancreas

Epidemiology: Accounts for ≤2% of all malignancy; highly lethal; 31,000 deaths in US in 2004. *Typical patient:* Male >60yrs old. *Risk factors:* Smoking, alcohol, diabetes, family history. *Pathology:* Most are ductal adenocarcinoma (metastasize early; late presentation). 60% arise in the pancreas head, 15% the tail, and 25% in the body. A minority arise from the ampulla of Vater (ampullary tumor) or pancreatic islet cells (insulinoma, gastrinoma, glucagonoma, somatostatinoma, VIPomas); these have a better prognosis.

Symptoms & signs Tumors in the head of the pancreas classically present with painless obstructive jaundice. Tumors in the body and tail present with epigastric pain, which typically radiates to the back and may be relieved by sitting forward. Either may cause anorexia, weight loss, diabetes or acute pancreatitis. Rare features include: Thrombophlebitis migrans; marantic endocarditis; hypercalcemia; Cushing's syndrome; ascites (peritoneal metastases); portal hypertension (splenic vein thrombosis); nephrotic syndrome (renal vein metastases). *Signs:* Jaundice + palpable gallbladder (Courvoisier's 'law': Painless jaundice + palpable GB implies a diagnosis other than gallstones); epigastric mass; hepatomegaly; splenomegaly; lymphadenopathy; ascites.

Tests *Blood:* Cholestatic jaundice. CA 19–9 is ↑ in pancreatic cancer but is non-specific and not indicated as a screening test. *Imaging:* Ultrasound or CT scan can show a pancreatic mass ± dilated biliary tree ± hepatic metastases. Staging CT or endoscopic ultrasound before stent placement in potential surgical candidates. ERCP delineates the biliary tree anatomy and localizes the site of obstruction. MRI is helpful: Sensitivity 84%, specificity 97% vs 70% and 94% for ERCP. *Histology:* Obtainable by ultrasound- and CT-guided percutaneous biopsy, or endoscopic ultrasound with fine-needle aspiration.

Treatment Most ductal carcinomas present with metastatic disease; <10% are suitable for radical surgery. *Surgery:* Consider pancreatoduodenectomy (Whipple's, p231 and p470) if fit and the tumor <3cm with no metastases. Post-op morbidity is high (mortality <5% in experienced hands). *Post-op chemotherapy* delays disease progression. *Palliation of jaundice:* Endoscopic (ERCP) or percutaneous stent insertion. Rarely, palliative bypass surgery is indicated for duodenal obstruction or unsuccessful ERCP. *Pain relief:* Disabling pain may be relieved by opiates or radiotherapy. Celiac plexus infiltration with alcohol may be done at the time of palliative surgery, percutaneously, or via endoscopic ultrasound.

Prognosis Mean survival <6 months. 5yr survival rate: <2%. Overall 5yr survival after Whipples' procedure 5–14%. Patients with the rarer ampullary or islet cell tumors have a better prognosis.

Management of IBS

The 1st step is to exclude other diagnoses, so:
- If young, with a classic history, CBC, ESR, LFT, celiac serology (p232), and urinalysis ± sigmoidoscopy with rectal biopsy is sufficient investigation.
- If the patient is aged ≥45yrs or has *any* marker or organic disease, request colonoscopy (barium enema if unavailable).
- If diarrhea is prominent, do: LFT; stool culture; B_{12}/folate; antiendomysial ab; TSH; consider referral ± rectal biopsy.
- Further investigation should be guided by symptoms and include:
  - Upper gi endoscopy (dyspepsia, reflux)
  - Duodenal biopsy (celiac disease), eg if anti-endomysial antibodies +ve.
  - Giardia tests (p544) (it often triggers IBS)
  - Small bowel radiology (Crohn's disease)
  - MRCP or EUS (chronic pancreatitis)
  - Transit studies and anorectal physiological studies—rarely used.

Refer if: (1) Equivocal diagnosis; (2) changing symptoms in 'known IBS'; (3) *to surgeon* if rectal prolapse; (4) *to dietitian* if food intolerances; (5) *to psychiatrists* if stress/depression is pronounced; (6) *to gynecologist* if cyclical pain (endometriosis) or if difficult pelvic infection.

Treatment Rarely 100% successful. Be realistic with patients. Careful explanation and reassurance are vital. *Create a good relationship with your patient.*
- *Food intolerance:* Try exclusion diets (difficult to maintain). Encourage patient to keep a food diary.
- *Constipation:* (p200) ↑Fiber intake gradually. Can lead to bloating.
- *Diarrhea:* Bulking agent ± loperamide 2mg after each loose stool; max 16mg/d; SE: Colic, nausea, dizziness, constipation, bloating, ileus.
- *Dyspeptic symptoms:* May respond to metoclopramide or antacids.
- *Psychological R:* Emphasize positive aspects and prognosis: In 50% symptoms go or improve after 1yr; <5% worsen. Symptoms are still troublesome in the rest at 5yrs. *Tricyclic antidepressants* (low dose) are often helpful, eg amitriptyline 10–50mg at night (SE: Constipation, dry mouth, etc.). *Psychotherapy, cognitive-behavioral therapy.* Explain that all forms of stress (sexual, physical, or verbal abuse) perpetuate IBS.

The future: Much interest is being expressed in modulating the 'brain-gut' axis by neurotransmitter manipulation. *Visceral hypersensitivity:* Those with IBS have lower visceral pain thresholds than others, and since 5HT antagonists ↑ pain tolerance, highly selective $5HT_3$-receptor antagonists (eg alosetron, tegaserod) are under trial and used clinically with discretion.

229

Nutritional disorders

Scurvy This is due to lack of vitamin C in the diet. *Is the patient poor, pregnant, or on an odd diet? Signs:* (1) Listlessness, anorexia, cachexia. (2) Gingivitis, loose teeth, and foul-smelling breath (halitosis). (3) Bleeding from gums, nose, hair follicles, or into joints, bladder, gut.

Diagnosis: No test is completely satisfactory. WBC ascorbic acid↓.

Treatment: Dietary education; ascorbic acid 250mg/d PO.

Beriberi There is heart failure with generalized edema (wet beriberi) or neuropathies (dry beriberi) due to lack of vitamin B_1 (thiamine).

Pellagra (Lack of nicotinic acid). *Classical triad:* Diarrhea, dementia, dermatitis (± neuropathy, depression, insomnia, tremor, rigidity, ataxia, fits). It may occur in carcinoid syndrome and anti-TB treatment. It is endemic in China and Africa. *Treatment:* Education, electrolyte replacement, nicotinamide. Look for other vitamin deficiencies.

Xerophthalmia This vitamin A deficiency is a major cause of blindness in the Tropics. Conjunctivae become dry and develop oval or triangular spots (Bitôt's spots). Corneas become cloudy and soft. Give vitamin A 200,000IU stat PO, repeat in 24h and a week later (halve dose if <1yr old; quarter if <6 months old); get special help if pregnant; vitamin A embryopathy must be avoided. Re-educate, and monitor diet.

Carcinoid tumors

A diverse group of tumors of argentaffin cell origin, by definition capable of producing 5HT. Common site: Appendix (25%) or rectum. They also occur elsewhere in the GI tract, ovary, testis, and bronchi. Tumors may be benign but 80% >2cm in size will metastasize. *Symptoms & signs:* Initially few. GI tumors can cause appendicitis, intussusception, or obstruction. Hepatic metastases may cause RUQ pain. Carcinoid tumors may secrete ACTH (∴ Cushing's syndrome); 10% are part of MEN-1 syndrome and 10% occur with other neuroendocrine tumors. Carcinoid *syndrome* occurs in 10%.

Carcinoid syndrome usually implies hepatic involvement. *Signs:* Paroxysmal flushing (± migrating wheals—bright-red color on the face, chest, trunk, and extremities lasting 10–30min), abdominal pain, tricuspid incompetence and pulmonary stenosis. *CNS effects:* Numerous, eg *enhanced* ability to learn new stimulus–response associations. *Carcinoid crisis:* When a tumor outgrows its blood supply, and mediators flood into vasculature; this is life threatening.

Diagnosis 24h urine 5-hydroxyindoleacetic acid↑ (5HIAA, a 5HT metabolite; levels change with drugs and diet: Discuss with lab). If liver metastases are not found, try to find the primary (CXR; chest/pelvis MRI/CT), as curative resection is possible. *New tests:* Plasma chromogranin A (reflects tumor mass); [111]Indium octreotide scintigraphy (octreoscan); positron emission tomography (PET).

Treatment *Carcinoid syndrome:* Octreotide (somatostatin analogue) blocks release of tumor mediators and counters peripheral effects. Effects lessen over time. Other options: Loperamide or cyproheptadine for diarrhea; ketanserin (experimental $5HT_2$ antagonist) for flushing; interferon-α. *Tumor therapy:* Surgical debulking (eg enucleation) or embolization of hepatic metastases can ↓symptoms. These must be done with octreotide on-board to avoid precipitating a massive carcinoid crisis. Crisis is treated with high-dose octreotide and careful management of fluid balance. *Median survival:* 5–8yrs; 38 months if metastases are present, but may be *much* longer (~20yrs).

Whipple's procedure

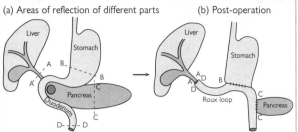

(a) Areas of reflection of different parts

Liver
Stomach
A   B
A'
Duodenum
Pancreas
C
C
D—   —D

(b) Post-operation

Liver
Stomach
A D   B
A
D
Roux loop
Pancreas
C
C

Whipple's procedure may be used for removing masses in the head of the pancreas—typically from pancreatic carcinoma, or less commonly, a carcinoid tumor.

Gastrointestinal malabsorption

Symptoms Diarrhea; ↓weight; steatorrhea (fatty stools, difficult to flush).

Deficiency signs: Anemia (↓Fe, B_{12}, folate); bleeding (↓vit K); edema (↓protein).

Common causes: Celiac disease, Crohn's, chronic pancreatitis. *Others causes include:*

↓Bile: 1° biliary cirrhosis; ileal resection; biliary obstruction; Rx: Eg cholestyramine.

Pancreatic insufficiency: Chronic pancreatitis; pancreas cancer; cystic fibrosis.

Small bowel mucosa: Celiac and Whipple's diseases; tropical sprue; radiation enteritis; small bowel resection; brush border enzyme deficiencies (eg lactase insufficiency); drugs (metformin, neomycin, alcohol); amyloid.

Bacterial overgrowth: Spontaneous (especially in elderly); in jejunal diverticula; post-op blind loops. Try fluoroquinolones, bactrim.

Infection: Giardiasis; diphyllobothriasis (B_{12} malabsorption); strongyloidiasis.

Intestinal hurry: Post-gastrectomy dumping; post-vagotomy; gastrojejunostomy.

Tests CBC (MCV↓, macrocytosis); ↓Ca^{2+}(↓vit D due to fat malabsorption); ↓Fe; ↓folate; ↑PT (↓vitamin K); celiac serology (below). *Stool:* Sudan stain for fat globules; stool microscopy for infestation. *Ba follow-through:* Diverticula; Crohn's; radiation enteritis. *Breath hydrogen analysis:* (bacterial overgrowth). Take samples of end-expired air; give glucose; take more samples at ½h intervals. If there is overgrowth there is ↑exhaled hydrogen. *Small bowel biopsy:* Use endoscopy. MRCP biliary obstruction; chronic pancreatitis.

Tropical malabsorption *Typical causes: Giardia intestinalis, Cryptosporidium parvum, Isospora belli, Cyclospora cayetanensis, and the microsporidia. Tropical sprue:* Villous atrophy and malabsorption occurring in the Far and Middle East and Caribbean (rare in Africa)—the etiology is unknown. Tetracycline and folic acid may be helpful.

Celiac disease is a T-cell mediated autoimmune disease of the small bowel in which gluten (alcohol-soluble proteins in wheat, barley, rye ± oats) intolerance causes villous atrophy and malabsorption. *Associations:* HLA DQ2 in 95%; the rest are DQ8; autoimmune disease; dermatitis herpetiformis.

Presentation: Steatorrhea/offensive stools; other abdominal pain; bloating; nausea/vomiting; aphthous ulcers, angular stomatitis; weight↓; fatigue; weakness; iron-deficiency anemia; osteomalacia; poor growth (children). One-third are asymptomatic, so have a low threshold for evaluating patients for celiac disease. Occurs at any age (peaks in infancy and 50–60yrs, ♀:♂ >1).

Diagnosis: Antibodies: (α-gliadin, transglutaminase, anti-endomysial—an IgA antibody; 95% specific, unless the patient is IgA-deficient). Duodenal biopsy done at endoscopy (as good as jejunal biopsy if ≥4 taken): Villous atrophy, reversing on gluten-free diet (along with ↓symptoms and antibodies).

Treatment: Lifelong gluten-free diet. Rice, maize, soya, potatoes, oats, and sugar are OK. Gluten-free biscuits, flour, bread, & pasta are prescribable. Verify diet by endomysial antibody tests. Refer to a nutritionist.

Complications: Anemia; 2° lactose-intolerance; GI T-cell lymphoma (rare; suspect if worsening despite diet); malignancy (gastric, esophageal, bladder, breast, brain); myopathies; neuropathies; hyposplenism; osteoporosis.

Chronic pancreatitis Epigastric pain 'bores' through to back; bloating; steatorrhea; ↓weight; diabetes.

Causes: Alcohol; rare: Familial; cystic fibrosis; hemochromatosis; pancreatic duct obstruction (stones or pancreatic cancer); hyperparathyroidism; hypertriglyceridemia, genetic mutations, cystic fibrosis, tropical pancreatitis, idiopathic.

Tests: Ultrasound (dilated biliary tree; stones); if normal consider CT/MRCP; *plain film:* Speckled pancreatic calcification; glucose↑; breath tests (above).

Drugs: • Give analgesia (± celiac-plexus block). • Lipase, eg Creon®; • Fat-soluble vitamins (eg Multivite®). *Diet:* Low fat (+ no alcohol) may help. Medium-chain triglycerides (MCT oil®) may be tried (no lipase needed for absorption, but diarrhea may be worsened). *Surgery:* For unremitting pain; narcotic abuse (beware of this); weight↓: Pancreatectomy or pancreaticojejunostomy.

Renal medicine

Michael J. Choi, M.D.

Contents

Web links for estimating glomerular filtration rate

The 4 variable MDRD equation estimates GFR based on age, sex, race, and serum creatinine (**www.nephron.com**). Another estimate of creatinine clearance uses serum creatinine (SCr), sex, and ideal body weight (IBW; muscle bulk is important). **www.globalrph.com/crcl.htm**. It is based on the Cockcroft & Gault equation:

$$CrCl \approx (140 - age) \times IBW/(SCr \times 72) \ (\times 0.85 \text{ for females}).$$

Ideal body weight in (kg) $\approx$ 50kg + 2.3kg for each inch of height over 5ft. ♀: IBW $\approx$ 45.5kg + 2.3kg for each inch over 5ft. *Units:* SCr (mcmol/L)/88.4 = SCr (mg/dL). *Example:* An 70-yr-old white woman with a serum creatinine of 1.3mg/dL has an estimated GFR of 43mL/min by the 4 variable MDRD equation.

R enal disease typically presents with one or more of a short list of clinical syndromes—listed below. One underlying pathology may have a variety of clinical presentations.

1 *Proteinuria and nephrotic syndrome:* Normal protein excretion is <150mg/d. In certain circumstances, this may rise to ~300mg/d—eg orthostatic proteinuria (related to posture); during fever, or after exercise. *Proteinuria* (excessive urine protein excretion) is a sign of glomerular or tubular disease. *Nephrotic syndrome* is the triad of proteinuria (>3g/d, p248), hypoalbuminemia (albumin <3.5g/dL) and edema. Hyperlipidemia is often seen.

2 *Hematuria and nephritic syndrome:* *Hematuria* (blood in the urine) may arise from anywhere in the renal tract. It may be *macroscopic* (visible to the naked eye), *microscopic,* or detected as *hemoglobinuria* (hemoglobin in the urine). *Nephritic syndrome* comprises hematuria and proteinuria. It may be associated with hypertension, peripheral edema, oliguria (urine output <400mL/d), and acute renal failure. The question of who to refer hematuria patients to (urologist or nephrologist) is answered on p236.

3 *Oliguria and polyuria: Oliguria* is a urine output of <400mL/d. It is a normal response to severe fluid restriction. *Abnormal causes:* ↓renal perfusion, renal parenchymal disease, urinary tract obstruction. *Polyuria* is the excretion of larger than normal volumes of urine, usually from high fluid or solute intake. Pathological causes include diabetes mellitus, diabetes insipidus p306, disorders of the renal medulla (resulting in failure to concentrate the urine), and supraventricular tachycardia.

4 *Flank pain and dysuria: Flank pain* is usually due to renal obstruction (look for swelling or tenderness), acute pyelonephritis, polycystic kidneys, or renal infarction. Severe flank pain (may be called renal colic) may be associated with fever and vomiting, and may radiate to the abdomen, groin, or upper thigh. It is usually caused by a renal calculus, clot, or sloughed papilla. Urinary *frequency & dysuria* (pain on passing urine) are symptoms of cystitis.

5 *Acute renal failure* (ARF) is significant decline in renal function occurring over hours to days, detected by a rising serum creatinine and urea nitrogen, with or without oliguria. ARF usually occurs secondary to ↓ blood flow to the kidneys (hypotension, hypovolemia, sepsis) urinary obstruction, or due to intrinsic renal disease.

6 *Chronic kidney disease* (CKD) Kidney damage ≥3 months as defined by structural or functional abnormalities of the kidney, with or without ↓ GFR or a GFR <60mL/min/1.73 meters squared body surface area. It is classified according to glomerular filtration rate (GFR) into 5 categories: Stage 1 (kidney damage with normal GFR >90mL/min), stage 2 (60–89mL/min); stage 3 (30–59mL/min); stage 4 (15–29mL/min) and stage 5 (<15mL/min). There is poor correlation between symptoms and signs of CKD. Progression may be so insidious that patients attribute symptoms to age or other illnesses. Severe CKD may not present with any symptoms. End-stage renal failure is a degree of renal failure that, without renal replacement therapy, would result in death.

7 *Microalbuminuria* is a silent harbinger of serious renal (and cardiovascular risk). In one study, 30% of those with type 2 diabetes mellitus died within ~5yrs of developing microalbuminuria.

Urine

Examine fresh urine whenever you suspect renal disease.

Dipsticks

• *Hematuria: Causes:* Infections (cystitis, pyelonephritis, prostatitis, TB, schistosomiasis, urethritis); calculi; neoplasia (bladder, prostate, urethra); trauma; glomerulonephritis; interstitial nephritis; polycystic kidney disease; papillary necrosis (sickle-cell disease, NSAIDs); medullary sponge kidney; vasculitis; vascular malformation; cyclophosphamide; hemophilia; anticoagulation should not cause hematuria at usual therapeutic goal levels. *Tests:* Urine dipstick and microscopic exam, culture, 24h urine collection (protein, creatinine clearance); CBC, ESR, CRP, BUN, creatinine. *Others:* Clotting, Hb electrophoresis; CT pyelogram with and without intravenous contrast or renal ultrasound, ± renal biopsy. *Management plan:* Usually refer to a urologist for urothelial malignancy evaluation if >40yrs old or other high risk (smoker, cyclophosphamide, dye worker). Refer to nephrologist if risk of urothelial malignancy is low and risk of glomerulonephritis is not negligible (eg <40yrs old; ↑ serum creatinine; ↑BP; proteinuria; systemic symptoms; family history of renal disease). *False +ve dipstick hematuria:* Free Hb; myoglobin; bacterial peroxidase *False negative:* Ascorbic acid, old dipsticks *Red urine:* Beets; porphyria; rifampin, phenindione, phenolphthalein.

• *Proteinuria:* Normal protein excretion is <150mg/d (may rise >300mg/d in fever, or with exercise). *Causes* UTI; orthostatic proteinuria; primary and secondary glomerular disease (SLE; amyloidosis; DM; pregnancy); interstitial disease; hemolytic-uremic syndrome; multiple myeloma. *Tests:* BP; urine diptick and microscopic exam; 24h urine collection (protein excretion, creatinine clearance); Spot urine protein: Creatinine ratio (ratio of 1 ≈ urine protein excretion of 1g/24h); renal ultrasound, serum complement or others (ANA; RPR; hepatitis C, hepatitis B, HIV, SPEP, UPEP). If abnormal, consider renal biopsy. *Microalbuminuria:* Albumin excretion 30–300mg/24h or spot urine sample value of 30–300mcg/mg creatinine. *Causes:* DM; ↑BP.

• *Other substances—Glucose:* DM; pregnancy; Fanconi's syndrome; proximal tubule damage. *Ketones:* Starvation; ketoacidosis. *Leukocytes:* UTI; vaginal discharge; interstitial nephritis. *Nitrites:* Enterobacteriaceae infection; high-protein meal. *Bilirubin:* Obstructive jaundice. *Urobilinogen:* Pre-hepatic jaundice. *Specific gravity:* Normal range: 1.000–1.030 (dilution and concentration). *pH:* Normal range: 4.5–8 (acid–base balance: lactose fermenting bacteria and distal RTA may cause alkaline urine).

Microscopy Put a drop of centrifuged urine sediment (centrifuge 10mL for 5min at 2000–3000 rpm and resuspend pellet in few drops after inverting tube) on a microscope slide, cover with a coverslip and examine under low (100x) and high (400x) power for leukocytes, RBCs, bacteria, crystals, and casts.

Leukocytes: >10/mm³ in an unspun urine specimen is abnormal. *Causes:* Cystitis; urethritis; prostatitis; pyelonephritis; interstitial nephritis; TB; renal calculi; glomerulonephritis.

Red cells: >3–5 RBCs/high powered field in 2/3 AM specimens. *Causes:* See hematuria.

Casts are cylindrical bodies formed in the lumen of distal tubules as cells or other elements are embedded in Tamm–Horsfall protein.

Finely granular and hyaline casts (clear, colorless) are found in: Concentrated urine, fever, after exercise, or with loop diuretics and pathologic conditions.

Densely granular casts: Acute tubular necrosis (ATN), GN, or interstitial nephritis.

Fatty casts: Heavy proteinuria. Under polarized light see Maltese cross appearance.

Red cell casts are a hallmark of glomerulonephritis (GN). May be seen with interstitial nephritis, or vasculitis.

White cell casts occur in pyelonephritis, interstitial nephritis and rarely proliferative glomerulonephritis.

Epithelial cell casts occur in ATN.

Crystals are common in old or refrigerated urine and may not signify pathology. Cystine crystals are diagnostic of cystinuria. (Oxalate crystals in fresh urine may indicate ethylene glycol poisoning in patients with severe metabolic acidosis). Medications (sulfonamides, indinivir, acyclovir).

24h urine for creatinine ± protein excretion. Take blood creatinine simultaneously to calculate creatinine clearance. Can check 24h urine for Na^+, K^+, for electrolyte disorders, or stone risk profile for recurrent stones.

Urine microscopy

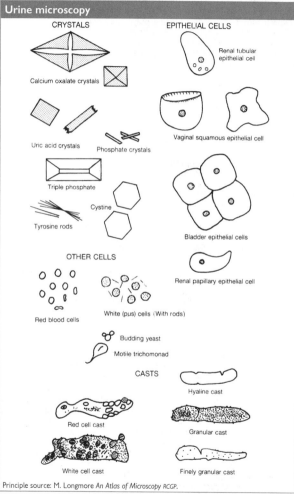

CRYSTALS

Calcium oxalate crystals

Uric acid crystals

Phosphate crystals

Triple phosphate

Cystine

Tyrosine rods

EPITHELIAL CELLS

Renal tubular epithelial cell

Vaginal squamous epithelial cell

Bladder epithelial cells

OTHER CELLS

Red blood cells

White (pus) cells (With rods)

Renal papillary epithelial cell

Budding yeast

Motile trichomonad

CASTS

Hyaline cast

Red cell cast

Granular cast

White cell cast

Finely granular cast

Principle source: M. Longmore *An Atlas of Microscopy RCGP*.

▶When you find red cells, consider their morphology to understand where in the GU tract they come from. If >80% of RBCs are dysmorphic G1 cells, suspect glomerular bleeding, and look hard for red cell casts. Acanthocytes are RBCs with donut shapes, target configurations, and membrane protrusions or blebs. Acanthocyturia >5% considered to be indicative of glomerularhematuria.
www.uninet.edu/cin2003/conf/nguyen/nguyen.html

Urinary tract imaging

Abdominal x-ray Look at kidneys, path of the ureters, and bladder. Abnormal calcification may be related to calculi (only 80% of stones are visible on plain films: See CT below), dystrophic calcification, eg in carcinomas or TB (uncommon), and nephrocalcinosis.

Ultrasound (US) is the usual initial image in renal medicine. May be performed with Doppler. Abnormal parenchyma if echogenicity > liver. It shows:
- Renal size—*small* (<9cm) implies CKD, *large* in renal masses, benign cysts,[1] hypertrophy if other kidney missing, polycystic kidney disease, amyloidosis, diabetes, HIV and lymphomatous infiltration.
- Hydronephrosis, which indicate renal obstruction or reflux.
- Perinephric collections (trauma, post-renal biopsy).
- Transplanted kidneys (collections, obstruction, color Doppler indicates perfusion).
- Bladder residual volume.
- Power Doppler ultrasound evaluates for renal artery stenosis.

Advantages: Fast; cheap; independent of renal function; no IV contrast or radiation risk. *Disadvantages:* Intraluminal masses such as transitional cell carcinomas (TCC) in the upper tracts may not be seen; not a functional study; only suggests obstruction when there is dilatation of the collecting system (~1–2% of obstructed kidneys have non-dilated systems).

Helical non-contrast/computer tomography (CT) is gold standard for diagnosis of renal colic. Non-contrast scans are 97% sensitive for calculi, and shows other pathologies. CT has a similar radiation dose as IVP. CT allows detailed characterization of: Masses (solid or cystic, contrast enhancement, calcification, local/distant extension, renal vein involvement); renal trauma (2 kidneys, hemorrhage, devascularization, laceration, urine leak); retroperitoneal lesions. CT urogram for hematuria uses IV contrast to visualize collecting system if non-contrast CT is negative.

Intravenous urogram/pyelogram (IVU = IVP) A study for defining anatomy (especially pelvi-calyceal), and for detecting pathology distorting the collecting system. It yields limited functional information. Abdominal films are taken before and after IV contrast, which is filtered by the kidney, reaching the renal tubules at ~1min (nephrogram phase). Later images show contrast in the system (pyelogram), ureters, and bladder. Detects papillary necrosis, medullary sponge kidney. SE: Flushing; nausea; rash; contrast nephropathy (caution: Risks include pre-existing CKD, DM).

Retrograde pyelography is good at showing anatomy of the pelvi-calyceal systems and ureters, and detecting pathology such as transitional cell carcinoma (TCC). Contrast is injected via a ureteric catheter.

Percutaneous nephrostomy The renal pelvis is punctured with imaging guidance. Diagnostic images are obtained following contrast injection. A nephrostomy tube may then be placed to allow drainage of an obstruction above the bladder.

Renal arteriography Still the gold standard for renal artery stenosis. Therapeutic indications include angioplasty and stenting and selective embolization (bleeding tumor, trauma, or AV malformations).

Magnetic resonance imaging (MRI/MRA) offers improved soft tissue resolution; it may be used to clarify equivocal non-contrast CT findings. Magnetic resonance angiography (MRA) is useful in imaging renal artery stenosis. Avoid gadolinium in severe CKD (p650).

Radionuclide imaging Scans quantify each kidney's contribution to renal function, and can detect renal scarring (^{99}Tc^{m}DTPA) (diethylenetriamine penta-acetic acid). Radiolabelled metal chelators, eg ^{51}Cr-EDTA (ethylenediaminetetraacetic acid), ^{125}I iothalamate, or ^{99}Tc^{m}DTPA can also measure glomerular filtration rate.

1 Cysts may be inherited, developmental, or acquired—eg polycystic kidney disease, medullary sponge kidney, multicystic dysplastic kidney, medullary cystic disease, tuberous sclerosis, renal sinus cysts, von Hippel-Lindau's disease.

Renal biopsy

Most acute renal failure is due to pre-renal causes or acute tubular necrosis, and recovery of renal function typically occurs over the course of a few weeks. Renal biopsy should be performed if knowing histology will influence management. Once CKD is long standing with small kidneys, risks of bleeding from biopsy may be ↑ and therapy may be limited.

Indications for renal biopsy:
• What is the cause of this acute renal failure p250?
• Investigating isolated hematuria with normal renal function and minimal proteinuria to rule out glomerulonephritis is nephrologist dependent. Is persistent hematuria in this scenario from IgA nephropathy, thin basement membrane disease, or hereditary nephropathy?
• What is the cause of this heavy proteinuria (eg >2–3g/d) when diabetic nephropathy is unlikely?
• Renal dysfunction post-transplantation: Is the cause rejection, drug toxicity, or recurrence of renal disease?

Pre-procedure: Check CBC, coagulation profile, bleeding time. Obtain written informed consent. Ultrasound (if only 1 kidney, many feel this is a contraindication).

Procedure: Biopsy may be performed with real time ultrasound using needle guides with the patient lying in the prone position and the breath held. May also be performed by radiology via transjugular approach or surgically via laproscopic or open techniques for those who are obese or who are at ↑ risk for bleeding. Samples should be sent to pathology for routine stains, immunofluorescence, and electron microscopy. A clear indication on the request form of why the test has been done, eg exclude amyloidosis, will help in the selection of special stains, immunofluorescence and use of electron microscopy.

Post procedure: Bed rest for 6–24h. Monitor pulse, BP, symptoms, and urine color. Bleeding is the main complication with nephrectomy and death ~1/1000 cases.

Urinary tract infection (UTI)

Definitions *Bacteriuria:* Bacteria in the urine; may be asymptomatic or symptomatic. *UTI:* The presence of a pure growth of 10^3 colony forming units (CFU)/mL or $>10^3$ of uropathogen with pyuria and symptoms. UTI sites: Bladder (*cystitis*); prostate (*prostatitis*); or kidney (*pyelonephritis*). Up to one-third of women with symptoms do not have bacteriuria; a condition known as *urethral syndrome. Classification:* UTIs may be classified as *uncomplicated* (normal renal tract and function) or *complicated* (most male patients, abnormal renal tract, impaired renal function, impaired host defenses, virulent organism). A *recurrent UTI* is a further infection with a new organism. A *relapse* is a further infection with the same organism.

Risk factors female sex; sexual intercourse; diaphragm or spermicide contraceptive; DM; immunosuppression; pregnancy; menopause; urinary tract obstruction p244, nephrolithiasis, instrumentation, or malformation.

Organisms E. coli is the commonest (~80% in the community but <41% in hospital). Others include Staphylococcus saprophyticus, Enterococcus fecalis, Proteus mirabilis, Klebsiella species, Enterobacter species, Acinetobacter species, Pseudomonas aeruginosa, and Serratia marcescens.

Symptoms *Cystitis:* Frequency; dysuria; urgency; hematuria; suprapubic pain. *Acute pyelonephritis:* Fever; rigors; vomiting; loin pain and tenderness. *Prostatitis:* Flu-like symptoms; low backache; few urinary symptoms; swollen, tender prostate.

Signs Fever; abdominal or flank tenderness; renal mass; distended bladder; enlarged prostate. **NB:** See also *vaginal discharge*, p528.

Tests Microscopic exam for leukocytes, or dipstick test for leukocyte esterase, or nitrites. May treat uncomplicated empirically if symptoms consistent with acute uncomplicated UTI. If complicated, UTI, pyelonephritis, uncertainty of diagnosis, child, pregnancy, ill appearing or if recent recurrence after therapy, send a fresh clean catch specimen to the lab for culture and sensitivity. A pure growth of $>10^5$CFU/mL is diagnostic for complicated UTIs or if bacteria is not always pathogenic. Two consecutive cultures with same bacteria are required for asymptomatic patients in complicated UTIs. If <10^3CFU/mL and pyuria, the result is significant. Cultured organisms are tested for sensitivity to a range of antibiotics.

Blood tests: CBC, BUN, creatinine, blood cultures, if systemically ill appearing.

Ultrasound, IVP, CT pyelogram/cystoscopy: Consider for: UTI in infants, children, or men; recurrent UTI; pyelonephritis; unusual organism; persistent fever; persistent or gross hematuria. *Ultrasound or IVP?* Ultrasound may miss stones, papillary necrosis, and clubbed calyces. Can do ultrasound first because it avoids contrast agents and radiation.

Treatment *Advice:* Drink plenty; urinate often; double voiding (going again after 5min); post-intercourse voiding; wipe front to back after micturition. *Antibiotics: Know your local pattern of resistance:* Increasingly, options are narrowing. *Cystitis:* Trimethoprim/sulfamethoxazole (TMP/SMX) 160/800mg bid PO x 3d). Alternative: Quinolone antibiotics (norfloxacin 400g PO bid: Or ciprofloxacin 250mg PO bid.). Longer courses (10–14d) may be needed in complicated UTI (see above) if fever present, sensitivity profile determines treatment although quinolones may be used empirically for severe symptoms.

Acute pyelonephritis: TMP/SMX or quinolones orally unless severe GI symptoms, hemodynamic instability, significant systemic symptoms, noncompliance.

Prostatitis: Ciprofloxacin 500mg/12h PO for ~4wks. *Pregnancy:* Ask OB.

Prevention: Antibiotic prophylaxis, either continuous or post-coital, ↑ infection rates in women with recurrent UTIs. Self-treatment with 1–3d course as symptoms start is an option. Effects of cranberry juice have not been fully assessed, but this may inhibit adherence of E. coli to bladder cells. Other studies are equivocal.

Causes of sterile pyuria

Renal TB (do 3 early morning urines). Other causes:
- Inadequately treated UTI
- Appendicitis
- Calculi; prostatitis
- Bladder tumor
- Papillary necrosis from DM, analgesic excess, sickle cell
- UTI with fastidious culture requirement
- Interstitial nephritis, polycystic kidney
- Chemical cystitis eg from cytotoxics

What is the predictive value of urinary symptoms and dipsticks for diagnosing UTI?

In one study of 343 women, the pre-test probability of having UTI if urinary symptoms were present was ~0.5. Positive likelihood ratios (LRs) for UTI were: Painful voiding (1.31), urgency (1.29), urinary frequency (1.16), and urinary tenesmus (1.16). Probability of UTI was lessened by presence of genital discomfort, dyspareunia, vaginal discharge, and perineal discomfort.

Nitrites on dipstick ↑ the probability of UTI 5-fold, moderate pyuria ↑ it by >1.5-fold, and the presence of both does so by >7-fold.[1]

1 Llobera J 2003 *Fam Practice* **20** 103. http://fampract.oupjournals.org/cgi/content/abstract/20/2/103

Renal calculi (nephrolithiasis)

Renal stones (calculi) consist mainly of crystal aggregates. Stones form in the collecting ducts and may be deposited anywhere from renal pelvis to urethra.

Epidemiology *Prevalence:* 0.2%. Lifetime incidence: Up to 12%. *Peak age:* 20–50yrs. M:F >4:1. *Risk factors:* Dehydration, UTI, hypercalcemia, hypercalciuria, hyperoxaluria, hypocitraturia, hyperuricosuria, small intestinal disease or resection, chronic diarrhea, cystinuria, distal renal tubular acidosis, gout, drugs (triamterine, indinivir), family history, anatomic abnormality (medullary sponge kidney).

Types of stone Calcium (usually oxalate ~75% with pure calcium phosphate rare (5%),) struvite (ammonium magnesium phosphate ± calcium phosphate ~15–20%), uric acid (~10%), cystine (~1%), other.

Clinical features Renal stones may be asymptomatic or present with a variety of symptoms. *Pain:* Stones in the kidney cause flank pain. Stones in the ureter cause renal (ureteric) colic. This classically radiates from the flank to the groin and is associated with nausea and vomiting. Bladder or urethral stones may cause pain on micturition, or interruption of urine flow. *Infection* may be acute, chronic, or recurrent. It may present with cystitis (frequency, dysuria), pyelonephritis (fever, rigors, flank pain, nausea, vomiting), or pyonephrosis (infected hydronephrosis). *Other:* Hematuria; sterile pyuria; anuria from obstructing bladder calculi or ureteral calculi with solitary functioning kidney.

Tests *Blood:* BUN, creatinine, electrolytes, Ca^{2+}, PO_4^{3-}, intact PTH if hypercalcemic, uric acid. *Urinalysis;* urine pH (normal range 4.5–8). Acid urine ↑uric acid stone formation and alkaline urine ↑ phosphate stone formation). *24h urine:* Ca^{2+}, sodium, sulfate/urea nitrogen reflects animal protein/protein intake, phosphate, uric acid, citrate, oxalate, pH, volume, creatinine for accuracy of collection.

Imaging: Non-contrast helical CT is the imaging modality of choice for stones. Renal ultrasound excludes hydronephrosis or hydroureter. Abdominal 'KUB' film (kidneys + ureters + bladder).

Management Stones not causing obstruction between attacks of renal colic may be managed conservatively. Advise to ↑ fluid intake and strain urine to retrieve stone for biochemical analysis. Note that stones often take ≥30d to pass. *Ureteric stones* <5mm in diameter usually pass spontaneously. They may need to be fragmented or removed endoscopically from below. If >5mm unlikely to pass spontaneously. *Pelvicalyceal stones* <5mm do not need treatment unless causing obstruction or infection. Stones <2cm in diameter are suitable for lithotripsy. Stones >2cm are usually removed by percutaneous or cystoscopic methods. *Renal colic:* Give IV fluids if unable to tolerate oral fluids, analgesia, and antibiotics if evidence of infection. *Seek urological help urgently if evidence of obstruction.* Procedures include retrograde stent insertion, nephrostomy, and antegrade pyelography p238. These may be combined with lithotripsy. Open surgery is rarely needed.

Prevention Drink plenty of fluid to keep urine output >2–3L/24h. It may be necessary to drink at night to cause voiding at night.

Calcium oxalate stones:

Hypercalciuria: Low salt (2g/d); watch animal protein intake; thiazide diuretic.

Hyperoxaluria: Calcium intake (dairy products) with meals; ↓oxalate intake (less tea, chocolate, nuts, strawberries, rhubarb, spinach, nuts); calcium supplements if enteric hyperoxaluria due to small bowel disease with colon hyperabsorption of oxalate.

Hyperuricosuria: Restrict dietary purine intake, allopurinol.

Hypocitraturia: Potassium citrate, lemonade.

Struvite: Antibiotics; urologic removal of stones.

Uric acid stones: Urinary alkalinization (to maintain pH >6); allopurinol (100–300mg/d). *Cystine stones:* Vigorous hydration to keep cystine concentration <250–300mg/L of urine, D-penicillamine, tiopronin, captopril; urinary alkalinization to achieve urine pH >7–7.5.

Questions for patients with stones

• *What is its composition?* In order of frequency, the likely answer is:
— Calcium oxalate stones: These are spiculated   (radiopaque)
— Calcium phosphate stones are smooth and may be large (radiopaque)
— Struvite staghorn stone: Large; spiculated   (radiopaque)
— Uric acid: (smooth, brown, and soft)   (radiolucent)
— Cystine stones: Yellow and crystalline   (semi-opaque)
• Risk factors?
— Diet: Excess salt and animal protien intake for hypercalciuria, calcium restriction with meals, ↑ oxalate intake (chocolate, tea, nuts, spinach) for hyperaxaluria, purine intake for calcium and uric acid stones
— Hypercalciuria/hypercalcemia (eg hyperparathyroidism, sarcoidosis, neoplasia, hyperthroidismn, Li$^+$, vit D excess)
— Dehydration: Diarrhea lose urine volume –all stones. Acidic urine can lead to uric acid stones
— Medullary sponge kidney
— Primary or secondary hyperoxaluria (excess oxalate gut reabsorption because of small bowel malabsorption)
— Gout and an ↑ urine uric acid: ↑ both calcium oxalate and uric acid stones
— UTI (predisposes to struvite stones with urea splitters and staghorn calculi)
— Distal renal tubular acidosis: Acidosis leads to low urine citrate and alkaline urine leads to calcium phosphate stones. (Sjögren's-secondary distal RTA)
— Cystinuria
— Family history? X-linked nephrolithiasis, or Dent's disease: Low molecular weight proteinuria, hypercalciuria, nephrocalcinosis?
Is there infection above the stone? Fever? Flank tender? Pyuria?

Urinary tract obstruction

Urinary tract obstruction is common, often reversible, and should be considered in any patient with impaired renal function due to bilateral or unilateral in solitary functioning kidney. It may occur from the renal calyces to the urethral meatus. It may be *partial* or *complete*, *unilateral* or *bilateral*. Obstructing lesions are *luminal* (stones, blood clot, sloughed papilla, tumor), *mural* (eg congenital or acquired stricture, neuromuscular dysfunction, schistosomiasis), or *extra-mural* (abdominal or pelvic mass/tumor, retroperitoneal fibrosis). Unilateral, partial, or slowly developing obstruction may be asymptomatic (ie normal urine output). Bilateral obstruction or obstruction + infection requires urgent treatment.

Clinical features *Acute upper tract obstruction:* Flank pain ± radiation to groin. There may be superimposed infection.

Chronic upper tract obstruction: Flank pain, renal failure, superimposed infection. Polyuria may occur due to impaired urinary concentration.

Acute lower tract obstruction: May be urinary retention usually presents with severe suprapubic pain, often preceded by symptoms of bladder outflow obstruction. Exam: Distended, palpable bladder.

Chronic lower tract obstruction: Symptoms: Urinary frequency, hesitancy, ↓stream, dribbling, overflow incontinence, nocturia, suprapubic fullness. *Signs:* Distended, palpable bladder; ↑prostate. Complications: UTI, urinary retention.

Tests *Blood:* Electrolytes, BUN, creatinine.

Urine: Dipstick and microscopic exam. Urine pH (may be ↑ from acidification defect—distal nephron damage). *Ultrasound* p238 is the imaging test of choice. If obstruction above the bladder, *antegrade or retrograde pyelography/ nephrostomy:* Offers therapeutic option of drainage. *Radionuclide imaging* enables functional assessment of collecting system dilation which may be from vesicoureteral reflux, chronic pyelonephritis, pregnancy (R > L), ↑ urine flow states, instead of true obstruction. *CT and MRI* may help identify location and etiology of obstruction.

Treatment ▶ *Drainage is urgent if there is infection above an obstruction.* Upper tract obstruction: Acute; nephrostomy. Chronic; ureteral stent or pyeloplasty. *Lower tract obstruction:* Urethral or suprapubic catheter. Treat the underlying cause if possible. Beware of large diuresis after relief of obstruction; a temporary salt-losing nephropathy may occur with the loss of several liters of fluid a day. Monitor vital signs for hypotension, weight, fluid balance, and electrolytes in case IV fluids (eg 0.045% NS) required.

Retroperitoneal fibrosis (part of chronic periaortitis which includes inflammatory abdominal aortic aneurysms, perianeurysmal retroperitoneal fibrosis)

In this rare autoimmune condition, there is vasculitis of adventitial aortic vaso vasorum and periaortic small vessels with fibrous tissue embedding the ureters resulting in progressive obstruction. Primary and secondary causes.

Associations: Drugs (eg beta-blockers, bromocriptine, methysergide, ergotamines); malignancy (carcinoid, lymphoma, sarcomas, carcinoma of colon, prostate, breast, stomach); infections (TB, histoplasmosis); radiation therapy; surgery (colectomy, hysterectomy); others (trauma, thyroiditis).

Typical patient: Middle-aged men with dull, non-colicky backache with constitutional symptoms of weight loss, fatigue, anorexia, ↑BP, ± edema.

Tests: Blood: anemia; uremia; ↑ESR; ↑CRP; ANA & few ANCA +ve.

Imaging: Ultrasound/IVP: Dilated ureters (hydronephrosis) + medial deviation of ureters with extrinsic compression, peri-aortic mass. Rarely, ultrasound may be negative. *CT/MRI:* Peri-aortic mass which entraps ureters (this allows biopsy, which confirms the diagnosis).

Treatment: Retrograde stent placement to relieve obstruction + steroids or other immunosuppressive medications (cyclosporine, mycophenlate mofetil) or tamoxifen ± surgery (open/laparoscopic ureterolysis).

Glomerulonephritis (GN)

Abbreviations: ANA = antinuclear antibody; ASO = anti-streptolysin O titer; BM = basement membrane (glomerular); EM = electron microscope; ESRD = end-stage renal disease; HCV = hepatitis C virus; IF = immunofluorescence.

Cardinal features Hematuria (microscopic/gross, dysmorphic red cells, ± red cell casts, p237) and/or proteinuria. Patients may be asymptomatic or present with hematuria, proteinuria, nephrotic syndrome, nephritic syndrome, renal failure, or hypertension. Diagnosis is usually made on renal histology, interpreted in the light of clinical, biochemical, and immunological features.

Tests *Blood:* CBC; electrolytes, BUN, creatinine; LFT; ESR; serum electrophoresis; complement (C3, C4); autoantibodies: ANA, ANCA p377, anti-dsDNA (*double stranded DNA*), anti-GBM (*glomerular basement membrane*); blood culture; ASO; HBsAg; anti-HCV, cryoglobulins. *Urinalysis:* To diagnose glomerular bleeding, look for RBC casts, dysmorphic RBCs, and acanthocyturia (≥5% of RBCs, p237). Urinalysis dipstick and microscopic exam. *24h urine* for protein and creatinine excretion/creatinine clearance. Spot urine protein to creatinine ratio for approximation. *CXR; renal ultrasound; renal biopsy.*

Management *Refer to a nephrologist for management.*

IgA nephropathy (Berger's disease) Commonest cause of GN

Typical patient: Children, young adults, males (2:1). *Presentations:* Episodic macroscopic gross hematuria 1–2d after precipitating URI (40–50%).

Diagnosis: Renal biopsy: Mesangial proliferation with +ve immunofluorescence (IF) for IgA and C3. *Prognosis:* 4–38% of adults develop end-stage renal failure (ESRF) over ~10yrs. Risk factors for progression include ↑ creatinine, BP and >1g/d proteinruia. *Treatment:* ACE inhibitors and /or ARB for hypertension or proteinuria. Consider fish oil supplementation. Immunosuppression if active crescents seen on biopsy.

Henoch–Schönlein purpura (HSP) can be regarded as a systemic variant of IgA nephropathy. *Clinical features:* Polyarthritis of the large joints; purpuric rash on the extensor surfaces; abdominal symptoms; GN. *Diagnosis:* Usually clinical. May be confirmed by finding positive IF for IgA and C3 in skin lesions or renal biopsy (identical to IgA nephropathy). *Prognosis:* 50% remission 15–20% impaired renal function; 3–5% renal failure.

Thin basement membrane nephropathy (Autosomal dominant). There is persistent microscopic hematuria ± minor proteinuria, with normal BP and renal function. *Diagnosis:* Positive family history. Renal biopsy: ↓width of glomerular BM. *Prognosis:* Benign.

Membranoproliferative GN Accounts 8% of children and 14% of adults with nephrotic syndrome. Variable presentation: Hematuria, non nephrotic proteinuria, slowly progressive glomerular disease, nephrotic syndrome

Diagnosis: Biopsy shows glomeruli with mesangial proliferation and 'double contoured' BM. 3 histological types: Type I (subendothelial and mesangial deposits) type II (intramembranous and mesangial deposits). Type III (subendothelial, mesangial, subepithelial deposits). ↓serum C3 and C3 nephritic factor are found in most patients (type II more than type I). *Associations:* Hep C; SLE; post-strep; endocarditis; visceral abscess; shunt nephritis; HBV; schistosomiasis; mixed cryoglobulinemia; carcinoma; α$_1$-antitrypsin deficiency; CLL partial lipodystropy; complement deficiency.

Treatment: In adults, long term benefit of ASA + dyridamole, or steroids, or other immuno-suppressive meds unclear. Hep C related tx (p516).

Prognosis: Risk factors for worse prognosis include nephrotic proteinuria ↑ Scr at presentation, HTN, interstitial fibrosis on box. 50% develop ESRD untreated.

Proliferative GN is classified histologically: Focal proliferative; diffuse proliferative; endocapillary proliferative; extracapillary proliferative; mesangial proliferative. The chief cause is post-streptococcal GN. *Clinical features:* Hematuria; proteinuria; nephritic syndrome; nephrotic syndrome; renal failure (rare). *Renal biopsy:* Hypercellularity, mesangial proliferation, inflammatory cell infiltrate, positive IF for IgG and C3 and subepithelial deposits on EM. Serology: ↑ASO; ↓C3. *Treatment:* Antibiotics, diuretics, and antihypertensives as necessary. Dialysis is rarely required. *Prognosis:* Good.

Rapidly progressive GN (RPGN) ESRD develops over weeks or months if untreated. *Causes:*
• Antiglomerular basement membrane (GBM) disease (Goodpasture's). Check anti-GBM titer.
• Immune complex disease: SLE, cryoglobulinemia; Henoch–Schönlein purpura/ IgA; rheumatoid arthritis; post infectious (post-streptococcal). Check complement levels and specific serologies. (ANA, anti-dsDNA, hep C, ASO, cryoglobulins).
• Pauci-immune glomerulonephritis (eg Wegener's granulomatosis, microscopic polyangiitis, Churg–Strauss syndrome. Check ANCA
• Other

Clinical features: Symptoms and signs of renal failure (oliguria, edema). Gross hematuria. There may be systemic symptoms (fever, malaise, myalgia, weight loss), hemoptysis, sinusitis, abdominal pain, purpura, mononeuritis multiplex.

Renal biopsy: Necrotizing GN with crescent formation (crescentic GN).

Treatment: High-dose corticosteroids (IV pulse followed by PO); cyclophosphamide for most (alternative mycophenolate mofetil for SLE) then consider change over to azathioprine or mycophenolate mofetil after 3–6m. Plasma exchange with anti-GBM disease for pulmonary hemorrhage or for severe renal failure if thought to be reversible (little fibrosis on renal biopsy, not dialysis dependent within 72h after treatment), and consider for severe renal failure (Scr >5.7mg/dL) in ANCA-related GN. Renal transplantation.

The nephrotic syndrome

When there is edema, check a urinalysis for protein to avoid missing this diagnosis.

Definition Nephrotic syndrome is the combination of edema, proteinuria (>3g/24h), hypoalbuminemia (albumin <3.5g/dL), and hyperlipidemia. In some cases, this is due to ↑urine protein loss resulting in ↓albumin, hence ↓plasma oncotic pressure (minimal change disease). However, most patients may have a normal or ↑plasma volume suggesting there is primary salt retention.

Causes Minimal change disease (common in children and young adults); focal segmental glomerulosclerosis (common in African Americans); membranous GN; (common in middle-aged/elderly); DM; amyloidosis; SLE; membranoproliferative GN.

Minimal change glomerulonephritis (MCGN) Commonest cause of nephrotic syndrome in children (76%—and 25% of nephrotic adults). *Associations:* Hodgkin's lymphoma; various drugs. *Clinical features:* Nephrotic syndrome; BP↑; usually little renal impairment; however acute renal failure in elderly from ATN or secondary to NSAIDs with interstitial nephritis. *Diagnosis:* Selective proteinuria (especially in children). Renal biopsy shows loss of podocyte foot processes on electron microscopy (EM). *Treatment:* Corticosteroids induce remission in >90% of children and 80% of adults (slower response). *Indications for other immunosuppression:* (cyclophosphamide, cyclosporine). *Prognosis:* 1% progress to ESRD.

Focal segmental glomerulosclerosis can be similar to MCGN as only some glomeruli have segmental sclerosis. It may be primary (idiopathic) or secondary (reflux, sickle-cell disease, obesity, HIV, heroin use, renal scarring after glomerulonephritis). *Clinical features:* Nephrotic syndrome; proteinuria; microscopic hematuria; ↓renal function; BP↑. *Renal biopsy:* Segmental areas of glomerular sclerosis, hyalinization of glomerular capillaries and positive IF for IgM and C3. *Treatment:* 35–60% complete and partial remission to steroids, but prolonged course of high dose (1mg/kg/d) for >4 months may be required. Cyclophosphamide or cyclosporin may be used in steroid-resistant cases. *Prognosis:* 10–40% if subnephrotic, 45–70% if nephrotic progress to ESRD in 10yrs.

Membranous nephropathy Accounts for 20–30% of nephrotic syndrome in adults; 2–5% in children. *Associations:* Malignancy (colon, lung, breast); drugs (gold, penicillamine); autoimmune (SLE, RA); infections (HBV; syphilis; leprosy). *Signs:* Nephrotic syndrome; proteinuria; hematuria; BP↑; renal impairment. Hypercoaguable state; see below.

Diagnosis: Renal biopsy shows thickened BM, IF +ve for IgG & C3 and subepithelial deposits on EM.

Prognosis: About 1/3 experience spontaneous remission, 1/3 has persistent proteinuria but not ESRD, 1/3 ESRD over 5–10yrs.

Treatment: Controversial because of variable natural history. If renal function deteriorates, persistent heavy proteinuria (eg >8g/d for 6m) consider corticosteroids + chlorambucil (Ponticelli regimen)/cyclophosphamide cyclosporine, others.

Clinical features of nephrotic syndrome Symptoms Ask about acute or chronic infections, drugs, allergies, systemic symptoms (SLE, malignancy).

Signs: Periorbital/peripheral edema (anasarca); hypertension; Rarely: Pleura effusions; ascites. Examine for signs associated with secondary causes hypercoaguable state.

Complications
- Thromboembolism especially membranous or MPGN (10–40%) with loss of anticoagulant proteins, ↑ of procoagualant proteins, ↑plt aggregation (DVT, PE, renal vein thrombosis; CNS vessels).
- Hyperlipidemia.
- Acute renal failure; overdiuresis; elderly with minimal change disease; renal vein thrombosis.
- ↑Susceptibility to infection (peritonitis, pneumococcus, eg in children).

Tests *Urine:* Dipstick (hematuria, proteinuria); microscopy (RBCs, casts); culture/sensitivity; 24h collection (protein excretion, creatinine clearance) or spot urine protein to creatinine ratio for approximation; urine protein electrophoresis. *Blood:* Electrolytes, BUN, creatinine; LFT; ESR; CRP; cholesterol; serum electrophoresis; complement (C3, C4); autoantibodies (ANA, anti-dsDNA); HEP B serology. *Imaging:* CXR; renal ultrasound. *Renal biopsy:* Usually do in all adults unless suspect diabetic nephropathy (and steroid unresponsive children, or if unusual features).

Treatment
- Monitor BUN, creatinine, electrolytes, BP, fluid balance, weight.
- Fluid restriction (1–1.5L/d), sodium-restriction (88mEq/d or 2g/d).
- Diet: Avoid excess protein: Aim for ≤0.8g/kg/d protein.
- Diuretics, eg furosemide eg 40–400mg/d in bid doses ± metolazone. *Aim for loss of 1kg/d.* Occasionally, to promote diuresis, you may need very high doses of furosemide (eg upto 200mg IV)± diuril (upto 500mg IV) or metolazone. (Salt-poor albumin used by some physicians in patients with albumin ≈1g/dL, evidence poor.)
- Treat hypertension with ACE inhibitors ± ARB.
- Persistent nephrotic syndrome: Immunosuppressive medications as above; ACE-I ± ARB to reduce proteinuria.
- Hypercoaguable state: Prophylactic warfarin advocated by some at high risk (membranous nephropathy with massive proteinruia >10g/d); warfarin for thrombosis.
- Hyperlipidemia improves with resolution of nephrotic syndrome. If unresponsive, treatment with a HMG-CoA reductase inhibitors + ACE inhibitor/ARB may reduce proteinuria further than ACE inhibitor/ARB alone.

249

Renal vein thrombosis Clinical prevalence: 6–8% with membranous GN; 1–3% of those with other forms of GN. Radiological prevalence: 10–40% of patients with membranous GN; 10% other causes. *Clinical features:* Flank pain (eg acute) hematuria, proteinuria, renal enlargement and deteriorating renal function. Usually asymptomatic and diagnosed incidentally. 35% have coincident PE. *Diagnosis:* Doppler ultrasound, renal angiography (venous phase), spiral CT, or MRI. *Treatment:* Anticoagulate with warfarin until non-nephrotic proteinuria achieved. Thrombolyitc treatment/mechanical thrombolysis for acute severe thrombosis. IVC/bilateral renal vein thrombosis with acute renal failure is reported.

Acute renal failure (ARF): Diagnosis

Definition A significant deterioration in renal function occurring over hours or days. ARF may lead to hyperkalemia, acidosis, pulmonary edema, and uremia. Clinically, there may be nausea, vomiting, fatigue, shortness of breath (crackles), chest pain (pericarditis), change in mental status (asterixis), seizures, ↓ urine volume (oliguria <400cc/d), or no symptoms or signs. Biochemically, ARF is detected by rising plasma urea nitrogen and creatinine. ARF may arise as an isolated problem; more commonly it occurs in the setting of circulatory disturbance, eg severe illness, sepsis, trauma, or surgery—or in the context of nephrotoxic drugs.

Causes: See various sections for details. ARF can be divided into three types
Pre-renal (renal hypoperfusion) is usually reversible. Causes are volume depletion, renal vasoconstriction due to medications (NSAIDS, ACE-i/ARB, calcinuerin inhibitors, amphotericin, iodinated contrast dye), hypercalcemia, sepsis, hepatorenal syndrome.

Intrinsic (intrarenal)

Tubular: Acute tubular necrosis (ATN) is associated with prolonged hypoperfusion (shock), nephrotoxins (aminoglycosides, amphotericin B, iodinated contrast dye, prolonged NSAIDS, ACE-i), rhabdomyolysis (see below). Complete recovery of renal function usually occurs within days or weeks.

Vascular: (renal artery/vein occlusion, renal infarction, malignant hypertension, atheroemboli).

Glomerular; Acute glomerulonephritis, small vessel vasculitis, hemolytic uremic syndrome—TTP.

Interstitial: Interstitial nephritis, tumor infiltration.

Intratubular obstruction (uric acid from tumor lysis syndrome, acyclovir, sulfonamides, indinavir).

Post renal due to urinary obstruction from nephrolithiasis, ↑prostate, pelvic masses, and dysfunctional bladder is a potentially treatable cause.

Assessment Make sure you know about the renal effects of *all* drugs taken.
1 *Is the renal failure acute or chronic?* Suspect chronic kidney disease if:
- History of chronic ill-health or signs of chronic kidney disease;
- Previously abnormal blood tests (previous records, laboratory results);
- Small kidneys (<9cm) on ultrasound.

The *presence* of anemia, Ca^{2+}↓ or PO_4^{3-} ↑ may not help to distinguish ARF from CKD, as these can occur subacutely, but their *absence* suggests ARF. Secondary hyperparathyroidism is suggestive of CKD

2 *Is there urinary tract obstruction?*
Obstruction should always be considered as a cause of ARF because it is reversible and prompt treatment is required to prevent permanent renal damage. Obstruction should be suspected in patients with a single functioning kidney, or in those with history of renal stones, anuria, prostatism, or previous pelvic/retroperitoneal surgery. Examine for a palpable bladder, pelvic or abdominal masses, or an enlarged prostate.

3 *Is there a rare cause of ARF?*—Eg glomerulonephritis, etc.—see above. These are usually associated with abnormal urinary sediment and warrant urgent renal referral for consideration of a renal biopsy and treatment.

Tests • *Urine: Dipstick* for leukocytes; nitrite; blood; protein; glucose; specific gravity. *Microscopy* for RBC, WBC; crystals; cellular or granular casts. *Culture and sensitivity. Chemistry:* Sodium, urea nitrogen, creatinine, osmolality; protein (spot/24h with urine creatinine measurement), UPEP—beware K$^+$↑; LFT; • *Blood tests* Electrolytes, BUN, CR, CBC; clotting; CPK; ESR; ABG; blood cultures. When glomerular disease suspected consider: Complement levels (C3/C4); autoantibodies (ANA; ANCA; anti-dsDNA; anti-GBM p377) & ASO. Suspect myeloma—serum electrophoresis; • *CXR:* Pulmonary edema/hemmorhage? • *ECG:* Signs of hyperkalemia? • *Renal ultrasound:* Renal size or obstruction?

Distinguishing pre-renal failure and ATN

	Pre-renal	ATN
Urine Na (mmol/L)	<20	>40
Urine osmolality (mosm/L)	>500	<350
Urine/plasma urea	>8	<3
Urine/plasma creatinine	>40	<20
Fractional Na excretion (%)	<1	>2
BUN/Cr	>20	≤20

These indices are of limited clinical use as intermediate values are common, they may be influenced by diuretics and pre-existing tubular disease and 'typical' values do not predict renal prognosis. Fractional excretion of urea nitrogen FeUN (<35% pre-renal vs. >50%) used for patients on diuretics. Both FeNa and FeUN are most accurate when patients are oliguric.

Acute renal failure (ARF): Management

Enlist nephrologist's help. While awaiting this, make sure that urine micros-copy results are available.
- If shock is the cause (↓intravascular volume, *below*), use protocol on p696
- Ultrasound; Check for a palpable bladder; but absence of this sign does not rule out obstruction. If it *is* palpable, insert a catheter.
- Stop nephrotoxic drugs—eg gentamicin; amphotericin B—*any* drug may be nephrotoxic: Peripheral eosinophilia is suggestive of allergic interstitial nephritis (unreliable).
- Any sign of a vasculitis? Arthralgias? Hemoptysis? Rash? ESR↑?
- Find and treat precipitating/exacerbating factors: Sepsis/UTI; ?CHF; BP↑↑.

NB: Assessing signs of ↓intravascular volume can be difficult: Look for ↓BP ↑pulse; urine volume↓; poor skin turgor; dry mucous membranes; ↓JVP When in doubt, insert a CVP line to measure central venous pressure. Signs of fluid overload: S3, ↑BP, ↑JVP, crackles, peripheral edema.

Monitoring Check pulse, BP, JVP, CVP (if available), & urine output frequently Daily fluid balance + weight chart. If euvolemic, match input to losses (urine vomit, diarrhea, drains) + 500mL for insensible losses (more if T°↑).
- Correct volume depletion with intravenous fluid—colloid, saline, or blood (watch plasma ↑K⁺) as appropriate.
- If the patient is septic, take appropriate cultures and treat empirically with antibiotics. Remove or change any potential sources of sepsis (eg central lines).
- Re-check about any nephrotoxic medications; adjust doses of renally excreted medications.
- Nutrition: Aim for calorie intake 35kcal/kg/d and protein intake ≈1–1.2g/dk/c although some recommend 0.8g/dk/d if uremic but not on renal replacement therapy. If oral intake is poor, consider nasogastric nutrition early (parenteral if NGT impossible). Restrict dietary sodium intake if volume overloaded to <2g/d, and if volume ↓ 2g/d. Oral potassium intake if hyperkalemic <50mEq/d Phosphate restriction 600–800mg/d if hyperphosphatemic.

Treat complications

Hyperkalemia may cause arrhythmias or cardiac arrest. *ECG changes:* Peaked T waves; small or absent P wave; ↑ P–R interval; widened QRS complex; 'sine wave' pattern; asystole. ECG p621.
1 Stabilize myocardium if severe hyperkalemia >7 or severe EKG changes (loss of P waves, QRS widening).
   - IV calcium, eg 10mL 10% calcium gluconate IV over 1min, repeat as neces-sary until ECG improves.
2 Shift potassium into cells
   - IV insulin + glucose, eg 10U regular insulin + 50mL of 50% glucose IV over 10min. if not diabetic, consider continuous infusion of D5 to prevent hy-poglycemia. Insulin stimulates the intracellular uptake of K⁺, lowering se-rum K⁺ by 1–2mmol/L over 30–60min.
   - *Beta* agonists. 10–20mg by albuterol nebulizer ↓ potassium within 30min 8 times usual dose and may not work if used alone.
   - Sodium bicarbonate if patient with severe metabolic acidosis to shift po-tassium in cells, otherwise unlikely benefit.
3 Remove potassium. Usually requires one of measures below
   - Sodium polystyrene sulfonate (kayexylate), eg 15–60g PO or PR to bind K⁺ in the gut. SE: Colonic necrosis of ileus (eg recent surgery).
   - Diuretics if responsive,
   - Hemodialysis (HD)/continuous renal replacement therapy (CRRT—see OPPO-SITE)—latter much slower potassium removal rate—is usually required if anuric CRRT will not remove potassium as quickly as HD.

Pulmonary edema p692. In summary:
- High-flow oxygen by face mask.
- IV furosemide 200mg IV as bolus, followed by continuous drip if some response with bolus ± IV diuril
- Consider inotropes in congestive heart failure due to systolic dysfunction.
- If no response, HD/CRRT is necessary.
- Other measeures:
- Consider continuous positive airways pressure ventilation (CPAP) therapy.
- Venous vasodilator, eg morphine 2.5mg IV.
- IV nitrates.

Bleeding: Impaired hemostasis due to uremic platelets may be compounded by the precipitating cause. In patients with ARF who are actively bleeding, give:
- Fresh frozen plasma, cryoprecipitate & platelets as needed—if there are clotting problems.
- Blood transfusion to maintain Hb >10g/dL and hematocrit >30%.
- Desmopressin to ↑factor VIII activity, normalizing bleeding time.

Indications for dialysis: • Severe hyperkalemia (K^+ >6.5–7mmol/L) • Refractory pulmonary edema • Severe or worsening metabolic acidosis (pH <7.2 or base excess <–10) • Uremic encephalopathy or other symptoms (nausea/vomiting) • Uremic pericarditis.

Prognosis for ARF. Mortality depends on cause: Burns (80%); trauma/surgery (60%); medical illness (30%); obstetric/poisoning (10%). ICU setting requiring renal replacement therapy (50–80%).

Continuous renal replacement therapy (CRRT)

CRRT may be preferable in an intensive care unit setting when sudden shifts in volume removal or osmolarity are undesirable. (HD is described in the next section, Chronic Kidney Disease.) Indications for CRRT include hemodynamic instability (vasopressors), ↑ intracranial pressure (eg acute hepatic encephalopathy to prevent ↑ intracranial pressure from conventional HD), large IV fluid requirements. Fluid intake requiring large fluid removal.

In continuous veno-venous hemodialysis (CVVHD), blood flows on one side of a semi-permeable membrane while dialysis fluid flows (1–2.5L/h) in the opposite direction on the other side much like conventional HD. Solute transfer occurs by diffusion. Ultrafiltration is the removal of excess fluid by creating –ve transmembrane pressure. In continous veno-venous hemofiltration (CVVH), blood is filtered across a filter (highly permeable synthetic membrane) allowing removal of waste products by a process of convection (not diffusion). The ultrafiltrate removed at high rates (1–2.5L/h) is substituted with an equal volume of replacement fluid which may remove larger molectular waste products (ideally cytokines in sepsis). The 2 modalities may be combined in continous veno-venous hemo diafiltration (CVVHDF). *Advantages:* Less hemodynamic instability. *Disadvantage:* More expensive than HD and requires intensive care unit setting and ↑ clotting.

Chronic kidney disease (CKD)

Definitions Kidney damage ≥3 months as defined by structural or functional abnormalities of the kidney, with or without ↓ GFR (proteinuria) or a GFR <60mL/min/1.73 meters squared body surface area.

It is classified according to glomerular filtration rate (GFR) into 5 categories: Stage 1 (kidney damage with normal GFR >90mL/min); stage 2 (60–89 –mL/min); stage 3 (30–59mL/min); stage 4 (15–29mL/min) and stage 5 (<15mL/min). End-stage renal disease (ESRD) is the degree of renal failure that, without renal replacement therapy, would lead to death.

Causes *Common:* BP↑; DM; chronic glomerulonephritis; chronic interstitial nephritis (pyelonephritis); polycystic disease, renal vascular disease, chronic obstruction. *Rare:* Myeloma, amyloidosis, SLE, scleroderma, vasculitis, thrombotic microangiopathy, nephrocalcinosis, renal tumor, Alport's syndrome, Fabry's disease.

History Ask about: Past and childhood UTI; known hypertension; DM. Any family history of renal disease? Take a careful medication history. Any fatigue, weakness, dyspnea, pleuritic chest pain, ankle swelling, restless legs, anorexia, vomiting, pruritus, concentration ↓, changes in sleep wake cycle, bone pain, nocturia, foamy urine, incontinence, ↓ urinary stream, dribbling, incomplete voiding?

Signs: BP↑; cardiomegaly; pericarditis; pleural effusion; pulmonary or peripheral edema; pallor; yellow skin pigmentation; easy bruising; epistaxis; calcifications of skin, eye, calciphylaxis; proximal myopathy; peripheral neuropathy; myoclonus; asterixis; encephalopathy; seizures; coma.

Tests • *Blood:* Hb↓ (normochromic, normocytic); ESR; ↑BUN, ↑creatinine, (electrolytes; ↓ bicarbonate, ↑potassium); glucose (DM); ↓Ca^{2+}, ↑PO$_4^{3-}$; ↑alk phos (renal osteodystrophy); ↑intact PTH (secondary hyperparathyroidism p284); urate↑. • *Urine:* Dipstick and microscopy; 24h urinary protein; creatinine clearance. • *Renal ultrasound* to exclude obstruction and look at renal size (usually small (<9cm) in CKD; normal or large in DM, HIV, polycystic kidney disease, amyloidosis, myeloma, and asymmetric in renovascular disease, chronic pyelo on small side.) Consider *MRA*, Doppler ultrasound to rule out renovascular disease. *CXR:* Cardiomegaly, pleural/pericardial effusions or pulmonary edema. *Bone x-rays* may show renal osteodystrophy, lytic lesions with multiple myeloma. • *Renal biopsy* should be considered if the process is felt to be reversible (normal sized kidneys may be one sign).

Treatment Refer early to a nephrologist. Treat reversible causes: Relieve obstruction, stop nephrotoxic medications, treat renal osteodystrophy, anemia, and acidosis.

- *Hypertension:* Controlling hypertension may save significant renal function. ACE-I/ARB can ↓rate of loss of function even if BP is normal if there is microalbuminuria. Aim for BP of <130/80. Watch serum creatinine and potassium after start of these meds.
- *Hyperlipidemia:* This may contribute to renal damage, and ↑ the risk of cardiovascular disease. Treat with HMG-CoA reductase inhibitors.
- *Edema:* This may require high doses of loop diuretics, furosemide, bumentanide, torsemide + metolazone 5–10mg/d.
- *Anemia:* If other causes are excluded, eg iron deficiency, chronic infection, etc. p557, consider erythropoietin to maintain Hb between 11–12g/dL.
- *Renal bone disease (osteodystrophy):* Treat as soon as ↑phosphate or ↑PTH. ↓Dietary PO$_4^{3-}$ (less milk, cheese, eggs). Phosphate binders calcium acetate or calcium carbonate for stages 3–5, sevelamer (Renagel) or lanthanum (non-calcium based phosphate binder) for stage 5 only. Use 1,25 dihydroxy vitamin D or analogs paracalcitol(zemplar); doxercalciferol (Hectoral) to treat secondary hyperparathyroidism with goal iPTH 150–300pg/mL stage 5 CKD, lower target values in earlier stages. Analogs cause less hypercalcemia and hyperphosphatemia. Calcimimetic drug cinacalcet ↓ PTH, calcium and phosphate.

- *Dietary advice:* Match dietary and fluid intake with excretory capacity. Protein restriction is reasonable. Na restriction may help to control BP and prevent edema. K⁺ restriction is required in hyperkalemia. Acidosis: treat with HCO_3^- supplements.
- *Preparing for dialysis:* KDOQI[1] guidelines suggests vascular access placement eg arterio–venous fistula when creatinine clearance is <25mL/min, serum creatinine >4mg/dL, or anticipate use within 1yr. These guidelines are difficult for patients to follow because of lack of referral or symptoms at this GFR. Insert a Tenchkoff catheter 4–6wks before anticipating need to start peritoneal dialysis. Refer for transplantation, if appropriate.

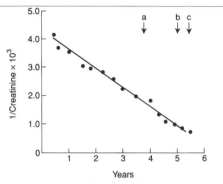

Plot of reciprocal plasma creatinine (mcmol/L) against time in a patient with adult polycystic disease. The letters represent life events: (a) work promotion, (b) arterio-venous fistula, and (c) hemodialysis.

Some patients with CKD lose renal function at a constant rate. Creatinine is produced at a fairly constant rate and rises on an exponential curve as renal function declines, so the reciprocal creatinine plot is a straight line, parallel to the fall in GFR. This is used to monitor renal function and to predict need for dialysis—but there is much individual variation in progression, so the plot has limited application. Rapid decline in renal function greater than that expected may be due to: Infection, dehydration, uncontrolled ↑BP, metabolic disturbance (eg Ca^{2+}↑), obstruction, nephrotoxins (eg drugs). Investigation and treatment at this point may delay ESRD.

Progression of CKD is sometimes slowed by using ACE-I *with* A2A (angiotensin-II blockers). In the COOPERATE randomized prospective trial (over 3yrs) the NNT was ~9 for preventing one case of ESRF (or a doubling of plasma creatinine)[2] by adding losartan (100mg/d) to trandolapril (3mg/d)—ie 11% progressed rather than 23% on ACE-I alone.

Prescribing in renal failure

Relate dose modification to creatinine clearance, and the extent to which a drug is renally excreted. This is significant for aminoglycosides (gentamicin), cephalosporins, and other antibiotics p493, lithium, opiates, and digoxin. Never prescribe in renal failure before checking how its administration should be altered through Micromedex or the Physician's Desk Reference. Loading doses should not be changed. If the patient is on dialysis (peritoneal or hemodialysis), dose modification depends on how well it is eliminated by dialysis. Some medications require supplementation after dialysis.

1 http://www.kidney.org/kidneydisease/ckd/index.cfm
2 Get expert advice. ↑Dose slowly. SE: BP↓↓ (esp if hypovolaemia); diarrhoea; odd taste; cough; myalgia; migraine; LFT↑; vasculitis. Monitor U&E. Cautions: aortic or mitral stenosis; cardiomyopathy.

Renal replacement therapy

The criterion for initiating dialysis in CKD patients is when GFR 10mL/min/1.73m^2 BSA by using the 4 variable MDRD formula or creatinine clearance estimated by the Cockcroft–Gault formula p234. *Early* psychological preparation is vital. Medical preparation involves hepatitis B vaccination and creating an arteriovenous fistula if hemodialysis is planned option. Choice of hemo- vs peritoneal dialysis depends on medical, social, and psychological factors. **NB:** Kidney function is only partly replaced by dialysis.

Hemodialysis (HD) Blood flows on one side of a semi-permeable membrane while dialysis fluid flows in the opposite direction on the other side. Solute transfer occurs by diffusion. Ultrafiltration is fluid removal from renal replacement therapy. In HD/CRRT, negative pressure across the dialysis membrane removes fluid from filtered blood. *Problems:* • Dialysis dysequilibrium syndrome (rapid shift in osmolality) • BP↓ • Infection • Vascular access (poor flow, infection, thrombosis, stenosis, bleeding, aneurysm, vascular steal syndrome, ischemia).

Peritoneal dialysis (PD) PD fluid is introduced into the peritoneal cavity *via* a Tenchkoff catheter and uremic solutes diffuse into it across the peritoneal membrane. Ultrafiltration may be achieved by using osmotic agents, eg glucose in the dialysis fluid of variable strengths. It is performed in those with low ejection fraction. Convection and diffusion both clear uremic toxins. As opposed to HD, PD clearance is significantly enhanced by residual renal function. Important to ask PD patients about ↓ urine output if uremic symptoms arise.

Continuous ambulatory peritoneal dialysis (CAPD) Patient performs manual exchanges of dialysate where fluid is continuously dwelling in the patient except for filling and draining of dialysate. 2–3L bags are exchanged usually 4 times a day to produce, with ultrafiltration, a total dialysate of >10L/d.

Automated PD Patient uses a cycler machine which automatically performs exchanges at night. Techniques include continuous cyclic peritoneal dialysis (CCPD) where there is fluid left in the abdomen during the day, night intermittent peritoneal dialysis (NIPD) where patient has no fluid in abdomen in the daytime. A manual exchange may have to be added to CCPD or NIPD patients if there is poor dialysis clearance.

Problems:
- Peritonitis (60% staphylococci, 20% Gram –ve organisms, <5% fungi)

• Exit-site infection	• Hernias
• Catheter malfunction	• Back pain
• Loss of ultrafiltration	• Hyperlipidemia.
• Obesity	

It may be difficult to achieve adequate clearance in larger patients who have lost residual renal function.

Complications in ESRD patients *Cardiovascular disease*, eg coronary heart disease, congestive heart failure, cerebrovascular disease is ↑↑ in dialysis patients and a major cause of mortality. *Hypertension* persists in 25–30% of patients on hemodialysis. *Anemia* is common and treated with erythropoietin and oral or IV iron supplements if deficient. *Bleeding tendency* is due to platelet dysfunction. Acute bleeding is treated with desmopressin and transfusion, as necessary. *Renal bone disease* is treated with phosphate binders calcium acetate or calcium carbonate, sevelamer or lanthanum. Secondary hyperparathyroidism with goal IPTH 150–300pg/mL treated with 1, 25 dihydroxy vitamin D, paracalcitol (zemplar) IV or PO (Hectoral) IV or PO, calcitriol PO or IV, or cinacalcet (Sensipar) PO. Calcitriol, and to lesser extents analogs paracalcitriol and doexercalciferol, may ↑ serum calcium and phosphate. Cinacalcet reduces serum calcium and phosphate. *Infections* non-sterility with exchanges during peritoneal dialysis or vascular access procedures with HD or may be related to UTI. *β_2-microglobulin amyloidosis* may cause carpal tunnel syndrome, arthralgia, and fractures. *Acquired renal cystic disease* is seen in patients with longstanding CKD (>90% incidence if on dialysis >5yrs) and there may be malignancy in 4–10%. *Malignancy* is more common in dialysis patients; some tumors are related to the cause of renal failure, eg urothelial tumors in analgesic nephropathy. *Aluminum toxicity* due to the use of aluminum based phophate binders is now rare (bone disease, dementia, anemia.)

Renal transplantation

This is the treatment of choice for ESRD. Each patient requires careful medical assessment and consideration of the advantages of dialysis vs transplantation.

Assessment *Note the following:* Pre-existing cardiovascular disease. CMV, zoster, HBV, Hep C, TB etc. may cause severe disease while immunocompromised requiring prophylaxis or other treatment.
• ABO blood group and HLA tissue typing are required.
• Urological assessment is made, where indicated.

Contraindications Active infection; recently treated cancer (<2yrs); severe heart disease; (HIV patients are being enrolled for transplantation).

Types of graft *Living related donor* (LRD) grafts offer the advantages of an optimally timed surgical procedure, HLA haplotype matching, and improved graft survival. *Live unrelated donation* is an option which is becoming commonplace. *Cadaveric grafts* are obtained from a brainstem dead donor and should ideally be transplanted within 24–36h. Grafts are inserted into an iliac fossa.

Immunosuppressants *Prednisone + cyclosporin/tacrolimus* (calcineurin inhibitors) + *mycophenolate mofetil/azathioprine*. Doses are slowly reduced over the 1st yr. *Others:* Sirolimus is an option for calcineurin inhibitor nephrotoxicity (CAN). Anti-T-cell antibodies. Antithymocyte globulin (polyclonal Ab)/OKT3 (monoclonal AB0, and anti IL-2 Ab to avoid CAN.

Complications Bleeding; thrombosis; infection; urinary leaks; oliguria; malignancy.

Acute rejection: (<3–6m post-op) This is characterized by rising serum creatinine ± fever and graft pain. Graft biopsy in acute cellular rejection shows an immune cell infiltrate and tubular damage. R: IV high-dose corticosteroids for 3–5d followed by PO. Cases with vascular component or resistant cases require antithymocyte globulin (ATG)(SE-fevers, chills , anaphylaxis) or monoclonal OKT3 (SE- 1st dose rxn, pulmonary edema, thrombic microangiopathy, lymphoprolifertive disease) antibody. Antibody mediated rejection: Plasma cell infiltrate with + CD4 staining, plasmapheresis ± IVIG.

Chronic allograft nephropathy: (>3m) Presents with a gradual rise in serum creatinine and proteinuria. Graft biopsy shows vascular changes, glomerular changes, fibrosis, & tubular atrophy. It is not responsive to ↑ immunosuppression.

Cyclosporin nephrotoxicity: Afferent arteriole vasoconstriction causes ↓renal blood flow and GFR. There is also chronic tubular atrophy and fibrosis.

Infection: Typically common community infections or those related to ↓T-cell immunity (∵ immunosuppression), eg skin infections (fungi, warts, HSV, zoster) and opportunistic (TB, fungi, *P. carinii* pneumonia, CMV), others (BK virus).

Malignancy: Immunosuppression causes ↑risk of neoplasia ± infection with viruses of malignant potential (EBV, HBV, HHV-8). Typical tumors are squamous cancers, lymphoma (EBV-related), and anogenital ca.

Atheromatous vascular disease: This is more common in transplant patients than in the general population and is a leading cause of death.

Hypertension: This occurs in >50% of transplant patients and may be due to diseased native kidneys, immunosuppressive drugs or dysfunction in the graft. Management is along standard lines p132. Use of ACE-I /ARB not contraindicated unless known renal artery stenosis of transplant kidney.

Diabetes: Estimated incidence 24% at 3yrs post transplant. Corticosteroids and calcineurin inhibitors are factors.

Prognosis 1yr graft survival: HLA identical 95%; 1 mismatch 90–95%; complete mismatch 75–80%. Average half-life of cadaveric grafts is 8yrs; 20yrs for HLA-identical living related donor grafts. Risk of neoplasia is ↑ x 5 from immunosuppression, eg skin cancers; lymphomas.

Interstitial nephritis and nephrotoxins

Interstitial nephritis is an important cause of both acute and chronic renal failure. *Acute interstitial nephritis (AIN): Typical cause:* Allergic reaction to antibiotics: Penicillins/cephalosporins, furosemide (sulfonamdies), NSAIDs, allopurinol, rifampin. Infection (staphylococci, streptococci, *Brucella, Leptospira*). Systemic disease- sarcoidosis, Sjögren's syndrome—or *no* obvious cause. *Clinical features:* Fever; arthralgia; rash (especially if drug related); eosinophilia; eosinophiluria; acute or chronic renal failure; rarely an associated uveitis (Tubulointerstitial nephrits uveitis syndrome TINU). *Diagnosis:* Biopsy: Mononuclear cell infiltration of the renal interstitium and tubules with eosinophils in drug induced causes.

Systemic features of fever, rash and eosinophilia or eosinophiluria are rarely present with NSAIDs, + in ~33–50% of non-penicillin drug induced causes.

Treatment: ARF p252; corticosteroids may be used with systemic disease, but use in drug induced causes is controversial. Nevertheless, many nephrologists will attempt its use. CKD: None. *Prognosis:* Favorable in ARF if etiology drug or treatment responsive systematic disease; may be gradual deterioration with chronic interstitial nephritis. *Chronic interstitial nephritis* may be a slowly evolving form of the acute disease, or caused by analgesic nephropathy (below), sickle-cell disease, chronic pyelonephritis/reflux nephropathy with secondary FSGS.

Analgesic nephropathy is associated with the prolonged, heavy ingestion of compound anti-pyretic analgesics. The incidence of analgesic nephropathy has fallen since the withdrawal of phenacetin. Use of acetaminophen has been associated, but controversial. *Signs:* Urinary abnormalities (proteinuria, hematuria, sterile pyuria); renal colic/obstruction; from sloughed papilla which may be infected casuing UTI/pyelonephritis; chronic kidney disease; hypertension. *Diagnosis* is based on a history of excess analgesic use, and demonstrating the characteristic renal lesion. *Tests:* CT scan reveals papillary calcifications, ↑ renal size, 'bumpy' contours. IVP shows cortical scarring/clubbed calyces/ shows papillary necrosis. Biopsy shows chronic interstitial nephritis or capillary sclerosis. *Treatment:* Stop analgesics; antibiotics for infection; drainage for obstruction; dialysis or transplantation for ESRD.

Urate nephropathy *Acute crystal nephropathy* may occur when insoluble purines deposit within the tubules causing blockage or inflammation of the tubules. It is caused by gross uric acid overproduction (eg treatment of myeloid tumors) or by inherited diseases (eg Lesch–Nyhan syndrome). Diagnosis by elevated serum uric acid levels ~15–20 and urine uric acid/ urine creatinine >1.

Treatment: Allopurinol, uricase (rasburicase) to ↓uric acid, good fluid intake, alkalinize urine, hemodialysis or CRRT if ↑uric acid levels and poor renal function. *Chronic urate nephropathy* typically affects middle-aged men with gout. May be secondary to lead exposure. Diagnosis: X-ray flourescence or ↑ urine lead levles after EDTA. Histologically, there is interstitial fibrosis with associated vascular changes; crystals are rarely found. *Treatment:* Allopurinol (↓dose in renal impairment), if lead nephropathy, can attempt EDTA to chlelate lead with moderate CKD.

Hypercalcemic nephropathy is caused by malignancy (commonest); hyperparathyroidism; multiple myeloma; sarcoidosis; vit. D intoxication. *Clinical features:* Nephrogenic diabetes insipidus (polyuria, polydipsia, dehydration, uremia); symptoms of hypercalcemia (nausea, vomiting, constipation, lethargy, weakness, confusion, coma); pancreatitis. *Investigations:* Creatinine↑; Ca^{2+}↑ (1, 25 OH vit D, intact PTH, PTH-related peptide, SPEP if clinical suspicion); proteinuria; hematuria; pyuria; hypercalciuria. AXR may show renal calculi/nephrocalcinosis. *Treatment:* IV fluids (3–6L 0.9% saline/24h); loop diuretics; IV bisphosphonates, p391. Steroids may be useful in sarcoidosis.

Radiation nephritis *Acute radiation nephritis* (within 1yr of radiotherapy) *Signs:* Hematuria, proteinuria, BP↑, anemia. *Chronic radiation nephritis* may occur after acute radiation nephritis or present with hypertension, proteinuria, anemia, or end-stage renal failure (ESRD 2–5yrs after exposure to radiation. *Treatment:* Control BP, renal replacement therapy for ESRD. *Prevention:* Exclusion or shielding of renal areas during radiotherapy.

Nephrotoxins

Many agents may be toxic to the kidneys and cause acute renal failure.

Exogenous nephrotoxins include:
- Analgesics: NSAIDs/COX-2 inhibitors
- Antimicrobials: ATN; gentamicin, amphotericin, pentamidine. AIN; (potentially all), penicillins, cephalosporins, sulfanamides. Tubular obstruction; acyclovir, indinavir. RTA; proximal—tenofovir, distal—amphoterecin, both—ifosfamide.
- Chemotherapeutic agents: Cisplatin- ATN; mitomycin C-TTP. Methotrexate—tubular obstruction.
- ACE-i and angiotensin II receptor antagonists (ARB) may cause glomerular hemodynamic changes
- Contrast agents: Especially in diabetic nephropathy, CKD, ARF. (myeloma)
- Organic solvents: Ethylene glycol; hippurate (glue sniffing- acidosis)
- Insecticides, herbicides, *Amanita* mushrooms, snake venom—all rare
- Immunosuppressants: Cyclosporin, tacrolimus.

Endogenous nephrotoxins include:
- Pigments (myoglobin, hemoglobin)
- Crystal deposition/precipitation (urate, phosphate)
- Tumors (immunoglobulin light chains)

Antimicrobials *Aminoglycosides* (eg gentamicin, amikacin) are well-recognized nephrotoxins. The typical clinical picture is of non-oliguric renal failure 1–2wks into therapy. The risk of nephrotoxicity is ↑ by old age, ↓ renal perfusion, pre-existing CKD, high dosage or prolonged treatment, and co-administration of other nephrotoxic drugs. These circumstances are common in severely ill patients. Recovery may be full, delayed, or incomplete.

Myoglobin Myoglobin from muscle injury or necrosis (rhabdomyolysis). *Causes:* Trauma; ischemia; immobility; excessive exercise; seizures; myositis; metabolic (K⁺↓, ↑ phosphate); medications (fibrates, statins); toxins (alcohol, ecstasy, snake bite, carbon monoxide); malignant hyperpyrexia; neuroleptic malignant syndrome; inherited muscle disorders. *Clinical features:* These may be absent or non-specific (muscle pain, swelling, or tenderness). *Tests:* Dark urine which is +ve for blood on dipstick but without RBCs on microscopy. Blood tests: ↑BUN; ↑creatinine; ↑K⁺; ↓Ca²⁺; ↓PO₄³⁻. ↑CK; ↑LDH; ↑urate. *Treatment:* Large volumes of IV fluids, urinary alkalinization with IV bicarbonate has been used. Hemodialysis/CRRT may be required.

Renal vascular diseases/secondary hypertension

Hypertension (HTN) may be a cause or consequence of renal disease. *Essential hypertension.* Investigations: p130. Treatment: p132. *Accelerated (malignant) hypertension* may cause renal failure. Treatment: p132. *Pregnancy-induced hypertension with proteinuria (pre-eclampsia):* Edema + proteinuria ± glomerula endothelisis/obliteration + deposition of fibrin and platelets. *May see:* Hemolysis, elevated liver enzymes, low platelet counts (=HELLP).

Renal diseases causing hypertension: Diabetic nephropathy; acute glomerulonephritis; chronic interstitial nephritis; polycystic kidneys; chronic kidney disease; renovascular disease; acute vasculitis; scleroderma renal crisis; hemolytic uremic syndrome- TTP (see below).

Renovascular disease *Causes:* Atherosclerosis (65–75%, age >50yrs, vascular disease); fibromuscular dysplasia (suspect in younger women). *History:* Coexistent cardiovascular, cerebrovascular, or peripheral vascular disease; deterioration in renal function after ACE-I/ARB, sudden ↑ in BP after stable baseline, HTN with asymmetric kidney sizes (>2cm), severe hypertension, recurrent unexplained flash pulmonary edema, proven onset later age (>50). *Examination:* Abdominal, carotid, or femoral bruits; absent leg pulses; grade III–IV hypertensive retinopathy. *Tests:* Renal angiography is gold standard. *Other tests:* MRA; CT angiography; Doppler ultrasound are currently used for screening tests for atherosclerotic renal artery disease. These test are poor for detecting fibromuscular dysplasia. CT angiography requires a large amount of potentially nephrotoxic contrast dye. *Treatment:* Percutaneous transluminal renal angioplasty ± stent or renal bypass surgery.

Thrombotic microangiopathy: Previously thought of as spectrum between Hemolytic uremic syndrome (HUS) and Thrombotic thrombocytopenic purpura (TTP). *It is a hematologic emergency: Get expert help.*

Thrombotic thrombocytopenic purpura (TTP) It is a pentad of: (1) Fever; (2) Fluctuating neurolgic signs (microthrombi, eg causing seizures ↓consciousness, ↓vision); (3) Microangiopathic hemolytic anemia; (4) Thrombocytopenia; (5) Renal failure. In TTP, there is ↓ADAMTS13 activity (inherited/Ab), leading to ↑unusually large Von Willebrand factor with ↑platelet clumping.

Hemolytic uremic syndrome (HUS) is characterized by a microangiopathic hemolytic anemia, thrombocytopenia, and ARF. Platelet aggregates stimulated by endothelial damage, causing release of ultra-large multimers of von Willebrand factor (vWf).

Thrombotic angiopathy other features: Purpura; GI or intracerebral bleeds; hematuria; proteinuria; BUN/CR↑.

Causes of thrombotic microangiopathy: Idiopathic, medications (cyclosporine, tacrolimus, OKT3, mitomycin C, 5-fluorouracil, ticlodipine, clopidogrel, quinine, gemcitabine); malignancy (adenocarcinomas); SLE; HIV; pregnancy; bone marrow transplant. Shigatoxin associated HUS: (*E. coli* 0157; *Shigella dysenteriae; Streptococcus pneumoniae*); atypical HUS (complement factor mutations). *Tests:* ↓Hb; ↓platelets; peripheral smear (fragmented RBC, ie schistocytes); ↑reticulocytes); ↑creatinine; ↑bilirubin; ↑LDH; ↓haptoglobin; hematuria; proteinuria.

Treatment: Plasma exchange may be life-saving with fresh frozen plasma (FFP) for idiopathic ttp, pregnancy, autoimmune disorders, adults with Shigatoxin, acute drug induced (quinine, clopidogrel). Cancer associated, post bone marrow transplant less likaly to respond. Immunosuppressive treatment may be used in some cases (idiopathic, autoimmune associated).

Prognosis: It may relapse (depends on underlying cause). Mortality: High.

Cholesterol emboli *Suspect in any patient with diffuse atherosclerosis. May have eosinophilia, cyanosis (eg of toes)* ± ↑creatinine. *Prevalence:* 0.3% in unselected autopsies. *Risk:* Atheroma; ↑cholesterol; aneurysms; thrombolysis; arterial procedures; spontaneous. *Signs:* Livedo reticularis, gangrenous lesion in toes, abdominal pain, Hollenhorst plaques in retinal vessels, *progressive renal failure, eosinophilia, eosinophiluria, hypocomplementemia. Urinalysis may be bland. Cholesterol clefts seen in renal biopsies; they induce inflammation, ischemia, and then fibrosis. *Treatment:* No proven medical therapy; avoid anticoagulants and instrumentation HMG-CoA reductase inhibitors. *Prognosis:* Often progressive and fatal. A few have regained renal function after dialysis.

Diabetes mellitus (type 2) and the kidney

Diabetes is a vascular disease—with the kidney as one of its chief targets for end-organ damage. An important intervention in the long-term care of DM is the control of BP, to protect the heart, the brain, and the kidney. Hypertensive type 2 DM patients with microalbuminuria (30–300mg albumin excreted per day)/overt nephropathy should either be on an ARB or ACE-i.

Microalbuminuria gives early warning to possible nephropathy. *SEs of ARB AND ACEIs* ↑K⁺ & ↑creatinine (close monitoring after starting/↑ dose); dry cough with ACEI>>ARB (rare). ARB or ACE-I are first-line. ARB for ACE-I intolerant individuals. Occasionally they may be combined, but only by specialists.

Example of target BP in DM *if no proteinuria:* 140/80 (educate patient; ensure he/she is well informed); *if proteinuric,* aim for <130/80mmHg.

Do targets work? Target-driven, long-term, intense therapy (including prophylactic aspirin) revolving around microalbuminuria and other risk factors can halve risk of macro- and microvascular events (MI etc.).

Is microalbuminuria reversible? Answer: Sometimes—and more likely if:
• Recent onset
• Hb$_{A1c}$ <8%
• Systolic <115mmHg.

Renal tubular disease

Nephrogenic diabetes insipidus is characterized by renal insensitivity to vasopressin resulting in ↓urinary concentration leading to polyuria, hypernatremia (if water access limited) and CKD. It may be *primary* (familial X-linked) or *secondary* to a number of causes:
• Drugs (lithium, ifosfamide, cidofovir, foscet, Amphotericin, democlocycline)
• Metabolic (hypercalcemia, hypokalemia)
• Tubulointerstitial disease (partial obstruction, renal amyloid, Sjogren's, sickle-cell disease).

Fanconi syndrome A disturbance of proximal renal tubular function resulting in:
• Generalized aminoaciduria
• Phosphaturia
• Glycosuria
• Rickets (children) or osteomalacia (adults)
• Renal tubular acidosis type 2 (proximal). Proximal tubular defect leads to inability to reclaim filtered bicarbonate.

Inherited causes: Cystinosis; galactosamia; glycogen storage disease type 1; fructose intolerance; Lowe's syndrome; tyrosinemia type 1; Wilson's disease. Idiopathic.

Acquired causes: Myeloma, medications (ifosfamide, tenofovir).

Type 1 (distal) renal tubular acidosis is characterized by an inability to generate acid urine in the distal nephron. There may be severe metabolic acidosis. *Causes:* Sjogren's, Amphoterecin B, idiopathic, familial, hypercalciuria, rheumatoid arthritis, SLE, ifosfamide, lithium, renal transplantation, obstruction, and sickle cell anemia (latter 2 may be hyperkalemic). *Signs:* Hyperventilation; muscle weakness (↓K^+); nephrocalcinosis; renal calculi. *Diagnosis:* Urinary pH >5.3; hypo/normo/hyperkalemia; hyperchloremic metabolic acidosis; hypercalciuria; nephrocalcinosis. *Treatment: Acute:* Correct hypokalemia if present and acidosis. *Chronic:* Oral bicarbonate (1–2mEq/kg/d) and K^+ supplements.

262

Type 2 (proximal) renal tubular acidosis may occur alone or with the Fanconi syndrome. It is characterized by a defect in H^+ secretion and thus defective HCO_3 reabsorption in the proximal tubule resulting in loss of HCO_3 in the urine. *Causes:* Idiopathic, sporadic, familial disorders (as in Fanconi's above), multiple myeloma, carbonic anhydrase inhibitors, ifosfamide, tenofovir, heavy metals, renal transplantation. *Clinical features:* Polyuria; polydipsia; proximal myopathy; osteomalacia; rickets. Nephrocalcinosis and renal calculi are virtually never seen. *Diagnosis:* Hypokalemia; hyperchloremic metabolic acidosis. **NB:** Inappropriately acid urine is present with metabolic acidosis. *Treatment:* High doses of bicarbonate (eg ≥3mmol/kg/d) are required. *Prognosis:* Good.

Type 4 (hyperkalemic) renal tubular acidosis occurs in diseases associated with hypoaldosteronism or failure of aldosterone action, eg Addison's disease; inborn errors of steroid metabolism; DM; chronic tubulointerstitial disease; drugs (ACE-i, β-blockers, K^+ sparing diuretics, NSAIDs). Mineralocorticoid deficiency ↓H^+ secretion in the distal nephron resulting in ↓NH_4^+ excretion. *Signs:* Urinary pH <5.4; K^+↑; hyperchloremic metabolic acidosis. *Treatment:* Fludrocortisone 0.05–0.15mg PO daily, if acidotic or hyperkalemic.

Hereditary hypokalemic tubulopathies *Bartter's syndrome:* Sodium reabsorption defect in ascending limb with mutations in the Na–K–2Cl co-transporter (NKCC2) ROMK channel, others; *Gitelman syndrome:* Sodium reabsorption defect in distal convoluted tubule; *Cause:* Mutations in the distal tubular Na–Cl co-transporter gene. Can see hypokalemia and metabolic alkalosis with both. Hypercalciuria with Bartter's and hypocalciuria with Gitelman's. Bartter's syndrome: May have growth/mental retardation. Gitelman syndrome: Autosomal recessive. Diagnosed later in life, may be asymptomatic.

Inherited kidney diseases

Autosomal dominant polycystic kidney disease (APKD) *Prevalence:* 1:1000. *Inheritance:* Autosomal dominant. Genes on chromosomes 16 (PKD1) and 4 (PKD2). *Signs:* Renal enlargement with cysts; abdominal pain; hematuria; UTI; renal calculi; BP↑; renal failure. Extrarenal: Liver cysts; intracranial aneurysms; subarachnoid hemorrhage; mitral valve prolapse; abdominal herniae. *Treatment:* Monitor U&E & BP: Treating ↑BP is most important. Treat infections; dialysis or transplantation for ESRD; genetic counseling. *Screening* (eg *magnetic resonance angiography*) eg for 1st-degree relatives.

Infantile polycystic kidney disease. Prevalence 1:40,000. Autosomal recessive (chromosome 6). *Signs:* Renal cysts; congenital hepatic fibrosis.

Nephronophthisis An inherited medullary cystic disease. The juvenile form (autosomal recessive) accounts for 10–20% of ESRD in children. *Signs:* Polyuria; polydipsia; enuresis; renal impairment; metabolic acidosis; anaemia; growth retardation; ESRD. Extrarenal signs: Retinal degeneration; retinitis pigmentosa; skeletal changes; cerebellar ataxia; liver fibrosis. The adult form (autosomal dominant; restricted to the kidney) is rare.

Renal phakomatoses *Tuberous sclerosis.* A complex disorder with hamartoma formation in skin, brain, eye, kidney, and heart caused by autosomal dominant genes on chromosomes 9 (TSC1) & 16 (TSC2). *Signs:* Skin: Adenoma sebaceum, angiofibromas, 'ash leaf' hypomelanic macules, sacral plaques of shark-like skin (shagreen patch), periungual fibromas; IQ↓; seizures. *von Hippel-Lindau syndrome* is the chief cause of inherited renal cancers. *Cause:* Germline mutations of the VHL tumor-suppressor gene (also inactivated in most sporadic renal cell cancers).

Alport's syndrome *Prevalence:* 1:5000. Inheritance: X-linked dominant, autosomal dominant, or rarely autosomal recessive. Genes code for type IV collagen molecules, eg *COL4A5, COL4A3, COL4A4.* Pathology: Thickened GBM with splitting of the lamina densa. *Signs:* Progressive hematuric nephritis, sensorineural deafness, and lenticonus (bulging of the lens capsule, seen on slit-lamp examination). *Treatment:* Control BP; supportive management of renal failure; dialysis; transplantation.

Anderson–Fabry disease X-linked recessive; intralysosomal deposits of trihexoside causing burning pain/parasthesia in the extremities and angiokeratoma corporis diffusum (blue-black telangiectasia in bathing trunk distribution).

Hyperoxaluria *Primary hyperoxaluria* is due to an autosomal recessive inherited enzyme defect (types I and II). Measure 24h urinary oxalate excretion and creatinine clearance (excretion ↓ in renal failure) for unexplained recurrent calcium oxalate stones. *Secondary hyperoxaluria* is due to small intestine disease/resection, ↓calcium intake, ↑↑oxalalte intake (diet, ethylene glycol poisoning), pyridoxine deficiency. *Signs:* Oxalate stones; nephrocalcinosis; renal failure; cardiac conduction defects; cardiomyopathy; subcutaneous calcinosis; peripheral neuropathy; mononeuritis multiplex; retinal changes; synovitis; osteodystrophy. *Treatment:* High fluid intake; restrict dietary oxalate (tea, chocolate, strawberries, rhubarb, beans, celery, nuts); pyridoxine (↓urinary oxalate excretion); hepatic ± renal transplantation.

Cystinuria The commonest aminoaciduria. *Clinical features:* Cystine stones; abdominal pain; hematuria; renal obstruction; UTI. *Treatment:* ↑Fluid intake; NaHCO$_3$ supplements (alkalinizes urine); penicillamine tiopronin (↓cystine excretion).

Renal manifestations of systemic disease

Amyloidosis AL (1°) or AA (2°) Proteinuria; nephrotic syndrome; progressive renal failure; renal tubular dysfunction. *Diagnosis:* p587. *Treatment* is of the cause—eg rheumatoid arthritis.

Diabetes 30–40% of patients on dialysis have diabetic nephropathy. *Pathology:* Nodular capillary glomerulosclerosis (Kimmelstiel–Wilson lesion). Early on there is renal hyperperfusion associated with ↑GFR and ↑renal size. *Microalbuminuria* (albumin excretion 30–300mg/d or 30–300mg/g Cr) occurs 5–15yrs post diagnosis and is associated with a normal GFR and a normal but rising BP.

Type 1 DM nephropathy occurs in 10–15yrs post diagnosis and is characterized by macroalbuminuria (albumin excretion >300mg/d or 30–300mg/g Cr), ↓GFR, and ↑BP. Renal failure occurs 15–30yrs post diagnosis (rare after 30yrs); there may be nephrotic range proteinuria (>3g/d).

Type 2 DM ('maturity onset') nephropathy: See p261 (box). >10–30% have nephropathy at diagnosis, and its prevalence ↑ linearly with time.

Treatment: Good glycemic control delays onset and progression of microalbuminuria, but has little effect on established proteinuria. Reducing BP reduces microalbuminuria and attenuates loss of GFR. ACE-I ± ARB reduce microalbuminuria and slow progression to CRF, even if normotensive.

Infection associated nephropathies are common causes of renal disease *Glomerulonephritis* is associated with hepatitis B (or C, or less commonly, HIV); SBE/IE, shunt nephritis, visceral abscess, septicaemia, typhoid fever, Legionnaire's disease, TB, leprosy, syphilis, malaria, schistosomiasis, and filiariasis.

Vasculitis p378—occurs with HBV, post-streptococcal, staphylococcal, or streptococcal septicaemia.

Interstitial nephritis is seen with *E. coli, Staphylococcus aureus, Proteus*, leptospirosis, hantavirus, and schistosomal infections.

Malignancy *Direct effects:* Renal infiltration (leukemia, lymphoma); obstruction (pelvic tumors); metastases. *Indirect:* Hypercalcemia; nephrotic syndrome; acute renal failure; amyloidosis; glomerulonephritis. *Treatment associated:* Nephrotoxic drugs; tumor lysis syndrome; radiation nephritis.

Multiple myeloma is characterized by excess production of monoclonal antibody and/or light chains. Bence Jones proteinuria is common. Myeloma kidney is characterized by accumulation of distal nephron casts. Light chain nephropathy is caused by direct toxic effects of light chains on nephrons. *Clinical features:* ARF; CRF; amyloidosis; nephrotic syndrome; tubular dysfunction; hypercalcaemic nephropathy. *Treatment:* Treat ARF p586 and hypercalcemia p391; chemotherapy; dialysis.

Rheumatological diseases *Rheumatoid arthritis (RA)* NSAIDs may cause ↓GFR or interstitial nephritis. Penicillamine and gold may induce membranous nephropathy. Amyloidosis occurs in 15% of RA patients. *SLE* involves the kidney in 40–60% of adults. *Clinical features:* Proteinuria; hematuria; ↑BP; renal impairment; ARF. Lupus nephritis shows a wide variety of histological patterns. *Treatment:* Corticosteroids; immunosuppressive meds (cyclophosphamide/myophenolate mofetil) p374. *Systemic sclerosis* p374 involves the kidney in 30% of patients. *Clinical features:* Proteinuria; hematuria; ↑BP; renal impairment; 'scleroderma crisis' (ARF + malignant hypertension) *Treatment:* Control BP (ACE inhibitors); dialysis; transplantation.

Hyperparathyroidism *Nephrocalcinosis:* Deposition of calcium in the renal medulla (seen on plain x-ray). *Renal stones* from associated hypercalciuria.

Sarcoidosis may involve the kidney in a number of ways. *Abnormal Ca^{2+} metabolism* may cause hypercalciuria, nephrocalcinosis, or nephrolithiasis. *Interstitial nephritis* may present with CKD or ARF. *Glomerular involvement* usually presents with the nephrotic syndrome and is due to membranous glomerulonephritis, other glomerulopathies, or amyloidosis.

Endocrinology

Matthew Kim, M.D.

Contents

The essence of endocrinology

- Define clinical syndromes associated with deficiencies of hormones (*hypo-* syndromes) and corresponding clinical syndromes associated with secretion of excessive amounts of hormones (*hyper-* syndromes).
- Measure levels of hormones or metabolites of hormones in blood or urine samples—be mindful of circadian variation in the secretion of specific hormones when planning measurements.
- Measure levels of stimulating or trophic hormones that serve as intrinsic assays of the function of specific endocrine glands—understand how these hormones may be used to diagnose and classify clinical syndromes (eg thyroid-stimulating hormone (TSH) to diagnose primary hypothyroidism and hyperthyroidism; adrenocorticotrophic hormone (ACTH) to distinguish between primary and secondary adrenal insufficiency).
- To confirm suspected deficiency of a hormone, administer an agent that stimulates secretion of that hormone before drawing samples for measurement.
- To confirm suspected secretion of excessive amounts of a hormone, administer an agent that suppresses secretion of that hormone before drawing samples for measurement.
- Use radiographic studies to evaluate the anatomic structure and physiologic function of specific endocrine glands.
- Treat conditions associated with deficiencies of hormones by administering a) pharmacologic preparations of hormone or hormone analogs, or b) agents that stimulate secretion of hormones from functional tissue.
- Treat conditions associated with secretion of excessive amounts of hormones by a) surgically resecting hyperfunctioning tissue, b) administering agents that target and destroy hyperfunctioning tissue, or c) administering agents that suppress secretion of hormones from hyperfunctioning tissue.

Type 1 diabetes mellitus

Definition Clinical syndrome precipitated by autoimmune destruction of pancreatic islet cells that is characterized by inadequate secretion of endogenous insulin. Type 1 diabetes mellitus usually presents during childhood or adolescence, but may occur at any age. Patients require treatment with insulin, and are prone to develop hypoglycemia and ketoacidosis. May be associated with specific HLA types (DR3 & DR4) and other autoimmune disorders. Anti-glutamic acid decarboxylase antibodies (anti-GAD) and anti-islet cell antibodies may be detectable at the time of diagnosis. Concordance is >30% in identical twins.

Presentation Usually acute with ketoacidosis characterized by progressive polyuria, polydipsia, weight loss, fatigue, lethargy, hyperventilation, and a distinctive odor of acetone on the breath. Subacute cases may present with more protracted courses of variable polyuria, polydipsia, and weight loss with associated lethargy and infectious complications (vaginal candidiasis, furunculosis).

Diagnosis A suspected diagnosis may be confirmed on the basis of 1) a random plasma glucose >200mg/dL with associated symptoms (polyuria, polydipsia, weight loss), 2) a fasting plasma glucose >126mg/dL, or 3) a 75-g oral glucose tolerance test with a 2-h plasma glucose >200mg/dL.[1] Positive results should be verified with repeat testing.

Treatment Insulin, administered as multiple daily injections or through a pump delivering a continuous subcutaneous infusion. Doses should be timed to reproduce normal patterns of basal and postprandial insulin secretion. Monitoring requires frequent self-measurement of blood glucose levels. Intensive control targeting normoglycemic preprandial and postprandial blood glucose levels reduces the risk of developing microvascular complications, but may be associated with more frequent episodes of hypoglycemia. Early on in the course of treatment, patients may experience a transient 'honeymoon phase' characterized by improved control with reduced daily insulin requirements. Hemoglobin A1C levels reflect average blood glucose control over the course of the previous 8–12wks. Clinical guidelines recommend intensifying treatment to target hemoglobin A1C levels <6.5–7.0%.

1 American Diabetic Association Position Statement 2005 *Diabetes Care* **28** S4.

Insulin

Available in 100U/mL preparations. May be drawn up and injected using special syringes (marked in units) or directly injected from preloaded adjustable pen injectors. Four major types available for use.

1 **Rapid-acting insulin analogs** *Insulin lispro* (Humalog®), *insulin aspart* (NovoLog®)—modified to promote rapid absorption, must be injected immediately before eating.
2 **Short-acting insulin** *Regular insulin*—must be injected 15–30min before eating.
3 **Intermediate-acting insulin** *NPH insulin*—peak effect at 4–10h, effective duration = 10–16h.
4 **Long-acting insulin analogs** *Insulin glargine* (Lantus®)—modified to promote steady absorption without peaks, administered once daily, effective duration = 24h, may not be mixed with other types of insulin or insulin analogs.

Premixed preparations combine intermediate-acting insulin with short-acting insulin or rapid-acting insulin analogs in specified fractions (eg 70/30 NPH insulin/regular insulin, 75/25 NPL/insulin lispro).

Insulin regimens used to treat type 1 diabetes

Two daily injections Comprised of (1) intermediate-acting insulin mixed with a rapid-acting insulin analog (or short-acting insulin) before breakfast; and (2) intermediate-acting insulin mixed with a rapid-acting insulin analog insulin (or short-acting insulin) before dinner. Often started by administering 2/3 of the estimated daily dose before breakfast and 1/3 before dinner.

Three daily injections Comprised of (1) intermediate-acting insulin mixed with a rapid-acting insulin analog (or short-acting insulin) before breakfast; (2) a rapid-acting insulin analog (or short-acting insulin) before dinner; and (3) intermediate-acting insulin at bedtime. May reduce the frequency and severity of overnight hypoglycemia.

Four daily injections Comprised of (1–3) a rapid-acting insulin analog (or short-acting insulin) before breakfast, lunch, and dinner; and (4) a long-acting insulin analog (or intermediate-acting insulin) at bedtime.

Prandial doses of rapid-acting insulin analogs and short-acting insulin may be administered as fixed doses or may be adjusted to account for a) estimated grams or exchanges of carbohydrate to be eaten, or b) sliding scale correction formulas based on preprandial blood glucose levels.

Intercurrent illnesses may ↑ daily insulin requirements, in spite of diminished appetite and reduced caloric intake. During the course of any moderate to severe illness, patients should be instructed to a) maintain caloric intake, b) drink large volumes of fluids, c) check blood glucose levels at least four times daily, and d) check for urine ketones with home dipstick tests if blood glucose levels are noted to be persistently elevated. Insulin doses may need to be transiently increased to prevent the onset of hyperglycemia, volume depletion, and ketoacidosis.

Type 2 diabetes mellitus

Definition Clinical syndrome characterized by insulin resistance that may precipitate endogenous hyperinsulinemia with eventual beta cell failure. Over time, the combined effects of insulin resistance and ↓ insulin secretion lead to persistent hyperglycemia. Strongly associated with obesity and physical inactivity. Higher prevalence among certain ethnic groups including African Americans, Latinos, Native Americans, Asian Americans, and Pacific Islanders. While long considered to be a disease of adults, the incidence of confirmed diagnoses of type 2 diabetes in children and adolescents appears to be ↑ with the expanding epidemic of obesity. Concordance is >80% in identical twins.

Presentation Highly variable. At one end of the spectrum, patients may present with mild asymptomatic hyperglycemia identified on routine screening or laboratory testing. At the other extreme, patients with unsuspected and untreated disease may present in advanced decompensated hyperosmolar states characterized by severe hyperglycemia, volume depletion, and mental status changes. The American Diabetes Association recommends that screening be considered in all individuals aged 45 and older (particularly those with a BMI ≥25kg/m^2), and in younger individuals with significant risk factors or findings consistent with the metabolic syndrome.

Diagnosis A suspected diagnosis may be confirmed on the basis of 1) a random plasma glucose >200mg/dL with associated symptoms (polyuria, polydipsia, weight loss), 2) a fasting plasma glucose >126mg/dL, or 3) a 75g oral glucose tolerance test with a 2-h plasma glucose >200mg/dL. Positive results should be verified with repeat testing. Pre-diabetes may be diagnosed when testing reveals a) a fasting plasma of 100–125mg/dL glucose (impaired fasting glucose), or b) a 2-h plasma glucose of 140–199mg/dL (impaired glucose tolerance). There is growing evidence that treatment of pre-diabetes with lifestyle modification and pharmacologic therapy may delay or prevent the progression of disease.

Treatment Must be tailored to the state of disease and the severity of hyperglycemia at the time of presentation. All patients should be counseled to exercise and lose weight. Asymptomatic patients with mild or intermittent hyperglycemia may be managed with medical nutrition therapy targeted to limit glycemic excursions. Patients with persistent hyperglycemia may need to be started on treatment with oral agents or insulin. Oral agents are generally preferred as first-line therapy. They may be used in different combinations to optimize glycemic control. Certain oral agents may be contraindicated in patients with impaired renal or hepatic function. Over time, most patients who have been maintained on regimens of oral agents eventually require the addition of insulin. In some cases, patients presenting with severe hyperglycemia who initially need to be treated with insulin may be successfully transitioned to oral agents as glucose toxicity subsides and beta cell function is restored. Monitoring requires self-measurement of blood glucose levels. Recommended frequency may vary depending on intensity of treatment. Hemoglobin A1C levels reflect average blood glucose control over the course of the previous 8–12wks. Clinical guidelines recommend intensifying treatment to target hemoglobin A1C levels <6.5–7.0%. This may be difficult to achieve in practice.

Oral agents

Five major classes.

Sulfonylureas Stimulate insulin secretion. Commonly prescribed preparations include *glipizide* (Glucotrol® 2.5–20mg qd-bid, GlucotrolXL® 5–10mg qd), *glyburide* (DiaBeta®, Micronase® 1.25–20mg qd, Glynase® 0.75–12mg qd), and *glimepiride* (Amaryl® 1–4mg qd). Often used in combination with biguanides and thiazolidinediones. Glimepiride may be associated with a lower incidence of hypoglycemia. Preparations are available that combine metformin with glyburide (Glucovance®) and glipizide (Metaglip®).

Biguanides Suppress hepatic gluconeogenesis. May help to increase insulin sensitivity. *Metformin* is the only biguanide available for use in the U.S. Available in regular and long-acting preparations (Glucophage® 500–1000mg bid, Glucophage XR® 1000–2000mg qpm). Usually started at a low dose with meals and titrated upward. Self-limited side effects may include nausea, abdominal cramping, and diarrhea. May help to promote weight loss. Contraindicated if creatinine is >1.5mg/dL. Must be held for 48h prior to and following exposure to intravenous contrast.

Thiazolidinediones PPAR gamma receptor agonists. ↑ insulin sensitivity. Available preparations include *rosiglitazone* (Avandia® 4–8mg qd) and *pioglitazone* (Actos® 15–45mg qd). May take 3–6wks to see full effect. Transaminase levels should be monitored regularly. May cause weight gain and lower extremity swelling. Contraindicated in patients with congestive heart failure or impaired hepatic function. Preparation available that combines metformin with rosiglitazone (Avandamet®).

Meglitinides Rapid-acting insulin secretagogues. Must be taken right before meals. May help to control postprandial hyperglycemia. Available preparations include *repaglinide* (Prandin® 0.5–4mg qac) and *nateglinide* (Starlix® 60–120mg qac).

Alpha-glucosidase inhibitors Limit glycemic excursions by inhibiting enzymatic breakdown of carbohydrates. Must be taken with meals. Available preparations include acarbose (Precose® 25–100mg qac) and miglitol (Glyset® 25–100mg qac). Limiting side effects include bloating and diarrhea. Contraindicated in patients with inflammatory bowel disease.

Insulin regimens used to treat type 2 diabetes

One daily injection May be added to supplement standing regimens of oral agents. Usually started as a fixed dose of a) intermediate-acting insulin at bedtime, b) a long-acting insulin analog at bedtime, or c) a long-acting insulin analog before breakfast.

Two daily injections May allow for greater flexibility in making adjustments to accommodate variations in blood glucose levels. Doses administered before breakfast and before dinner may be comprised of a) intermediate-acting insulin, b) intermediate-acting insulin mixed with a rapid-acting insulin analog (or short-acting insulin), or c) premixed preparations combining intermediate-acting insulin with short-acting insulin or rapid-acting insulin analogs.

Multiple daily injection regimens similar to those used to treat patients with type 1 diabetes may also be employed to target more intensive control. Total daily insulin requirements tend to be much higher in patients with type 2 diabetes. Some patients may require >100U daily to achieve and maintain adequate glycemic control.

Diabetic retinopathy

Microvascular complication of diabetes mellitus that represents the sequelae of changes in retinal blood vessels caused by prolonged exposure to elevated blood glucose levels. Affects most patients with type 1 diabetes, though manifestations are usually not detectable until 5yrs after initial diagnosis. May be detectable in up to 25% of patients with type 2 diabetes at time of presentation. Leading preventable cause of blindness in adults between 20–74yrs of age.

Stages of diabetic retinopathy

Preretinopathy Subtle dilation of the retinal veins.

Non-proliferative retinopathy Also known as background retinopathy. Weakened areas of the walls of retinal capillaries form outpouchings that may be visible as microaneurysms. Bleeding from these weakened areas in the superficial layer of the retina may produce flame-shaped hemorrhages. Bleeding in deeper layers may produce dot-blot hemorrhages. Leakage of plasma from retinal capillary may lead to formation of yellowish hard exudates. If this leakage occurs near the macula, it may lead to swelling identifiable as macular edema.

Preproliferative retinopathy Closure of retinal capillaries leads to focal hypoxia visible as poorly defined soft exudates or cotton wool spots. Retinal veins develop irregular contours.

Proliferative retinopathy Neovascularization with growth of vessels into the vitreous humor. New vessels are weak and prone to rupture. Vitreous hemorrhages may obscure vision. Reabsorption of blood may lead to scarring and traction that may cause retinal detachment. Growth of vessels into the anterior chamber may cause a painful ↑ in intraocular pressure.

Evaluation Should be performed by an experienced provider. Comprehensive evaluation requires pupillary dilation, slip-lamp examination, and indirect ophthalmoscopy. Examinations limited to direct ophthalmoscopy often miss key findings. Type 1 diabetics should be referred for evaluation within 3–5yrs of initial diagnosis. Type 2 diabetics should be referred at the time of presentation. Pregnancy may ↑ the risk of development or progression of diabetic retinopathy. Comprehensive evaluation should be performed prior to conception and during the first trimester.

Prevention and treatment Intensive control of blood glucose levels may delay the onset or progression of diabetic retinopathy. Adjunctive treatment should target aggressive control of hypertension and hyperlipidemia. Laser photocoagulation treatment may help to arrest identified proliferative retinopathy and macular edema. Symptoms or signs concerning for vitreous hemorrhage, retinal detachment, or changes in intraocular pressure should prompt urgent referral.

Other complications Elevated glucose levels in the aqueous humor may draw fluid out of the lens causing ↑ stiffness and myopia. Changes are reversible with improved blood glucose control. Patients with diabetes are more prone to develop cataracts.

Diabetic nephropathy

Microvascular complication that develops as a result of changes in glomerular function precipitated by prolonged exposure to elevated blood glucose levels. Similar risk in patients with type 1 and type 2 diabetes. Proximate cause of almost 50% of cases of end-stage renal disease requiring renal replacement with dialysis. Progression may be exacerbated by concomitant hypertension or preexisting renal disease.

Stages of diabetic nephropathy

Stage I Marked by onset of disease. Characterized by 30–40% increase in glomerular filtration rate (GFR) with enlargement of kidneys.

Stage II Normal urinary excretion of albumin (<30mg/24h).

Stage III Incipient diabetic nephropathy. Microalbuminuria with urinary excretion of 30–300mg albumin/24h. Approximately 20% of patients with type 1 diabetes who reach this stage will progress to end-stage renal disease within 10yrs.

Stage IV Overt diabetic nephropathy. Proteinuria with urinary excretion of >0.5g protein/24h. Corresponds to urinary excretion of >300mg albumin/24h. Protein is usually detectable on urine dipstick testing. Marks the beginning of a progressive decline in GFR.

Stage V End-stage renal disease.

Detection Initial evaluation with urine dipstick testing. Detectable protein indicates the presence of proteinuria consistent with stage IV overt diabetic nephropathy. If protein is undetectable on urine dipstick, further evaluation should focus on quantification of urinary excretion of albumin. This can be assessed by measuring albumin in a 24-h urine collection, or by measuring the albumin/creatinine ratio in a random urine specimen. An albumin/creatine ratio >30mcg/mg has been proven to be a sensitive and specific predictor of microalbuminuria. Results that are consistent with microalbuminuria or proteinuria should be confirmed on repeat testing within 3 months.

Treatment of hypertensive patients In patients with concomitant hypertension, aggressive control of blood pressure may help to forestall the progressive decline in GFR. Clinical guidelines recommend targeting systolic blood pressures <130mmHg and diastolic blood pressures <80mmHg. Whenever possible, an ACE inhibitor (ACEi) should be selected as a first line antihypertensive agent. ACEi have been proven to effectively reduce urinary protein excretion in patients with type 1 and type 2 diabetes. Persistent cough may be a limiting side effect. ACEi may precipitate a) hyperkalemia, which may be particularly severe in patients with hyporeninemic hypoaldosteronism, and b) acute renal failure in patients with renal artery stenosis. Serum potassium and creatinine levels should be checked 2–3wks after starting treatment. Patients who cannot tolerate ACEi should be treated with angiotensin receptor blockers (ARBs). Additional antihypertensive agents may need to be added in a stepwise fashion to achieve target levels of blood pressure control. Thiazide diuretics may provide an additive effect in patients with preserved renal function (GFR>50mL/min). A range of different preparations combining ACEi and ARBs with thiazide diuretics in varying doses are available. Other classes of agents may be used as well, though attention should be paid to potential complicating side effects (beta blockers may impair recognition of hypoglycemia; alpha blockers and centrally acting agents may exacerbate orthostatic hypotension).

Treatment of normotensive patients In patients with type 1 diabetes, confirmed microalbuminuria, and normal blood pressure, treatment with an ACEi may delay the onset of proteinuria marking a progression to overt diabetic nephropathy. Similar benefits may accrue in patients with type 2 diabetes.

Diabetic neuropathy

Complication that develops as a result of irreversible damage to nerve fibers precipitated by prolonged exposure to elevated blood glucose levels. Classification schemes differentiate between peripheral neuropathy and autonomic neuropathy.

Peripheral neuropathy Most common type is distal symmetric polyneuropathy. Manifestation of progressive damage to sensory and motor nerve fibers that may be detected in up to 30% of patients with diabetes. Usually begins in the distal lower extremities, extending proximally in a stocking-and-glove distribution. Asymptomatic involvement may be suspected when physical examination of the feet reveals diminished or absent ankle jerk reflexes, diminished proprioception, or diminished sensation to light touch with 10g monofilament testing. Symptomatic involvement may present with pain characterized as paresthesias, hyperesthesias, or burning sensations. May spontaneously resolve or progress to a state of numbness. Other variants include focal mononeuropathy (commonly involving oculomotor nerves), radiculopathy (involving thoracic or lumbar nerve roots), and mononeuropathy multiplex (presenting with asymmetric involvement of multiple peripheral nerves). Intensive control of blood glucose levels may delay progression of peripheral neuropathy. Pain may respond to staged treatment with tricyclic antidepressants (*desipramine* or *amitriptyline* 25–200mg qhs), *topical capsaicin cream* (Zostrix® 0.075% cream qid), *gabapentin* (Neurontin® 300–600mg tid), *carbamazepine* (Tegretol® 200–600mg bid), or *tramadol* (Ultram® 50–100mg q6).

Autonomic neuropathy Variable manifestations, depending on distribution and extent of disruption in function of sympathetic and parasympathetic nerve fibers. Cardiovascular involvement may present with evidence of resting tachycardia, exercise intolerance, or orthostatic hypotension (defined as a 20mmHg drop in systolic blood pressure or a 10mmHg drop in diastolic blood pressure after standing for 2min). Patients with orthostatic hypotension may report dizziness, weakness, and nausea when standing. Treatment with *fludorocortisone* (Florinef® 0.05–0.1mg qd) may help to relieve symptoms by augmenting intravascular volume. Peripheral edema may be a limiting side effect. Gastrointestinal involvement may present with symptoms reflecting variable degrees of gastropathy, diarrhea, or constipation. Diabetic gastroparesis is an extreme form of gastropathy that presents with marked dilation and hypotonia of the stomach with delayed transit of food into the small intestine that may lead to early satiety, regurgitation of undigested food, and problems with coordination of preprandial insulin injections. Delayed transit may be confirmed on gastric emptying studies. Prokinetic agents used to treat persistent diabetic gastroparesis include *metoclopramide* (Reglan® 5–20mg 15–60min qac) and *erythromycin* (50mg suspension qac). Severe diabetic diarrhea may respond to treatment with *clonidine* or *octreotide*. Genitourinary involvement may lead to development of a neurogenic bladder. Urinary retention may respond to treatment with *bethanechol* (Urecholine® 10–50mg tid). Self-catheterization may be necessary in extreme cases. Erectile dysfunction is a common complication that may be exacerbated by a range of contributing factors (atherosclerotic disease, treatment with antihypertensive agents). Affected patients may respond to treatment with phosphodiesterase inhibitors (*sidenafil* (Viagra® 25–50mg x 1), *vardenafil* (Levitra® 2.5–20mg x 1), and *tadalafil* (Cialis® 5–20mg x 1)). These agents may be contraindicated in patients with known or suspected orthostatic hypotension or coronary artery disease. Type 1 diabetics with significant autonomic neuropathy may have blunted or absent counterregulatory responses to treatment-induced hypoglycemia, a complication identified as hypoglycemic unawareness.

The diabetic foot

Combined effects of distal symmetric polyneuropathy and peripheral vascular disease restricting blood flow to the lower extremities may predispose patients to develop significant complications related to foot injuries. Damage to motor nerve fibers may lead to atrophy and weakness of muscles in the distal lower extremities. Progressive changes may lead to deformities that ↑ pressure at prominent points on the soles of the feet. This may lead to the development of thick calluses that may eventually ulcerate. Damage to sensory nerve fibers may make it difficult for patients to detect foot ulcers and other traumatic injuries that may damage the joints and soft tissues in the foot and ankle. If left untreated, foot ulcers may lead to the development of polymicrobial cellulitis and osteomyelitis that may be difficult to eradicate in devitalized sites exposed to persistently elevated blood glucose levels. Serious life-threatening infections in limbs compromised by restricted blood flow may require treatment with surgical amputation. More than 60% of lower extremity amputations are performed to treat complications of diabetic foot infections.

Prevention Close inspection of the feet should be performed on an annual basis to check for evidence of diminished sensation, altered peripheral pulses, joint deformities, signs of tissue damage, or calluses that may be forming at points of direct pressure. Patients with identifiable risk factors should be counseled to a) perform regular self-inspection to check for signs of unsuspected trauma or injury, b) trim toenails to recommended lengths, and c) wear fitted shoes that provide adequate support without binding or constricting the feet. Patients with progressive distal symmetric polyneuropathy may benefit from regular foot care under the direction of a podiatric specialist.

Treatment Superficial diabetic foot ulcers that do not appear to be infected should be treated with aggressive debridement. Casting may help to promote healing by relieving direct pressure. Deep ulcers may be cultured and probed to check for signs of osteomyelitis. Radiographic evaluation with MRI scanning and tagged WBC studies may help to confirm a suspected diagnosis. Cellulitis and osteomyelitis require treatment with bed rest, surgical debridement, and prolonged courses of IV antibiotics. In cases complicated by peripheral vascular disease, revascularization may help to promote resolution and healing. Amputation may be necessary if deep infections fail to resolve, or if a spreading anaerobic infection or gangrene supervenes.

Hypoglycemia

Strict definition based on confirmation of 1) a plasma glucose level ≤50mg/dL 2) hyperadrenergic or neuroglycopenic symptoms that occur at the time th low plasma glucose level is detected, and 3) relief of those symptoms corresponding to an ↑ in the plasma glucose level after administration of oral or I' glucose. Hyperadrenergic symptoms may include palpitations, tremulousness nausea, diaphoresis, and anxiety. Neuroglycopenic symptoms may include dizziness, drowsiness, confusion, and dysarthria. Severe neuroglycopenia may result in loss of consciousness and seizures. Symptoms may develop in variable combinations and sequences.

Causes Most common cause by far is treatment with insulin or with insulin secretagogues. In patients who are not being treated with these agents hypoglycemia may be classified as fasting (occurring at any time of day) o postprandial (occurring reproducibly after meals).

Fasting hypoglycemia Distinction must be made between insulin-mediated and non-insulin-mediated mechanisms. Disorders associated with insulin mediated mechanisms include insulinoma, insulin autoantibody production and factitious administration of insulin or insulin secretagogues. Disorders associated with non-insulin-mediated hypoglycemia include chronic renal failure, hepatic failure, sepsis, primary adrenal insufficiency, hypopituitarism neoplasms that produce insulin-like growth factor 2 (IGF-2), and a range of inherited metabolic defects. Mechanisms underlying hypoglycemia associated with exposure to specific pharmacologic agents (quinolones, quinine, intravenous pentamidine, aminoglutethimide) are less clear. Investigation usually focuses on sequentially 1) ruling out disorders associated with non-insulin mediated hypoglycemia, 2) conducting a monitored fast to confirm insulin-mediated hypoglycemia, and 3) determining whether detectable insulin is endogenously secreted or factitiously administered.

Monitored fast

May be conducted in any inpatient or outpatient setting that allows for monitoring of intake and activity. The patient may drink sugar-free and non-caffeinated beverages. Physical activity should be encouraged.

Protocol

Draw blood samples every 6h to measure plasma glucose, insulin, C-peptide, and proinsulin. Once plasma glucose drops to ≤60mg/dL, ↑ frequency of blood draws to every 1–2h. Terminate the fast once a) plasma glucose drops to <45mg/dL, b) the patient develops hyperadrenergic or neuroglycopenic symptoms, or c) 72h have elapsed. Before feeding the patient, administer glucagon 1mg IV, then draw blood samples to measure plasma glucose at 10, 20, and 30min. Insulin, C-peptide, and proinsulin levels should only be measured in blood samples collected at times when plasma glucose is ≤60mg/dL.

Interpretation

In a blood sample collected when plasma glucose is ≤55mg/dL, an insulin level >4mcU/mL may be considered to be inappropriately elevated. An insulinoma may be suspected when a concomitant C-peptide level is >1ng/mL with a proinsulin level >5pmol/L. Plasma glucose levels should increase by >25mg/dL following administration of glucagon in a patient with a true insulinoma. Factitious administration of insulin may be suspected when C-peptide and proinsulin levels are lower than these thresholds. In situations where factitious administration of insulin secretagogues may be suspected, blood samples can be checked to screen for sulfonylurea exposure.

Insulinoma Very rare. May develop in the setting of multiple endocrine neoplasia type 1 (MEN 1) syndrome. The majority of confirmed insulinomas represent isolated benign neoplasms. Less than 10% eventually prove to be malignant. Principal treatment is surgical enucleation. Preoperative localization may be difficult. Imaging modalities include CT scanning, MRI scanning, transabdominal ultrasound, endoscopic ultrasound, and octreotide scanning. Measurement of insulin levels drawn from hepatic veins after arterial administration of calcium gluconate may help to localize regions of excessive secretion. In cases where imaging fails to identify a suspicious mass, intraoperative localization may be attempted through exploration, palpation, and direct ultrasonography. Distal or partial pancreatectomy may be considered as an empiric measure when a suspicious mass cannot be localized. Persistent or malignant disease may require treatment with diazoxide to suppress insulin secretion.

Postprandial hypoglycemia Recurrent episodes may occur in patients who have undergone upper gastrointestinal surgical procedures. Transient episodes related to excessive physiologic insulin secretion may occur during the initial onset of type 2 diabetes mellitus. Self-identified 'reactive' hypoglycemia in otherwise healthy individuals is considered to be a controversial diagnosis. Experimental attempts to provoke and correlate symptoms have reported conflicting results. Oral glucose tolerance testing has not proven to be reliable in this setting. Anecdotally, some patients report improvement in symptoms after altering diets to ↑ intake of protein and complex carbohydrates in smaller feedings distributed throughout the course of the day.

Thyroid function tests

Physiology Thyrotropin releasing hormone (TRH) secreted by the hypothalamus stimulates secretion of thyroid stimulating hormone (TSH) from thyrotroph cells in the anterior pituitary. TSH binds to receptors on thyrocytes in the thyroid gland, stimulating a) uptake of iodine, b) organification of iodine with thyroid peroxidase and thyroglobulin (TG) to produce thyroxine (T4) and triiodothyronine (T3), and c) secretion of T4 and T3 from the thyroid gland. Most of the T4 and T3 secreted by the thyroid gland binds to transport proteins in the circulation. Free (unbound) T4 is converted to T3 by deiodinase enzymes. Free T3 is the active form of thyroid hormone that binds to nuclear receptors to exert different regulatory effects. Free T4 and T3 exert negative regulatory feedback on the secretion of TRH from the hypothalamus and the secretion of TSH from the anterior pituitary. There is a log-linear relationship between thyroid hormone levels and TSH levels. The vast majority of functional abnormalities stem from disorders that primarily involve the thyroid gland itself. As such, TSH may serve as an intrinsic assay that provides the most sensitive index of thyroid gland function.

Evaluation of suspected hypothyroidism

1 Check a TSH level
  • Normal = euthyroid
  • Elevated = likely primary hypothyroidism
  • Low = possible secondary hypothyroidism
2 If the TSH level is elevated, check a total (T4) or unbound (free T4) thyroxine level
  • Elevated TSH + low T4 or free T4 = primary hypothyroidism
  • Elevated TSH + normal T4 and free T4 = subclinical hypothyroidism
3 If the TSH level is low, check an unbound (free T4) thyroxine level
  • Low TSH + low free T4 = possible secondary hypothyroidism
4 If no obvious underlying cause for primary hypothyroidism is evident, check anti-thyroid peroxidase and anti-thyroglobulin antibody titers
  • Elevated anti-thyroid peroxidase and/or anti-thyroglobulin antibody titers = autoimmune thyroiditis

Evaluation of suspected hyperthyroidism

1 Check a TSH level
   - Normal = euthyroid
   - Low = thyrotoxicosis
2 If the TSH level is low, check a total (T4) or unbound (free T4) thyroxine level and a total triiodothyronine (T3) level
   - Low TSH + elevated T4, free T4, or T3 = thyrotoxicosis
   - Low TSH + normal T4, free T4, and T3 = subclinical thyrotoxicosis
3 Check for findings consistent with manifestations of Graves' disease (goiter, dermopathy, symptoms and signs of thyroid eye disease)
4 If no findings consistent with manifestations of Graves' disease are evident, check a radionuclide thyroid uptake study and a thyroglobulin level
   - ↑ uptake = hyperthyroidism
   - Low uptake + elevated or normal thyroglobulin = thyroiditis
   - Low uptake + low thyroglobulin = ingestion of thyroid hormone
5 If ↑ uptake indicates the presence of hyperthyroidism, consider checking a radionuclide thyroid scan—patterns of tracer uptake may provide clues to underlying causes
   - Diffuse bilateral uptake with a visible pyramidal lobe = Graves' disease
   - Single focus of intense uptake (a 'hot' nodule) with suppression of uptake in the remainder of the thyroid gland = toxic adenoma
   - Patchy uptake with foci of ↑ and diminished uptake = toxic multinodular goiter

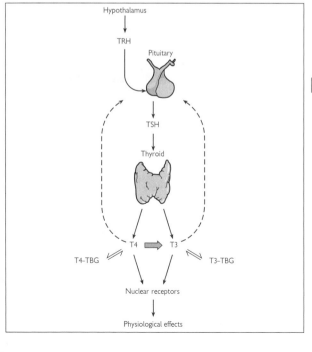

Hyperthyroidism

Definitions Thyrotoxicosis is defined as a systemic syndrome that represents the manifestations of exposure to excessive levels of thyroid hormone. Hyperthyroidism is defined as thyrotoxicosis caused by ↑ production and secretion of thyroid hormone from functional thyroid tissue.

Symptoms of thyrotoxicosis May include weight loss, heat intolerance, diaphoresis, palpitations, ↑ appetite, ↑ frequency of bowel movements, oligomenorrhea, tremulousness, anxiety, and irritability.

Signs of thyrotoxicosis May include resting tachycardia, atrial arrhythmias, warm moist skin, thinning of the hair, onycholysis, osteopenia, proximal muscle weakness, hyperreflexia, a resting tremor, lid lag (defined as a delay in the descent of the upper eyelids on downward gaze), and hypercalcemia.

Causes of hyperthyroidism Common causes include Graves' disease, toxic multinodular goiter, toxic adenoma, and exposure to large amounts of iodine (IV contrast loads, amiodarone). Rare causes include struma ovarii, metastatic thyroid cancer, and TSH-secreting pituitary adenoma.

Graves' disease Autoimmune disorder characterized by production of antibodies that bind to and stimulate TSH receptors (also knows as thyroid stimulating immunoglobulins). Marked female predominance. Stimulation of TSH receptors may cause significant enlargement of the thyroid gland evident as a goiter with a palpable pyramidal lobe. ↑ vascularity of the thyroid gland may be detected as an audible bruit or palpable thrill. Complications believed to be caused by inflammation and antibody-mediated stimulation of fibroblast growth include dermopathy (pretibial myxedema), acropachy, and thyroid eye disease (Graves' ophthalmopathy). Associated hyperthyroidism may be effectively treated with anti-thyroid drugs, radioactive iodine ablation, or subtotal thyroidectomy. Radioactive iodine treatment may exacerbate active thyroid eye disease. Pretreatment with systemic glucocorticoids may reduce risk.

Thyroid eye disease

Complication of Graves' disease believed to be caused by inflammation and antibody-mediated stimulation of fibroblast growth in soft tissues in the orbits and eyelids. Inflammation may cause swelling of the eyelids, conjunctival injection, and chemosis. Affected patients may report excessive tearing, ocular irritation, and persistent foreign body sensations. Swelling of the soft tissues in the orbits may cause protrusion of the eyeballs (proptosis), entrapment of the extraocular muscles, and compression of the optic nerve. Affected patients may report problems with excessive dryness of the eyes, diplopia, and disruptive changes in visual acuity. Risk of developing thyroid eye disease may be ↑ in patients who smoke. Imaging with orbital CT scanning may help to define degree of proptosis and extent of extraocular muscle involvement. Treatment of mild symptoms focuses on protecting the corneas from exposure and abrasion while using artificial tears and ointments to provide adequate lubrication. High-dose systemic glucocorticoids may help to attenuate active inflammation. Progressive diplopia and disruptive changes in visual acuity may require surgical decompression of the orbits. Staged strabismus surgery and eyelid surgery may be considered. Treatments based on the use of orbital irradiation, immunosuppressive agents, and plasmapheresis have been tried with varying degrees of success. Patients with persistent diplopia may need to wear glasses with corrective prismatic lenses.

Toxic multinodular goiter Growth of multiple autonomously functioning hyperplastic thyroid nodules. More common among older individuals. May develop in the setting of a previously euthyroid multinodular goiter. May extend substernally, causing compressive thoracic outlet symptoms. Hyperthyroidism may be precipitated by exposure to large amounts of iodine. May be treated with radioactive iodine ablation, surgical resection, or anti-thyroid drugs.

Toxic adenoma Progressive growth of a single autonomously functioning thyroid nodule. Usually quite large. May be treated with surgical resection, anti-thyroid drugs, or radioactive iodine ablation.

Treatment of hyperthyroidism

Beta-blockers May help to attenuate symptoms of thyrotoxicosis while other treatment modalities are being planned or taking effect. Commonly used preparations include *propranolol* (Inderal® 10–40mg tid, Inderal LA® 60–120mg qd) and *atenolol* (Tenormin® 25–100mg qd). Should be titrated to relief of symptoms (palpitations, tremulousness) instead of resting heart rate.

Anti-thyroid drugs Thionamides that inhibit thyroid hormone production. Available preparations include *methimazole* (Tapazole 10–40mg qd) and *propylthiouracil* (PTU 50–200mg bid-tid). Methimazole offers the advantage of once-daily dosing. PTU may be safer during pregnancy, and may reduce peripheral conversion of T4 to T3. Doses should initially be titrated to reduce T4 and T3 levels to within normal ranges. Return of suppressed TSH levels to normal range may be delayed. Limiting side effects may include pruritic rash and hepatotoxicity with elevated transaminase levels or jaundice. Reversible agranulocytosis may develop as a rare complication. Patients should be instructed to stop treatment pending further evaluation if they develop a fever or severe pharyngitis.

Radioactive iodine ablation Administration of a single oral dose of iodine-131. Isotope is taken up and organified by hyperfunctioning thyroid tissue. Over time, locally acting beta radiation gradually destroys thyrocytes. Calculated doses used to treat Graves' disease based on thyroid gland volume and uptake. High incidence of postablative hypothyroidism. Calculated doses may be used to treat toxic adenomas. Higher-range empiric doses are usually used to treat toxic multinodular goiters.

Thyroid surgery Procedures vary depending on indication. Toxic adenomas may be resected, leaving the remainder of the thyroid intact. Toxic multinodular goiters usually require total thyroidectomy, especially when substernal extension may be contributing to compressive symptoms. Subtotal thyroidectomy may be considered in cases of Graves' disease when anti-thyroid drugs and radioactive iodine are contraindicated.

Causes of non-hyperthyroid thyrotoxicosis Include ingestion of pharmacologic and non-pharmacologic preparations of thyroid hormone, subacute thyroiditis, and autoimmune thyroiditis.

Subacute thyroiditis Granulomatous inflammation of thyroid tissue. Onset often preceded by a non-specific viral illness. Patients present with pain localized to the thyroid gland that may radiate upwards to the neck and jaw. The thyroid gland may be slightly enlarged and exquisitely tender to palpation. Inflammation may spread from one lobe to the other. Lab tests may reveal an elevated erythrocyte sedimentation rate (ESR). Thyroid function test profiles typically reveal a hyperthyroid phase lasting 1–4wks caused by release of thyroid hormone, followed by a resolving hypothyroid phase lasting 1–3 months caused by impaired production of thyroid hormone. May require treatment with a) beta-blockers to attenuate thyrotoxicosis, and b) systemic glucocorticoids to alleviate discomfort associated with inflammation.

Hypothyroidism

A systemic syndrome caused by a deficiency of thyroid hormone. Primary hypothyroidism represents a deficiency of thyroid hormone caused by intrinsic dysfunction of the thyroid gland itself. Secondary hypothyroidism represents a deficiency of thyroid hormone caused by dysfunction of the hypothalamus or pituitary gland.

Symptoms May include weight gain, cold intolerance, dyspnea, constipation, myalgias, arthralgias, fatigue, lethargy, and amenorrhea.

Signs May include bradycardia, pericardial effusion, cool dry skin, brittle nails, delayed terminal relaxation of peripheral reflexes, non-pitting edema caused by deposition of glycosaminoglycans(myxedema), anemia, and hyponatremia.

Causes of primary hypothyroidism Common causes include autoimmune thyroiditis, radioactive iodine or external beam radiation-induced ablation of thyroid tissue, surgical removal of thyroid tissue, and drug-mediated inhibition of thyroid hormone production and release. Rare causes include congenital absence of thyroid tissue and resistance to thyroid hormone. Most common cause worldwide is iodine deficiency (rare in the US due to abundant dietary supplementation).

Autoimmune thyroiditis Also known as Hashimoto's thyroiditis. Chronic lymphocytic inflammation that is often associated with progressive destruction of functioning thyroid tissue. Marked female predominance. ↑ prevalence with age. Proximate cause of 95% of cases of primary hypothyroidism. Elevated titers of anti-thyroid peroxidase and anti-thyroglobulin antibodies may confirm a suspected diagnosis (measurement may not be necessary, given prevalence of disorder). May be associated with other autoimmune disorders including type 1 diabetes mellitus, autoimmune adrenalitis, and vitiligo.

Treatment Thyroid hormone replacement based on administration of pharmacologic preparations of *levothyroxine* (brand name versions include Levothroid®, Levoxyl®, Synthroid®, Unithroid®; taken qd; available in 25, 50, 75, 88, 100, 112, 125, 137, 150, 175, 200, and 300mcg color-coded preparations). Usual daily replacement dose is approximately 1.6mcg/kg body weight. Elderly patients may only require 1mcg/kg body weight due to ↓ clearance of thyroid hormone. Levothyroxine may be started at full replacement doses in patients under age 50 without evidence of heart disease. In patients with known or suspected heart disease, treatment should be started at a dose of 12.5–25mcg daily, and should be ↑ gradually by 12.5–25mcg increments at 4-wk intervals based on changes in TSH levels. A TSH level should be checked 6wks after starting a dose or 4wks after adjusting a dose to assess the adequacy of replacement. Treatment should target maintenance of TSH levels within reference ranges. Co-administration of large doses of calcium supplements, iron supplements, and bile acid resins may inhibit absorption of levothyroxine.

Subclinical hypothyroidism Profile of thyroid function test results characterized by an elevated TSH level with normal T4 and T3 levels. Indications for treatment are controversial. Concomitant evidence of hypercholesterolemia or underlying autoimmune thyroiditis may provide a rationale for starting treatment with thyroid hormone replacement.

Non-thyroidal illness

When thyroid function tests are checked in the setting of severe non-thyroidal illness, secondary changes in TSH and thyroid hormone levels that reflect the impact of the illness itself may return profiles that appear to be consistent with primary thyroid dysfunction. T3 levels usually decline during the early stages of severe non-thyroidal illness. As illness progresses, T4 levels may also decline. TSH levels are usually normal or suppressed during the early stages of severe non-thyroidal illness. They may rise above the upper limit of the normal range during recovery, producing a profile that may be mistaken for primary hypothyroidism. If thyroid function tests are checked in severely ill patients, clinical correlation is important. The presence of a goiter, history of radioactive iodine treatment, history of pituitary disease, or findings consistent with prior thyroid surgery may help to establish a correct diagnosis. For patients without findings consistent with underlying thyroid dysfunction, re-testing 6–8wks after recovery may be recommended.

Hyperparathyroidism

Physiology Parathyroid hormone (PTH) secreted by the parathyroid gland stimulates a) ↑ breakdown of bone through secondary activation of osteoclasts, b) ↑ reabsorption of calcium (Ca^{2+}) and ↓ reabsorption of phosphate (PO_4^-) in the distal tubule, and c) ↑ production of 1,25-hydroxyvitamin D. The overall effect is to ↑ Ca^{2+} levels while ↓ PO_4^- levels. Negative feedback exerted by ↑ Ca^{2+} levels regulates secretion of PTH.

Primary hyperparathyroidism Inappropriate autonomous secretion of PTH due to hyperplastic growth of one or more parathyroid glands. Approximately 80% of cases are associated with growth of a solitary adenoma, 15% with hyperplasia of all four glands, 4% with growth of multiple adenomas, and 1% with malignant growth of parathyroid carcinoma. Patients often present with asymptomatic hypercalcemia. Confirmation based on finding an elevated Ca^{2+} level in conjunction with an elevated or inappropriately normal PTH level. Complications associated with progressive disease may include a) osteoporosis, b) nephrolithiasis, c) precipitation or exacerbation of psychiatric symptoms, and d) gastrointestinal symptoms. Variants presenting with hyperplasia of all four glands associated with specific multiple endocrine neoplasia (MEN) syndromes. Treatment involves surgical resection of autonomously functioning parathyroid tissue. Surgery is indicated in patients presenting with severe or life-threatening hypercalcemia, osteoporotic fractures, impaired renal function, or recurrent nephrolithiasis. In asymptomatic cases, evaluation based on quantitation of 24-h urine calcium excretion, measurement of creatinine clearance, and DEXA scanning with measurement of distal forearm bone mineral density may help to determine which patients should be referred for surgery.[1]

Indications for treatment of asymptomatic primary hyperparathyroidism

- Calcium level >11.4mg/dL
- 24-h urine calcium excretion >400mg
- DEXA scan with measurement of distal forearm bone mineral density with Z-score <2.0
- Creatinine clearance <70% age-matched normal range
- Age <50yrs

Planned operations may involve exploration and comparison of all four glands to identify hypertrophic tissue, or targeted resection of specific glands based on attempted pre-operative localization. Studies commonly utilized for pre-operative localization include sestamibi scans, MRI scans, CT scans, and cervical ultrasonography. Intraoperatively, PTH levels may be measured to track changes following resection of suspect tissue. Solitary adenomas are usually resected in isolation. Confirmed hyperplasia of all four glands may require resection of up to three and a half glands with reimplantation of residual tissue in an accessible location.

Secondary hyperparathyroidism Presents with a profile of an elevated PTH level in conjunction with a low or normal Ca^{2+} level. Precipitated by ↓ conversion of 25-hydroxyvitamin D to 1,25-hydroxyvitamin D that leads to ↓ intestinal absorption of Ca^{2+}. Relative hypocalcemia stimulates ↑ secretion of PTH to restore and maintain normal Ca^{2+} levels. Usually develops in patients with chronic renal failure once creatinine clearance declines to <40mLmin. May respond to treatment with calcium supplementation, phosphate restriction, and administration of potent 1,25-hydroxyvitamin D analogs. Secondary hyperparathyroidism may also develop in the setting of osteomalacia associated with vitamin D deficiency.

1 NIH Consensus Statement 82. Diagnosis and Management of Asymptomatic Primary Hyperparathyroidism.

Tertiary hyperparathyroidism In patients with chronic renal failure, prolonged severe secondary hyperparathyroidism may lead to growth of autonomously functioning parathyroid tissue. Inappropriate secretion of PTH in this setting may lead to hypercalcemia with extracellular Ca^{2+} deposition evident as cutaneous calcification. In extreme cases, this may precipitate digital gangrene as part of a life-threatening syndrome known as calciphylaxis. Urgent parathyroidectomy may be required.

Multiple endocrine neoplasia syndromes

Multiple endocrine neoplasia type 1 (MEN 1) Clinical manifestations include primary hyperparathyroidism, pancreatic tumors, and pituitary adenomas. Autosomal dominant loss-of-function mutation of the MENIN tumor suppressor gene. Penetrance of primary hyperparathyroidism characterized by four-gland hyperplasia is 95%. Most common pancreatic tumors are gastrinomas (associated with the Zollinger-Ellison syndrome) and insulinomas. Pituitary adenomas may secrete prolactin or growth hormone, or may be non-functional.

Multiple endocrine neoplasia type 2a (MEN 2a) Clinical manifestations include medullary thyroid carcinoma (MTC), pheochromocytoma, and primary hyperparathyroidism. Autosomal dominant mutation of the RET proto-oncogene. Different mutations identified in different kindreds. MTC may be diagnosed in 80–100% of affected individuals. Tends to be multicentric. Preceded by hyperplasia of parafollicular C-cells. Pheochromocytomas may develop in 50% of affected individuals. Often bilateral. Rarely malignant. RET proto-oncogene screening is available as a commercial test.

Multiple endocrine neoplasia type 2b (MEN 2b) Clinical manifestations include MTC, pheochromocytoma, and mucosal neuromas (lesions that may be discernable as submucosal masses on the lips, cheeks, tongue, glottis, eyelids, and visible corneal nerves). Affected individuals may present with a characteristic marfanoid habitus. MTC tends to be more aggressive than in MEN 2a, mandating earlier diagnosis and treatment.

285

Hypoparathyroidism

Characterized by decreased secretion of PTH. Patients may present with symptoms and signs of hypocalcemia including perioral numbness, digital paresthesias, carpopedal spasm, and tetany. Confirmation based on finding a ↓ Ca^{2+} level in conjunction with a low or inappropriately normal PTH level. May develop as a complication of surgical procedures that inadvertently lead to removal or destruction of a critical mass of parathyroid tissue. Idiopathic hypoparathyroidism caused by autoimmune destruction of parathyroid tissue may develop in conjunction with autoimmune adrenalitis and mucocutaneous candidiasis as part of the type I polyglandular autoimmune syndrome.

Treatment Acute hypocalcemia may require treatment with IV infusions of *calcium chloride* (272mg of elemental calcium per 10mL) or *calcium gluconate* (90mg of elemental calcium per 10mL). Doses of 200mg of elemental calcium may be administered over several minutes. Prolonged infusions of 400–1000mg of elemental calcium may be administered over 24h. Chronic hypocalcemia may require treatment with calcium supplementation and vitamin D analog therapy. Patients may require 1500–3000mg of elemental calcium daily in divided doses. Vitamin D analogs that may be used to promote absorption of elemental calcium include *calcitriol* (Rocaltrol® 0.25–1.0mcg qd–bid) and *ergocalciferol* (50,000–200,000IU qd) Treatment should target maintenance of calcium levels in low normal ranges.

Osteoporosis

Characterized by a loss of bone mass associated with an ↑ risk of fracture. Proximate cause of 1.5 million fractures annually in the US. Most common sites of fracture are the vertebral bodies, wrist, and hip.

Risk factors Principal risk factors associated with development of osteoporosis are female sex and advancing age. More common in Caucasians and Asians than other ethnic groups. Other risk factors include small frame, early menopause, amenorrhea, smoking, alcohol abuse, family history, and a history of minimally traumatic fractures. Iatrogenic risk factors include immobilization, treatment with anticonvulsants, and treatment with supraphysiologic doses of glucocorticoids. Disorders associated with development of osteoporosis include primary hyperparathyroidism, thyrotoxicosis, Cushing's syndrome, hypogonadism, and connective tissue disorders that disrupt synthesis of bone matrix (osteogenesis imperfecta, Ehlers–Danlos syndrome, Marfan's syndrome).

Diagnosis Usually suspected when an individual presents with a minimally traumatic hip, wrist, or vertebral compression fracture. Asymptomatic presentation may be associated with progressive height loss attributed to vertebral compression fractures. Plain films may reveal osteopenia and anterior wedging of vertebral bodies. Reliable diagnosis and quantification of bone loss relies on direct measurement of bone density with DEXA scanning.

DEXA scanning

Provides an estimate of areal density of bone measured in g/cm^2. Most commonly scanned sites are the lumbar verterbrae and hip. Scoliotic changes, hardware, and verterbral compression fractures may distort lumbar vertebral readings. Generates actual measurements along with T-scores that represent number of standard deviations above or below the mean for healthy young adults. Z-scores represent number of standard deviations above or below mean for representative age group. T-scores have been correlated with associated fracture risk to assign classifications.

WHO definitions

T-score –1.0 to –2.5 = osteopenia

T-score ≤ –2.5 = osteoporosis

Screening The National Osteoporosis Foundation recommends screening with DEXA scanning be considered for a) all women aged 65 and older, and b) younger postmenopausal women with more than one predisposing risk factor.

Preventive measures Include regular weight-bearing exercise, adequate calcium intake (>1200mg elemental calcium daily), adequate vitamin D intake (400–800IU daily), smoking cessation, and moderation of alcohol intake are recommended. Postmenopausal estrogen replacement therapy is no longer recommended as a preventive measure.

Treatment of osteoporosis

Available agents include bisphosphonates, raloxifene, teriparatide, and calcitonin.

Bisphosphonates Agents that bind to hydroxyapatite crystals in mineralized bone. Act to inhibit bone resorption. Oral bisphosphonates include *alendronate* (Fosamax® 10mg qd or 70mg once a week), *risedronate* (Actonel® 5mg qd or 35mg once a week), and *etidronate*. Weekly dosing may improve compliance and limit risk of side effects. May cause severe esophageal irritation. Should be swallowed with 8oz of water with directions to remain in an upright position for 30min afterwards. Lower-range doses (Fosamax® 5–10mg qd or 35mg once a week, Actonel® 5mg qd) may help to prevent steroid-induced osteoporosis. Patients who cannot tolerate oral bisphosphonates may be treated with doses of intravenous *pamidronate* (Aredia® 30mg in 250mL NS infused over 4h) administered every 3 months.

Raloxifene (Evista® 60mg qd). Selective estrogen receptor modulator (SERM). May be used to prevent and treat osteoporosis. Often precipitates hot flashes. Associated with an increased risk of deep venous thrombosis.

Teriperitide (Forteo®). Recombinant form of the N-terminal segment of PTH that must be administered as a daily subcutaneous injection. An anabolic agent that promotes new bone formation. Often considered when patients have continued to lose bone or sustain fractures during treatment with bisphosphonates.

Calcitonin (Miacalcin® 100U qd). Pharmacologic preparation of salmon calcitonin. Can be administered subcutaneously or as an intranasal spray. May help to relieve bone pain after an acute osteoporotic fracture. Tachyphylaxis limits long-term utility in prevention and treatment of osteoporosis.

DEXA scanning may be repeated after 1–2yrs to assess responses to treatment. Comparisons should be based on measurements taken with similar types of equipment loaded with valid databases. Bone mineral density changes that are >2% in the lumbar spine and >3% in the hip may be considered significant. Changes in urinary bone turnover markers (N-telopeptides, pyridinoline) tracked over time may reflect degrees of bone loss.

Paget's disease of the bone

Disorder characterized by focally accelerated remodeling of bone that disrupts normal architecture. Commonly involves the sacrum, spine, femur, skull, and pelvis. May present with bone pain, fractures, deformities, or manifestations of associated neurologic, rheumatologic, or metabolic complications. Examination may reveal cutaneous erythema, warmth, and tenderness localized to the soft tissue overlying affected regions. Characteristic findings may include enlargement of the skull, frontal bossing, and bowing of the lower extremities. Associated with an ↑ risk of sensorineural deafness, osteoarthritis, spinal stenosis, and development of osteosarcoma. Extensive involvement with hypervascularity of remodeled bone may lead to high-output heart failure.

Diagnosis Often detected when localized symptoms prompt evaluation with plain films that reveal characteristic ragged lytic lesions. Bone scanning may reveal other sites of involvement that may be confirmed with dedicated plain films. Laboratory testing often reveals moderately elevated alkaline phosphatase levels. Calcium and phosphorus levels are usually normal. Urinary bone turnover markers (N-telopeptides, pyridinoline) are usually elevated.

Treatment Bone pain may respond to treatment with NSAIDs. Intranasal calcitonin (Miacalcin® 100U qd) may provide effective analgesia. Limited courses of treatment with bisphosphonates may help to alleviate symptoms and stabilize deformities. Alendronate (Fosamax® 40mg qd for 6 months) and risedronate (Actonel® 30mg PO qd for 2 months) may be equally effective. Patients who cannot tolerate oral bisphosphonates may respond to treatment with IV pamidronate (Aredia® 30mg qd x 3d). Changes in alkaline phosphatase levels and urinary bone turnover markers may be tracked over time to assess responses to treatment. Patients who continue to manifest symptoms after an initial course of treatment with a bisphosphonate may respond to subsequent courses of treatment with the same agent.

Osteomalacia

Condition characterized by ↓ mineralization of bone matrix. May be precipitated by disorders that limit effective reserves of circulating calcium and phosphorus. Impairment of mineralization that occurs during growth may lead to development of rickets associated with short stature, proximal muscle weakness, and bony deformities. Demineralization that occurs after the epiphyses have fused may give rise to bone pain and tenderness.

Vitamin D deficiency Most common cause of osteomalacia in adults. Pure nutritional deficiency is rare, due to adequate supplementation of dairy products. May still occur with adherence to a strict vegan diet. Malabsorption of vitamin D may occur in the setting of disorders associated with pancreatic insufficiency, impaired biliary secretion, or intestinal malabsorption. Treatment with anticonvulsants may enhance metabolism of vitamin D in the liver, diminishing effective stores of 25-hydroxyvitamin D. In rare instances, severe liver disease may diminish stores of 25-hydroxyvitamin D. In cases where no obvious underlying cause is evident, a confirmed diagnosis of vitamin D deficiency may prompt serologic or endoscopic evaluation to check for evidence of unsuspected celiac disease.

Evaluation Should initially focus on measurement of Ca^{2+}, PO_4^-, PTH, alkaline phosphatase, and 25-hydroxyvitamin D levels. Moderate-to-severe cases of vitamin D deficiency may present with secondary hyperparathyroidism characterized by low Ca^{2+} and PO_4^- levels in conjunction with elevated PTH and alkaline phosphatase levels. Mild cases may present with normal Ca^{2+}, PO_4^-, and alkaline phosphatase levels in conjunction with normal or slightly elevated PTH levels. Confirmation of a suspected diagnosis based on documentation of a low 25-hydroxyvitamin D level. Population studies have shown that normal ranges reported for some commercial assays may be too low. A 25-hydroxyvitamin D level that is <10ng/dL may be considered deficient, while a level that is between 10–20ng/dL may be considered insufficient.

Treatment Vitamin D deficiency repletion requirements may vary depending on the underlying cause and severity of the disorder. Mild cases may respond to repletion with *ergocalciferol* 50,000IU weekly for 6wks, followed by daily administration of a multivitamin containing 400–800IU of cholecalciferol. Severe cases associated with persistent malabsorption may require long-term treatment with a combination of calcium supplements and ergocalciferol administered in doses ranging from 50,000–100,000IU daily. Patients with underlying liver disease may require treatment with *calcifediol*. Ca^{2+} levels should be monitored during treatment, as vitamin D toxicity may precipitate hypercalcemia.

Hypophosphatemic disorders Persistent renal phosphate wasting may lead to hyphosphatemia with associated osteomalacia. Familial X-linked hypophosphatemic rickets is the most common inherited disorder associated with renal phosphate wasting. Affected males present with in early childhood with poor growth complicated by severe rickets, hypophosphatemia, phosphaturia, and low or inappropriately normal 1,25-vitamin D levels. Treatment involves administration of large amounts of supplemental phosphate along with calcitriol taken to prevent secondary hyperparathyroidism. Oncogenic osteomalacia represents an acquired form of renal phosphate wasting that may develop in patients diagnosed with benign and malignant mesenchymal tumors. It appears to be caused by the synthesis and secretion of an associated humoral factor that induces phosphaturia. In most cases, resection of neoplastic tissue has proven to be curative.

Cushing's syndrome

Physiology Corticotropin-releasing hormone (CRH) secreted by the hypothalamus stimulates secretion of adrenocorticotrophic hormone (ACTH) from corticotroph cells in the anterior pituitary. ACTH binds to receptors on cells in the zona fasciculata and zona reticularis of the adrenal cortex, stimulating the production and secretion of cortisol and androgens. Basal secretion of cortisol follows a circadian pattern. Cortisol levels fall to nearly undetectable levels in the late evening, and then gradually ↑ to peak after 6–8h of sleep. Physiologic stress may stimulate ↑ secretion of cortisol. Most of the cortisol secreted by the adrenal cortex binds to transport proteins in the circulation. Free (unbound) cortisol, binds to cytosolic receptors to exert different regulatory effects. Free cortisol exerts negative regulatory effects on the secretion of CRH from the hypothalamus and the secretion of ACTH from the anterior pituitary.

Cushing's syndrome Represents the sequelae of prolonged exposure to chronically elevated glucocorticoid levels. Endogenous Cushing's syndrome is caused by the ↑ production and secretion of cortisol (hypercortisolemia). Underlying causes may be mechanistically classified as ACTH-dependent (hypercortisolemia driven by ↑ secretion of ACTH from a pituitary or non-pituitary source) or ACTH-independent (hypercortisolemia that develops as a result of the growth of autonomously functioning adrenal cortex tissue). Iatrogenic Cushing's syndrome may be caused by prolonged exposure to supratherapeutic doses of a range of different pharmacologic glucocorticoid preparations.

ACTH-dependent Cushing's syndrome Most common cause is growth of an ACTH-secreting pituitary adenoma (Cushing's disease). May also be caused by ectopic secretion of ACTH from other identified or occult neoplasms including small cell lung carcinoma, carcinoid tumors, pancreatic islet cell tumors, medullary thyroid carcinoma, and pheochromocytomas. Rare cases caused by ectopic secretion of CRH.

ACTH-independent Cushing's syndrome Most common cause is growth of an isolated cortisol-secreting adrenal adenoma. May also be caused by secretion of cortisol from functional adrenal carcinomas. Rare cases caused by growth of pigmented micronodules (Carney complex) or macronodular adrenal hyperplasia.

Symptoms May include weight gain, weakness, fatigue, oligomenorrhea, impotence, easy bruising, anxiety, irritability, depression, and impaired concentration.

Signs Most common manifestation is fat deposition in a central distribution with relative sparing of the limbs. Central fat deposition may lead to expansion of the cheeks (producing characteristic 'moon' facies), protrusion of supraclavicular fat pads, protrusion of the dorsocervical fat pad (producing a 'buffalo hump'), and truncal obesity. Atrophy of connective tissue in the dermis may lead to facial plethora and development of expanding darkened striae (>0.5cm wide) in the axillae and lower abdominal quadrants. Other manifestations may include hypertension, osteopenia, proximal muscle weakness, and evidence of hirsutism or virilization.

Treatment of ACTH-dependent Cushing's syndrome Depends on underlying cause and rate of progression. Whenever feasible, confirmed ACTH-secreting pituitary adenomas should be surgically resected. Microadenomas (<1cm in diameter) can usually be removed via transsphenoidal approaches. Removal of larger macroadenomas may require craniotomy. Success rates following initial surgery vary. Persistent disease may require repeat surgery or treatment with external beam radiation. Successful treatment of ectopic secretion of ACTH depends on accurate localization and surgical resection of functional tissue. In either setting, severe refractory hypercortisolemia may lead to consideration of bilateral surgical adrenalectomy or temporizing use of adrenolytic agents (*ketoconazole, metyrapone, aminoglutethimide*) to inhibit excessive cortisol production.

Treatment of ACTH-independent Cushing's syndrome Principal treatment is surgical resection of cortisol-secreting neoplastic adrenal tissue.

Evaluation of suspected Cushing's syndrome

1 Check a urine free cortisol level, a salivary cortisol level, or an overnight low-dose dexamethasone suppression test to confirm the presence of hypercortisolemia
   • Urine free cortisol level—measured in a 24-h urine collection—concomitant measurement of creatinine may confirm adequate collection volume (>1g/24h)—upper limit of normal range may vary depending on assay used—may want to perform up to 3 collections for verification
   • Salivary cortisol level—measured by having the patient chew a cotton pledget to collect 2.5mL sample of saliva at 11:00 PM—upper limit of normal range may vary depending on assay used—an elevated level may reflect an abnormal pattern of secretion—may want to check several samples for verification
   • Overnight low-dose dexamethasone suppression test—in the normal state, dexamethasone should suppress ACTH secretion, suppressing cortisol secretion in turn—performed by having the patient take 1mg of *dexamethasone* (Decadron®) at 11:00 PM, then measuring a cortisol level at 8:00 AM the next morning
      • Cortisol <3mcg/dL = normal response
      • Cortisol >3mcg/dL = hypercortisolemia
2 If hypercortisolemia has been confirmed, check a plasma ACTH level to distinguish between ACTH-dependent and ACTH-independent Cushing's syndrome
   • Plasma ACTH >10pg/mL = ACTH-dependent Cushing's syndrome
   • Plasma ACTH <5pg/mL = ACTH-independent Cushing's syndrome
3 If ACTH-dependent Cushing's syndrome is suspected, check an overnight high-dose dexamethasone suppression test or a CRH stimulation test to distinguish between an ACTH-secreting pituitary adenoma and non-suppressible ectopic secretion of ACTH
   • Overnight high-dose dexamethasone suppression test—performed by measuring a baseline cortisol level at 8:00 AM, having the patient take 8mg of *dexamethasone* (Decadron®) at 11:00 PM, then measuring a repeat cortisol level at 8:00 AM the next morning
   • Suppression of cortisol by > 50% = ACTH-secreting pituitary adenoma
   • CRH stimulation test—performed by measuring a baseline plasma ACTH level, administering 100mcg of synthetic ovine CRF intravenously, then measuring plasma ACTH levels at 5, 10, 15, and 30min marks
      • Progressive ↑ in plasma ACTH levels = ACTH-secreting pituitary adenoma

4 If an ACTH-secreting pituitary adenoma is suspected, consider pituitary MRI scanning or inferior petrosal sinus sampling as a confirmatory study
   • Inferior petrosal sinus sampling—performed by measuring baseline peripheral and petrosal sinus plasma ACTH levels, administering *synthetic ovine CRF*, then measuring peripheral and petrosal sinus plasma ACTH levels at defined intervals
      • Stimulated petrosal sinus/peripheral plasma ACTH ratio >3.0 = ACTH-secreting pituitary adenoma
5 If ectopic secretion of ACTH is suspected, consider targeted imaging with high-resolution thoracic CT scanning, thoracic MRI scanning, or octreotide scanning to attempt to localize an ACTH-secreting neoplasm
6 If ACTH-independent Cushing's syndrome is suspected, consider targeted imaging with abdominal CT scanning, abdominal MRI scanning, or iodo-cholesterol scintigraphy scanning to identify and characterize adrenal abnormalities.

Adrenal insufficiency

A systemic syndrome caused by deficiency of hormones secreted by the adrenal cortex. Primary adrenal insufficiency represents a deficiency of cortisol and aldosterone caused by intrinsic dysfunction of the adrenal cortex. Secondary adrenal insufficiency represents a deficiency of cortisol caused by dysfunction of the hypothalamus or pituitary gland.

Symptoms May vary depending on specific deficiencies. Symptoms associated with deficiency of cortisol may include weight loss, fatigue, weakness, anorexia, nausea, and vomiting. Deficiency of aldosterone may precipitate orthostatic dizziness and lightheadedness with positional changes.

Signs Deficiency of cortisol may present with orthostatic hypotension, hypoglycemia, and hyponatremia. Deficiency of aldosterone may present with hyperkalemia, metabolic acidosis, and exacerbation of orthostatic hypotension and hyponatremia. Prolonged primary adrenal insufficiency may eventually cause diffuse hyperpigmentation of the skin and mucous membranes.

Causes of primary adrenal insufficiency Common causes include autoimmune adrenalitis, bilateral adrenal hemorrhage, disseminated tuberculosis, and HIV infection. Rare causes include disseminated histoplasmosis, bilateral adrenal metastases, lymphoma, and adrenoleukodystrophy. Most clinically significant cases are associated with destruction of >90% of functioning adrenal cortical tissue. In undiagnosed cases, physiologic stress associated with acute illness, infection, trauma, or surgery may precipitate an adrenal crisis characterized by fever, refractory hypotension, volume depletion, severe weakness, nausea, vomiting, abdominal pain, and delirium leading to obtundation and coma.

Autoimmune adrenalitis Also know as Addison's disease. Lymphocytic infiltration associated with progressive destruction of functioning adrenal cortical tissue. May be associated with other autoimmune disorders including autoimmune thyroiditis, type 1 diabetes mellitus, vitiligo, and idiopathic hypoparathyroidism.

Adrenal crisis Treatment of a suspected adrenal crisis should not be delayed for any reason. Confirmatory testing may be performed once a patient has been stabilized. Effective therapy incorporates a) IV volume repletion with large volumes of isotonic fluid (D5 NS administered as rapidly as possible), b) concomitant administration of *dexamethasone* (Decadron®) 4mg IV every 12h (other glucocorticoid preparations may interfere with plasma cortisol assays used to confirm diagnosis), and c) identification and treatment of precipitating causes.

Evaluation of suspected adrenal insufficiency

1 Perform a cosyntropin stimulation test to evaluate the intrinsic function of the adrenal cortex
- Cosyntropin stimulation test—performed by measuring a baseline cortisol level, administering 250mcg of *cosyntropin* (Cortrosyn®) IV, and measuring cortisol levels at 30 and 60 minutes
  - Peak cortisol >18mcg/dL = normal response
  - Peak cortisol <18mcg/dL = adrenal insufficiency
2 If adrenal insufficiency has been confirmed, check a plasma ACTH level to distinguish between primary and secondary adrenal insufficiency
- Plasma ACTH >50pg/mL = primary adrenal insufficiency
- Plasma ACTH <30pg/mL = secondary adrenal insufficiency

Treatment Primary and secondary adrenal insufficiency require treatment with glucocorticoid replacement therapy. One commonly employed regimen is based on twice-daily administration of *hydrocortisone* (Cortef® 7.5–30mg daily split into two doses with 2/3 of the daily dose taken before breakfast and 1/3 taken in the late afternoon). Other regimens are based on once-daily administration of *prednisone* (2.5–10mg taken before breakfast or at bedtime), or *dexamethasone* (Decadron® 0.25–0.75mg taken at bedtime). There are no specific tests or assays that provide an accurate index of the adequacy of glucocorticoid replacement. Clinical assessment is required to identify doses that strike a balance between inadequate replacement with residual symptoms and signs of adrenal insufficiency and over-replacement predisposing to iatrogenic Cushing's syndrome. Intercurrent illness, trauma, or planned surgery may require transient doubling of doses of pharmacologic glucocorticoid preparations to meet the demands of superimposed physiologic stress. Patients should be provided with prefilled syringes containing *dexamethasone* (4mg Decadron® in 1mL NS) that can be administered intramuscularly or subcutaneously in emergency situations. Primary adrenal insufficiency may also require treatment with mineralocorticoid replacement therapy. *Fludrocortisone* (Florinef® 0.1–0.2mg qd) is usually the agent of choice. Orthostatic vital signs, serum potassium levels, and plasma renin activity levels may be measured and tracked to assess the adequacy of mineralocorticoid replacement.

Hyperaldosteronism

Primary aldosteronism Secretion of aldosterone from the zona glomerulosa of the adrenal cortex is mediated by the renin-angiotensin axis. Excessive secretion of aldosterone leads to ↑ uptake of sodium (Na^+) and ↑ excretion of potassium (K^+) in the distal tubules of the kidney. Over time, this may lead to development of hypertension and hypokalemia.

Symptoms Tend to be non-specific. May include fatigue, weakness, headaches, polydipsia, and polyuria.

Signs Hypertension and concomitant hypokalemia.

Causes of primary aldosteronism Approximately 75% of all cases are caused by growth of an autonomously functioning aldosterone-producing adrenal adenoma (also known as Conn's syndrome). The remainder are caused by idiopathic hyperaldosteronism, a condition characterized by bilateral micronodular or macronodular hyperplasia of the adrenal cortex. Rare causes include adrenal carcinoma and glucocorticoid-remediable hypertension.

Evaluation of suspected primary aldosteronism

1 Screen for inappropriate aldosterone secretion by checking a plasma aldosterone level and a plasma renin activity level*
  - Plasma aldosterone >20ng/dL + plasma aldosterone/plasma renin activity ratio >30 = inappropriate aldosterone secretion consistent with possible primary aldosteronism
2 If primary aldosteronism is suspected, check a urine aldosterone level and urine Na^+ level after volume expansion
  - Volume expansion—may be accomplished by liberalizing Na^+ intake to a level of at least 5000mg daily for 3 days—alternatively, NaCl may be administered in tablet form as 2000mg qac— K^+ levels should be monitored and repleted as necessary
  - Urine aldosterone and Na^+ levels—measured in 24-hr urine collections— urine aldosterone >14mcg/24h + urine Na^+ >200meq/24h = primary aldosteronism
3 If primary aldosteronism is confirmed, consider targeted adrenal imaging with abdominal CT scanning , abdominal MRI scanning, or iodocholesterol scintigraphy scanning to identify and characterize adrenal abnormalities
4 If targeted imaging is unrevealing or equivocal, consider bilateral adrenal vein sampling to determine whether lateralization of aldosterone secretion consistent with an aldosterone-producing adrenal adenoma is present

* If the patient is being treated with an aldosterone receptor blocker (spironolactone or eplerenone), discontinue treatment and wait at least 6wks before testing

---

Treatment of aldosterone-producing adrenal adenomas Principal treatment is surgical resection. Pre-treatment with *spironolactone* (Aldactone® 12.5–200mg bid) or *eplerenone* (Inspra® 25–50mg bid) titrated to control blood pressure for 2–4wks prior to surgery may reduce risk of perioperative complications associated with changes in blood pressure.

Treatment of idiopathic hyperaldosteronism Long-term medical therapy based on treatment with aldosterone receptor blockers titrated to control blood pressure and normalize serum K^+ levels. Available agents include *spironolactone* (Aldactone® 12.5–200mg bid) and *eplerenone* (Inspra® 25–50mg bid). Patients who cannot tolerate aldosterone receptor blockers may be treated with *amiloride* (Midamor® 5–15mg bid) in combination with other antihypertensive agents. Surgery is not indicated.

Pheochromocytoma

Represents a rare catecholamine-secreting neoplasm. Approximately 85% develop within the adrenal medulla, with 5–10% presenting in bilateral distributions and 10% ultimately proving to be malignant. Catecholamine-secreting neoplasms that are identified in extra-adrenal locations are called paragangliomas. Associated with the MEN 2 syndromes and von Hippel–Lindau syndrome. Overall, pheochromocytomas account for <0.2% of all cases of newly diagnosed hypertension.

Symptoms Episodic paroxysms that may present with varying constellations of symptoms including palpitations, diaphoresis, headache, anxiety, tremulousness, fatigue, nausea, vomiting, abdominal pain, chest pain, and visual disturbances.

Signs Severe hypertension is characteristic. Peripheral vasoconstriction during paroxysms may produce transient pallor. Resultant ↑ core body temperature may lead to subsequent flushing.

Evaluation of suspected pheochromocytoma

1 Screen for ↑ catecholamine secretion by checking a plasma free metanephrine levels* or urine metanephrine levels
   • Plasma free metanephrine levels—screening test of choice when available sensitivity is >99%, specificity is 89%[1] • Urine metanephrine levels—based on 24-h urine collection—labetalol and buspirone may artifactually ↑ levels
   • Normal plasma free metanephrine or urine metanephrine levels = excluded
   • Markedly elevated plasma free metanephrine or urine metanephrine levels = pheochromocytoma • Marginally elevated plasma free metanephrine or urine metanephrine levels = ↑ catecholamine secretion consistent with a possible pheochromocytoma

2 If a possible pheochromocytoma is suspected, check repeat plasma free metanephrine levels or urine metanephrine levels and plasma catecholamine levels • Normal repeat plasma free metanephrine or urine metanephrine levels + normal plasma catecholamine levels = excluded • Marginally elevated repeat plasma free metanephrine or urine metanephrine levels + marginally elevated plasma catecholamine levels = ↑ catecholamine secretion consistent with a possible pheochromocytoma—consider performing a clonidine suppression test or a glucagon stimulation test for confirmation
   • Positive clonidine suppression test or glucagon stimulation test = pheochromocytoma

3 If a pheochromocytoma is confirmed, consider targeted adrenal imaging with abdominal CT scanning or abdominal MRI scanning to identify and characterize adrenal abnormalities—pheochromocytomas may show a characteristic bright intensity on T2-weighted MRI images

4 If targeted imaging is unrevealing or equivocal, consider whole-body imaging with metaiodobenzylguanidine (MIBG) scanning to attempt to localize a suspicious focus of increased catecholamine secretion

* If the patient is being treated with acetaminophen, discontinue treatment and wait at least 48h before testing

Treatment Surgical resection of benign pheochromocytomas and paragangliomas may be curative. Patients require pre-operative treatment with alpha blockers started at least 1wk prior to planned procedures. Agents used for this purpose include *phenoxybenzamine* (Dibenzyline® 10–100mg qd) and *doxazosin* (Cardura® 2–8mg qd). Doses should be titrated every few days to target normotensive blood pressures. Intraoperative hypertensive crises may require treatment with *phentolamine* or *nitroprusside*. Postoperatively, patients may require volume repletion and monitoring for symptoms and signs of incipient hypoglycemia.

1 K Pacak, W Linehan, G Eisenhofer (2001) Recent advances in genetics, diagnosis, localization, and treatment of pheochromocytoma. *Annals of Internal Medicine* **134**(4) 315.

Hirsutism

Defined as new or ↑ abnormal growth of thick, coarse, pigmented terminal hair in females. May be distributed in regions commonly associated with the development of male secondary sexual characteristics including the face, chest, back, lower abdomen, and inner thighs. May be caused by a) ↑ secretion of androgens from the ovaries, b) ↑ secretion of androgens from the adrenal cortex, or c) ↑ 5α-reductase activity leading to conversion of testosterone to dihydrotestosterone.

↑ **secretion of androgens from the ovaries** Most common cause is polycystic ovary syndrome. May also be associated with ovarian hyperthecosis or growth of androgen-secreting ovarian neoplasms.

↑ **secretion of androgens from the adrenal cortex** Most common cause is late-onset congenital adrenal hyperplasia associated with 21-hydroxylase deficiency. May also be caused by Cushing's syndrome, growth of androgen-secreting adrenal adenomas, or growth of adrenal carcinomas.

Evaluation Should initially focus on identification and quantification of abnormal terminal hair growth. Patients may need to limit cosmetic treatment for a period to allow for accurate assessment. Reproductive history should focus on identification of significant menstrual irregularities and problems with infertility.

Evaluation of hirsutism

1 Check total testosterone and dehydroepiandrosterone-sulfate (DHEA-S) levels
   - Total testosterone >150ng/dL + DHEA-S <700mcg/dL = possible androgen-secreting ovarian neoplasm—consider targeted imaging with pelvic ultrasonography
   - Total testosterone >150ng/dL + DHEA-S >700mcg/dL = possible Cushing's syndrome, androgen-secreting adrenal adenoma, or adrenal carcinoma—consider formal evaluation for hypercortisolemia or targeted imaging with abdominal CT scanning or abdominal MRI scanning
2 If late-onset congenital adrenal hyperplasia is suspected, check a baseline 17-hydroxyprogesterone level, administer 250mcg of *cosyntropin* (Cortrosyn®) IV, then check repeat 17-hydroxyprogesterone levels at 30 and 60min
   - Baseline 17-hydroxyprogesterone >200ng/dL + stimulated 17-hydroxyprogesterone >1500ng/dL = late-onset congenital adrenal hyperplasia

---

Polycystic ovary syndrome Clinical diagnosis based on identification of a history of significant menstrual irregularities in conjunction with findings consistent with exposure to ↑ levels of circulating androgens (hirsutism, comedonal acne). May be caused by relative ↑ secretion of luteinizing hormone (LH) leading to increased production and secretion of androgens from the ovaries. May lead to enlargement and polycystic thickening of the ovarian capsule. Subsequent conversion of androgens to estrogen may lead to endometrial hyperplasia. Frequently associated with infertility. May be associated with insulin resistance. Patients who are trying to conceive may be treated with *clomiphene* (Clomid® 50–100mg qd x 5d starting on the 5th day of the menstrual cycle) or *metformin* (Glucophage® 500–1000mg bid, Glucophage XR® 1000–2000mg qpm). These agents may be used in combination to help to induce ovulation. Patients who do not desire fertility may be treated with oral contraceptives that combine 30–35mcg of ethinyl estradiol with progestins known to demonstrate minimal androgenic activity (desogestrel, norethindrone). Patients who cannot take oral contraceptives may be treated with cycles of *medroxyprogesterone* (Provera® 10mg qd x 7d) to promote withdrawal bleeding on a monthly basis.

Late-onset congenital adrenal hyperplasia

Condition associated with ↓ production and secretion of glucocorticoids that leads to ↑ secretion of ACTH. ↑ ACTH levels stimulate ↑ secretion of androgens from the adrenal cortex. Findings consistent with exposure to ↑ levels of circulating androgens may first become evident during the onset of puberty. Confirmation based on measurement of baseline and stimulated 17-hydroxyprogesterone levels. Treatment usually involves use of *dexamethasone* (Decadron® 0.25–0.75mg qhs) at doses targeted to suppress ACTH levels.

Antiandrogen therapy *Spironolactone* (Aldactone 50–200mg qd) acts to inhibit binding of dihydrotestosterone to target receptors. It may be used as a principal agent or in conjunction with other therapies. Continuous treatment for up to 6 months may be necessary before efficacy can be determined. Cosmetic treatments involving shaving, plucking, waxing, bleaching, electrolysis, or use of depilatories may still be required to achieve desired appearances.

Virilization Constellation of findings that reflect exposure to markedly ↑ levels of circulating androgens. Patients may present with frontal balding, deepening of the voice, clitoral enlargement, and ↑ muscle mass. Presence should raise suspicion of an underlying androgen-secreting ovarian or adrenal neoplasm.

Gynecomastia

Defined as enlargement of breast tissue in males. Transient self-limited gynecomastia may be evident in up to 70% of males during puberty. Enlargement that persists or presents as a new development in adult males may be considered abnormal. May develop as a result of a range of different underlying disorders that mechanistically promote relative imbalances between circulating levels of estrogens and androgens. Continued exposure to relatively ↑ circulating levels of estrogens may promote growth of ductal and stromal elements in breast tissue. Usually bilateral. Discernable as a firm concentric ridge of tissue that extends beyond the perimeter of the areola. May be painful with associated tenderness to palpation.

Mechanisms of disorders associated with gynecomastia

- ↑ production of sex hormone-binding globulin—leads to ↑ binding of testosterone that ↓ circulating free testosterone levels—may occur in the setting of thyrotoxicosis or chronic liver disease
- Excessive stimulation of Leydig cells due to exposure to ↑ LH levels—leads to ↑ secretion of estrogens—may develop as a complication of primary hypogonadism associated with Klinefelter's syndrome or adult Leydig cell failure—may also occur as part of the refeeding syndrome
- Excessive stimulation of Leydig cells due to exposure to ↑ human chorionic gonadotropin (hCG) levels—leads to ↑ secretion of estrogens—may be associated with the growth of germ cell testicular neoplasms that secrete excessive amounts of hCG
- Inhibition of binding of dihydrotestosterone to target receptors—may be associated with treatment with spironolactone or cimetidine
- Direct binding of estrogen receptors—may be associated with treatment with digoxin—may also occur as a result of exposure to phytoestrogens present in marijuana

Evaluation Should focus on a) quantification of extent of breast tissue, b) documentation of any history of exposure to possible offending agents, and c) measurement of testosterone, estradiol, LH, hCG, and TSH levels. If findings consistent with undetected Klinefelter's are evident on exam, a karyotype may be performed to confirm a suspected diagnosis. If a suspiciously firm or enlarged breast mass is detected on exam, a mammogram may be considered to check for possible male breast cancer.

Treatment Should be centered on identification and treatment of underlying disorders. Gynecomastia may persist long after relative balance between circulating levels of estrogens and androgens has been restored. In cases presenting with significant pain, tenderness, or cosmetic deformity, surgical bilateral reduction mammoplasty may be indicated.

Pituitary adenomas

The incidence of detection of sellar masses has increased with more widespread use of neuroradiographic imaging to evaluate a range of symptoms. Dedicated pituitary MRI scanning with gadolinium may provide the most accurate assessment of the size and location of a suspected pituitary adenoma. The maximum diameter may be used to classify a suspected pituitary adenoma as a microadenoma (<10mm) or a macroadenoma (≥10mm). A key question to address is determining whether a suspected pituitary adenoma is functional, secreting stimulating or trophic hormones that may lead to development of characteristic clinical syndromes. Some functional pituitary adenomas may be treated medically, while others require surgery.

Clinical syndromes associated with functional pituitary adenomas

- Prolactin-secreting pituitary adenoma (prolactinoma) = hyperprolactinemia
- ACTH-secreting pituitary adenoma (Cushing's disease) = ACTH-dependent Cushing's syndrome
- GH-secreting pituitary adenoma = acromegaly
- TSH-secreting pituitary adenoma = hyperthyroidism

* FSH and LH-secreting pituitary adenomas do not appear to correlate with specific clinical syndromes

Evaluation Comprehensive functional evaluation of a suspected pituitary adenoma may incorporate a) static testing based on measurement of TSH, free T4, prolactin, and IGF-1 levels, and b) dynamic testing based on performance of an overnight low-dose dexamethasone stimulation test and a GH suppression test. 24-h urine free cortisol levels or salivary cortisol levels may be measured as well.

Non-functional pituitary adenomas If a suspected pituitary adenoma proves to be non-functional, further evaluation should focus on determining whether its growth may be associated with a) hypopituitarism, b) hyperprolactinemia, c) visual field deficits caused by upward growth with compression of the optic chiasm, d) cranial nerve palsies caused by lateral extension into the cavernous sinuses, or e) severe headaches caused by pressure and traction on meningeal structures. Symptomatic non-functional pituitary adenomas may require surgery to preserve eyesight or alleviate headaches. Asymptomatic non-functional pituitary adenomas may often be followed with serial imaging and visual field testing.

Pituitary apoplexy Hemorrhage into an undetected or previously identified pituitary adenoma may cause sudden expansion that may provoke a severe headache. Upward expansion may lead to compression of the optic chiasm with loss of visual acuity. Lateral expansion may lead to compression of cranial blood vessels and herniation. Expansion within the constrained space of the sella may lead to rapid development of secondary adrenal insufficiency that may provoke an adrenal crisis. Suspected cases may require a) treatment with stress-dose glucocorticoids, b) urgent assessment of visual acuity, and c) urgent neurosurgical decompression.

Hypopituitarism

Condition characterized by deficiency of one or more of the stimulating or trophic hormones secreted by the anterior pituitary. May be caused by disorders that disrupt the function of the anterior pituitary itself, or by disorders that disrupt the function of the hypothalamus to interrupt secretion of releasing hormones that bind to receptors on cells in the anterior pituitary. The principal stimulating and trophic hormones secreted by clusters of cells in the anterior pituitary include adrenocorticotrophic hormone (ACTH), thyroid stimulating hormone (TSH), growth hormone (GH), follicle stimulating hormone (FSH), and luteinizing hormone (LH).

Causes of hypopituitarism Common causes include pituitary surgery, cranial irradiation, head trauma, and compression due to growth of pituitary adenomas. Rare causes include hypovolemic pituitary infarction (Sheehan syndrome), hemochromatosis, disseminated tuberculosis, pituitary abscess, pituitary metastases, lymphocytic hypophysitis, and compression due to growth of suprasellar masses.

Evaluation Comprehensive evaluation of suspected hypopituitarism may incorporate a) targeted imaging with dedicated pituitary MRI scanning, b) static testing based on measurement of ACTH, TSH, free T4, FSH, LH, testosterone, and insulin-like growth factor 1 (IGF-1) levels, and c) dynamic testing based on performance of a cosyntropin stimulation test and a GH stimulation test.

Component disorders Variable clinical manifestations reflect relative deficiencies of hormones produced by the tissues and endocrine glands targeted by stimulating and trophic hormones. Associated disorders may be identified as central or secondary forms of clinical syndromes.

Secondary adrenal insufficiency Presentation may vary, depending on underlying cause. Patients may present in adrenal crisis or with insidious nonspecific weight loss, fatigue, and weakness. Diagnosis based on confirmation of a stimulated plasma cortisol <18mcg/dL in conjunction with a plasma ACTH <30pg/mL. Treated with glucocorticoid replacement therapy. Mineralocorticoid replacement therapy is usually not necessary.

Secondary hypothyroidism Patients may present with characteristic symptoms and signs reflecting deficiency of thyroid hormone. Diagnosis based on confirmation of a low or inappropriately normal TSH level in conjunction with a low free T4 level. In some cases it may be prudent to check a free T4 level measured by equilibrium dialysis to provide verification. Treated with thyroid hormone replacement. TSH levels do not provide an accurate index of replacement in this setting. Doses of levothyroxine should be adjusted to target normal free T4 levels

Secondary hypogonadism Often classified as hypogonadotropic hypogonadism. Manifestations may vary depending on age of onset. Sex steroid deficiency that develops during childhood may lead to delayed or absent onset of puberty. Premenopausal adult females may present with oligomenorrhea or amenorrhea. Diagnosis in females is based on confirmation of low or inappropriately normal FSH and LH levels in conjunction with previously normal menstrual and reproductive history. Treatment usually involves estrogen replacement with cyclic oral contraceptives. Conception may require successive courses of ovulation induction and in vitro fertilization. Adult males may present with variable symptoms that may include diminished libido, erectile dysfunction, impotence, and an appreciable decline in muscle strength. Examination may reveal diminished growth of facial hair and body hair, ↓ muscle mass, osteopenia, and fine wrinkles at the corners of the eyes and mouth. Diagnosis in males is based on confirmation of a low or inappropriately normal LH level in conjunction with a low testosterone level. Treatment involves androgen replacement therapy with *testosterone* administered as a 1% topical gel (Androgel® 5–10g qam, Testim® 5–10g qam), a transdermal patch (Androderm® 2.5–10mg qhs), or an intramuscular depot injection (testosterone cypionate 50–400mg IM every 2–4wks). Doses may be adjusted to target testosterone levels in the normal range.

Growth hormone deficiency Manifestations may vary depending on age of onset. Growth hormone deficiency that develops during childhood may lead to short stature. Adults may present with osteopenia and changes in body composition discernable as an ↑ in fat mass and ↓ in lean body mass. Diagnosis based on confirmation of a low IGF-1 level by itself or in conjunction with an abnormal growth hormone stimulation test. Growth hormone stimulation tests are performed by measuring GH levels before and after administration of provocative agents that may include arginine, levodopa, clonidine, or a combination of arginine and growth hormone releasing hormone (GHRH). A peak GH level <5ng/mL may be consistent with growth hormone deficiency. Treatment involves daily administration of subcutaneous injections of *recombinant human growth hormone*. Doses may be adjusted to target normal IGF-1 levels.

Arginine-GHRH stimulation test Performed by measuring a baseline GH level, administering an IV bolus of GHRH (1mcg/kg body weight) and an infusion of arginine (0.5g/kg body weight, maximum 30g) over 30min, and measuring GH levels at 30, 60, 90, and 120min.

Hyperprolactinemia

Physiology Prolactin is constitutively secreted by lactotroph cells in the anterior pituitary. Dopamine secreted by the hypothalamus travels along the pituitary stalk through the hypophyseal portal circulation to bind to dopamine receptors on lactotroph cells. This binding inhibits the secretion of prolactin. A range of different underlying mechanisms may lead to ↑ secretion of prolactin with resultant hyperprolactinemia.

Mechanisms of disorders associated with hyperprolactinemia

- Proliferation of lactotroph cells in the form of a prolactin-secreting pituitary adenoma (prolactinoma)—leads to ↑ constitutive secretion of prolactin
- Exposure to agents that inhibit binding of dopamine to dopamine receptors—most commonly implicated agents are phenothiazines used to treat psychosis (haloperidol, risperidone), and prokinetic agents used to treat diabetic gastroparesis (metaclopramide, domperidone)
- Compression of the pituitary stalk—may interrupt passage of dopamine through the hypophyseal portal system—may be associated with growth of non-functional pituitary adenomas or other sellar and suprasellar masses
- ↑ secretion of prolactin caused by ↑ secretion of thyrotropin releasing hormone (TRH)—precise mechanism is unclear—may develop in cases of untreated primary hypothyroidism

Symptoms Hyperprolactinemia may suppress secretion of gonadotropin releasing hormone (GnRH), effectively inhibiting secretion of FSH and LH. This may lead to development of hypogonadotropic hypogonadism. Premenopausal adult females may present with oligomenorrhea, amenorrhea or infertility. Elevated prolactin levels in premenopausal females may also stimulate abnormal secretion of milk from one or both breasts, a condition known as galactorrhea. Adult males may present with a diminished libido, erectile dysfunction, or impotence.

Evaluation Initial evaluation should focus on a) documenting a recent medication history to check for exposure to specific agents, and b) measuring a TSH level to check for primary hypothyroidism. Further evaluation may require dedicated pituitary MRI scanning with gadolinium to check for the presence of a sellar mass that may represent a prolactin-secreting pituitary adenoma or a non-functional pituitary adenoma.

Treatment of prolactin-secreting pituitary adenomas Many prolactin secreting pituitary adenomas prove to be exquisitely responsive to treatment with dopamine agonists. Reduction in size with diminished secretion of prolactin may be confirmed in up to 90% of successfully treated patients. When available, *cabergoline* (Dostinex® 0.5mg) may be preferred as a first line agent. Usual starting dose is 0.25mg twice a week. May be advanced as tolerated to 1mg twice a week. Dose-limiting side effects may include nausea, orthostasis, and cognitive impairment. *Bromocriptine* (Parlodel® 2.5mg bid-tid) may also be considered as an alternative agent when cost, availability, or tolerance of side effects present difficulties. Prolactin levels may be checked 2–3wks after starting treatment or adjusting a dose of a dopamine agonist to gauge efficacy. Changes in size may be detected on pituitary MRI scan checked 6–8wks after starting treatment. In cases where patients require treatment but cannot tolerate therapeutic doses of dopamine agonists, surgery may be considered. Microadenomas can usually be removed via transsphenoidal approaches. Removal of larger macroadenomas may require craniotomy. Success rates following initial surgery vary. Persistent disease may require repeat surgery or treatment with external beam radiation.

Treatment of prolactin-secreting pituitary adenomas during pregnancy

Increased production and secretion of estrogen during pregnancy may promote growth and expansion of prolactin-secreting pituitary adenomas. Macroadenomas may expand to the point where they cause visual field deficits or severe headaches. As the effects of cabergoline on fetal development are unknown, expectant management may focus on a) considering surgery prior to conception to prevent potential complications, or b) carefully monitoring visual acuity and neurologic symptoms during pregnancy to detect changes that may prompt evaluation with dedicated pituitary MRI scanning and visual field testing. Expanding macroadenomas may be treated with bromocriptine. If it proves to be necessary, surgery may be considered during the second trimester.

Acromegaly

A rare systemic syndrome that represents the manifestations of exposure to excessive levels of growth hormone (GH). The most common cause is proliferation of somatotroph cells in the form of a GH-secreting pituitary adenoma. GH stimulates ↑ production and secretion of IGF-1 in the liver. Over time, exposure to excessive levels of IGF-1 may lead to growth and enlargement of somatic tissues.

Signs Changes in appearance may be insidious, developing gradually over the course of several years. Review of older photographs may help to establish timing and extent of changes. Overgrowth of soft tissues may lead to striking coarsening of facial features. Patients and observers may note bossing of the frontal bones, expansion of the nose, enlargement of the tongue (macroglossia), and increased prominence of the jaw with resultant spacing of the teeth. Spade-like enlargement of the hands and feet may prompt successive changes in ring and shoe sizes. Findings consistent with left ventricular hypertrophy may be evident.

Complications Untreated acromegaly may be associated with the development of hypertension, type 2 diabetes mellitus, hypertrophic cardiomyopathy, colonic neoplasia, and obstructive sleep apnea.

Evaluation of suspected acromegaly

1 Screen for ↑ GH secretion by checking an IGF-1 level
2 If the IGF-1 level is elevated, check a GH suppression test
  • GH suppression test—performed by measuring a baseline GH level, administering a 75g oral glucose tolerance test load, then measuring GH levels at 30, 60, 90, and 120min marks
  • Peak GH <1ng/mL = normal response
  • Peak GH >2ng/mL = acromegaly
3 Consider dedicated pituitary MRI scanning with gadolinium to check for the presence of a sellar mass that may represent a GH-secreting pituitary adenoma

---

Treatment Principal treatment is surgical resection. Smaller macroadenomas can usually be removed via transsphenoidal approaches. Removal of larger macroadenomas may require craniotomy. Success rates following initial surgery vary. Documentation of cure may depend on demonstrating a) normal post-surgical IGF-1 levels, and b) a post-surgical GH suppression test with a peak GH <1ng/mL. Persistent disease may require repeat surgery, treatment with external beam radiation, or initiation of medical therapy targeted to a) inhibit secretion of GH from residual tissue, or b) inhibit production and secretion of IGF-1.

Medical therapy targeted to inhibit secretion of GH In some cases, dopamine agonists may inhibit secretion of GH from residual tissue. *Cabergoline* (Dostinex® 0.5mg) has proven to be more effective than other agents when used for this purpose. Usual starting dose is 0.25mg twice a week. May be advanced as tolerated to 1mg twice a week. Dose-limiting side effects may include nausea, orthostasis, and cognitive impairment. Patients who fail to respond to cabergoline or cannot tolerate its side effects may respond to treatment with somatostatin analogs. These agents act by binding to somatostatin receptors on target tissues. *Octreotide* is a somatostatin analog that is commercially available in a short-acting subcutaneous preparation (Sandostatin®) and a long-acting IM preparation (Sandostatin LAR®). A starting test dose of 100mcg of the short-acting preparation can be administered three times daily to assess tolerance. Limiting side effects may include nausea, abdominal discomfort, hyperglycemia, and cholelithiasis. Patients who tolerate test doses may be continued on escalating doses of the short-acting preparation, or may be switched to the long-acting preparation at a starting dose of 20mg every 4wks. Doses may be adjusted every 6–8wks to target normalization of IGF-1 levels.

Medical therapy targeted to inhibit production and secretion of IGF-1 Pegvisomant (Somavert®) is a modified form of GH that acts by competitively binding to GH receptors, inhibiting the production and secretion of IGF-1 in the liver. Clinical trials have shown that it may effectively normalize IGF-1 levels in patients who have failed to respond to treatment with somatostatin analogs.

Diabetes insipidus

Physiology of water balance ↑ serum osmolality and ↓ effective circulating volume stimulate release of antidiuretic hormone (ADH) from the supraoptic and paraventricular nuclei in the hypothalamus. Circulating ADH binds to receptors in the distal tubules of the kidney, activating aquaporin channels that mediate ↑ reabsorption of free water. Diabetes insipidus is a disorder characterized by ↓ reabsorption of free water in the distal tubules. It may be precipitated by disorders that interrupt the release of ADH from the hypothalamus (central diabetes insipidus), or by disorders that inhibit the action of ADH in the distal tubules (nephrogenic diabetes insipidus). Patients present with severe polyuria (urine output >3000mL/day) and polydipsia associated with the excretion of large volumes of dilute urine.

Causes of central diabetes insipidus Include neurosurgery, head trauma, growth of suprasellar masses, histiocytosis, neurosarcoidosis, hypothalamic metastases, and idiopathic central diabetes insipidus

Causes of nephrogenic diabetes insipidus Include exposure to lithium, hypercalcemia, hypokalemia, and hereditary nephrogenic diabetes insipidus.

Evaluation of polyuria Principal goal is to determine whether ↑ urine output is primarily driven by ↑ intake of free water (primary polydipsia) or by ↓ reabsorption of free water (central or nephrogenic diabetes insipidus). Performance of a water deprivation test may clarify this distinction while providing clues to the root cause of diabetes insipidus.

Water deprivation test

1 Starting after breakfast, hold all intake of fluids—check the patient's baseline weight, pulse, and blood pressure, and measure a baseline serum osmolality and serum sodium level
   - Every hour, check the patient's weight, pulse, and blood pressure
   - Every two hours, measure a serum osmolality and serum sodium level
   - With each urine void, measure the urine volume and urine osmolality
2 Consider terminating the test when one of the following endpoints has been reached*
   - Urine osmolality >600mosm/kg
   - Serum osmolality >295–300mosm/kg
   - Serum sodium >150meq/dL
   - Weight loss >5% of baseline body weight
   - Signs of volume depletion
3 Interpretation
   - Determine the maximum urine osmolality and calculate the percentage increase in urine osmolality following administration of vasopressin
     - Maximum urine osmolality >500mosm/kg = primary polydipsia
     - Maximum urine osmolality <500mosm/kg = central or nephrogenic diabetes insipidus
     - Maximum urine osmolality <300mosm/kg + 100%–800% ↑ in urine osmolality = complete central diabetes insipidus
     - Maximum urine osmolality <300mosm/kg + 15–50% ↑ in urine osmolality = partial central diabetes insipidus
     - Maximum urine osmolality >300mosm/kg + 15–50% ↑ in urine osmolality = partial nephrogenic diabetes insipidus
     - Maximum urine osmolality >300mosm/kg + <15% ↑ in urine osmolality = complete nephrogenic diabetes insipidus

* If the serum osmolality has increased to >295mosm/kg, administer 5U of *vasopressin* subcutaneously, then measure the urine volume and urine osmolality with the next urine void before allowing resumption of fluid intake

Treatment of central diabetes insipidus Identify and treat any reversible conditions that may be interrupting the release of ADH from the hypothalamus. Persistent central diabetes insipidus may require long-term treatment with *desmopressin* (DDAVP®), an ADH analog that has minimal vasopressor activity. Desmopressin is available as a 10mcg metered nasal spray and in 0.1mg tablet form. The usual starting dose is one spray intranasally or 0.05mg orally taken at bedtime. Doses may be increased incrementally with expansion to twice daily administration to attenuate nocturia and daytime polyuria.

Treatment of nephrogenic diabetes insipidus Identify and treat any reversible conditions that may be inhibiting the action of ADH in the distal tubules. Persistent nephrogenic diabetes insipidus may respond to treatment with *hydrocholorothiazide* (12.5–25mg bid), *amiloride* (Midamor® 5–20mg qd), or NSAIDs. Amiloride may be particularly effective in attenuating polyuria in patients who develop nephrogenic diabetes insipidus associated with exposure to lithium used to treat affective disorders.

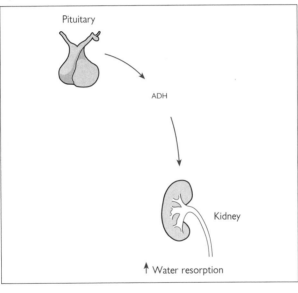

Pituitary

ADH

Kidney

↑ Water resorption

Neurology

Benjamin Greenberg, M.D., M.H.S.

Contents

Approach to the neurology patient

Localization

Diagnosing patients with neurologic conditions begins with localization. Individual symptoms can be caused by dysfunction in a variety of structures. For example, a patient complaining of weakness might have a cerebral, cerebellar, myelopathic, neuropathic, neuromuscular junction, or myopathic pathology. Identifying the location of dysfunction within the central or peripheral nervous system is critical for developing an appropriate differential. The diseases that affect the brain are quite different than the diseases that affect the spinal cord which are distinctly different from peripheral nervous system pathologies.

Where is the lesion? Localizing the site of the lesion depends on recognizing the pattern of cognitive, cranial nerve, motor, and sensory deficits which occur following lesions at different sites within the nervous system. Weakness associated with aphasia or agnosia localizes the motor lesion to the cortex. Weakness associated with double vision or an asymmetric gag reflex signifies a brainstem lesion. An associated sensory level identifies a spinal cord pathology. Weakness in the distribution of a single nerve localizes the dysfunction to the peripheral nervous system as does symmetric, bilateral patterns of weakness. A complete neurologic exam is essential for adequately localizing the site of pathology.

Patterns of motor deficits: Localizing the lesion that is responsible for weakness is dependent on identifying whether the pattern of motor weakness is consistent with lower or upper motor neuron dysfunction (LMN or UMN; see BOXES). Lesions within the cortex, subcortex, internal capsule, basal ganglia, and brainstem will cause contralateral weakness. While, classically, the weakness is described as having UMN qualities (↑ tone, ↑ reflexes, and no atrophy or fasiculations), early on these features may be absent. Lesions within the spinal cord will cause UMN type weakness ipsilateral to the lesion (as the corticospinal tracts deccusate within the medulla oblongata). Similar to lesions within the cerebrum, acute spinal cord lesions causing weakness may have variable UMN findings. Lesions of the motor neurons within the anterior horn of the spinal cord or within the periphery will always cause weakness with LMN features (↓ tone, ↓ reflexes and over time the development of atrophy and fasiculations). Neuromuscular junction pathologies typically cause variable weakness that may wax and wane in severity, but is often worse with activity ('fatigueability'). Due to the variability in UMN findings early on in central nervous system pathologies it is necessary for clinicians to recognize associated findings and patterns of weakness in order to localize lesions correctly.

LMN lesions

These are caused by damage anywhere from anterior horn cells in the cord, nerve roots, plexi, or peripheral nerves. The distribution of weakness corresponds to those muscles supplied by the cord segment involved, nerve root, part of plexus, or peripheral nerve. A combination of anatomical knowledge, good muscle testing technique, and experience is needed to distinguish them, eg a radial nerve palsy from a C7 root lesion, or a common peroneal nerve palsy from an L5 root lesion. The relevant muscles show *wasting* ± spontaneous involuntary twitching (*fasiculation*)—and provide little resistance to passive stretch (*hypotonia/flaccidity*). *Reflexes are reduced* or absent, the *plantars remain flexor*.

UMN lesions

These are caused by damage to motor pathways anywhere from the motor nerve cells in the precental gyrus of the frontal cortex, through the internal capsule, brainstem, and spinal cord. Typical characteristics are the so-called 'pyramidal' distribution of preferential weakness involving physiological extensors of the upper limb (shoulder abduction; elbow, wrist, and finger extension; and the small muscles of the hand) and the flexors of the lower limb (hip flexion, knee flexion, and ankle dorsiflexion and everters). It is little muscle wasting and *loss of skilled fine finger movements* may be greater than expected from the overall grade of weakness. ↑ tone, (spasticity) develops in stronger muscles (eg arm flexors and leg extensors). It is manifest as resistance to passive movement that can suddenly be overcome (clasp-knife feel). There is *hyperreflexia:* Reflexes are brisk; *plantars are upgoing* (+ve Babinski sign) ± *clonus* (elicited by rapidly dorsiflexing the foot) is more suggestive of an UMN lesion (3 rhythmic, downward beats of the foot are normal); a positive *Hoffman's reflex*—passive flicking of a finger (examiner rapidly flexes a DIP joint) causes neighboring digits to flex. UMN weakness affects *muscle groups* not individual muscles.

Muscle weakness grading (MRC classification)

Grade 0 no muscle contraction	*Grade 3* active movement against gravity
Grade 1 flicker of contraction	*Grade 4* active movement against resistance
Grade 2 some active movement	*Grade 5* normal power (allowing for age)

Grade 4 covers a big range: *4-*, *4*, and *4+* denote movement against slight, moderate, and stronger resistance.

Sensory deficits Information about the site of a lesion is confirmed by the distribution of the sensory loss, although the range of sensory modalities involved (pain, temperature, light touch, vibration, and joint position sense) may add information, as pain and temperature sensations travel along small fibers in peripheral nerves and spinothalamic tracts in the cord and brainstem and are distinct from joint position and vibration sense (travelling in fast fibers in the dorsal columns of the cord). Distal sensory loss suggests a neuropathy and may involve all sensory modalities or be more selective, depending on the nerve fiber size involved. Individual nerve lesions are identified by the anatomic territories they innervate, which are more defined than those of root lesions (dermatomes; refer to figure p318, 319), which often show considerable overlap. The hallmark of a cord lesion is a sensory level, ie an area of ↓ or absent sensation below the lesion (eg the legs) with normal sensation above this level (eg in abdomen, trunk, and arms). Lateralized cord lesions give a Brown-Séquard syndrome with dorsal column loss on the side of the lesion and spinothalamic loss on the contralateral side. In cortical lesions, sensory loss is contralateral to the lesion and can be confined to more subtle and discriminating sensory functions (graphesthesia, stereognosis).

Nervous system anatomy

The elegance of clinical neurology is a product of nervous system anatomy. Understanding the functions associated with various locations within the central and peripheral nervous system is critical for localization. While some person-to-person variability exists, most higher cortical functions can be mapped to specific locations within the cortex. Within the white matter, brain stem, spinal cord and peripheral nervous system there is limited variability among patients, making localization extremely reliable.

Higher functions of the cortex

Hemispheric dominance is defined by the location of Broca's area, which is responsible for the production of speech. The vast majority of right-handed individuals have their speech production area within the left hemisphere, while left handed individuals are split ~50–50 between right and left hemisphere dominance. The frontal lobes anteriorly have both the orbitofrontal and dorsolateral regions. These areas are involved in olfaction, visual interpretation, executive planning, and memory. Also within the frontal lobes are the frontal eye fields responsible for initiating saccadic eye movements. On the dominant side Broca's area is responsible for the motor production of speech while on the non-dominant side the frontal lobe controls prosody (voice inflections with questions and statements). Posteriorly in the frontal lobe are the premotor and motor strips. These structures are the control center for voluntary face, head, neck, body, and limb movements.

The parietal lobes are primarily sensory structures, acting as the primary input for various somatosensory systems and providing significant networks for the interpretation of the incoming information. A significant portion of parietal lobe function is dedicated to developing a visuo-spatial map of ourselves and surroundings. Hence, a non-dominant hemisphere parietal lobe lesion will often cause hemineglect syndromes, in which patients do not attend to the contralateral side (ie dressing one half of their body, only speaking to people on one side of the room, etc.).

The temporal lobes have a variety of functions including language, memory, behavior, interpretation of visual inputs, and hearing. Within the temporal lobes are the hippocampi which are responsible for solidifying new memories. Seizures located within the temporal lobe often present as complex partial seizures with patients appearing confused and acting strangely.

The occipital lobes are dedicated to visual pathways. Information from the retina is carried via the optic nerves and optic tracts to the lateral geniculate nuclei of the thalami. From there optic radiations transmit the information to the occipital lobes. Primary visual information is translated into more intricate forms within the occipital lobes. The temporal and parietal lobes assign significance to the structures perceived by the occipital lobes. Occipital lobe lesions cause loss of vision.

Spinal cord anatomy

Unlike the brain where the grey matter lines the outer layer, the spinal cord has white matter tracts coursing along the outer portions. The grey matter of the spinal cord forms the anterior horn, which houses the motor neuron cell bodies that will project into the periphery. Important to understanding anatomic-clinical correlations is keeping track of where specific white matter tracts decussate. Ultimately, all motor and sensory information will be generated or interpreted within the contralateral brain, but while the corticospinal tracts (motor pathways) and ascending dorsal columns (vibration and proprioceptive information) decussate within the medulla. The spinothalamic tracts (pain and temperature information) cross over within the spinal cord shortly after entering.

The corticospinal tracts run along the posterio-lateral portions of the spinal cord. The cell bodies are located within the precentral gyrus and project their axons down to the appropriate level of the spinal cord, crossing over to the contralateral side within the medulla. Within the spinal cord, the fibers travelling down to the legs are located along the outer portions of the corticospinal tract. Thus, extramedullary spinal processes within the cervical or thoracic spine can present with ipsilateral leg weakness.

The dorsal columns which carry vibratory and proprioceptive information, are located along the posterio-medial aspects of the spinal cord. Lesions of these afferent pathways cause ipsilateral symptoms. These pathways will decussate within the medulla, such that lesions above the medulla cause contralateral symptoms. The dorsal columns have two distinct pathways, the fasciculus cuneatus and gracilis. Fibers entering the spinal cord below T6 utilize fasciculus gracilis, while fibers at T6 and above utilize fasciculus cuneatus. Above T6 fasciculus gracilis is located within the medial portion of the dorsal columns.

The spinothalamic tracts occupy the anterior-lateral portions of the spinal cord and convey pain and temperature information from the contralateral portion of the body to the post-central gyrus. Within the spinothalamic tracts information from the legs are carried along the outer portions of the tracts. The decussation of the white matter tracts occurs along the most medial anterior portion of the spinal cord, anterior to the central canal. Thus, central spinal cord pathologies (eg syringomyelia) can cause a band-like pattern of sensory loss due to disruption of the crossing fibers at that level.

Blood is supplied to the spinal cord via a singular anterior spinal artery and paired posterior spinal arteries. The anterior spinal artery is derived from branches of the vertebral arteries and is supplemented by the artery of Adamkewicz off of the abdominal aorta. The anterior spinal artery supplies blood flow to the anterior two-thirds of the spinal cord, such that occlusion or hypoperfusion of this artery causes ischemia to the spinothalamic tracts and corticospinal tracts, but spares the dorsal columns. Clinically, patients with anterior spinal artery syndromes will have paraplegia, with loss of temperature and pain below the level of the lesion, but vibration and proprioception are spared.

Cerebral artery territories

A basic knowledge of the anatomy of the blood supply of the brain is helpful in the diagnosis and management of cerebrovascular disease. It is important to be able to identify the area of brain that correlates with a patient's symptoms and identify the affected artery.

Cerebral blood supply The brain is supplied by the 2 internal carotid arteries and the basilar artery (formed by the joining of the 2 vertebral arteries). These 3 vessels feed into an anastomotic ring at the base of the brain called the circle of Willis. This arrangement may lessen the effects of occlusion of a feeder vessel proximal to the anastomosis by allowing collateral supply from unaffected vessels. The anatomy of the circle of Willis is, however, highly variable and in many people it cannot provide much protection from ischemia due to carotid, vertebral, or basilar artery occlusion. Collateral supply from other vessels in the neck may mitigate occlusions of feeder vessels (eg occlusion of the internal carotid in the neck may not cause infarction if flow from the external carotid artery enters the circle of Willis via the facial artery and its anastomosis with the ophthalmic artery).

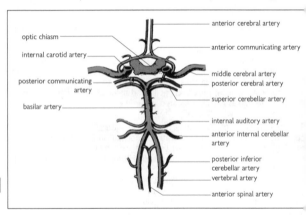

Arteries and CNS territories

Carotid artery Internal carotid artery occlusion may cause total infarction of the anterior two-thirds of the ipsi-lateral hemisphere and basal ganglia (lenticulostriate arteries). More often, the picture is similar to a middle cerebral artery occlusion (below).

The cerebral arteries 3 pairs of arteries leave the circle of Willis to supply the cerebral hemispheres; the anterior, middle, and posterior cerebral arteries. The anterior and middle cerebrals are branches of the carotid arteries; the basilar artery divides into the 2 posterior cerebral arteries. These arteries are essentially end arteries (there is no significant anastomosis between them), and ischemia due to occlusion of any one of them may be reduced, if not prevented, by retrograde supply from meningeal vessels.

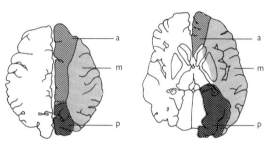

Anterior cerebral artery: ('a' above) Supplies the frontal and medial part of the cerebral hemispheres. Occlusion may cause a weak, numb contralateral leg ± similar, if milder, arm symptoms. The face is spared. Bilateral infarction is associated with an akinetic mute state due to damage to the cingulate gyri (also a rare cause of paraplegia).

Middle cerebral artery: ('m') Supplies the lateral (external) part of each hemisphere. Occlusion may cause: Contralateral hemiplegia, hemisensory loss mainly of face and arm; contralateral homonymous hemianopia due to involvement of the optic radiation, cognitive change including aphasia if the dominant hemisphere is affected, and visuo-spatial disturbance (eg cannot dress; gets lost) with non-dominant lesions.

Posterior cerebral artery: ('p') Supplies the occipital lobe. Occlusion causes contralateral homonymous hemianopia.

Vertebrobasilar circulation Supplies the cerebellum, brainstem, and occipital lobes. *Occlusion may cause:* Hemianopia; cortical blindness; diplopia; vertigo; nystagmus; hemi- or quadriplegia; unilateral or bilateral sensory symptoms; cerebellar symptoms; hiccups; dysarthria; dysphagia; and coma. Infarctions of the brainstem can produce various syndromes, eg *Lateral medullary syndrome* (occlusion of 1 vertebral artery or the posterior inferior cerebellar artery). It is due to infarction of the lateral medulla and the inferior surface of the cerebellum causing vertigo with vomiting, dysphagia, nystagmus ipsilateral ataxia, and paralysis of the soft palate, ipsilateral Horner's syndrome, and a crossed pattern sensory loss (analgesia to pinprick on ipsilateral face and contralateral trunk and limbs).

Subclavian steal syndrome: Subclavian artery stenosis proximal to the vertebral artery may cause blood to be *stolen* by retrograde flow down this vertebral artery down into the arm, causing brainstem ischemia after exertion. Suspect if the BP in each arm differs by >20mmHg.

Peripheral nerves

The peripheral nervous system is made up of sensory and motor nerves that form from the dorsal and anterior horns of the spinal cord. Pathologies can affect the nerve root, plexus, or peripheral nerve itself. Thus, identifying the root and the nerve that is responsible for each area of sensation and each muscle is vital for localizing peripheral nervous system pathologies. The following table summarizes nerve root innervation and individual peripheral nerve innervation patterns. When trying to discern a C7 lesion from a radial nerve lesion an examiner could test muscles innervated by the radial nerve, but not C7 such as brachioradialis. Also, an examiner could test C7 innervated muscles that are not innervated by the radial nerve, such as flexor carpi radialis which is innervated by the median nerve.

Nerve root	Muscle	Test—by asking the patient to:
C3, 4	Trapezius	Shrug shoulder (via accessory nerve).
C5, 6	Serratus anterior	Push arm forward against resistance; look for winging of the scapula, if weak.
C5, 6	Pectoralis major (p major) clavicular head	Adduct arm from above horizontal, and push it forward.
C6, **7**, 8	P major sternocostal head	Adduct arm below horizontal.
C**5**, 6	Supraspinatus	Abduct arm the first 15°.
C**5**, 6	Infraspinatus	Externally rotate arm, elbow at side.
C6, **7**, 8	Latissimus dorsi	Adduct arm from horizontal position.
C5, 6	Biceps	Flex supinated forearm.
C**5**, 6	Deltoid	Abduct arm between 15° and 90°.

Radial nerve

C6, **7**, 8	Triceps	Extend elbow against resistance.
C5, **6**	Brachioradialis	Flex elbow with forearm half way between pronation and supination.
C5, **6**	Extensor carpi radialis longus	Extend wrist to radial side with fingers extended.
C6, 7	Supinator	Arm by side, resist hand pronation.
C**7**, 8	Extensor digitorum	Keep fingers extended at MCP joint.
C**7**, 8	Extensor carpi ulnaris	Extend wrist to ulnar side.
C**7**, 8	Abductor pollicis longus	Abduct thumb at 90° to palm.
C**7**, 8	Extensor pollicis brevis	Extend thumb at MCP joint.
C**7**, 8	Extensor pollicis longus	Resist thumb flexion at IP joint.

Median nerve

C6, 7	Pronator teres	Keep arm pronated against resistance.
C6, 7	Flexor carpi radialis	Flex wrist towards radial side.
C7, **8**, T1	Flexor digitorum superficialis	Resist extension at PIP joint (with proximal phalanx fixed by the examiner).
C7, **8**	Flexor digitorum profundus I & II	Resist extension at index DIP joint of index finger.
C7, **8**, T1	Flexor pollicis longus	Resist thumb extension at interphalangeal joint (fix proximal phalanx).
C8, **T1**	Abductor pollicis brevis	Abduct thumb (nail at 90° to palm).
C8, **T1**	Opponens pollicis	Thumb touches base of 5th finger-tip (nail parallel to palm).
C8, **T1**	Lumbrical/interosseus (median & ulnar nerves)	Extend PIP joint against resistance with MCP joint held hyperextended.

Ulnar nerve

C7, **8**, T1	Flexor carpi ulnaris	Flex wrist to ulnar side; observe tendon

C7, **C8**	Flexor digitorum profundus III and IV	Resist extension of distal phalanx of 5th finger while you fix its middle phalanx.
C8, **T1**	Dorsal interossei	Finger abduction: Cannot cross the middle over the index finger (tests index finger adduction too).
C8, **T1**	Palmar interossei	Finger adduction: Pull apart a sheet of paper held between middle and ring finger DIP joints of both hands; the paper moves on the weaker side
C8, **T1**	Adductor pollicis	Adduct thumb (nail at 90° to palm).
C8, **T1**	Abductor digiti minimi	Abduct little finger.
C8, **T1**	Flexor digiti minimi	Flex the little finger at MCP joint.

Lower limb

Nerve root   *Muscle*   *Activity to test:*

L4, **5**, S1	Gluteus medius & minimus (superior gluteal nerve)	Internal rotation at hip, hip abduction.
L5, S1, 2	Gluteus maximus (inferior gluteal nerve)	Extension at hip (lie prone).
L2, **3**, 4	Adductors (obturator nerve)	Adduct leg against resistance.

Femoral nerve

| **L1**, **2**, 3 | Iliopsoas (also supplied via L1, 3, & 3 spinal nerves) | Flex hip against resistance with knee flexed and lower leg supported: Patient lies on back. |
| L2, **3**, 4 | Quadriceps femoris | Extend at the knee against resistance. Start with the knee flexed. |

Obturator nerve

| L2, **3**, 4 | Hip adductors | Adduct the leg against resistance. |

Inferior gluteal nerve

| **L5**, S1, S2 | Gluteus maximus | Hip extension ('bury heal into the couch')—with knee in extension. |

Superficial gluteal nerve

| **L4**, **5**, S1 | Gluteus medius & minimus | Abduction and internal hip rotation with leg flexed at hip and knee. |

317

Sciatic (and common peroneal*) and sciatic (and tibial**) nerves

*L**4**, 5	Tibialis anterior	Dorsiflex ankle.
*L**5**, S1	Extensor digitorum longus	Dorsiflex toes against resistance.
*L**5**, S1	Extensor hallucis longus	Dorsiflex hallux against resistance.
*L5, S1	Peroneus longus & brevis	Evert foot against resistance.
*L5, S1	Extensor digitorum brevis	Dorsiflex proximal phalanges of toes.
L5, **S1, 2	Hamstrings	Flex the knee against resistance.
L4**, 5	Tibialis posterior	Invert the plantarflexed foot.
S1**, 2	Gastrocnemius	Plantarflex ankle or stand on tiptoe.
L5, **S1, **2**	Flexor digitorum longus	Flex terminal joints of the toes.
**S1, 2	Small muscles of foot	Make the sole of the foot into a cup.

Quick screening test for muscle power

Shoulder	Abduction	C5	*Hip*	Flexion	L1–L2
	Adduction	C5–C7		Adduction	L2–3
Elbow	Flexion	C5–C6		Extension	L5–S1
	Extension	C7	*Knee*	Flexion	L5–S1
Wrist	Flexion	C7–8		Extension	L3–L4
	Extension	C7	*Ankle*	Dorsiflexion	L4
Fingers	Flexion	C8		Eversion	L5–S1
	Extension	C7		Plantarflexion	S1–S2
	Abduction	T1	*Toe*	Big toe extension	L5

Dermatomes

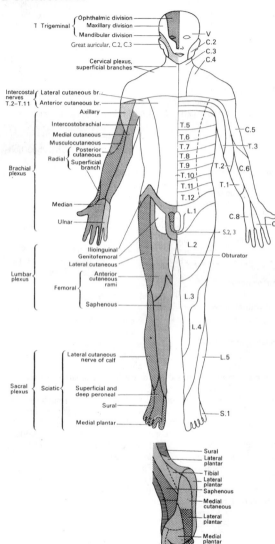

T Trigeminal {
Ophthalmic division
Maxillary division
Mandibular division
}

Great auricular, C.2, C.3

Cervical plexus,
superficial branches

V

C.2
C.3
C.4

Intercostal nerves T.2–T.11 {
Lateral cutaneous br.
Anterior cutaneous br.
}

Axillary

Intercostobrachial

Medial cutaneous

Musculocutaneous

Radial {
Posterior cutaneous
Superficial branch
}

Brachial plexus

Median

Ulnar

T.5
T.6
T.7
T.8
T.9
T.10
T.11
T.12

C.5
T.3
T.2
C.6
T.1
C.8
C.7

L.1

S.2, 3

Ilioinguinal
Genitofemoral
Lateral cutaneous

L.2

Obturator

Lumbar plexus

Femoral {
Anterior cutaneous rami
Saphenous
}

L.3

L.4

Lateral cutaneous nerve of calf

L.5

Sacral plexus

Sciatic {
Superficial and deep peroneal
Sural
Medial plantar
}

S.1

Sural
Lateral plantar
Tibial
Lateral plantar
Saphenous
Medial cutaneous
Lateral plantar
Medial plantar

ANTERIOR ASPECT

318

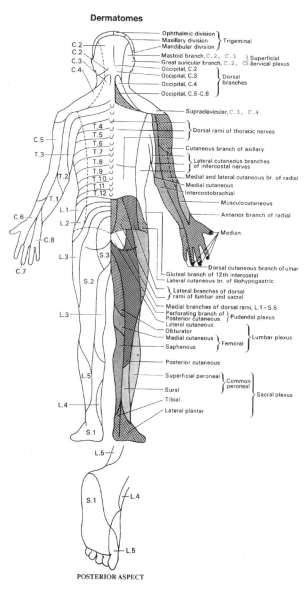

Dermatomes

Ophthalmic division ⎫
Maxillary division ⎬ Trigeminal
Mandibular division ⎭

Mastoid branch, C.2, C.3 ⎫ Superficial
Great auricular branch, C.2, C.3 ⎬ cervical plexus
Occipital, C.2
Occipital, C.3 ⎫ Dorsal
Occipital, C.4 ⎬ branches
Occipital, C.5–C.8 ⎭

Supraclavicular, C.3, C.4

Dorsal rami of thoracic nerves

Cutaneous branch of axillary

Lateral cutaneous branches of intercostal nerves

Medial and lateral cutaneous br. of radial

Medial cutaneous

Intercostobrachial

Musculocutaneous

Anterior branch of radial

Median

Dorsal cutaneous branch of ulnar

Gluteal branch of 12th intercostal

Lateral cutaneous br. of iliohypogastric

Lateral branches of dorsal rami of lumbar and sacral

Medial branches of dorsal rami, L.1–S.6
Perforating branch of ⎫ Pudendal plexus
Posterior cutaneous ⎬
Lateral cutaneous
Obturator
Medial cutaneous ⎫ Femoral ⎫ Lumbar plexus
Saphenous ⎬

Posterior cutaneous

Superficial peroneal ⎫ Common
peroneal ⎫ Sacral plexus
Sural
Tibial
Lateral plantar

POSTERIOR ASPECT

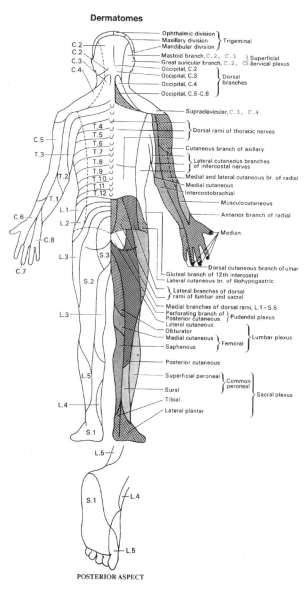

Headache

Every day, *thousands* of patients visit doctors complaining of headache. There are a variety of pathologies that can cause *cephalgia* (head pain), most of which are benign. Recognizing common syndromes as well as indications for evaluating patients for more serious conditions is extremely important for every physician. There are a variety of ways to approach the differential diagnosis for headache, but the most useful focuses on the time-course of head pain as acute headaches get evaluated very differently than chronic headaches. The following tables outline a small differential for headache syndromes based on how they present.

Acute single episode

Meningitis	Fever, photophobia, stiff neck, rash, coma
Encephalitis	Fever, odd behavior, seizures or ↓ consciousness
Subarachnoid	*Sudden* headache ± stiff neck
Sinusitis	Tender face + coryza + post-nasal drip
Head injury	Cuts/bruises, ↓consciousness; lucid interval, amnesia

Acute recurrent attacks

Migraine	Any pre-attack aura? Visual aura? Vomiting? Sensitivity to light, noise, or movement
Cluster headache	Typically nightly pain in 1 eye for ~8wks then OK for the next few months—then intermittently repeated
Glaucoma	Red eye; sees haloes, fixed big oval pupil; ↓acuity

Subacute onset

Giant cell arteritis	Tender scalp; >50yrs old; vision changes

Chronic headache (pain for >15d/month for longer than 3 months.)

Tension headache	'A tight band round my head'; stress at work /home
Chronically elevated ICP	Worse on waking, focal signs
Chronic daily headache	Analgesic overuse

Acute single episode

Meningitis, encephalitis, subarachnoid hemorrhage:

If the headache is acute, severe, felt over most of the head and accompanied by meningeal irritation (neck stiffness) ± drowsiness you must think of meningitis, encephalitis, or a subarachnoid hemorrhage. Emergent head imagining with a CT scan and possible lumbar puncture is indicated to confirm the appropriate diagnosis.

After head injury: Headache is common after minor trauma. It may be at the site of trauma or be more generalized. It lasts approximately 2wks and is often resistant to analgesia. Bear in mind subdural or extradural hemorrhage. Sinister signs are drowsiness, focal signs.

Sinusitis: Presents with dull, constant, aching pain over the affected frontal or maxillary sinus, with tender overlying skin ± post-nasal drip. Ethmoid or sphenoid sinus pain is felt deep in the midline at the root of the nose. Pain is worsened by bending over. Often accompanied by coryza, the pain lasts only 1–2wks.

Acute glaucoma: Mostly observed in elderly, far-sighted people. Constant, aching pain develops rapidly around 1 eye and radiates to the forehead. *Symptoms:* Markedly reduced vision in affected eye, nausea, and vomiting. *Signs:* Red, congested eye; cloudy cornea; dilated, non-responsive pupil. Attacks may be precipitated by sitting in the dark, eg at the movies, dilating eye-drops or emotional upset. Seek expert help immediately. If delay in treatment of >1h is likely, start IV acetazolamide (500mg over several minutes).

Recurrent acute attacks of headache

Cluster headache Pain occurs once or twice every 24h, each episode lasting 15–160min. Clusters typically last 4–12wks and are followed by pain-free periods of months or even 1–2yrs before another cluster begins. Sometimes there are no remissions. Men outnumber women 5 to 1. Classically, patients are writhing in pain, unlike migraneurs who usually remain quite still and quiet during a headache. *Symptoms:* Rapid onset severe pain around 1 eye which may become watery and bloodshot with lid swelling, lacrimation, facial flushing, and rhinorrhoea. Miosis ± ptosis (20% attacks), remaining permanent in 5%. Pain is strictly unilateral and almost always affects the same side. *Treatment: Acute attack:* 100% O₂ (7–15L/min for 20min) often helps—or *sumatriptan* SC 6mg at attack's onset. Indomethacin and intranasal lidocaine are also effective abortive agents. *Preventives:* Verapamil; lithium; steroids.

Trigeminal neuralgia: Paroxysms of intense, stabbing pain, lasting seconds, in the trigeminal nerve distribution eg from anomalous intracranial vessels compressing the trigeminal root. It is unilateral, affecting the mandibular and maxillary divisions most often. The face may twist with pain (hence *tic douloureux*). Pain may recur many times a day and night and can often be triggered by touching the skin of the affected area, by washing, shaving, eating, or talking. Typical patient is a man over 50yrs. *Treatment:* Carbamazepine (start at 100mg/12h PO; max 400mg/6h; lamotrigine; phenytoin 200–400mg/24h PO; or gabapentin. If drugs fail, surgery may be necessary. This may be directed at the peripheral nerve, the trigeminal ganglion or the nerve root. *Microvascular decompression:* Anomalous vessels are separated from the trigeminal root.

Headaches of subacute onset

Giant cell arteritis: Exclude in all patients greater than 50 years of age presenting with a headache that has lasted a few weeks. Look for tender, thickened, pulseless temporal arteries with an extremely elevated ESR. *Ask about:* Jaw claudication during eating. Prompt diagnosis and immediate treatment with steroids are essential for avoiding blindness. The temporal arteries should be biopsied to confirm the diagnosis.

Chronic headaches

Raised intracranial pressure: Headache is a complaint of ~50% patients. Although variable in nature, headaches are characteristically present on waking or may awaken the patient. They are generally not severe and are worse lying down. If accompanied by other signs of ↑ ICP, such as vomiting, papilledema, seizures, focal deficits, or mental status change, admit the patient urgently for diagnostic imaging. Any space-occupying lesion (neoplasm, abscess, subdural hematoma) may present in this way, as may pseudotumor cerebri. Patients with pseudotumor are classically overweight women who have constant dull head pain and vision changes. Lumbar puncture is the diagnostic test of choice, as an elevated opening pressure will be noted. Often patients' symptoms improve after CSF drainage. The mainstay of medical management are carbonic anhydrase inhibitors.

Chronic daily headache from medication overuse: Culprits are mixed analgesics containing codeine, ergotamine, triptans and most over the counter 'headache medications'. It is a common reason for episodic headaches becoming daily headache. The culprit must be withdrawn, and a preventive added (eg tricyclics, valproate, gabapentin).

Migraine

Migraine is the most common cause of recurrent headaches.

Symptoms *Classically:* Visual (or other) aura lasting 15–30min followed within 1h by unilateral, throbbing headache. *Other patterns:* Aura with no headache. Episodic (often premenstrual) severe headaches, often unilateral, with nausea, vomiting ± photophobia/phonophobia but no aura; may have allodynia (all stimuli produce pain)—'I can't brush my hair/wear earrings or glasses/shave because it's so painful'

Aura Visual chaos (cascading, distortion, 'melting' and jumbling of print lines, dots, spots, zig-zag fortification spectra); hemianopia, hemiparesis, aphasia, dysarthria, ataxia (basilar migraine). Mood or appetite change may occur hours before the aura. *Sensory auras:* Eg parasthesia spreading from fingers to face, or *speech auras:* (8% of auras; eg aphasia; dysarthria; paraphasia, eg phoneme substitution). *Criteria for diagnosis if no aura:* 5 headaches lasting 4–72h with either nausea/vomiting or photophobia/phonophobia *and* 2 of these 4 features: Unilateral/pulsating/interferes with normal life/aggravated by routine activity.

Triggers— eg CHOCOLATE or: Cheese, oral contraceptives, caffeine (or its withdrawal), alcohol, anxiety, travel, or exercise. In ~50%, no trigger is found, and in only a few does avoiding triggers prevent *all* attacks.

Differential Cluster or tension headache, cervical spondylosis; hypertensive headache; intra-cranial pathology, sinusitis/otitis media. TIAs may mimic migraine auras.

Prophylaxis (If frequency is greater than twice a month).

Propranolol 40–120mg/12h PO or amitriptyline 25–75mg per night; *Side effects include:* Drowsiness, dry mouth, blurred vision. Valproate 400–600mg/12h. Calcium channel blockers (specifically verapamil) and SSRIs also have some evidence for efficacy in migraine. Gabapentin and topiramate show promise in recent trials.

Treating attacks Aborting migraine attacks is related to 3 factors: Speed of administration of the agent (how long from first symptom does it take for medication to be administered), absorption/bioavailability of the agent, and the efficacy of the medication. In general, abortive medications are more efficacious the sooner they are taken. A medication taken during the aura of a migraine works significantly better than one taken an hour into the painful portion. Secondly, there is evidence indicating that many migraneurs have delayed gastric emptying times (related to their nausea), thus pills may not achieve the same bioavailability as injections, nasal sprays, or wafers that dissolve under the tongue. Finally, medications can be compared based on their relative efficacy, time to onset of analgesia, and half life. The following is a partial list of the medications that can be utilized as abortive agents for migraine headaches.

The triptans are serotonergic *agonists*, constricting cranial arteries. There are a variety of formulations including pills, wafers, injections and nasal sprays. Rare side effects include arrhythmias or angina ± MI, even if no pre-existing risk. Ergotamine (a 5HT agonist, constricting cranial arteries), acetaminophen, NSAIDs and aspirin have all been effectively utilized in the past for migraines

Altered mental status

Delirium (acute confusional state) Common in hospitalized patients (5–15% patients in general medical or surgical wards) so consider any unexplained behavior change in a hospital patient as possible delirium and look for an organic cause. There are 7 signs:

1 *Consciousness* is impaired (onset over hours or days). This has been described as an impairment of thinking, attention, and concentration—or more simply as a mild global impairment of cognitive processes associated with a reduced awareness. Level of consciousness fluctuates throughout the day with confusion typically worsening in the late afternoon and at night.

2 *Disorientation* in time (does not know time, day, or year) and place (often more marked) is the rule.

3 *Behavior:* Inactivity, quietness, reduced speech, and perseveration (repetition of words) or else hyperactivity, noisiness, and irritability.

4 *Thinking:* Slow and confused, commonly with ideas of reference or delusions (eg accusing staff of plotting against them).

5 *Perception:* Disturbed, often with illusions and visual hallucinations (unlike in schizophrenia, where auditory modality dominates) or tactile.

6 *Mood:* Lability, anxiety, perplexity, fear, agitation, or depression.

7 *Memory:* Impaired. Later, patients may be amnesic for this episode.

Causes (Pain and other psychological states are important co-factors.)
• Infections: Pneumonia, UTI, wounds; IV lines. • Drugs: Opiates, anticonvulsants, L-dopa, sedatives, recreational, post-anesthesia. • Alcohol withdrawal (2–5d post-admission; may or may note be associated with elevated LFTs and raised MCV; history of alcohol abuse), also drug withdrawal. • Metabolic: Hypoglycemia, uremia, liver failure, anemia. • Hypoxia: Respiratory or cardiac failure. • Vascular: Stroke, MI. • Intracranial infection: Encephalitis, meningitis.
• Raised intracranial pressure/space occupying lesions. • Epilepsy: Status epilepticus (see BOX), post-ictal states. • Trauma, head injury: Especially subdural hematoma. • Nutritional: Thiamine, nicotinic acid, or B_{12} deficiency.

Evaluation and work up: Once the diagnosis of delirium is established a thorough attempt to identify the cause should be undertaken. Obtaining vital signs, including oxygen saturation and blood glucose, performing a thorough general physical and neurologic exam, obtaining appropriate lab tests (ie electrolytes, ABG) and possibly an electrocardiogram are warranted first steps in the evaluation of a delirious patient. Reviewing medication administration records can be extremely helpful in identifying causes of altered mental status.

Management: After identifying and treating the underlying cause, aim to:

1 Reduce distress and prevent accidents. Close monitoring is prudent. Repeated reassurance and orientation to time and place can help.

2 Minimize medication (especially sedatives). If agitated and disruptive, however, some sedation may be necessary. Use haloperidol 0.5–2mg IM/PO, judiciously. Wait 20min to judge effect, further doses can be given if needed. Benzodiazepines may be used for night-time sedation, but can worsen delirium.

Non-convulsive status epilepticus (NCSE) as a cause of confusion

NCSE is under-diagnosed, and may manifest itself as confusion, impaired cognition/memory, odd behavior, dreamy derealization, aggression, or psychosis ± abnormalities of eye movement, eyelid myoclonus, or odd postures. It may or may not occur in the context of classic seizures or ischemic brain injury. Other causes and associations: Drugs (eg antidepressants), infections (eg, arboviruses; HIV; syphilis), neoplasia, dementias, sudden changes in calcium levels, renal failure. *Diagnosis:* EEG *Treatment:* Valproate, ethosuximide, or IV benzodiazepines may be indicated (get expert help). In general, non-convulsive status epilepticus is not considered to be as dangerous as generalized convulsive status epilepticus. Thus, the treatment algorithm is quite different: Trying to avoid the need for intubation.

Dizziness

Dizziness and vertigo

Complaints of 'dizzy spells' are very common and are used by patients to describe many different sensations. The key to making a diagnosis is to find out exactly what the patient means by 'dizzy' and then decide whether or not this represents vertigo.

Does the patient have vertigo? *Definition:* An illusion of movement, often rotatory, of the patient or their surroundings. In practice, straightforward 'spinning' is rare—the floor may tilt, sink, or rise. Vertigo is always worsened by movement. *Associated symptoms:* Difficulty walking or standing; relief on lying or sitting still; nausea; vomiting; pallor; sweating. Attacks may even cause patients to fall suddenly to the ground. Associated hearing loss or tinnitus implies labyrinth or 8th nerve involvement. *What is not vertigo:* Faintness may be described as dizziness but is often due to anxiety with associated palpitations, tremor, and sweating. Anemia can cause light-headedness as can orthostatic hypotension but in all of these there is no illusion of movement or typical associated symptoms. Loss of consciousness during attacks should prompt thoughts of epilepsy or syncope rather than vertigo.

Causes Disorders of the labyrinth, vestibular nerve, vestibular nuclei, or their central connections are responsible for practically all vertigo. Only rarely are other structures implicated (see BOX).

Labyrinthine vertigo *Benign paroxysmal positional vertigo:* Displacement of the otoconia (otoliths) from the maculae (the receptor for sensing acceleration in the semicircular canals). Otoconia then settle on the lowest part of the labyrinth. This is curable by the Epley maneuver which repositions the particles. Classically, patients describe vertigo with head movement (eg rolling over in bed or looking up). The Dix–Hallpike maneuver can be used to establish the diagnosis. *Ménière's disease:* Recurrent, spontaneous attacks of vertigo, hearing loss, tinnitus, and a sense of aural fullness caused by endolymphatic hydrops. Vertigo is severe and rotational, lasts 20min to hours and is often accompanied by nausea and vomiting. Hearing loss is sensorineural, affects primarily low frequencies, fluctuates and is progressive; often to complete deafness of the affected ear. Drop attacks may rarely be experienced (no loss of consciousness or vertigo, but sudden falling to one side).

Vestibular nerve Damage in the petrous temporal bone or cerebellopontine angle often involves the auditory nerve, causing deafness or tinnitus. Causes: Trauma and vestibular schwannomas (acoustic neuromas).

Acoustic neuromas: Usually present with hearing loss, vertigo coming only later. With progression, ipsilateral cranial nerves V, VI, IX, and X may be affected (also ipsilateral cerebellar signs). Paradoxically, there is rarely VII nerve involvement pre-operatively. Signs of ↑ ICP occur late, and indicate a large tumor.

Vestibular neuronitis: Abrupt onset of severe vertigo, nausea, and vomiting, with prostration and immobility. No deafness or tinnitus. May be from a virus in the young, or a vascular lesion in the elderly. Severe vertigo subsides in days, complete recovery takes 3–4wks.

Herpes zoster: Herpetic eruption of the external auditory meatus; facial palsy ± deafness, tinnitus, and vertigo (Ramsay Hunt syndrome).

Brainstem Infarction of the brainstem (vertebrobasilar circulation) may produce marked vertigo but other lesions may also be responsible (see BOX). Vertigo is protracted as are the associated nausea, vomiting, and nystagmus. It is exceptional for vertigo to be the only symptom of brainstem disease; multiple cranial nerve palsies and sensory and motor tract defects are commonly also seen. Hearing is spared.

Causes of vertigo

Vestibular end-organs and vestibular nerve
  Ménière's disease
  Vestibular neuronitis (acute labyrinthitis)
  Benign positional vertigo
  Motion sickness
  Trauma
  Ototoxicity (aminoglycosides)
  Herpes zoster oticus (Ramsay Hunt syndrome)

Brainstem, cerebellum, and cerebello-pontine angle
  MS
  Infarction/TIA
  Hemorrhage
  Migraine (very rarely)
  Vestibular schwannoma (acoustic neuroma)

Cerebral cortex
  Vertiginous epilepsy

Alcohol intoxication

Cervical vertigo (controversial—neck symptoms are more commonly a result of a patient keeping the neck stiff to avoid exacerbating vertigo).

Deafness

Simple hearing tests To establish deafness, the examiner should whisper a number increasingly loudly in one ear while blocking the other ear with a finger. The patient is asked to repeat the number. Make sure that failure is not from misunderstanding.

Rinne's test Place the base of a vibrating 256 (or 512) Hz tuning fork on the mastoid process. When the patient no longer perceives sound move the fork so that the prongs are 4cm from the external acoustic meatus. The energy in the fork will be lessening, but the sound will be heard again if air conduction (AC) is better than bone conduction (BC). AC is normally better than BC. If not, then it is either conductive deafness or a false negative due to sensorineural deafness with 'hearing' of sound in the other ear. Distinguish from Weber's test (below). If there is hearing loss and AC is better than BC, this suggests sensorineural deafness, ie a cause central to the oval window (eg presbyacusis from aging or excess noise) or ototoxic drugs, or post-meningitis.

Weber's test Place a vibrating tuning fork in the middle of the forehead. Ask which side the patient localizes the sound to—or is it heard in the middle? In unilateral sensorineural deafness, the sound is located to the good side. In conduction deafness, the sound is located to the bad side (as if the sensitivity of the nerve has been turned up to allow for poor AC). Neither of these tests is completely reliable.

Conductive deafness Usually due to wax, otosclerosis, or otitis media.

Causes of sensorineural deafness Presbyacusis (senile deafness), Ménière's disease, causing paroxysmal vertigo, deafness ± tinnitus due to dilatation of the endolymphatic sac). *Other:* Meningitis; acute labyrinthitis; head injury; acoustic neuroma; MS; Paget's disease; excessive noise; aminoglycosides; several rare congenital syndromes; maternal infections during pregnancy.

Tinnitus

This is ringing or buzzing in the ears. It is a common phenomenon.

Causes Unknown; hearing loss (20%); wax; viral; presbyacusis; noise (eg gunfire); head injury; suppurative otitis media; post-stapedectomy; Ménière's; head injury; anemia; hypertension (found in up to 16%, but it may not be causative). *Drugs:* Aspirin; loop diuretics; aminoglycosides (eg gentamicin).

Causes of pulsatile tinnitus: (eg audible with stethoscope; do MRI) Carotid artery stenosis/dissection; AV fistula; glomus jugulare tumors. *Treatment:* Underlying conditions should be treated if possible (ie vascular lesions). Causative medications should be stopped if possible. There is no specific treatment for tinnitus.

Abnormal movements

Dyskinesia (abnormal involuntary movements)

Tremor *Rest tremor* is rhythmic, present at rest, and abolished on voluntary movement. It occurs in Parkinsonism (with rigidity/bradykinesia). *Intention tremor* is an irregular, large-amplitude shaking worse on reaching out for something. It is typical of cerebellar disease, (eg MS). *Postural tremor* is absent at rest, present on maintained posture (eg arms outstretched) and may persist (but is not exaggerated) on movement. *Causes:* Familial essential tremor (autosomal dominant; helped by alcohol); thyrotoxicosis; anxiety. Parkinsonian tremors are treated with dopaminergic medications. Beta blockers can be used for postural tremors. Intention tremors are extremely difficult to treat and are usually refractory to a variety of medications.

Chorea, athetosis, and hemiballismus *Chorea:* Non-rhythmic, jerky, purposeless movements which flit from one part of the body to another. *Causes* are Huntington's and Sydenham's chorea (choreoathetoid movements)—a rare complication of strep infection. The anatomical basis of chorea is uncertain but it is thought of as the pharmacological mirror image of Parkinson's disease (L-dopa worsens chorea). *Hemiballismus:* Large-amplitude, flinging hemichorea (affects proximal muscles) contralateral to a vascular lesion of the subthalamic nucleus (often elderly diabetics). Recovers spontaneously over months. *Athetosis:* Slow, sinuous, confluent, purposeless movements (esp. digits, hands, face, tongue), often difficult to distinguish from chorea. Commonest cause is cerebral palsy.

Tics Brief, repeated, stereotyped movements which patients are able to suppress for a while. Tics are common in children, but usually resolve. In *Gilles de la Tourette's syndrome*, multiple motor and vocal tics occur. Consider psychological support, clonazepam or clonidine if tics are severe.

Myoclonus Sudden involuntary focal or general jerks arising from cord, brainstem, or cerebral cortex, seen in neurodegenerative disease (eg lysosomal storage enzyme defects), CJD, and myoclonic epilepsies (infantile spasms). *Benign essential myoclonus:* General myoclonus begins in childhood as muscle twitches (eg autosomal dominant and has no other consequences). *Asterixis:* Jerking of outstretched hands (metabolic flap) from loss of extensor tone. Myoclonus may respond to valproate, or clonazepam.

327

Dystonia Prolonged muscle contraction causing abnormal posture or repetitive movements due to many causes. *Idiopathic torsion dystonia* (ITD), the commonest, starts in adulthood as a focal dystonia (eg *spasmodic torticollis:* The head is pulled to one side and held there by a contracting sternomastoid). It is worse in conditions of mental or emotional stress. Patients <40yrs old need a trial of L-dopa to rule out *dopa-responsive dystonia* (rare). A few ITD patients respond to high-dose trihexyphenidyl. *Blepharospasm*, involuntary contraction of orbicularis oculi) and *writer's cramp* are other focal dystonias. *Acute dystonia* may occur in young men starting neuroleptics (head pulled back, eyes drawn upward, trismus). Use anticholinergics (benzatropine 1–2mg IV). Disabling focal dystonias *may* respond to botulinum toxin injected into the muscle.

Tardive dyskinesia Involuntary chewing and grimacing movements due to long-term neuroleptics (eg metoclopramide and prochlorperazine). *Treatment:* Withdraw neuroleptic and wait 3–6 months. The dyskinesia may fail to resolve or even worsen. If so, consider tetrabenazine 25–50mg/8h PO.

Ischemic stroke

Stroke: Clinical features and investigations

Strokes result from ischemic infarction or bleeding into part of the brain, manifest by rapid onset (over minutes) of focal CNS signs and symptoms. It is the major neurological disease of our times.

Incidence: There are 700,000 strokes each year within the US. It is the third leading cause of death behind heart disease and cancer.

Causes:
- Thrombosis-in-situ
- Heart emboli (atrial fibrillation, infective endocarditis, MI)
- Atherothromboembolism (eg from carotids)
- Ischemia due to hypoperfusion distal to an intracranial stenosis
- CNS hemorrhage (hypertension; trauma; cocaine use)

Rare causes: Sudden hypotension; vasculitis; venous sinus thrombosis. *In young patients suspect:* Thrombophilia; vasculitis; venous-sinus thrombosis; carotid artery dissection (spontaneous or from neck trauma or fibromuscular dysplasia).

Risk factors Hypertension, smoking, diabetes mellitus; heart disease (valvular, ischemic, atrial fibrillation, peripheral vascular disease, past TIA, carotid bruit, hyperlipidemia, excess alcohol; hypercoaguable states.

Signs Sudden onset, or a step-wise progression over hours is typical. In theory, focal signs relate to distribution of the affected artery, but collateral supplies can cloud the issue. *Cerebral hemisphere infarcts* (50%) may cause: Contralateral hemiplegia which is initially flaccid (floppy limb, falls like a dead weight when lifted), then becomes spastic (UMN); contralateral sensory loss; homonymous hemianopia; dysphasia. *Brainstem infarction* (25%): Wide range of effects which include quadriplegia, disturbances of gaze and vision, locked-in syndrome (aware, but unable to respond), ataxia, vertigo and possibly dysphagia. *Lacunar infarcts* (25%): Small infarcts around basal ganglia, internal capsule, thalamus, and pons. May cause pure motor, pure sensory, mixed motor and sensory signs, but has intact cognition/consciousness.

Evaluation of acute strokes The approach to emergent stroke management has changed dramatically with the advent of thrombolytic therapy. Establishing the diagnosis of ischemic stroke and the time of onset has become critical for identifying patients who could benefit from the IV or intra-arterial administration of thrombolytics. Thus, the evaluation of a patient presenting with new onset stroke symptoms includes the following: ABCs, evaluation of vital signs, assessment of blood glucose (as hypo- and hyperglycemia can cause focal neurologic deficits), a thorough history and physical, and a non-contrast CT scan of the brain to rule out intracranial hemorrhage. If a patient presents early enough (such that a workup can be completed and therapy initiated within 3h of onset of symptoms), meets inclusion criteria and has no exclusion criteria then they are a candidate for IV thrombolytics. If the patient presents in such a way that therapy cannot be administered within 3h of symptoms onset then there can be consideration for intra-arterial thrombolytics (if administration will occur within 6h of symptoms). After the acute management stage, physicians need to pursue appropriate evaluations to identify modifiable patient risk factors for future strokes. These tests are meant to improve secondary prevention. They include evaluations for:

Hypertension: Look for retinopathy and a big heart on CXR. Acutely raised BP is common in early stroke. In general, don't treat the elevated pressure acutely. This elevation of BP may be responsible for collateral flow to at risk brain tissue (an ischemic penumbra).

Cardiac source of emboli: Atrial fibrillation (AF): Emboli from the left atrium may have caused the stroke. Look for a big left atrium (CXR; echo). *Post-MI:* Mural thrombus is best seen by echocardiography. In stroke from AF or mural thrombus do CT to exclude a hemorrhagic stroke, then start aspirin;

wait before commencing full anticoagulation to avoid bleeds into infarcts.
SBE/IE: 20% of those with endocarditis present with CNS signs due to septic emboli from valves. Treat as endocarditis; ask a cardiologist's opinion.

Carotid artery stenosis: In carotid territory stroke/TIA, 2 randomized trials show clear benefit of carotid surgery, so expert bodies affirm that 80% stenoses (on Doppler) merit angiography ± surgery—in fit patients.

Diabetes mellitus.

Hyperlipidemia.

Giant cell arteritis If ESR is extremely elevated, or there is a story of headache or tender scalp (not necessarily temporal). Give steroids promptly.

Syphilis: Look for active, untreated disease.

Cardiac causes of stroke

Cardioembolic causes are the source of stroke in >30% of patients in population studies. If identified, cardioembolic sources can dramatically change secondary prevention strategies.

- Atrial fibrillation (AF) ↑ risk of stroke 5-fold (5 to 12% per year, depending on comorbidities). This risk rises with age, duration of AF, hypertension, and heart failure—and if the AF follows rheumatic fever. Left ventricular dilatation, left atrial enlargement with stasis, and mitral valve disease particularly ↑ risk for stroke; this risk can be largely reduced by anticoagulation. Aspirin may be preferable for those at low risk of stroke (<65yrs old, no concurrent vascular risk factors, no history of cerebral events), or for those with high risk of hemorrhage. Aim for an INR of 2.0–3.0 (stroke risk is twice as much for those with an INR of 1.7 as opposed to 2).
- External cardioversion is complicated in 1–3% by peripheral emboli: Pharmacological cardioversion may carry similar risks.
- Prosthetic valves risk major emboli; anticoagulate (INR 2.5–3.5).
- Acute myocardial infarct with large left ventricular wall motion abnormalities on echocardiography predispose to left ventricular thrombus. Emboli arise in 10% of these patients in the next 6–12 months; risk being reduced by two-thirds by anticoagulation.
- Paradoxical systemic emboli via the venous circulation in those with patent foramen ovale, atrial and ventricular septal defects can occur.

329

The treatment of stroke will vary somewhat depending on the etiology, but in almost all cases patients will be started on an anti-platelet agent (aspirin), a statin, and possibly an ACE inhibitor or angiotensin receptor blocking agent. DVT prophylaxis is indicated during hospitalization and rehabilitation. Dysphagia screens for anyone with facial weakness or cognitive impairments should be done upon admission in order to identify patients at ↑ risk for aspiration. Based on numerous large studies, there is no indication for empiric anticoagulation or 'heparinization' in stroke patients. The addition to heparin in all stroke patients seems to help as many individuals as it harms, making its 'standard' use impractical and unwarranted.

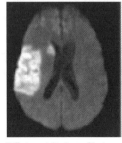

Diffusion-weighted MRI of brain revealing right sided, MCA territory infarct

Transient ischemic attack (TIA)

The sudden onset of focal CNS signs or symptoms due to temporary occlusion, usually by emboli, of part of the cerebral circulation is termed a TIA if symptoms fully resolve within 24h (TIAs are often much shorter) and there is no evidence of infarct on MRI. They are the harbingers of stroke and MI. If they are recognized for what they are, and preventive measures are prompt, a disastrous stroke may be averted.

Symptoms Attacks may be single or many. Symptoms may be the same or different on each occasion. *Carotid territory ischemia:* Contralateral weakness/numbness; dysphasia; dysarthria; homonymous hemianopia; amaurosis fugax (one eye's vision is blotted out 'like a curtain descending over my field of view') represents a transient occlusion of the ophthalmic artery (the first branch of the internal carotid). *Vertebrobasilar territory:* Hemiparesis; hemisensory loss; bilateral weakness or sensory loss; diplopia; homonymous hemianopia in cortical blindness; vertigo; deafness; tinnitus; vomiting; dysarthria; ataxia.

Signs *(No CNS signs 24h after an attack):* Listen for carotid bruits; their absence does not rule out a carotid source of emboli. Tight stenoses often have *no* bruit. Listen for cardiac murmurs suggesting valve disease and identify AF.

Causes *Atherothromboembolism* from the carotid emboli from the heart (AF, mural thrombus post-MI, valvular disease, prosthetic valves). *Hyperviscosity*, eg polycythemia, sickle-cell anemia.

Differential diagnosis of brief focal CNS symptoms: *Migraine* (symptoms spread and intensify over minutes, often with visual scintillations before headache); *focal epilepsy* (symptoms spread over seconds and often include twitching and jerking). Sometimes the problem lies in the peripheral nerves. Rare mimics of TIAs: *Malignant hypertension; hypoglycemia; MS; intracranial lesions; somatization.*

Tests TIAs should be evaluated in a manner similar to strokes, since they can be thought of as 'near misses'. Thus, carotid artery imaging (Doppler, MRA, or CTA) should be obtained. Echocardiography to look for cardioembolic sources and prolonged cardiac rhythm monitoring should be obtained to look for paroxysmal atrial fibrillation.

Treatment Begin after the first attack—don't wait for another; it could be a stroke. Control risk factors for stroke (eg smoking, hypertension, hypercholesterolemia, etc.) and MI. An inpatient admission should be considered if the TIA was recent, given the 12% rate of stroke within 30d following a TIA. Based on the workup, stroke prevention strategies will be determined. Regardless of findings all patients should initiate therapy with an antiplatelet therapy (eg aspirin). If an indication for anticoagulation is found then warfarin should be instituted. Carotid endarterectomy should be undertaken if the patient is found to have a 70% or greater stenosis on the symptomatic side and the surgical team has a stroke/mortality rate of <5%.

Intracerebral hemorrhage

10–20% of all strokes are hemorrhagic. The pathophysiology and management of hemorrhagic strokes is completely different than ischemic strokes, yet initial clinical presentations can be identical. Thus, it is imperative that all patients presenting with symptoms of an acute stroke have a non-contrast head CT in order to quickly diagnose intracerebral hemorrhages. Hypertension, drug use, head trauma, and vascular malformations are risk factors for ICH, with hypertension being the most common cause of spontaneous intracerebral hemorrhage.

The treatment of patients with intracerebral hemorrhages begins with evaluation of the airway, breathing, and cardiovascular status. If the patient is stable then directed therapy for the hemorrhage is initially focused on preventing expansion of the hematoma. Two factors, if left uncontrolled, can lead to dramatic worsening of the patient—hypertension and coagulopathies. Patients who present with an ICH and elevated BP should have a careful, but rapid reduction in their BP following the guidelines used to treat hypertensive emergencies. If the patient is known to be on anticoagulation, has a known bleeding disorder or has coagulation profiles that are noted to be abnormal then transfusion with fresh frozen plasma should be instituted (specific coagulopathies can be treated differently).

In general patients with larger intracerebral hemorrhages, unstable vitals at presentation, diminished level of consciousness (as measured by the Glasgow Coma Scale) and the presence of intraventricular extension do much worse. If patients survive the initial hemorrhage and do not suffer further bleeding than the outcome will dictated by the amount of ↑ intracranial pressure and tissue damaged.

Subarachnoid hemorrhage (SAH)

Spontaneous bleeding into the subarachnoid space is often a catastrophic event. Incidence: 8/100,000/yr; typical age: 35–65. *Causes:* Rupture of saccular aneurysms is the most common cause (80%) with arterio-venous malformations accounting for 15%. No cause is found in <5%. *Associations:* Smoking; hypertension; alcohol abuse; bleeding disorders; mycotic aneurysm post infective endocarditis. Lack of estrogen (post-menopausal) has been cited *Genetics:* Close relatives of those with SAH have a 3–5-fold ↑ in risk of SAH.

Berry aneurysms Common sites: Junction of the posterior communicating with the internal carotid (or of the anterior communicating with the anterior cerebral) or bifurcation of the middle cerebral artery. 15% are multiple. Some are hereditary. Skin biopsy may show type 3 collagen deficiency and identify relatives at risk. *Associations:* Polycystic kidneys, coarctation of the aorta, Ehlers–Danlos syndrome (hypermobile joints + ↑ skin elasticity).

Clinical features *Symptoms:* Sudden (within a few seconds) devastating headache 'The worst headache of my life', often occipital. Vomiting, collapse (± seizures), and coma frequently follow. Coma/drowsiness may last for days. *Signs:* Neck stiffness; retinal and subhyaloid hemorrhage, or focal neurologic findings.

Differential In primary care, only 25% of those with severe, sudden 'thunderclap' headache have SAH. In most, no cause is found; the remainder have meningitis, migraine, intracerebral bleeds, or cerebral venous thrombosis.

Sentinel headache SAH patients may earlier have experienced a sentinel headache, perhaps due to a small warning leak from the offending aneurysm (~6%), but the picture is clouded by recall-bias. As corrective surgery is more successful in the least symptomatic, be suspicious of any *sudden* headache, particularly if associated with neck or back pain.

Tests CT (early) shows subarachnoid or ventricular blood but misses approximately 2% of small bleeds. If a CT scan is negative, then a lumbar puncture should be performed to analyze the CSF for red cells. Always send 2 tubes (the first and last) for cell counts in order to help differentiate traumatic taps from SAH. The CSF in SAH is uniformly bloody in the early stages of SAH and xanthochromic (yellow) after a few hours. The supernatant from spun CSF is looked at photometrically in the lab to find breakdown products of hemoglobin. Finding bilirubin confirms SAH, and shows that the LP was not a 'bloody tap'.

Management Get a neurosurgical opinion (immediately if ↓level of consciousness, progressive focal deficit, or cerebellar hematoma suspected). Bed rest, BP control (maintain within normal range). Repeat CT if deteriorating. Re-examine CNS often. Prevent the need for straining with stool softeners. Maintain euvolemia. *Vasospasm:* Nimodipine (60mg/4h PO for 3wks, or 1mg/h IVI) is a Ca^{2+} antagonist that improves outcome (give to all if blood pressure allows). The definitive management of a cerebral aneurysm involves either surgical clipping of the aneurysm or intravascular coiling of the aneurysm lumen.

Rebleeding is a common mode of death in those who have had a subarachnoid hemorrhage. Rebleeding occurs in 30%, often in the first few days.

Vasospasm follows a bleed, often causing ischemia ± permanent CNS deficit. Treatment includes nimodipine, induced hypertension, hypervolemia, and hemodilution ('triple H therapy').

Mortality in subarachnoid hemorrhage based on Hunt and Hess grading

Grade:	Signs:	Mortality: (%)
I	None	0
II	Neck stiffness and cranial nerve palsies	11
III	Drowsiness	37
IV	Drowsy with hemiplegia	71
V	Prolonged coma	100

Almost all the mortality occurs in the 1st month. Of those who survive the 1st month, 90% survive a year or more.

Unruptured aneurysms

The management of unruptured cerebral aneurysms is controversial, based on conflicting data series. In general the risk of rupture is felt to be between 0.5 and 1.5% per year. There is some data to suggest that aneurysms larger than 10mm in diameter have a higher rate of rupture than smaller aneurysms, but this is not absolute. Careful consultation with a neurosurgeon and interventional neuroradiologist is warranted when unruptured aneurysms are discovered.

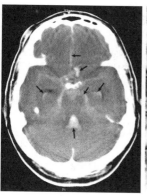 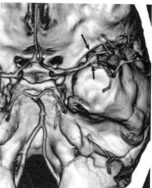

Blood from a ruptured aneurysm occupies the interhemispheric fissure (top arrow), a crescentic intracerebral area presumably near the aneurysm (2nd arrow), the basal cisterns, the lateral ventricles (temporal horns), and the 4th ventricle (bottom arrow).

CT images can be manipulated to show only high-density structures such as bones and arteries containing contrast. Here is a middle cerebral artery aneurysm.

We thank Professor Peter Scally for these CT images and the commentaries on them.

Intracranial venous thrombosis

Isolated sagittal sinus thrombosis (47% of patients) *Presentation:* Headache, vomiting, seizures, papilledema (one cause of intracranial hypertension and is in the differential diagnosis of pseudotumor cerebri). If venous infarction supervenes, focal neurologic deficit will be seen, eg hemiplegia. Sagittal sinus thrombosis is usually accompanied by thrombosis of other sinuses, eg *lateral sinus thrombosis* (35%—eg with VI and VII cranial nerve palsies, field defect, ear pain), *cavernous sinus thrombosis* (central retinal vein thrombosis, grossly edematous eyelids, chemosis), *sigmoid sinus thrombosis* (cerebellar signs, lower cranial nerve palsies), *inferior petrosal sinus* (V and VI cranial nerve palsies—Gradenigo's syndrome).

Cortical vein thrombosis This may cause venous infarcts (± focal signs), encephalopathy, seizures, and headache (eg thunderclap headache, ie sudden and severe). It usually coexists with sinus thromboses, but may be an isolated event.

Predisposing factors In 30%, no cause is found. Hypercoaguable states, genetic and acquired, such as pregnancy and the postpartum period are risks factors for cerebral vein thrombosis.

Systemic diseases	*Infections*	*Drugs*
Dehydration; diabetes	Meningitis	Oral contraceptives
Neoplasms; heart failure	Cerebral abscess	Androgens
Renal/hematological disease	Septicemia	Antifibrinolytics
Crohn's/UC	Fungal infections	
Hyperviscosity	Otitis media	*Pregnancy/postpartum*
Behçet's disease		
Activated protein C resistance		

Differential diagnosis (See subarachnoid differential diagnosis list) Pseudotumor cerebri, thunderclap headaches also occur in dissection of a carotid or vertebral artery, as well as in *benign thunderclap headache*.

Evaluation

Check that there are no signs of meningitis. Do an emergency MRI or CT scan. If CT normal, do LP. Measure the opening CSF pressure. If high, and the headache is persisting, and no subarachnoid bleed, suspect cerebral vein thrombosis if predisposing factors. Get further imaging. While angiography is the gold standard, MRV is being utilized as a non-invasive screening tool with variable success. CT may be normal at first and then at 1wk develop the delta sign, where a transversely cut sinus shows a contrast filling defect (dark). This may also be an early sign. CSF may be normal, or show RBCs and elevated bilirubin with an elevated opening pressure.

Management While there is a paucity of good trials on the treatment of intracerebral venous thrombosis, the standard of care is to anticoagulate with heparin, *even in the setting of intracerebral hemorrhage.* Manage ↑ intracranial pressure as needed.

Subdural hemorrhage

Consider this very treatable condition in all whose conscious level fluctuates, and also in those having an 'evolving stroke'—especially if on anticoagulants. Bleeding is from bridging veins between cortex and venous sinuses (vulnerable to deceleration injury), resulting in accumulating hematoma between dura and arachnoid. This gradually raises ICP, shifting midline structures away from the side of the clot and, if untreated, eventual tentorial herniation and coning.

Most subdurals are secondary to trauma but they can occur without. The trauma may have been so minor or have happened so long ago that it is not recalled. The elderly are particularly susceptible, as brain atrophy makes bridging veins more vulnerable. Others at risk are those prone to falls (epileptics, alcoholics) and those on long-term anticoagulation.

Symptoms Development of a subdural hemorrhage may be insidious so be alerted by a fluctuating level of consciousness (present in 35%). Typical complaints are of physical and intellectual slowing, sleepiness, headache, personality change, and unsteadiness.

Signs ↑ ICP. Localizing neurological symptoms (eg unequal pupils, hemiparesis) occur late and often long after the injury (63d average).

CT Shows clot ± midline shift (but beware bilateral isodense clots). Look for crescent-shaped collection of blood over 1 hemisphere. The sickle-shape differentiates subdural blood from epidural hemorrhage.

Differential Evolving stroke, cerebral tumor, dementia.

Treatment Evacuation via burr holes usually leads to full recovery.

Epidural hemorrhage

Suspect this if, after head injury, conscious level falls or is slow to improve. Extradural bleeds are commonly due to a fractured temporal or parietal bone causing laceration of the middle meningeal artery and vein, typically after trauma to a temple just lateral to the eye. Any tear in a dural venous sinus will also result in an extradural bleed. Blood accumulates between bone and dura.

Symptoms and signs Look out for a deterioration of consciousness after any head injury that initially produced no loss of consciousness or after initial drowsiness post-injury seems to have resolved. This 'lucid interval' pattern is typical of extradural bleeds. It may last a few hours to a few days before a bleed declares itself by a deteriorating level of consciousness caused by a rising ICP. Increasingly severe headache, vomiting, confusion, and seizures can follow, accompanied by a hemiparesis with brisk reflexes and an upgoing plantar. If bleeding continues, the ipsilateral pupil dilates, and coma deepens, a bilateral spastic paraparesis develops, and breathing becomes deep and irregular. Death follows a period of coma and is due to respiratory arrest. Bradycardia and raised BP are late signs.

Tests CT shows a hematoma which is often lens-shaped (biconvex; the blood forms a more rounded shape because the tough dural attachments to the skull tend to keep it more localized). Skull x-ray may be normal or show fracture lines crossing the course of the middle meningeal vessels. Skull fracture after trauma greatly ↑ the risk of an extradural hemorrhage, and should lead to prompt CT.

Management Stabilize and transfer promptly (with skilled medical and nursing escorts) to a neurosurgical unit for clot evacuation. Care of the airway in an unconscious patient, and measures to ↓ ICP often mandate intubation, hyperventilation and administration of intravenous mannitol.

Meningitis

Meningitis, an inflammation of the lining surrounding the brain can be caused by a variety of pathologies. Bacteria, viruses, fungi, mycobacteria, medications, and tumors can all cause acute meningitis. Depending on the etiology the presentation will vary dramatically. Bacterial meningitis classically causes fulminant illnesses with severe headaches, photophobia, and meningeal symptoms, viral and drug related etiologies tend to have milder symptoms, fungal and mycobacterial infections can be indolent, while meningeal carcinomatosis is often accompanied by radicular or cranial nerve findings.

The evaluation of suspected meningitis (fever, headache, stiff neck, nausea, photophobia) is centered around the lumbar puncture. A significant amount of time has been spent trying to identify patients who require a head CT prior to lumbar puncture in order to better identify patients who are at risk of herniating. There is an abundance of data identifying time to antibiotic administration as being critical for successful treatment of bacterial meningitis. There is, however, concern that a significant delay between antibiotic administration and CSF acquisition can diminish the diagnostic capabilities of the CSF. The delay involved while waiting for a CT scan could dramatically alter clinicians' ability to appropriately care for patients. Thus, the Infectious Disease Society of America has formulated a consensus statement regarding management of patients with suspected bacterial meningitis. If a patient is immunocompromised, has a CNS disease, develops a seizure during presentation, has papilledema, alteration of conciousness, or a focal neurologic deficit then they should have blood cultures drawn, therapy initiated, and a head CT performed *before* the lumbar puncture is performed. If all of those features are absent then the patient should have urgent blood cultures drawn, an urgent lumbar puncture performed, and therapy initiated.

Empiric therapy for bacterial meningitis includes dexamethasone and an antibiotic regimen based on the patients age and risk factors (see TABLE)

Predisposing factor	Common organisms	Empiric antibiotics
Age <1 month	*Streptococcus agalactiae, Eschericia coli, Listeria monocytogenes, Klebsiella species*	Ampicillin plus cefotaxime or ampicillin plus an aminoglycoside
Age 1–23 months	*Streptococcus pneumoniae, Neisseria meningitidis, S. agalactiae, Haemophilus influencae, E. coli*	Vancomycin plus a third generation cephalosporin
Age 2–50yrs	*N. meningitides, S. pneumoniae*	Vancomycin plus a third generation cephalosporin
Age >50yrs	*S. pneumoniae, N. meningitides, L. monocytogenes,* aerobic Gram-negative bacilli	Vancomycin plus ampicillin plus a third generation cephalosporin
Basilar skull fracture	*S. pneumoniae, H. influenzae,* group A β-hemolytic streptococci	Vancomycin plus a third generation cephalosporin
Penetrating head trauma	*Staphylococcus aureus,* coagulase-negative staphylococci, aerobic Gram-negative bacilli (including *Pseudomonas aeruginosa*).	Vancomycin plus cefepime, vancomycin plus ceftazidime, or vancomycin plus meropenem

Post neurosurgery	Aerobic Gram-negative bacilli (including *P. aeruginosa*), *S. aureus*, coagulase-negative staphylococci	Vancomycin plus cefepime, vancomycin plus ceftazidime, or vancomycin plus meropenem
CSF shunt	Coagulase-negative staphylococci, *S. aureus*, aerobic Gram-negative bacilli, *Propionibacterium acnes*	Vancomycin plus cefepime, vancomycin plus ceftazidime or vancomycin plus meropenem

Once the CSF is obtained it can be analysed to determine if it is consistent with a bacterial, viral, fungal, mycobacterial, neoplastic, or drug related etiology. This interpretation *must* include an assessment of the clinical situation as the patterns of CSF findings are never observed in 100% of cases.

In general bacterial meningitis is associated with higher white blood cell counts with a predominance of polymorphonuclear cells while viral meningitides have predominantly lymphocytes. The typical features of CSF in a variety of pathologies are summarized in the following table.

	Cell count	Differential	Protein	Glucose
Bacterial	++++	Polys	++	Low
Viral	+++	Lymphocytes	+	Low to normal
Fungal	+++	Monocytes	+++	Low
Mycobacterial	++	Variable	+++	Low
Neoplastic	+	Variable	++	Very low
Drug related	++	Variable	+	Normal

Encephalitis

While meningitis is caused by inflammation within the lining around the brain (the meninges), encephalitis is caused by inflammation within the brain parenchyma. Encephalitis can be caused by both infectious and non-infectious etiologies, but classically the term encephalitis refers to infectious causes while the term cerebritis is used to identify non-infectious inflammatory processes within the brain.

Infectious causes of encephalitis include viral, bacterial, fungal, and mycobacterial pathogens, but viruses are by far the most common cause of acquired encephalitis in the world. The differential of viruses varies depending on geography with arboviral pathogens (mosquito borne viruses) changing dramatically from country to country. Within the US the most common identifiable cause of non-epidemic encephalitis is herpes (HSV 1).

Typically, encephalitis presents with fever, photophobia, altered sensorium or behavior, and variable degrees of meningeal symptoms. In this setting a patient should be initiated on IV acyclovir therapy for possible HSV encephalitis while a lumbar puncture is performed. Besides testing for cell count, protein, glucose, Gram stain and bacterial culture, a HSV PCR should be sent. This highly sensitive and specific test is the gold standard for identifying patients with HSV encephalitis. Caution should be taken, however, due to the false negative rate that occurs within the first 3 to 4 days of symptoms. In the appropriate clinical setting, when a high pre-test probability occurs, a negative HSV PCR should not be an indication to stop acyclovir therapy, but rather a second lumbar puncture should be performed and a second HSV PCR obtained.

Multiple sclerosis (MS)

This relapsing/remitting disorder consists of plaques of demyelination (and axon loss) at sites throughout the CNS (but not peripheral nerves). Pathogenesis involves focal disruption of the blood–brain barrier and associated immune response and myelin damage as well as neurodegenerative processes

Epidemiology MS effects approximately 350,000 people within the US with a female:male ratio of 2:1. The peak age of onset is in the 20s and 30s, making MS one of the most common causes of disability in young adults. MS is more common in temperate climates with some data suggesting an ↑ prevalence as you move further away from the equator. There is a strong genetic influence within MS with monozygotic twins having a 30% concordance rate and dizygotic twins having a 5% concordance rate. Children of patients with multiple sclerosis have a 3–5% rate of MS, compared to the background rate of 0.2% in Caucasion populations.

Presentation is usually monosymptomatic: Unilateral optic neuritis (pain or eye movement and rapid deterioration in central vision); numbness or tingling in the limbs; leg weakness or brainstem or cerebellar symptoms such as diplopia or ataxia. Less often there may be more than 1 symptom. Uthoff's phenomenon, symptoms worsening with heat (eg a hot bath) or exercise may be present.

Progression/prognosis: Early on, relapses may be followed by remission/full recovery. With time, remissions are incomplete, so disability accumulates This form of *Relapsing Remitting Multiple Sclerosis* (RRMS) occurs in 80% of patients. *Poor prognostic signs:* Older males; motor signs at onset; many relapses early on; many MRI lesions.

Examination Look carefully for CNS deficits other than the presenting problem. Lhermitte's symptom (paresthesia/pain in the back or limbs on flexing of the neck) may be positive (also in cervical spondylosis or B_{12} deficiency).

Diagnosis This is clinical, requiring demonstration of lesions disseminated in time and space, unattributable to other causes. Isolated CNS deficits are never diagnostic, but may become so if a careful history reveals previous episodes, eg unexplained blindness for a week. Before the advent of MRI making the diagnosis of clinically definite multiple sclerosis required more than one clinical episode. Utilizing MRI techniques, the diagnosis of clinically definite MS can be made after only one clinically apparent demyelinating event. This ability is important due to data that suggests early immunomodulatory treatment can alter the course of the disease.

Tests None is pathognomonic. *CSF:* Typically, the CSF of patients with MS have normal cell counts or a mild pleocytosis (up to 50 lymphocytes/mm³) but, rarely there can be more profound elevations. A white blood cell count above 50 cells/mm³ should prompt considerations for alternate diagnoses The protein level is usually normal or mildly elevated, but rarely above 100mg/L. Evidence of inflammation restricted to the CNS can be tested for by examining the CSF for oligoclonal bands of IgG on electrophoresis. More than two oligoclonal bands within the CSF, but not identified within the serum is consistent with intrathecal IgG production. While not specific for multiple sclerosis, the presence of oligoclonal bands in the CSF of a patient in the right clinical setting ↑ one's confidence in the diagnosis. Delayed visual auditory, and somatosensory evoked potentials can provide information regarding previous demyelinating events that are not identified on clinical exam. *MRI* is sensitive but not specific for plaque detection and may exclude other causes, eg cord compression. Correlation of MRI with clinical condition is poor. Some studies have identified *antibodies to myelin oligodendrocyte glyco protein* (MOG) and *myelin basic protein* (MBP) in patients with a single MS-like clinical lesion as being predictive of conversion to clinically definite MS.

Treatment *Methylprednisolone* 1g/d for 3–5d given IV shortens relapses, but does not alter the overall prognosis.

Disease-modifying agents: Interferon beta (infβ-1b; infβ-1a): Trials show that these can ↓ relapses by 30% in active RRMS. They also ↓ lesion accumulation in MRI. Their power to diminish disability remains controversial, as does benefit in secondary and primary progressive MS. Side effects include flu-like symptoms (low grade fevers, myalgias, fatigue), depression, and site reactions. Monitoring of liver functions tests is indicated. *Glatiramer acetate:* Is a copolymer comprising a random mix of four amino acids, glutamate, lysine, alanine, and tyrosine. Some data suggests that glatiramer acetate exerts its therapeutic effect by shifting a patient's immune system from predominately a Th1 response to a more protective Th2 response. Side effects include site reactions and an idiosyncratic episode of flushing, palpitations and chest pain that can last for 20min after injection. This response is not an allergy and it is safe to continue treatment. No blood tests need to be followed on this therapy.

McDonald criteria for diagnosing MS

Clinical presentation	*Additional data needed*
2 or more attacks (relapses) with 2 or more objective clinical lesions	None; clinical evidence will do (imaging evidence desirable; must be consistent with MS)
2 or more attacks with 1 objective clinical lesion	Dissemination in space, shown by: • MRI or • positive csf and 2 MRI lesions consistent with MS or • Further attack involving different site
1 attack with 2 or more objective clinical lesions	Dissemination in time, shown by • MRI OR 2nd clinical attack
1 attack with 1 objective clinical lesion (monosymptomatic presentation)	Dissemination in space: • MRI OR positive CSF if 2 MRI lesions consistent with MS • AND dissemination in time shown by MRI or 2nd clinical attack[3]
Insidious neurological progression suggestive of MS (primary progressive MS)	Positive CSF AND Dissemination in space shown by: • MRI evidence of 9 T2 brain lesions • or 2 or more cord lesions • or 4–8 brain and 1 cord lesion • or positive visual evoked potential (VEP) with 4–8 MRI lesions • or positive VEP + <4 brain lesions + 1 cord lesion • AND dissemination in time shown by MRI or continued progression for ≥1yr

Attacks: These must last >1h, eg motor weakness etc.
Time between attacks: 30d. *MRI abnormality:* 3 out of 4:
1 1 Gadolinum (Gd)-enhancing or 9 T2 hyperintense lesions if no Gd-enhancing lesion
2 1 or more infratentorial lesions
3 1 or more juxtacortical lesions
4 3 periventricular lesions (1 spinal cord lesion = 1 brain lesion)
CSF: Oligoclonal IgG bands in CSF (and not serum) or ↑ IgG index.
Evoked potentials: This counts if delayed but well-preserved waveform.
What provides MRI evidence of dissemination in time? A Gd-enhancing lesion demonstrated in a scan done at least 3 months following onset of clinical attack at a site different from attack, OR

In absence of Gd-enhancing lesions at a 3-month scan, follow-up scan after an additional 3 months showing Gd-lesion or new T2 lesion.

Transverse myelitis

Transverse myelitis is a demyelinating disease restricted to the spinal cord. Patients present with acute to subacute onset of myelopathic symptoms. There are usually prominent motor, sensory, and bowel/bladder symptoms. This disease is usually monophasic, but some patients experience recurrences. Risk factors for recurrence include underlying autoimmune conditions such as Sjögren's or serology suggestive of an underlying condition (ie positive SSA/anti-Ro or SSB/anti-La antibodies). In the appropriate clinical setting of a acute subacute myelopathy imaging (MRI with gadolinium) must be obtained to rule out compressive lesions, intrinsic masses, or vascular lesions and a lumbar puncture should be obtained to confirm evidence of inflammation (ie mild pleocytosis or elevated IgG index). Absence of an enhancing lesion on MRI or pleocytosis within the CSF should prompt concern about the diagnosis.

Differential diagnosis A MRI of the brain should be obtained to evaluate the patient for possible MS. White matter lesions within the brain in association with a spinal cord demyelinating event could indicate that the myelopathy is in fact the first symptom of MS. Other pathologies that should be considered include neuromyelitis optica (see below), dural AV fistula, sarcoidosis, spinal cord tumor, spinal cord infarct (venous and arterial) and compressive myelopathies.

Treatment Treatment of transverse myelitis has two components, specific treatments to ↓ the degree of inflammation and supportive care given to all patients with spinal cord pathology. Specifically for the transverse myelitis high dose IV steroids (1g of methylprednisolone a day for 5d) is the standard of care. For patients not improving on this therapy plasmapheresis and/or pulse dose cyclophosphamide is indicated.

Neuromyelitis optica (Devic's)

Neuromyelitis optica (Devic's syndrome) is a demyelinating condition that is limited to the optic nerves and the spinal cord. Clinically, it presents as either an optic neuritis (diminished vision in one eye accompanied by pain with movement of that eye) or as an episode of transverse myelitis. Some patients diagnosed as having transverse myelitis will actually go on to have the diagnosis of Devic's syndrome after they have an episode of optic neuritis. After presentation a patient should have a MRI of the entire CNS with gadolinium to evaluate for evidence of MS. Patients with neuromyelitis optica (NMO) tend to progress more rapidly than MS patients and do not respond to interferons or glatiramer acetate. A circulating IgG has been identified in a large number of NMO patients suggesting a humoral etiology. Thus, these patients may respond best to plasmapheresis, IVIG or immunosuppressants with humoral activity.

Dementia

Dementia, which has many causes, entails *impaired cognition with intact consciousness* (unlike delirium). The key is a good history: Ask spouse, relatives, or friends about *progressively* impaired cognition/memory. Get *objective* evidence. Histories usually go back months or years. There is ↑forgetfulness, and normal tasks of daily living are done with ↑ incompetence, eg going to the store several times in a day, and then being baffled as to why there is a great quantity of food in the kitchen. Sometimes the patient appears to have changed personality, eg apathy, uncharacteristically rude or literalness. For objective evidence, do tests of cognitive functioning.

Epidemiology Rare below 55yrs of age. 5–10% prevalence above 65yrs. 20% prevalence above 80yrs, and 70% of those over 100yrs.

Commonest causes *Alzheimer's disease (AD)—see below. Vascular dementia:* ~25% of all dementias. It represents the cumulative effects of many small strokes. Look for evidence of vascular pathology (hypertension; past strokes; focal CNS signs). Onset is sometimes sudden, and deterioration is often stepwise (versus slowly progressive).

Lewy body dementia: Characterized by Lewy bodies in brainstem *and* neocortex, *fluctuating* cognitive loss, alertness and attention; parkinsonism; detailed visual hallucinations; falls; loss of consciousness/syncope. It is the 3rd commonest dementia (15–25%) after AD and vascular causes. Neuroleptics in these patients *often* cause neuropsychiatric symptoms.

Fronto-temporal dementia: (Frontal and temporal atrophy) without Alzheimer histology. *Signs:* Behavioral/personality change; early preservation of episodic memory & spatial orientation; disinhibition; hyperorality, stereotyped behavior, and emotional unconcern.

Ameliorable causes Hypothyroidism; vitamin B$_{12}$ deficiency; thiamine deficiency (eg as seen in alcoholics); syphilis; some cerebral tumors (eg parasagittal meningioma); subdural haematoma; normal pressure hydrocephalus (dilatation of ventricles without signs of ↑ pressure, possibly due to obstructed CSF flow from subarachnoid space; CSF shunts help; it is suggested by incontinence early-on and gait apraxia). *Rarer causes:* Alcohol/drug abuse; pellagra, Huntington's; CJD; Parkinson's; Pick's disease; HIV; cryptococcosis; SSPE; progressive leukencephalopathy.

Tests Make absolutely certain that no treatable cause is missed. Complete blood count, ESR, electrolyes, liver function tests, TSH, B$_{12}$, RPR/FTA, HIV, CT/MRI and consider EEG.

Alzheimer's disease (AD)

This leading cause of dementia is currently having a large impact on our health care system, nursing home system, and society. As our population continues to live longer a greater portion of our society will suffer from this disease, requiring ↑ attention from their children and families. *Mean survival:* 7 to 10 years from onset. Suspect Alzheimer's in adults with enduring, acquired deficits of visual-spatial skill ('he gets lost easily'), memory, and cognition, eg tested by mental test scores + other neuropsychometric tests. *Cause:* Accumulation of β-amyloid peptide, a degradation product of amyloid precursor protein, resulting in progressive neuronal damage, neurofibrillary tangles, ↑ numbers of senile plaques, and loss of the neurotransmitter acetylcholine from damage to an ascending forebrain projection (nucleus basalis of Meynert; connects with cortex).

Risk factors *Defective genes* on chromosomes 1, 14, 19, 21; the apoE4 variant is linked to earlier age of onset.

Presentation Decline in memory capabilities and cognition; behavioral change (eg aggression, wandering, disinhibition); delusions; apathy; depression; irritability. There is no standard natural history. Cognitive impairment is progressive, but behavioral/psychotic symptoms may change after a few months or years. Towards the end, often but by no means invariably, patients become sedentary, taking little interest in anything. Wasting, mutism, incontinence ± seizures may occur.

Diagnosis The absolute diagnosis of Alzheimer's is based on pathology on biopsy or autopsy. Clinically, neurocognitive testing can identify patients with dementia that is consistent with an Alzheimer's type.

Treatment The standard of care for AD is cholinergic therapy with cholinesterase inhibitors. These medications do not cure or reverse the effects of this dementing illness, but rather, slow the progression and delay nursing home placement. A new class of drug, NMDA receptor antagonist, has also shown efficacy for delaying the cognitive decline seen in AD.

Epilepsy

Epilepsy is a recurrent tendency to spontaneous, intermittent, abnormal electrical activity in part of the brain, manifest as *seizures*. These may take many forms: For a given patient they tend to be stereotyped. *Convulsions* are the motor signs of electrical discharges. Many of us would have seizures in abnormal metabolic circumstances—eg hyponatremia, hypoxia (reflex anoxic brief convulsions after syncope), but some patients have a lowered threshold for having seizures and do not require metabolic stresses to have a convulsion.

Presentation There may (rarely) be a *prodrome* lasting hours or days preceding the seizure. It is not part of the seizure itself: The patient or others notice a change in mood or behavior. An *aura*, which is part of the seizure, may precede its other manifestations. The aura may be a strange feeling in the gut, or a sensation or an experience such as *déja vu* (disturbing sense of familiarity), or strange smells, or flashing lights. It implies a partial seizure (a focal event), often, but not necessarily, caused by temporal lobe epilepsy. After a partial seizure involving the motor cortex (Jacksonian convulsion) there may be temporary weakness of the affected limb(s) (Todd's palsy). After a generalized seizure, patients experience a headache, myalgias, confusion, and lethargy.

Diagnosis First, since most seizures are not witnessed by medical personel, confirming that a reported event was a seizure is important. A detailed description from a witness of the event is crucial. While a diagnosis based on history is never 100% accurate, certain historical features can ↑ the odds that an event was epileptic versus syncopal. The presence of prolonged tonic–clonic activity, automatisms, or tongue biting is suggestive of an ictal event. Syncopal events are often preceded by feelings of lightheadedness, vision changes, and/or diaphoresis. One or two clonic movements after syncope is not abnormal and can be confused for an epileptic event. A more complete differential of recurrent movements include non-epileptic (psychogenic) seizures, tetanus, posturing, rigors, neuroleptic malignant syndrome, myoclonic jerks, tremors, and hemiballismus. The attack's *onset* is the key for determining what type of seizure is occurring: Partial or generalized? If the seizure begins with focal features, it is a partial seizure, however rapidly it generalizes.

Types *Partial onset seizures:* Simple partial seizures, complex partial seizures, and secondary generalized seizures. *Generalized onset seizures:* Absence seizures, myoclonic seizures, clonic seizures, tonic seizures, tonic–clonic seizures and atonic seizures.

Causes Often none is found. *Physical:* Trauma, space occupying lesions, stroke, hypertension, tuberous sclerosis, SLE, PAN, sarcoid, vascular malformations. *Metabolic:* Alcohol or benzodiazepine withdrawal; hyperglycemia or hypoglycemia, hypoxia, uremia, hypernatremia, hyponatremia, hypercalcemia, liver disease, drugs (eg phenothiazines, tricyclics, cocaine). *Infections:* Encephalitis, syphilis, cysticercosis, HIV.

Evaluation of an adult who has just had a first-ever seizure

Obtain as much history as possible from patient and witnesses. Try to form an opinion as to whether the witness is reliable.

You must attempt to establish a cause. Adult-onset seizures particularly with focal features are often 'symptomatic', ie secondary to another structural pathology (or cardiac, metabolic, or drug-related problem).

Clues from the history may point to an obvious illness or other toxic/metabolic cause for the seizure. If not, then these tests may help: Urine, electrolytes, liver function tests, glucose, calcium, phosphorous, coagulation profiles, serum and urine toxicology screens. Measure serum levels of medications. If the patient is not alert on presentation, consider screening for common anti-epileptics in case the patient is a known seizure patient on medication and subtherapeutic.

Consider LP if CT shows no signs of ↑ ICP and there are signs or symptoms of a CNS infection.

Imaging: Don't assume that if one CT scan is normal, there is no structural lesion. MRI/MRA should be obtained to find small areas of cortical dysgenesis, tumors, vascular malformations, and cavernomas.

Emergency EEG only if concerned about non-convulsive status.

You must give advice against driving, occupational hazards, bathing, swimming, and reproductive issues if the patient is a woman of child-bearing age. Document your discussion.

The decision to initiate anti-epileptic therapy after a first, unprovoked seizure should be individualized to the patient. Neurologic consultation is indicated.

Epilepsy: Management

Involve patients in all decisions. Compliance depends on communication and doctor–patient concordance issues. Living with epilepsy creates many problems (eg inability to drive, or operate machinery) and fears (eg of sudden death), and drug issues.

Therapy Treat with 1 drug (with 1 doctor in charge) only. ↑ doses until seizures are controlled, or toxic effects are manifest, or maximum drug dosage reached. Beware of drug interactions. Most specialists would not recommend treatment after 1 seizure but would start treatment after 2. Discuss options with the patient. If your patient has only 1 seizure every 2yrs, he or she may accept the risk (particularly if there is no need to drive or operate machinery) rather than have to take drugs every day.

Commonly used drugs

Carbamazepine: Has indications for partial epilepsy. Starting dose is 400mg a day (divided into bid dosing) with a maximum dose of 2400mg a day (in divided doses). Side effects include rash, nausea, diplopia, dizziness, fluid retention, hyponatremia, blood dyscrasias.

Gabapentin: Has indications for partial epilepsy as an adjunctive agent. Typical doses begin at 300mg/d and can be titrated to a maximum dose of 3600mg/d (divided into tid dosing). Side effects include weight gain, edema, somnolence and rarely heart failure.

Lamotrigine: Has indications for generalized and partial epilepsy. Usual starting dose for adults is 25mg twice a day, titrating to a maximum of 400mg a day (total dose). Side effects include rash, Stephens–Johnson syndrome, dizziness, headaches, aplastic anemia, and toxic epidermal necrosis. Caution when used in conjunction with valproate as this will reduce the clearance of lamotrigine.

Levetiracetam: Has indications for partial epilepsy and myoclonic epilepsy, but is also useful for seizure disorders with secondary generalization. Usual dosing begins at 250mg or 500mg twice a day and can be titrated to a maximum dose of 1500mg twice a day. Side effects can include irritability and rarely psychosis.

Oxcarbazepine: Has indications for partial epilepsy. Starting doses are between 300 and 600mg a day with a maximum dose of 2400mg a day (divided into bid dosing). Side effects include headaches, dizziness, hyponatremia and ataxia.

Phenytoin: Has indications for generalized or partial epilepsy. Initial maintenance doses are around 300mg per day with dosing being altered based on presence or absebce of side effects, efficacy, and serum levels of the drug. Side effects include coarsening of facial features, gum hypertrophy, blood dyscrasias, nystagmus and ataxia.

Topiramate: Has indications for generalized and partial seizures. Starting doses are between 25 and 50mg a day with a maximum dose of 400mg a day (divided into bid dosing). Side effects include cognitive slowing, weight loss, renal stones, glaucoma, acidosis and parasthesias (related to the drugs partial carbonic anhydrase inhibition activity).

Valproate: Has indications for generalized and partial epilepsy. Starting dose is approximately 250mg tid with a maximum daily dose of 3000mg per day (in divided doses). Side effects: Sedation, tremor, weight gain, hair thinning, ankle swelling, hyperammonemia (causing encephalopathy) and hepatic failure.

Changing drugs *Indications:* On inappropriate drug; side-effects unacceptable; treatment failure. *Method:* Begin new drug at its starting dose. At the same time, withdraw the old drug, eg over 6wks (sooner if toxicity). Slowly ↑ new drug to middle of its therapeutic range.

Status epilepticus

Management

Status epilepticus (SE) has traditionally been defined as continuous seizure activity for 20 to 30min or two seizures occurring without improvement in between. While more than 90% of all seizures will stop within 2min, some are prolonged. No emergent therapy is needed for a normal seizure. Prolonged seizures, however, are medical emergencies given the risk of death with status epilepticus. Once identified, the management of a patient with SE begins with assessment of the airway, acquisition of a rapid blood glucose determination (to rule out hypo- and hyperglycemia as easily treatable causes of SE), and establishment of IV access. Labs should be sent for a complete blood count, electrolytes including calcium, arterial blood gas, liver function tests, toxicology, renal function, and antiepileptic drug concentrations. While labs are being analysed treatment of SE is initiated with the administration of 0.1mg/kg of lorazepam intravenously at a rate of 2mg/min. If seizures continue the patient should be loaded with phenytoin or fosphenytoin at a dose of 20mg/kg or 20 PE/kg[1], respectively. If seizures continue despite this load an additional 10mg/kg of phenytoin or 10PE/kg of fosphenytoin should be administered. At this stage the use of anesthesia should be considered in conjunction with continuous EEG monitoring. Remember that once a patient is paralysed for intubation the clinical signs of seizures are lost and an EEG is needed to guide therapy.

[1] PE = phenytoin equivalents

Parkinson's disease (PD) and parkinsonism

Parkinsonism is a syndrome of *tremor, rigidity, bradykinesia (slowness)*, and loss of postural reflexes. *Prevalence*: 1 : 200 in people over 65yrs of age.

Tremor: 3–6Hz (cycles per sec). It is most marked at rest and coarser than cerebellar tremor. It is typically a 'pill rolling' tremor of thumb over fingers.

Rigidity: ↑ resistance to passive stretch of muscles throughout range of movement (*lead-pipe*); tone may be broken-up by tremor (*cogwheel rigidity*). Unlike in spasticity, rigidity is present equally in flexors and extensors.

Bradykinesia: Slowness of movement initiation with progressive reduction in speed and amplitude of repetitive actions; also monotonous speech. Expressionless face. Short shuffling steps with flexed trunk as if forever a step behind one's center of gravity (*festinating gait*). Feet as if frozen to the ground. ↓ blink rate. Micrographia (small writing).

Parkinson's disease is one cause of parkinsonism (due to degeneration of substantia nigra dopaminergic neurons. Symptoms usually start between 50 and 70yrs old.

Other causes of parkinsonism include neuroleptics (eg metoclopramide, prochlorperazine, haloperidol) rarely postencephalitis; supranuclear palsy (Steele-Richardson–Olszewski syndrome with absent vertical gaze, both upward and downward, and dementia); multisystem atrophy (MSA) (formerly Shy-Drager syndrome) with prominent orthostatic BP; carbon monoxide poisoning; Wilson's disease; communicating hydrocephalus.

Management of Parkinson's disease:

The goal of therapy is to treat symptoms, restore function, and avoid side effects. The mainstay of this approach utilizes dopamine and dopamine agonists. Start drugs when PD is seriously interfering with life (not too soon, as L-dopa's effects wear off with time; explain this to patients, and let them choose). Use the lowest dose giving symptom relief, without troublesome SEs. While L-dopa remains the most potent treatment for the symptoms of Parkinson's disease, a significant portion of patients will develop dyskinesias over time with prolonged use. Thus, many neurologists take the approach of utilizing dopamine agonists in younger patients in order to 'save' L-dopa for later. The dopamine agonists currently used are either ergotamine derivatives (pergolide and bromocriptine) or non-ergotamines (pramipexole and ropinirole). While these have a lower rate of dyskinesias than L-dopa, they tend to be less effective for severe symptoms. Anticholinergic agents can be added to PD therapy regimens in an attempt to improve tremor control. Drugs utilized for this include trihexiphenidyl, benztropine and biperiden. Amantadine has been show to be useful in PD by helping early mild symptoms and later by controlling some dyskinesias. As PD progresses, strategies that augment delivery of L-dopa into the nervous system can be utilized to improve therapeutic effects. Catechol-o-methyl transferase (COMT) inhibitors (tolcapone and entacapone) can be used to reduce the peripheral and central degradation of L-dopa. In patients with symptoms refractory to medical management, surgical interventions are available. These include implantable stimulators and lesional surgery (thalamotomy, pallidotomy, subthalamotomy).

Tremor

Tremors can be classified based on when they appear—ie at rest, during assumption of a posture, or with activity. Classically, rest tremors are seen in PD and parkinsonian states. Postural and action tremors include essential tremor, metabolic disorders (eg hyperthyroidism, hypoglycemia, pheochromocytoma) and medication related tremors (eg lithium). One of the most common neurologic causes of tremor is essential tremor.

Essential tremor (ET) is a kinetic/postural tremor usually seen in the upper extremities. Generally, it is characterized by low amplitude, high frequency movement that can be disabling in its most severe forms. Often, patients identify other family members with similar tremors. More than half of patients will report improvement in the tremor after consumption of alcoholic beverages. Primidone and propranolol are the mainstays of therapy for patients with ET. Responses are seen in 50–75% of patients.

Neuromuscular disease

Neuromuscular diseases involve pathologies of the nerve roots, plexuses, nerve axons, myelin sheaths, neuromuscular junctions, and muscles. Patients will complain of weakness, numbness, or both. The pattern of dysfunction is the clinical key to identifying neuromuscular conditions. Electrophysiology (nerve conduction studies and electromyography) serve as an extension of the clinical exam, *they do not replace it!*

For example, once a peripheral neuropathy is identified, there is no way to determine if the pathology is demyelinating or axonal. A variety of different diseases cause demyelinating conditions and would be treated quite differently than axonal pathologies. A conduction study would identify if there were reduced conduction velocities (indicative of demyelination) versus low amplitudes (signifying axonal loss).

The pattern of nerve weakness and numbness is crucial for determining where within the peripheral nervous system pathology exists. A mononeuropathy will give symptoms confined to one nerve distribution. A systemic condition causing a polyneuropathy classically affects the longest nerves first giving predominantly distal symptoms. The following section reviews neuromuscular disease from a clinical standpoint. Thus, when a polyneuropathy is identified in clinic an evaluation and management plan can be produced.

Mononeuropathies

These are lesions of individual peripheral and cranial nerves. There are a variety of causes, including trauma, diabetes, heavy metal exposure, infections such as leprosy, and vasculitides. If more than one peripheral nerve is affected, the term *mononeuritis multiplex* is used. Causes include diabetes, vasculitis, infections, amyloidosis, rheumatoid arthritis, paraneoplastic syndromes, and a variety of hereditary diseases.

Median nerve C6–T1 *At the wrist:* (eg lacerations; carpal tunnel syndrome—see BOX) Weakness of abductor pollicis brevis and sensory loss over the radial 3½ fingers and palm. Lesions confined to the anterior interosseous nerve: Weakness of flexion of the distal phalanx of the thumb and index finger. *Proximal lesions* (eg at the elbow) may show combined defects.

Ulnar nerve C7–T1 Vulnerable to elbow trauma. *Signs:* Weakness/wasting of medial (ulnar side) wrist flexors; weakness/wasting of the interossei (cannot cross the fingers) and medial 2 lumbricals (claw hand); wasting of the hypothenar eminence which abolishes finger abduction and sensory loss over the medial 1½ fingers and the ulnar side of the hand. Flexion of 4th & 5th DIP joints is weak. Treatment: See BOX. With lesions at the wrist (digitorum profundus intact), claw hand is more marked.

Radial nerve C5–T1 This nerve opens the fist. Damaged by compression against the humerus (commonly seen with humeral fractures). Test for wrist and finger drop with elbow flexed and arm pronated. Sensory loss: Variable; test dorsal aspect of root of thumb.

Sciatic nerve L4–S2 Damaged by pelvic tumors or fractures to pelvis or femur. Lesions affect the hamstrings and all muscles below the knee (foot drop), with loss of sensation below the knee laterally.

Common peroneal nerve L4–S2 Frequently damaged as it winds round the fibular head by trauma or tight-fitting casts. Lesions lead to inability to dorsiflex the foot (foot drop), evert the foot, extend the toes—and sensory loss over dorsum of foot.

Tibial nerve S1–3 Lesions lead to an inability to stand on tiptoe (plantarflexion), invert the foot, or flex the toes. Sensory loss over the sole.

Carpal tunnel syndrome: The commonest mononeuropathy

Nine tendons and the median nerve compete for space within the wrist. Compression is common, especially in women who have narrower wrists but similar-sized tendons to men.

The patient: Aching pain in the hand and arm (especially at night), and paraesthesias in the thumb, index, and middle fingers, all relieved by dangling the hand over the edge of the bed and shaking it. Some patients experience referred pain into the forearm and shoulder. There may be sensory loss and weakness of abductor pollicis brevis with or without wasting of the thenar eminence. Light touch, 2-point discrimination, and sweating may be impaired.

Associations: Pregnancy, rheumatoid, DM, hypothyroidism, dialysis, trauma.

Tests: Neurophysiology helps by confirming the lesion's site and severity (and likelihood of improvement after surgery). Maximal wrist flexion for 1min (Phalen's test) may elicit symptoms but is unreliable. Tapping over the nerve at the wrist induces tingling (Tinel's test; also rather non-specific).

Treatment: Splinting of the wrist for 3–6 months may help. If not, local steroid injection with or without decompression surgery may be indicated.

Managing ulnar mononeuropathies from entrapments

The ulnar nerve is in an anatomic precarious position and is subject to compression at multiple sites around the elbow. Most commonly compression occurs at the epicondylar groove or at the point where the nerve passes between the 2 heads of the flexor carpi ulnaris muscle (true *cubital tunnel syndrome*). Trauma can easily damage the nerve against its bony confines (the medial condyle of the humerus—the 'funny bone'). Normally, the ulnar nerve suffers stretch and compression forces at the elbow that are moderated by its ability to glide in its groove. When normal excursion is restricted, irritation ensues. This may cause a vicious cycle of perineural scarring, consequent loss of excursion, and progressive symptoms—without there being any antecedent trauma.

Rest and avoiding pressure on the nerve helps but if symptoms continue, night-time soft elbow splinting (to prevent flexion to >60°) is warranted, eg for 6 months. For chronic neuropathy associated with weakness, or if splinting fails, a variety of surgical procedures have been tried. For moderately severe neuropathies, decompressions *in situ* may help, but often fail. Medial epicondylectomies are effective in 50% (there is a high rate of recurrence). SC nerve re-routings (transpositions) may be tried. IM and submuscular transpositions are more complicated, but the latter may be preferable.

Compressive ulnar neuropathies at the wrist (*Guyon's canal*—between the pisiform and hamate bones) are less common, but they can also result in disability. *Thoracic outlet compression* is another cause of a weak numb hand. Electromyography (EMG) helps define the anatomic site of lesions.

Polyneuropathies

Polyneuropathies are generalized disorders of peripheral nerves (including cranial nerves) whose distribution is usually bilaterally symmetrical and widespread—usually a distal pattern of muscle weakness and sensory loss (known as 'stocking-glove anesthesia'). They may be classified by time course (acute or chronic); by the functions disturbed (motor, sensory, autonomic, mixed); or by the underlying pathology (demyelination, axonal degeneration, or both). Guillain–Barré syndrome, for example, is a subacute, predominantly motor, demyelinating neuropathy, whereas chronic alcohol abuse leads to a chronic, initially sensory then mixed, axonal neuropathy. Causes of polyneuropathies appear below.

Mostly motor	Mostly sensory
Guillain–Barré syndrome	Diabetes mellitus
Lead poisoning	Uremia
Charcot–Marie–Tooth syndrome	Leprosy

Symptoms *Sensory neuropathy:* Numbness; 'feels funny'; tingling or burning sensations often affecting the extremities first ('stocking-glove' distribution). There may be difficulty handling small objects such as a needle.

Motor neuropathy: Often progressive (may be rapid) weakness or clumsiness of the hands; difficulty walking (falls; stumbling); respiratory difficulty. Signs are those of LMN lesion: Wasting and weakness most marked in the distal muscles of hands and feet (foot or wrist drop). Reflexes are reduced or absent. Involvement of the respiratory muscles may be shown by a diminished vital capacity.

Cranial nerves: Difficulties swallowing; speaking; double vision; changes in facial sensation, facial weakness.

Diagnosis The history is vital; make sure you are clear about the illness's time course; the precise nature of the symptoms; any preceding or associated events (eg gastrointestinal or respiratory symptoms preceding Guillain–Barré syndrome; weight loss in cancer; arthralgia from a connective tissue disease); travel; sexual history (infections); alcohol use; medications; and family history. Pain is typical of neuropathies due to DM or alcohol. *Examination:* Do a careful neurological examination looking particularly for lower motor signs (weakness, wasting, reduced or absent reflexes) and sensory loss which should be carefully mapped out for each modality. Do not forget to assess the autonomic system and cranial nerves. Look also for signs of trauma (eg finger burns) indicating reduced sensation. Scuff marks on shoes suggest foot drop. If there is nerve thickening think of leprosy or Charcot–Marie–Tooth. Examine other systems for clues to the cause, eg signs of alcoholic liver disease.

Tests complete blood count, glucose, hemoglobin A1C, LFT, thyroid function tests, B_{12}, protein electrophoresis, ANCA(P&C), ANA, CXR, urinalysis, and consider a lumbar puncture in the appropriate clinical setting (concern for GBS or CIDP). In a patient with a distal sensory neuropathy and no clear cause, obtain a glucose tolerance test to identify patients in a 'pre-diabetic' state (which is a significant cause of peripheral neuropathy). Consider specific genetic tests for inherited neuropathies (eg Charcot–Marie–Tooth syndrome), lead levels, and antiganglioside antibodies. Nerve conduction studies are necessary for distinguishing demyelinating from axonal neuropathies.

Treatment Treat the cause if possible (eg withdraw precipitating drug). Involve physical therapists and occupational therapists. Care of the feet and shoe choice is important in sensory neuropathies to minimize trauma and subsequent disability. In Guillain–Barré syndrome and chronic inflammatory demyelinating polyradiculoneuropathy (CIDP), IV immunoglobulin helps. Steroids and other immunosuppressants may help vasculitic neuropathy.

Causes of polyneuropathies

Inflammatory
Guillain–Barré syndrome, CIDP, sarcoidosis

Metabolic
Diabetes mellitus, renal failure, hypothyroidism, hypoglycemia, mitochondrial disorders

Vasculitides
Polyarteritis nodosa, rheumatoid arthritis, Wegener's granulomatosis

Malignancy
Paraneoplastic syndromes (especially small cell lung cancer), polycythemia vera

Infections
Leprosy, syphilis, Lyme disease, HIV

Vitamin deficiencies and excesses
Lack of B_1, B_6, B_{12} (eg alcoholic), folate; also *excess* vit B_6 (100mg/d)

Inherited
Refsum's syndrome; Charcot–Marie–Tooth syndrome, porphyria, leukodystrophy (and many more)

Toxins
Lead, arsenic

Drugs
Alcohol, cisplatin, isoniazid, vincristine, nitrofurantoin. Less frequently: Metronidazole, phenytoin

Others
Paraproteinemias, eg multiple myeloma, amyloidosis, pre-diabetic states (impaired glucose tolerance)

Bell's palsy

An *idiopathic* palsy of the facial nerve (VII) resulting in a unilateral facial weakness or paralysis. Other causes of a facial palsy must be excluded before a diagnosis of Bell's palsy is made. Possible etiologies for Bell's palsy include a viral neuropathy—(HSV-1 has been implicated) and idiopathic inflammation.

Incidence ~20/100,000/yr; risk ↑ in pregnancy (3-fold) and diabetes (~5-fold)

Symptoms Onset of facial weakness is rapid and may occur with or be preceded by pain below the ear. Weakness worsens for 1 to 2d before stabilizing, and pain resolves within a few days. Symptoms and signs are unilateral If bilateral, consider other diagnoses (eg sarcoidosis; Lyme disease). Patients will experience weakness of the face, including the periocular muscles (difficulty closing the eye), drooling, impaired taste on the anterior tongue and hyperacusis (the perception of loud sounds due to a paralysis of the stapedius muscle which normally dampens down sounds).

Natural history Those with incomplete paralysis and no axonal degeneration typically recover completely within a few weeks (approximately 85% of patients with Bell's Palsy). Those with complete paralysis nearly all fully recover too but ~15% have axonal degeneration (recovery frequently begins only after 3 months, may be incomplete, fail to happen at all, or else will be complicated by the formation of aberrant reconnections). These produce synkinesis, eg eye blinking is accompanied by synchronous upturning of the mouth. Misconnection of parasympathetic fibers can produce so-called crocodile tears when eating stimulates unilateral lacrimation. Cutting the tympanic branch of IX solves this problem (rarely needed).

The House-Brackmann scale is commonly used to score patients with Bell's Palsy and can prognosticate recovery. The scale has six grades (1 through 6), with grade 1 being normal and grade 6 describing a patient with no movement whatsoever.

Tests *Electroneurography* at 1–3wks can predict delayed recovery by identifying axonal degeneration but does not influence management.

MRI and *LP* help rule out other diagnoses (only needed in atypical presentations such as bilateral Bell's palsy or a facial nerve palsy in the presence of other concominant cranial neuropathies).

Management If presentation is within 6d of onset, prednisone (eg 1mg/kg per day for 5 to 10d) is relatively safe and probably effective in improving facial function outcomes in patients, but data is not conclusive. Acyclovir, however, is considered by the American Academy of Neurology Practice Guidelines to be safe (in combination with prednisone) and *possibly* effective in treating Bell's palsy. Protect the eye with artificial tears if there is any evidence of drying. Encourage regular eyelid closure by pulling down the lid by hand Use tape to close the eyes at night. If ectropion is severe, lateral tarsorrhaphy (partial lid-to-lid suturing) can help.

Other causes of a VII nerve palsy

Infection
  Ramsay Hunt syndrome (cephalic herpes zoster). This is peripheral facial
    nerve palsy accompanied by an erythematous vesicular rash on the ear
    (zoster oticus) or in the mouth. (Famciclovir 500mg/8h PO + predniso-
    lone may be indicated.)
  Lyme disease
  HIV
  Meningitis
  Polio
  TB
  Chronic meningitis (eg fungal)
Brainstem lesions
  Brainstem tumor
  Stroke
  MS
Cerebello-pontine angle lesions
  Acoustic neuroma; meningioma
Systemic disease
  Diabetes mellitus
  Sarcoidosis (facial palsy is the most common CNS sign of sarcoidosis)
  Guillain–Barré syndrome
ENT and other rare causes
  Orofacial granulomatosis—recurrent VII palsies
  Parotid tumors
  Cholesteatoma
  Otitis media
  Trauma to skull base
  Pregnancy/delivery, via intracranial hypotension

Neuromuscular junction disorders

Myasthenia gravis (MG)

This is an antibody-mediated, autoimmune disease with too few functioning acetylcholine receptors on muscle, leading to muscle weakness. Anti-acetylcholine receptor antibodies are detectable in 80–90% of patients, and cause depletion of functioning postsynaptic receptor sites.

Presentation Can present at any age with ↑ muscular fatigue. If less than 50yrs old, myasthenia is more common in women, associated with other autoimmune diseases and thymic hyperplasia. Over 50yrs old, it is more common in men, and associated with thymic atrophy or, rarely, a thymic tumor. Muscle groups commonly affected (most likely first): Extraocular; bulbar; face; neck; limb girdle; trunk. Look especially for: Ptosis; diplopia; 'myasthenic snarl' on smiling. On counting aloud to 50, the voice weakens. Reflexes are normal. Weakness may be exacerbated by pregnancy, infection, overtreatment, change of climate, emotion, exercise, gentamicin, opiates, tetracycline, quinine, quinidine, procainamide and many other medications. *Associations:* Thymic tumor; hyperthyroidism; rheumatoid arthritis; SLE.

Diagnosis In the clinically appropriate situations, obtain an anti-acetylcholine receptor antibody titer. While the titer itself does not correlate with disease severity, a positive test is highly suggestive and the rise or fall in titer can be used to track the success of treatment. Additional tests include a single fiber repetitive stimulation EMG to look for decremental responses and, more rarely, the tensilon test. This pharmacologic test uses the administration of edrophonium (an anticholinesterase) to determine if a patients symptoms would improve with more acetylcholine at a neuromuscular junction. The test is difficult to assess and has significant risks associated with it, hence it is rarely used. Once the diagnosis of MG is established a CT scan of the chest is obtained to rule out thymic tumors. In patients with MG and thymic tumors, thymectomy can cause remission in a third of patients and significant improvement in another third of patients.

Treatment options

Symptomatic control with an anticholinesterase eg *pyridostigmine* 60–450mg/24h PO taken through the day. Side effects include diarrhea, salivation, lacrimation, vomiting, and miosis. Immunosuppression with prednisone, azathioprine, cyclosporin, and mycophenylate have all been utilized with success. Also, both plasmapheresis and IVIg have been used on 2–4wk schedules for patients with difficult to control symptoms or in patients suffering from myasthenic crises.

Myasthenic crisis is characterized by weakness significant enough to cause respiratory compromise. This occurs in 10–20% of patients at some time in the course of their disease and can be triggered by preceeding infections. Plasmapharesis is commonly used to treat patients in crisis.

Lambert–Eaton myasthenic syndrome

This typically occurs in association with small cell lung cancer (Lambert–Eaton syndrome) or, less commonly, with other autoimmune disease. Unlike true MG, it: Affects especially proximal limbs and trunk (rarely the eyes); there is *hypo*reflexia, only a slight response to edrophonium, repeated muscle contraction may lead to ↑ muscle strength and reflexes and it is the presynaptic membrane which is affected (the carcinoma provokes production of antibodies to Ca^{2+} channels).

Other causes of muscle fatigability Polymyositis; SLE; botulism; Takayasu's disease (fatigability of the extremities due to ischemia from the vasculitis).

Myopathies

Signs and symptoms *Muscle weakness* Rapid onset suggests a toxic, drug, or metabolic cause. *Excess fatigability* (weakness ↑ with exercise) may suggest MG versus storage disease myopathy. *Myotonia* (delayed muscular relaxation after contraction, eg on shaking hands) is characteristic of myotonic disorders. Spontaneous *pain* at rest occurs in inflammatory disease as does local tenderness. Pain on exercise suggests ischemia or metabolic myopathy (eg McArdle's disease). *Fasciculation* (spontaneous, irregular, and brief contractions of part of a muscle) suggest anterior horn cell or root disease. Look carefully for evidence of systemic disease. *Tests:* Consider EMG with or without muscle biopsy; and investigations relevant to systemic causes (eg TSH). Many genetic disorders of muscle can be detected by DNA analysis, and muscle biopsy is now reserved for when genetic tests are non-diagnostic (eg Duchenne's or myotonic dystrophy). *There are 5 main categories of myopathy:*

1 Muscular dystrophies are a group of genetic diseases with progressive degeneration and weakness of specific muscle groups. The primary abnormality may be in the muscle membrane. Secondary effects are marked variation in size of individual fibres and deposition of fat and connective tissue. The commonest is *Duchenne's muscular dystrophy* (sex-linked recessive—30% from spontaneous mutation) and is (almost always) confined to boys. The Duchenne gene is on the short arm of the X chromosome, and its product, dystrophin, is absent (or present in only very low levels). Serum creatine kinase is raised greater than 40-fold. It presents usually around 4yrs of age with increasingly clumsy walking, progressing to difficulty in standing and respiratory failure. Some survive beyond 20yrs. There is no specific treatment. Genetic counselling is vital. *Fascioscapulohumeral muscular dystrophy* (Landouzy–Dejerine) is almost as common. *Inheritance:* Autosomal dominant (4q35). *Typical age of onset:* 12–14yrs. *Early symptoms:* Inability to puff out the cheeks, difficulty raising the arms above the head (eg changing light-bulbs). *Signs:* Weakness of face, shoulders, and upper arms (often asymmetric with deltoids spared), with or without foot-drop and/or winging of the scapula. Twenty percent of patients will need a wheelchair by 40yrs old.

2 Myotonic disorders are characterized by myotonia (tonic spasm of muscle). Muscle histology shows long chains of central nuclei within the fibres. The chief disorder is *myotonic dystrophy* (autosomal dominant). Typical onset: 25yrs with weakness (hands, legs, sternocleidomastoids) and myotonia. Muscle wasting and weakness in the face gives a long, haggard appearance. Other features: Cataracts; frontal baldness (men); atrophy of testes or ovaries; cardiomyopathy; mild endocrine abnormalities (eg DM); and mental impairment. Most patients die in middle age of intercurrent illness. Genetic counselling is important.

3 Acquired myopathies of late onset are often a manifestation of systemic disease. Look carefully for evidence of: Carcinoma; thyroid disease (especially hyperthyroidism); Cushing's disease; hypo- and hypercalcaemia.

4 Inflammatory disorders: Inclusion-body myositis, polymyositis.

5 Toxic myopathies: Alcohol; statins; steroids; chloroquine; colchicine; procainamide; zidovudine; vincristine; cyclosporin; hypervitaminosis E; cocaine.

Myelopathies

The time course of symptom onset is critical for evaluating patients with myelopathic symptoms (UMN weakness, a sensory level, and/or bowel/bladder dysfunction). In the acute setting compressive lesions must be ruled out because of the urgent indication for surgical intervention. Traumatic spinal cord injuries are currently treated with massive doses of steroids, while non-traumatic, non-compressive myelopathies are evaluated and treated very differently. Certain facts about the patient's history is critical for determining the etiology of the myelopathy. For example, a patient that has a T10 sensory level and spinal cord dysfunction after an angiogram most probably has suffered an anterior spinal artery occlusion and spinal infarct due to disruption of blood supply in the artery of Adamkewicz.

Differential of non-compressive myelopathy: Acute and subacute pathologies include arterial infarct, venous hypertension (with or without infarct), transverse myelitis, MS, neuromyelitis optica, spinal cord ischemia related to spinal AV malformations and various spinal tumors (primary and metastatic). A gadolinium enhanced MRI of the spine and brain and lumbar puncture can be used to identify to causative process. Evidence of inflammation (enhancing lesion on MRI, pleocytosis, elevated protein, oligoclonal bands or IgG Index) supports the diagnosis of TM, MS, or NMO. In cases where an acute myelopathy has no clear cause, a spinal angiogram must be considered if a vascular malformation is suspected

Space-occupying lesions

Signs: Features of ↑ intracranial pressure, evolving focal neurologic symptom, seizures, false localizing signs, cognitive or behavioral change and local effects (eg proptosis). *Raised ICP:* Headache, vomiting, papilledema (only in 50% of tumors), altered consciousness (the most common finding in patients with ↑ ICP). *Seizures:* Seen in about 50% of tumors. Suspect in all adult-onset seizures especially if focal, or with a localizing aura or post-ictal weakness (Todd's palsy). *False localizing signs:* These are caused by ↑ ICP. Cranial nerve VI palsy is commonest due to its long intracranial course. *Subtle personality change.* Irritability, lack of application to tasks, lack of initiative, socially inappropriate behavior may be seen early in the process, but are non-specific.

Causes: Tumor (primary or secondary), aneurysm, abscess (25% multiple) chronic subdural hematoma, granuloma, (eg tuberculoma), cyst (eg cysticercosis). *Tumor histology:* 30% secondaries (breast, lung, melanoma; 50% multiple). Primaries include: Astrocytoma, glioblastoma multiforme, oligodendroglioma, ependymoma (all <50% 5yr survival), cerebellar hemangioblastoma (40% 20yr survival); meningioma (generally benign).

Differential diagnosis: Stroke, head injury, vasculitis, eg SLE, syphilis, PAN, giant cell arteritis, MS, encephalitis, post-ictal (Todd's palsy), metabolic, or electrolyte disturbances. Also colloid cyst of the 3rd ventricle and benign intracranial hypertension.

Tests: CT; MRI (good for posterior fossa masses). Consider biopsy. Extreme caution with lumbar punctures (performed only if absolutely necessary) due to risks of cerebellar herniation through the foramen magnum).

Tumor management: *Benign:* Complete removal if possible but some may be inaccessible. *Malignant:* Complete removal of gliomas is difficult as resection margins are rarely clear, but surgery does give a tissue diagnosis and allows debulking pre-radiotherapy. If a tumor is inaccessible but causing hydrocephalus, a ventriculo-peritoneal shunt can help. Radiotherapy is used post-op for gliomas or metastases and as sole therapy for some tumors if surgery is impossible. Chemotherapy is used in gliomas with limited benefit. Intracranial, chemotherapy impregnated wafers have improved outcome omewhat. Dexamethasone 4mg/8h PO for cerebral edema. Prophylatic dministration of antiepileptics in patients with newly diagnosed brain tumors s not recommended due to a lack of efficacy and the presence of side effects.

Prognosis: Complete removal of a benign tumor achieves cure but the rognosis of those with malignant tumors is poor.

Benign intracranial hypertension (pseudotumor cerebri) Think of this in hose presenting as if with a mass (headache, ↑ ICP and papilledema)—*when o mass is found.* Typical patients are obese women with blurred vision, and n enlarged blind spot, if papilledema is present (it usually is). Consciousness nd cognition are preserved. The opening pressure during lumbar punctures s usually elevated. *Cause:* Often unknown, or secondary to venous sinus hrombosis, or drugs, eg tetracycline, minocycline, nitrofurantoin, vitamin A, sotretinoin, danazol, and somatropin.

Treatment: Urgent lumbar punctures (with measurement of the opening ressure) may be indicated in patients with worsening symptoms. Aceta-zolamide, loop diuretics, advise weight loss. Consider optic nerve sheath enestration if drugs fail and visual loss is progressing. *Prognosis:* Often self-miting. Permanent significant visual loss in 10% (ie not so benign). CSF shunt-ng with or without optic nerve sheath fenestration can help vision.

Localizing signs

Temporal lobe Seizures (complex partial ± automatisms); hallucinations (smell, taste, sound, *déja vu*); complex partial with automatisms; dysphasia; field defect (contralateral upper quadrantanopia); forgetfulness; psychosis; fear/rage; hypersexuality.

Frontal lobe Hemiparesis; seizures (focal motor seizures, eg aversive seizures involving head and eyes); personality changes (indecent; indolent; indiscreet); positive grasp reflex (fingers drawn across palm are grasped) significant only if unilateral; aphasia (Broca's area); loss of smell unilaterally. *Orbitofrontal syndrome:* Lack of empathy; disinhibition; diminished social skills; over-eating; rash actions (mania); unconscious imitation of postures (eg when you put your feet on the desk, or sit on the floor).

Parietal lobe Hemisensory loss; diminished 2-point discrimination; astere-ognosis (inability to recognize object in hand by touch alone); sensory inattention; aphasia; Gerstmann's syndrome ie left–right disorientation, finger agnosia, acalculia, and agraphia).

Occipital lobe Contralateral visual field defects (homonymous hemiano-pia); hallucinations such as palinopsia (persisting or recurring images, once the stimulus has left the field of view).

Cerebellum ('DASHING') **D**ysdiadochokinesis; **a**taxia (truncal); **s**lurred speech; **h**ypotonia; **i**ntention tremor; **n**ystagmus; **g**ait abnormality.

Dysdiadochokinesis is impaired *rapidly alternating* movements, eg pronation–supination.

Cerebellopontine angle (Usually vestibular schwannoma). Ipsilateral deafness; nystagmus; reduced corneal reflex, facial weakness; ipsilateral cerebellar signs, papilledema, and cranial nerve VI palsies.

Midbrain (eg pineal gland tumors or midbrain infarction) Failure of up or down gaze; light/near dissociated pupil responses, with convergence retrac-tion nystagmus—upward saccadic retracting pulses from co-contraction of opposing horizontal muscles, precipitated by attempted up-gaze. The eyes retract in their sockets because of contraction of the medial recti, eg while looking at a down-moving target.

Neuroradiology

Computer tomography (CT) works by identifying x-ray attenuation of materials, measured in Hounsfield units (HU), eg bone +1000, water 0, and air −1000 HU. You see the x-ray attenuation of an area as a shade of gray. At the extremes, high attenuation is white and low attenuation is black. The attenuation of biological soft tissues is in a narrow range from about +80 for blood and muscle, to 0 for CSF, and down to −100 for fat. IV contrast may be given demonstrating initially an angiographic effect, the high attenuation contrast in the vessels making them appear white. Later, if there is a defect in the blood-brain barrier, as with neoplasms or infection, contrast will extravasate, giving an enhancing, white area in the cerebrum or cerebellum. Some intracranial components do not have a blood–brain barrier and enhance normally: Eg the pituitary gland and choroid plexus.

Compared with MRI, CT is good at showing acute hemorrhage and fractures, and is much easier to do in ill or anesthetized patients—so it is invaluable in emergencies. Fresh blood is of higher attenuation (ie whiter) than brain tissue. Attenuation of hematomas declines as hemoglobin breaks down so that a sub-acute subdural hematoma at 2wks may have an attenuation same as adjacent brain, making it difficult to detect. A chronic subdural hematoma will be of relatively low attenuation.

CT is commonly performed in acute stroke to exclude hemorrhage (eg pre-thrombolytics). An area of ischemia will not show up for a day or so, and will be low-attenuation cytotoxic edema (intracellular edema mainly confined to the grey matter).

Tumors and abscesses can have common features, eg ring enhancing mass, surrounding vasogenic edema, and mass effect. Vasogenic edema is extracellular and spreads through the white matter. Mass effect can cause compression of the sulci and ipsilateral ventricle. It may also cause subfalcine, transtentorial or tonsillar herniation.

One indication for CT scan is acute, severe headache. If there is concern about subarachnoid hemorrhage, a non-contrast CT may show acute blood. Even if it does not, it will show if the basal cisterns are normal and therefore lumbar puncture is probably safe.

Magnetic resonance imaging (MRI) An image is made by disturbing a nucleus in a strong magnetic field by using a radiofrequency pulse at the resonant frequency, and detecting the signal as the nucleus (usually hydrogen) returns to equilibrium. The chief image sequences are:

- *T1 weighted images:* Give good anatomical detail to which the T2 image can be compared/related. Fat is brightest (↑ signal intensity) other tissues are darker to varying degrees. Flowing blood appears black ('flow voids')
- *T2 weighted images:* These provide the best detection of pathology, most pathology having some edema fluid, therefore appearing white. Fat and fluid appear brightest.

Advantages of MRI:
Non-ionizing radiation
Shows vasculature without contrast
Images can easily be produced in any
plane, eg sagital or coronal
Visualization of posterior fossa and
other areas prone to bony artifact
on CT, eg at the cranio-cervical
junction. MRI images the posterior
fossa extremely well.
High inherent soft tissue contrast
Precise staging of malignancy, eg
involvement of bone marrow

Disadvantages of MRI:
High cost
Claustrophobia (in magnet tunnel
for 15–60min—sedation may be
needed)
Motion artifact and longer time for
image acquisition
Unhelpful in imaging calcium
Unsuitable for those with ferromag-
netic foreign bodies (pacemakers,
CNS vascular clips, cochlear
implants, valves, shrapnel, etc.)
Difficult in anesthetized patients
Gadolinium may be harmful in
patients with renal failure p650

Rheumatology and musculoskeletal conditions

John A. Flynn, M.D., M.B.A.

Contents

Important points in assessing for rheumatic disease

Is there a history to suggest inflammation?
• Morning stiffness (>30min)
• Joint swelling, warmth, or redness
• Loss of function.

How many joints are involved?
• One → monoarthritis
• Several (2–4) → oligoarthritis
• Many (>4) → polyarthritis.

Are there any extra-articular manifestations?

Also consider: age, gender, occupation, family history, ancestry (eg SLE more common in women and African-Americans).

	• Presenting symptoms	• Rheumatological and related
Joints:	Morning stiffness (eg RA)	diseases: eg Crohn's/UC in ankylosing spondylitis; psoriasis; gonorrhea, or reactive arthritis
	Pattern of distribution; mono vs. polyarticular	
	Swelling; loss of function	• Current & past drugs: Disease modifying drugs, eg methotrexate et al
Extra-articular:	Rashes, photosensitivity (SLE)	
	Raynaud's (SLE; CREST; poly- and dermatomyositis)	• Family history: Arthritis; psoriasis (psoriatic arthritis, ankylosing spondylitis)
	Dry eyes or mouth (Sjögren's)	
	Diarrhea/urethritis (Reactive arthritis)	• Social history: Functioning, eg dressing, writing, walking, ADLs, social support, home adaptations
	Red eyes, eg ank. spond., Nodules or nodes (RA, sarcoid, SLE, TB, and gouty tophi)	
	Mouth/genital ulcers (Behçet's)	
	Weight loss (eg TB arthritis)	

Features of inflammatory arthritis Pain, stiffness (especially morning), loss of function, and signs of inflammation at 1 or more joints.

Causes—Monoarthritis	Polyarthritis (eg >4 swollen painful joints)
Septic arthritis (eg staph, strep, Gram −ve bacilli, gonococci, TB)	Viruses, eg mumps, rubella, parvovirus B19, EBV, hepatitis B, enteroviruses, HIV, α-viral arthropathy
Psoriatic and reactive arthritides	Rheumatoid (RA) or osteoarthritis (OA)
Trauma (hemarthrosis)	Spondyloarthritis
Calcium pyrophosphate dihydrate (CPPD) crystals; gout	Connective tissue diseases (eg scleroderma, SLE)
Osteoarthritis	Crystal arthropathies (gout, CPPD)
Monoarthritic presentation of a polyarticular disease (eg RA).	Post-streptococcal reactive arthritis
	Sarcoidosis.

Assess Extent of joint involvement (include spine), symmetry, disruption of joint involvement, limitation of movement, effusions and peri-articular involvement. Associated features: Dysuria or genital ulcers, skin or eye involvement, lungs, kidneys, heart, GI (eg mouth ulcers, bloody diarrhea), and CNS

Urine: Dipstick urine for blood and protein. If +ve, arrange urgent microscopy (?casts), culture, and Gram stain.

Radiology: Look for erosions, calcification, loss of joint space, changes in underlying bone (eg periarticular osteoporosis, sclerotic areas, osteophytes) of affected joints. Image sacroiliac joints if considering a spondyloarthritis (irregularity of lower third); CXR in RA, SLE, vasculitis, and TB. In septic arthritis x-rays may be normal, as may be ESR and CRP (if CRP ↑, expect it to fall with treatment).

Septic arthritis Consider septic arthritis in any acute monoarthritis. Features may be less overt if immunosuppressed or if underlying joint disease. Aspirate the joint. Look for blood, crystals, and pus (polarized light microscopy, culture, Gram stain). Sepsis may damage a joint within 24h. If in doubt, treat initially for sepsis, as described below.

Joint aspiration: Microscopy (+culture): Any blood, crystals, or pus? Do polarized light microscopy for urate or CPPD crystals (p370).

Blood: Culture if sepsis is possible. CBC, ESR, uric acid, urea, and creatinine if systemic disease. Rheumatoid factor, antinuclear antibody, and other autoantibodies (p377). Consider HIV serology.

Treatment is determined by the cause. If *septic arthritis* is suspected, provide analgesia and immediate antibiotics. Oxacillin or cefazolin for meth sensitive staph; vancomycin if meth resistance is suspected, 3rd generation cephalosporin if Gram – is suspected, until sensitivities are known. Look for atypical mycobacteria and fungi if HIV +ve. Request ID consultant for how long to continue treatment (eg. 2wks IV, then 3wks PO).

Repeat aspiration (arthrocentesis), if no improvement (falling joint WBCs and culture becoming sterile) then consider lavage, and arthroscopic debridement—(eg for knee) or open (eg for hip or shoulder; this allows biopsy—helpful for TB). Ask for orthopedic consult. If a joint prosthesis is *in situ*, get orthopedic consult before aspiration. Try to determine the source of infection. Is there immunosuppression, or a focus of infection (eg pneumonia, in 50% of those with pneumococcal arthritis)?

Synovial fluid analysis

Aspiration of synovial fluid is primarily used to look for infection or crystal (gout and CPPD crystal arthritis.

	Appearance	Viscosity	WBC/mm³	Neutrophils
Normal	Clear, colorless	↑	≤200	None
Non-inflammatory[1]	Clear, straw	↑	≤5000	≤25%
Hemorrhagic[2]	Bloody, xanthochromic	Varies	≤10,000	≤50%
Acutely inflamed[3]	Turbid, yellow	↓		
• Crystal			~14,000	~80%
• Rheumatic fever			~18,000	~50%
• RA			~16,000	Varies
Septic	Turbid, yellow	↓		
• Tb			~20,000	~70%
• Gonorrheal			~10,000	~60%
• Septic (non-gonococcal)[4]			~50,000	~95%

1 Eg degenerative joint disease.
2 Eg tumors, hemophilia, trauma.
3 Eg Reactive arthritis, CPPD crystals, SLE.
4 Includes staphs, streps, and *Pseudomonas* (eg post-op).

Back pain

This is very common, and often self-limiting; *but be alert to 'red flags' that may indicate serious underlying causes.* Key points in the history: (1) Onset: Sudden (related to trauma?) or gradual? (2) Are there motor or sensory symptoms? (3) Is bladder or bowel affected? Pain worse with movement and relieved by rest is often mechanical. If it is worse after rest, an inflammatory cause should be considered like ankylosing spondylitis. (4) Constitutional symptoms (fever, weight loss, night sweats)

Examination: (1) With the patient standing (legs straight), gauge the extent and smoothness of lumbar forward/lateral flexion and extension. (2) Neurological deficits: Peri-anal sensation; upper and lower motor neuron (UMN & LMN) signs in legs (p310); (3) Signs of generalized disease suggest malignancy.

Nerve root impingement causes pain in relevant dermatomes, and can be worsened by bending forward. A positive straight leg raising sign occurs when a supine patient experiences pain in buttock/back/other leg when lifting leg to <45°. It suggests lumbar disc herniation impinging on nerve roots. (Its sensitivity is ~0.9 and its specificity is 0.2.)

Neurosurgical emergencies • *Acute cauda equina compression:* Alternating or bilateral root pain in legs, saddle anesthesia (ie bilaterally around anus), and disturbance of bladder or bowel function • *Acute cord compression:* Bilateral pain, LMN signs at level of compression, UMN and sensory signs below, sphincter disturbance. Causes (same for both types of compression): Bony metastasis (look for missing pedicle on x-ray), myeloma, cord or paraspinal tumor, TB (p506), abscess. Urgent treatment needed to prevent irreversible loss: Laminectomy for disc protrusions; decompression for abscess; radiotherapy for tumors.

Tests MRI is the best way to image cord compression, myelopathy, spinal neoplasms, cysts, hemorrhages, and abscesses. CBC, ESR (↑ in myeloma, infections, tumors), PSA, and bone scan 'hot spot' suggest neoplastic diagnoses.

Causes Age determines the most likely causes.
• 15–30yrs: Herniated disc, trauma, fractures, ankylosing spondylitis (AS) (p372), spondylolisthesis (eg L5 shifts forward on S1).
• 30–50yrs: Degenerative spinal disease, herniated disc, malignancy (lung, breast, prostate).
• >50yrs: Degenerative, osteoporosis compression fracture, Paget's, malignancy, myeloma (request serum electrophoresis), lumbar spinal stenosis.

Rarer causes: Cauda equina tumors, spinal infection (usually staphylococcal, also TB).

Treatment Specific causes need specific treatment. For most back pain a specific cause is not found, so treat empirically: Avoid precipitants; arrange physical therapy. Analgesia and normal activities is better than bed rest. In certain patients there are roles for disc, epidural or nerve root injections and surgical procedures: Foramenotomy, stabilization, or laminectomy.

Features of serious causes of back pain
• Young (<20yrs) or old (>55yrs)
• Trauma
• Alternating sciatica
• Bilateral sciatica
• Weak legs
• Weight loss
• FUO; ESR↑ (>25mm/h)
• Systemic steroids or immuno-suppressive use
• Progressive, continuous, non-mechanical pain
• Constitutionally ill; drug abuse; HIV +ve
• Spine pain in *all* directions of movement
• Localized bony tenderness
• CNS deficit at more than one root level
• Pain or tenderness of thoracic spine
• Bilateral nerve impingement
• Past history of malignancy.

Rheumatoid arthritis (RA)

Typically a persistent, symmetrical, deforming, polyarthritis often affecting hands and feet. Peak onset: 5th decade. ♀:♂ > 2:1. Prevalence: 0.5–1% (higher in smokers). Genetics: HLA DR4 linked in caucasians.

Presentation Typically with swollen, painful, and stiff hands and feet, especially in the morning. This can fluctuate and larger joints become involved. Less common presentations are:

1 Recurring monoarthritis of various joints (*palindromic*).
2 Persistent monoarthritis (often of 1 knee).
3 Systemic illness (pericarditis, pleurisy, weight↓) with minimal joint problems at first. (More common in men.)
4 Sudden onset of widespread arthritis.

Signs At first, swollen fingers and MCP joint swelling. Later, ulnar deviation at MCPS and dorsal wrist subluxation. Boutonnière and swan-neck deformities of fingers (see BOX) or Z-deformity of thumbs. Hand extensor tendons may rupture and adjacent muscles waste. Foot changes are similar. Larger joints may be involved. Atlanto-axial joint subluxation may threaten the cervical spinal cord.

Extra-articular Anemia; nodules; lymphadenopathy; vasculitis; carpal tunnel syndrome; multifocal neuropathies; splenomegaly (5%; but only 1% have Felty's syndrome: Splenomegaly & granulocytopenia). Eyes: Episcleritis; scleritis; kerato-conjunctivitis sicca. Other signs: Pleurisy; pericarditis. Pulmonary fibrosis. Osteo-porosis. Amyloidosis. Associated with ↑ risk of ischemic heart disease and lymphomas.

X-rays ↑Soft tissue; juxta-articular osteoporosis; ↓joint space. Later: Bony erosions ± subluxation ± complete carpal destruction.

Blood tests ESR↑; HB↓; MCV ↔; WBC↓; platelets↑. *Rheumatoid factor* often –ve at start, becoming +ve in 80% (also +ve in: Sjögren's: 80%; SLE: 30%; mixed connective tissue disease (MCTD): 30%; systemic sclerosis: 30%); ANA +ve in 30%.

Anti-CCP (cyclic citrullinated peptide) can be seen in early polyarthritis when RF negative indicating early RA.

Treatment Encourage regular exercise, physio- and occupational therapy.
• Assistive devices and appropriate orthotics, eg wrist splints. • Intra-articular steroids. • Oral drugs: If no contraindication (asthma, active peptic ulcer) start an NSAID: Often, NSAIDs, such as ibuprofen 400mg/8h, after food do not control symptoms or are not tolerated (GI bleeds). Consider COX II selective NSAID if needing maximum dose regular NSAID or age >65; celecoxib 200mg/12h PO. Patients who need low dose aspirin ± prednisone may also need regular proton pump inhibitor. One cannot predict which NSAID a patient will respond to: Different ones can be tried. Disease-modifying anti-rheumatic drugs (DMARDS) should be considered early (see BOX). Regular monitoring is vital.
• Steroids may ↓joint damage and control difficult symptoms—eg prednisone 7.5mg/d PO, but place in treatment schema is controversial. One problem is ↓ bone density over long periods.
• Manage cardiovascular risk factors (p106) as atherosclerosis is accelerated. • Surgery—to relieve pain, improve function, and to prevent disease complications (eg radial-carpal fusion; joint replacements).

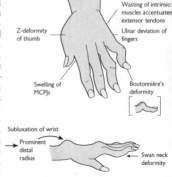

Z-deformity of thumb

Wasting of intrinsic muscles accentuates extensor tendons

Ulnar deviation of fingers

Swelling of MCPJs

Boutonnière's deformity

Subluxation of wrist

Prominent distal radius

Swan neck deformity

Influencing biological events in RA

The chief biological event is inflammation. Monocytes traffic into joints, cytokines are produced, fibroblasts and endothelial cells are activated, and tissue proliferates. Inflammatory fluid is generated (synovial effusion) and cytokines and cellular processes erode cartilage and bone. Cytokines also produce systemic effects: Fatigue, accelerated atherosclerosis, and accelerated bone turnover.

Disease-modifying drugs (DMARDs) Start DMARDs if there is persisting synovitis for >6wks. Sulfasalazine and methotrexate are typical 1st choices and are often used together.

- *Sulfasalazine:* Common SE: Nausea, headaches, diarrhea, marrow↓, reversible sperm count↓, rash, oral ulcers.
- *Methotrexate:* Avoid in liver disease and pregnancy and if alcohol consumption↑; caution if pre-existing lung disease. SE: Mucositis, nausea, fatigue/lethargy, pneumonitis (rare; can be life-threatening), AST & ALT↑. Give concurrent folate supplements, eg folic acid 1mg/d, PO.
- *Cyclosporin:* SE: Nausea, tremor, gingival hypertrophy, hypertension, renal impairment/hypertension.
- *Leflunomide* ↓ autoimmune effects (takes months to work). For 1st 6 months, do CBC & chemistry monthly. Stop if: Platelets <150×10⁹/L; WBC <4×10⁹/L, or AST↑ by >3-fold or rashes.
- *Gold:* SE: Marrow↓, proteinuria, rash, hepatitis.
- *Azathioprine:* SE: Marrow↓, nausea, LFT↑, oncogenic (do TPMT† test 1st).
- *Hydroxychloroquine:* SE: Rash, diarrhea, rarely retinopathy, tinnitus, headache.

Anti-cytokine therapy *Tumor necrosis factor α (TNFα)* is a key cytokine over-produced in RA synovium. Infliximab (chimeric murine/human anti-TNF antibody given IV every 8wks), etanercept (TNFα receptor/Ig Fc fusion protein given 25mg SC twice weekly or 50mg weekly), and *adalimumab* (fully human anti-TNF monoclonal given as 40mg SC every 2wks). SE: Rashes, nausea, diarrhea, and infections (eg reactivation of TB). ANA and even SLE-type illness can evolve. Long-term safety issues are unclear (?↑risk of cancer, multiple sclerosis) but responses can be striking compared with other DMARDs.

Immune modulator therapy Abatacept (binds to CD86 and CD80 receptors on antigen presenting cells with down-regulation of T cell activation given IV every 4 weeks). SE: exacerbation of COPD, headaches, nausea. Rituximab (a monoclonal antibody that binds to CD20 antigen on B lymphocytes reducing B cell function). Given in combination with methotrexate and prednisone as two separate IVs 2 weeks apart. SE: fevers, chills, headache, rash, nausea, hepatitis B reactivation and progressive multifocal leukoencephalopathy (PML) reported.

Forms of arthritis not associated with rheumatoid factor (sero −ve)

Lyme disease, Behçet's, leukemia, pulmonary osteoarthropathy, endocarditis, acromegaly, Wilson's disease, familial Mediterranean fever, sarcoid, hemophilia, sickle-cell, hemochromatosis, and infections, eg from:

Post-streptococcal	Hepatitis B	Rubella
Parvovirus B19	Chl pneumoniae	Ureaplasma; HIV
Vibrio parahemolyticus	Borrelia burgdorferi	Clostridium difficile

Chronic arthritis in children (ie before 16yrs) takes several forms, and is classified into juvenile idiopathic arthritis (JIA) subforms:

- Systemic arthritis (or Still's disease)
- Oligoarthritis (1–4 joints affected in first 6 months)
- Polyarthritis (RhF −ve, ANA +ve)
- Polyarthritis (RhF +ve)
- Psoriatic arthritis
- Enthesitis-related arthritis at ligament/tendon insertion into bone.

NB: JIA shares only some features with RA:

JIA shares these in common with RA:	*JIA and RA differ in these ways:*
Both display destructive arthritis	RA is more likely to run in families
Autoimmune with autoantibodies	RA is more homogeneous than JIA
Both have HLA associations	RA has poorer outcomes than JIA

Children with chronic arthritis need regular ophthalmic review to detect occult uveitis—and regular monitoring of growth and development.

Thiopurine methyl transferase—deficiency of this enzyme can lead to bone marrow suppression in the setting of azathioprine use.

Osteoarthritis (OA)

OA is the commonest joint condition. Women are prone to symptomatic OA ($\varphi:\sigma \approx 3:1$). *Mean age at onset:* 50yrs. OA is usually primary, but may be secondary to any joint disease/injury or some diseases (eg hemochromatosis).

Signs & symptoms In single joints, pain on movement, worse at end of day; background pain at rest; minimal stiffness; joint instability. In polyarticular OA with Heberden's nodes ('nodal OA'), the most commonly affected joints are DIP, thumb metacarpophalangeal joints, cervical and lumbar spine, and knee. There may be joint tenderness, derangement, ± bony swelling (eg Heberden's nodes, ie bony lumps at DIP joints), poor range of movement, and some (usually limited) synovitis.

Imaging/tests *Radiology:* Loss of joint space, subchondral sclerosis and cysts, osteophytes. *CRP* usually normal.

Treatment Acetaminophen for pain. If no good, try NSAIDs (see BOX). Reduce weight; walking aids; supportive footwear; physical therapy. Do exercises (eg regular quadriceps exercises in knee OA) and keep active. Joint replacement for end-stage OA.

Crystal-induced arthritis   PLATE 16

Gout In the acute stage there is severe pain, redness, and swelling of the joint—often the metatarsophalangeal joint of the big toe (podagra). Attacks are due to the deposition of monosodium urate crystals in and around joints and may be precipitated by trauma, surgery, starvation, infection, or diuretics. With long-term hyperuricemia, after repeated attacks, urate deposits (tophi) develop, eg finger pads, tendons, joints, pinna. 'Secondary' causes: Polycythemia, psoriasis, leukemia, cytotoxics, renal impairment, long-term alcohol excess.

Diagnosis depends on finding urate crystals in tissues and synovial fluid (serum urate not always↑). Synovial fluid microscopy: Negatively birefringent crystals; neutrophils (+ingested crystals). X-rays may show only soft-tissue swelling in the early stages. Later, well-defined 'punched out' lesions are seen in juxta-articular bone. Sclerotic reaction develops later creating an 'overhanging edge' or 'rat-bite' erosion. Joint spaces are preserved until late. *Prevalence:* ~½–1%. $\sigma:\varphi \approx 5:1$.

Treating acute gout: Use a NSAID unless contraindicated (eg peptic ulcer, renal insufficiency): Steroids are effective (40–60mg PO with rapid taper over 6–10d) Oral colchicine has a narrow therapeutic window. Avoid IV colchicine (get expert help). *Preventing attacks:* Avoid prolonged fasts, alcohol excess, and high purine food. Lose weight. Avoid low-dose aspirin (it ↑ serum urate). Consider reducing serum urate with long-term allopurinol, but not until 3wks after an attack. Start with regular NSAID or colchicine cover (0.6mg PO q day) as introduction of allopurinol may cause gout attack. *Allopurinol dose:* Start at low dose (100mg/24h PO), adjust monthly in the light of serum urate levels to achieve <6mg/dL. Haste makes waste! (typically 300–400mg/24h max 300mg/8h). SE: Rash, fever, WBC↓. If simple treatment fails, refer to a rheumatologist.

Calcium pyrophosphate dihydrate (CPPD) arthritis Risk factors:
• Dehydration • Intercurrent illness • Hyperparathyroidism   • Myxedema
• PO_4^{3-}↓; Mg^{2+}↓ • Osteoarthritis   • Hemochromatosis   • Acromegaly

Acute CPPD monoarthritis (pseudogout): Similar to gout; affects different joints (mainly wrist or knee). *Chronic CPPD:* Destructive changes like OA, but more severe; affecting knees (also wrists, shoulders, hips). Can present as polyarthritis (pseudo-rheumatoid) *Tests:* Polarized light microscopy of joint fluid Crystals are weakly positively birefringent. Associated with soft-tissue calcium deposition on x-ray, eg triangular ligament in wrist or in knee cartilage (chondrocalcinosis). *Treatment:* NSAIDs help but are rarely sufficient and often contraindicated in the elderly; consider steroid joint injection for mono-arthritis, oral or parenteral administration for greater that 2 joints with taper over 1–2wks. For chronic disease, consider colchicine 0.6mg/d.

Prescribing NSAIDs: Patient education

Most patients prescribed NSAIDs do not need them all the time, but some patients obediently take them continuously, as prescribed, with potential serious side-effects, such as GI bleeding. So explain to your patients that:
- Drugs are for relief of symptoms: *On good days none may be needed.*
- Abdominal pain may be a sign of impending problems: Stop the medication and notify your physician.
- Ulcers may occur with no warning: *Report black stool or lightheadedness at once.*
- Don't supplement prescribed NSAIDs with ones bought over the counter (eg ibuprofen): Mixing NSAIDs can ↑ risks greatly.
- Smoking and alcohol ↑NSAID risk.

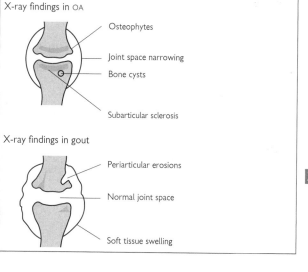

X-ray findings in OA

- Osteophytes
- Joint space narrowing
- Bone cysts
- Subarticular sclerosis

X-ray findings in gout

- Periarticular erosions
- Normal joint space
- Soft tissue swelling

Spondyloarthritis

Ankylosing spondylitis (AS) *Prevalence:* 0.25–1%. *Men present earlier:* ♂:♀ ≈ 6:1 at 16yrs old, and ≈ 2:1 at 30yrs old. >85% are HLA B27 +ve.

Symptoms: The typical patient is a young man presenting with low back pain, spinal morning stiffness, progressive loss of spinal movement (spinal ankylosis) who later develops kyphosis and cervical ankylosis. Other features and associations:

- Chest wall expansion ↓
- Chest pain
- Hip involvement
- Knee involvement
- Enthesitis[1] of calcaneal, tibial or ischial tuberosities, or plantar fascia
- Crohn's/UC
- Amyloid
- Carditis; iritis; recurrent sterile urethritis
- Aortic valve disease
- Psoriaform rashes
- Osteoporosis

Investigations: Diagnosis is clinical, supported by radiology findings (may be normal in early disease). Look for irregularities, erosions, or sclerosis affecting both sides of the lower third of the sacroiliac joints. Later: Squaring of the vertebra, 'bamboo spine', erosions of the apophyseal joints, obliteration of the sacroiliac joints (sacroiliitis also occurs in reactive arthritis, Crohn's disease, psoriatic arthritis, Brucella arthritis). Other tests: CBC (normochromic anemia); ESR↑; ↑CRP.

Treatment: Exercise, not rest, for backache; physical therapy regimens to maintain posture and mobility. NSAIDs may help pain and stiffness. Sulfasalazine and methotrexate help peripheral arthritis and enthesitis, but not spinal inflammation. Efficacy is proved with anti-TNF therapies. Rarely, spinal osteotomy is useful. Difficult-to-fix osteoporotic spinal fractures can occur (long term bisphosphonates may prevent this).

Enteropathic spondyloarthritis Inflammatory bowel disease (Crohn's and UC) are associated with spondyloarthritis.

Psoriatic arthritis Often asymmetrical, involves DIP joints, spine, typically causing dactylitis (sausage digits). X-ray changes can be misinterpreted as OA. Associated with synovitis, acneiform rashes, palmo-plantar pustulosis, hyperostoses and (sterile) osteomyelitis (SAPHO). Responds to NSAIDs, methotrexate, cyclosporin, and anti-TNFα therapy (p369).

Reactive arthritis *Presentation:* Secondary to *Chlamydia trachomatis* urethritis, *Campylobacter jejuni*, *Salmonella*, *Shigella*, and *Yersinia* species. A typical story: A young man with recent non-specific urethritis which may be asymptomatic; it may also follow dysentery. Often large joint, lower limb mono- or oligoarthritis or enthesitis; it may be chronic or relapsing. *Also:* Iritis, keratoderma blenorrhagica (brown, aseptic abscesses on soles and palms) and circinate balanitis—painless serpiginous penile rash; mouth ulcers; enthesitis (plantar fasciitis, Achilles tendonitis) and aortic regurgitation. *Tests:* ESR & CRP ↑ or ↔. Culture stool if diarrhea. Obtain sexual history. X-rays: Periostitis at ligamentous entheses; enthesopathic erosions. *Management:* Rest; splint affected joints; NSAIDs or steroids. Consider sulfasalazine or methotrexate. Treating the original infection makes little difference on outcome.

---

1 Enthesitis ≈ painful inflammation/fasciitis where bone meets a ligament, or tendon.

Spondyloarthritis typically hold these features in common

1 Seronegativity (rheumatoid factor –ve).
2 Pathology in spine (spondylo-) and sacroiliac (SI) joints, ie 'axial arthritis'.
3 Asymmetrical large-joint oligoarthritis (ie few joints) or monoarthritis.
4 Inflamed tendon ligament union sites (enthesitis), eg plantar fasciitis, Achilles tendonitis, costochondritis, or digit (finger and toe) tendon sheaths (dactylitis).
5 Extra-articular manifestations eg: Uveitis, psoriaform rashes, Crohn's, UC.
6 HLA B27 association (84–96% of those with AS).

Different forms of spondyloarthritis show much overlap with one another. They are treated with physical and occupational therapy, advice on posture, NSAIDs, sulfasalazine, methotrexate, and TNF inhibitors.

Autoimmune connective tissue diseases

Included under this heading are: SLE, diffuse/limited cutaneous systemic sclerosis, primary Sjögren's syndrome, idiopathic inflammatory myopathies, MCTD, and relapsing polychondritis. They overlap with each other, may affect many organ systems, and often respond to immunosuppressives.

Systemic lupus erythematosus (SLE)

SLE is a non-organ-specific, autoimmune disease in which autoantibodies are produced against a variety of autoantigens (ANA). Immunopathology results in polyclonal B-cell secretion of pathogenic autoantibodies and subsequent formation of immune complexes which deposit in sites such as the kidneys. $\female : \male \approx 9:1$. *Prevalence:* ~0.2%. *Common in:* Pregnancy; African-Americans; Asians—and if HLA B8, DR2 or DR3 +ve. ~10% of relatives of SLE patients are affected. It is a remitting and relapsing illness, with peak age at diagnosis being 30–40yrs. *Clinical features:* See BOX. In addition: $T° \uparrow$ (77%); splenomegaly; lymphadenopathy; alopecia (in 70%) recurrent abortion; retinal exudates; fibrosing alveolitis; myalgia (50%); anorexia (40%); myositis; migraine (40%); $ESR \uparrow$ (CRP often $\leftrightarrow$: Think of SLE whenever someone has a multisystem disorder and $ESR \uparrow$ but $CRP \leftrightarrow$).

Immunogenetics >95% are ANA +ve. High titer of antibodies directed against double-stranded DNA is nearly exclusive to SLE. Its absence does not exclude it. 11% have false +ve syphilis serology from IgG anticardiolipin antibodies. Antibodies to Ro (SS-A), La (SS-B), and U1 ribonuclear protein help define overlap syndromes (eg with Sjögren's).

Monitoring activity *3 best tests:* (1) ESR (2) Complement: $C3 \downarrow$, $C4 \downarrow$; $C3d \uparrow$ (denotes degradation products of C3, hence it moves in the opposite way) (3) Double-stranded (anti-DS) DNA antibody titers. *Others:* Urinalysis, electrolytes, CBC.

Drug-induced lupus This can be caused by isoniazid, hydralazine (in slow acetylators), procainamide, chlorpromazine, minocycline, TNF inhibitors. Lung and skin signs prevail over renal and CNS signs. It remits if the drug is stopped. Sulfonamides and birth control pills may exacerbate idiopathic SLE.

Antiphospholipid syndrome SLE may occur with arterial or venous thrombosis, livedo rash, stroke, adrenal hemorrhage, migraine, miscarriages, myelitis, myocardial infarct, multi-infarct dementia, and cardiolipin antibodies. *Presentation:* Abdominal pain (55%); $BP \downarrow$ (54%); fever (40%); nausea (31%); weakness (31%), altered mental status (19%). Venous thrombi occur more often if lupus anticoagulant is +ve, and arterial thrombi if IgG or IgM antiphospholipid antibody +ve. $R:$ Long-term warfarin (INR $\approx$ 3) may be used.

Treatment Refer to a rheumatologist. NSAIDs. Sun-block creams.
- *Hydroxychloroquine* if joint or skin symptoms are uncontrolled by NSAIDs, 200mg BID. SE: Irreversible retinopathy—annual ophthalmic referral is recommended.
- *High-dose prednisone* is kept for severe episodes of SLE (~1mg/kg/24h PO for 6wks or pulse IV methylprednisolone), may be combined with other immunosuppressive agents (eg cyclophosphamide), or 'steroid-sparing agents', eg azathioprine, methotrexate, or mycophenolate.
- *Low-dose steroids* may be of value in chronic disease.
- *Cyclophosphamide* is indicated for some nephritides. Dose example: 0.5–3mg/kg/d PO; intermittent pulses of 20mg/kg/month IV—give fewer SE.
- *Azathioprine* 1–2.5mg/kg/d PO can be a 'steroid-sparer'. SE: Lymphoma.
- *Renal transplantation* may be needed; nephritis recurs in ~50%, on biopsy, but is a rare cause of graft failure (graft survival 87% at 1yr and 60% at 5yrs).

Systemic sclerosis The 2 main forms:
- *Limited cutaneous systemic sclerosis:* (of which CREST syndrome is part) **c**alcinosis (subcutaneous tissues), **R**aynaud's, **e**sophageal dysmotility, **s**clerodactyly, and **t**elangiectasia. 'Limited' to face and limbs distal to elbows

or knees. Often associated with anticentromere antibodies and pulmonary hypertension.

- *Diffuse cutaneous systemic sclerosis:* 'Diffuse' defines skin involvement. More profound internal organ involvement. Often associated with lung (anti-Topo I [scl-70] antibodies), cardiac, and renal changes. *Prognosis:* Often poor.
- *Therapy:* Calcium antagonists, ACE-i and ARB for Raynaud's. Prostacyclin by IVI is being evaluated. Consider cyclophosphamide for lung disease. Meticulous BP control (ACE-i) if any renal crisis. Endothelin-1 receptor blockade (bosentan) if pulmonary hypertension and renal crisis.

Sjogren's syndrome results in dry mouth (xerostomia), dry eyes (keratoconjunctivitis sicca) due to chronic lymphocytic infiltration of salivary and lacrimal glands. Can also cause polyarthritis and can develop into lymphoma. Will have autoantibodies SSA/anti-Ro and/or SSB/anti-La.

Mixed connective tissue disease (MCTD) combines features of SLE, systemic sclerosis, and polymyositis. Renal & CNS signs are rare. Anti-RNP (ribonuclear protein) antibody is present (without other types of ANA).

Relapsing polychondritis attacks the pinna, nasal septum ± larynx (∴ stridor). *Association:* Aortic valve disease; arthritis; vasculitis. *R:* Steroids.

Revised criteria for diagnosing SLE

1 *Malar rash (butterfly rash):* Fixed erythema, flat or raised, over the malar eminences, tending to spare the nasolabial folds.

2 *Discoid rash:* Erythematous raised patches with adherent keratotic scaling and follicular plugging ± atrophic scarring. Think of it as a 3-stage rash affecting ears, cheeks, scalp, forehead, and chest: Erythema → pigmented hyperkeratotic edematous papules → atrophic depressed lesions.

3 *Photosensitivity* on exposed skin representing unusual reaction to light.

4 *Oral ulcers:* Oral or nasopharyngeal ulceration.

5 *Arthritis:* Non-erosive arthritis involving 2 or more peripheral joints, characterized by tenderness, swelling, or effusion. Joint involvement is seen in 90% of patients. Deforming arthropathy may occur due to capsular laxity (Jaccoud's arthropathy). Aseptic bone necrosis also occurs.

6 *Serositis:* (a) Pleuritis (pleuritic pain or rub—80% of all patients have lung function abnormalities; 40% have dyspnea) pleural effusion OR (b) *Pericarditis* (ECG or pericardial rub or evidence of pericardial effusion).

7 *Renal disorders:* (a) Persistent proteinuria >0.5g/d (or >3+ on dipstix) OR (b) *Cellular casts*—may be red cell, granular, or mixed.

8 *CNS disorders:* (a) Seizures, in the absence of causative drugs or known metabolic imbalance, eg uremia, ketoacidosis, OR (b) *Psychosis* in the absence of causative drugs/metabolic derangements, as above.

9 *Hematological disorders:* (a) *Hemolytic anemia* with reticulocytosis OR (b) *Leukopenia*, ie WBC <4 ×10⁹/L on ≥2 occasions OR (c) *Lymphopenia*, ie <1.500 ×10⁹/L on ≥2 occasions OR (d) *Thrombocytopenia*, ie platelets <100 ×10⁹/L in the absence of a drug effect.

10 *Immunological disorders:* (a) *Anti-DNA* antibody to native DNA in abnormal titer OR (b) *Anti-Sm* antibody to Sm nuclear antigen OR (c) Antiphospholipid antibody +ve based on:

   (1) an abnormal serum level of IgG or IgM anticardiolipin antibodies,
   (2) positive result for lupus anticoagulant using a standard method, or
   (3) false positive serological test for syphilis +ve for >6 months and confirmed by *Treponema pallidum* immobilization or fluorescent treponemal antibody absorption tests.

11 *Antinuclear antibody:* Positive in 95%.

Diagnose SLE in the appropriate clinical setting if ≥4 out of the 11 criteria are present, serially or simultaneously.

Polymyositis and dermatomyositis

Both conditions cause symmetrical, proximal muscle weakness from muscle inflammation. Can be associated with malignancy (in 9–23%). Dysphagia, dysphonia, facial edema, or respiratory weakness may develop.

Skin signs Macular rash (if over back & shoulder the *shawl sign* is +ve). A lilac-purple *(heliotrope rash)* on cheeks, eyelids and light-exposed areas in 25%, ± nail-fold erythema *(dilated capillary loops)*, and erythematous papules over extensor surfaces of phalanges (*Gottron's papules*—pathognomonic if CK↑ + muscle weakness). Also *mechanic's hands* (rough, cracked skin on the lateral and palmar surfaces of the fingers and hands, with irregular 'dirty' lines—particularly in the antisynthetase syndrome [anti-Jo1]).

Systemic signs Fevers, Raynaud's; lung involvement (20%); polyarthritis/arthralgia (40%); calcifications; retinitis (like cotton-wool patches); myocardial involvement (myocarditis; arrhythmias); dysphagia and gut dysmotility.

Diagnosis Muscle enzymes (ALT, CK & aldolase) ↑ in plasma; electromyography (EMG: Shows fibrillation potentials); muscle biopsy. *Autoantibody (ab) associations:* Myositis-specific: Anti-Mi-2, anti-Jo1 (look for lung fibrosis too). *Overlap syndromes:* Scleroderma with dermatomyositis (eg anti-PM-Scl +ve) or polymyositis/alveolitis (eg anti-Jo1 +ve). *Differential diagnosis:* Subacute weakness from: Inclusion-body myositis; muscular dystrophies; SLE myositis; polymyalgia; systemic sclerosis; endocrine/metabolic myopathies; rhabdomyolysis.

Management Investigate extensively for malignancy; get expert help; rest and prednisone help (start with 1mg/kg/24h PO). Immunosuppressives (p591) and cytotoxics are also used early, eg azathioprine, methotrexate, cyclophosphamide, or cyclosporin. High-dose immune globulin has a role. Dapsone can help skin disease.

A more aggressive form with prominent vasculitis occurs in children.

Plasma autoantibodies: Disease associations

Antinuclear antibody (ANA)	+ve in (%)
SLE	95
RA	32
JIA (p369)	76
Chronic active hepatitis	75
Sjögren's syndrome	68
Systemic sclerosis	64
'Normal' controls	0–2

Gastric parietal cell antibody

Pernicious anemia (adults)	>90%
Atrophic gastritis:	
Females	60%
Males	15–20%
Autoimmune thyroid disease	33%
'Normal' controls	2–16%

Antibody to reticulin

Celiac disease	37%
Crohn's disease	24%
Dermatitis herpetiformis	17–22%
'Normal' controls	0–5%

Smooth muscle antibody (SMA)	+ve in(%)
Chronic active hepatitis	40–90
Primary biliary cirrhosis	30–70
Idiopathic cirrhosis	25–30
Viral infections (low titers)	80
'Normal' controls	3–12
(↑ with age: 20% at 70yrs)	

Mitochondrial autoantibodies, AMA

Primary biliary cirrhosis	60–94%
Chronic active hepatitis	25–60%
Idiopathic cirrhosis	25–30%
'Normal' controls	0.8%

Thyroid antibodies

	Microsomal (%)	Thyroglobulin (%)
Hashimoto's thyroiditis	70–91	75–95
Graves' disease	50–80	33–75
Myxedema	40–65	50–81
Thyrotoxicosis	37–54	40–75
Juvenile lymphocytic thyroiditis	91	72
Pernicious anemia	55	
'Normal' controls (50% in older women)	10–13	6–10

Rheumatoid factor +ve in (%)

RA	70–80	Juvenile arthropathy	
Sjögren's syndrome	≤80	Infective endocarditis	≤50
Felty's syndrome	≤100	SLE	≤40
Systemic sclerosis	30	'Normal' controls	5–10

ANCA-associated vasculitis: 2 types:
- Classical antineutrophil cytoplasmic antibody (c-ANCA): Target: Serine protease 3: +ve in Wegener's disease (p378) in >90% of patients.
- Perinuclear antineutrophil cytoplasmic antibody (p-ANCA): Target: Myeloperoxidase; +ve in ~80% pauci-immune crescentic GN (p246) and systemic vasculitides, eg microscopic polyangiitis (a vasculitis of kidney ± lung, pANCA +ve in ~75%).

NB: Churg-Strauss may be associated with p- and cANCA.

Vasculitis

Vasculitis, defined as any inflammatory disorder of blood vessels (typically non-infectious), can affect vessels of any organ. It may be occlusive (necrotizing, as in SLE) or non-occlusive, as in Henoch–Schönlein purpura (p246). It can occur *de novo*, eg polyarteritis (see BOX), Churg–Strauss, Behçet's, giant cell arteritis (GCA), Takayasu's, and Wegener's, or be from drugs or infection (syphilis is an endarteritis obliterans)—or be mediated by complement activation induced by immune complexes in autoimmunity (eg SLE, RA). *Consider vasculitis as a diagnosis for any unidentified multisystem disorder.* Organ involvement can be from acute vasculitis or end-organ damage resulting from recurrent vasculitis. *Features seen in many vasculitides:*

- General: Fever; malaise; weight↓; arthralgia; myalgia; ESR↑.
- Skin: Purpura; ulcers; livedo reticularis; nailbed infarcts; digital gangrene.
- Eyes: Episcleritis; ulceration; visual loss.
- ENT: Epistaxis; nasal crusting; stridor; deafness.
- Pulmonary: Hemoptysis; dyspnea.
- Cardiac: Loss of pulses; heart failure; myocardial infarction; angina.
- GI: Abdominal pain (any viscus may infarct); malabsorption because of chronic mesenteric ischemia.
- Renal: BP↑ hematuria; proteinuria; casts; acute/chronic renal failure.
- Neurological: Mononeuritis multiplex; sensorimotor neuropathy; hemiplegia; seizures; psychoses; confusion; cognition↓; mood↑↓; odd behavior.

Diagnosis: This is based on clinical findings, supported by histological and occasionally angiographic findings. ANCA may be +ve (p377).

Treatment: Treat hypertension meticulously. Refer to experts. Use high-dose prednisone, and cyclophosphamide if major organ involvement.

Polyarteritis nodosa (PAN)

PAN is a necrotizing vasculitis that causes aneurysms of medium-sized arteries. ♂:♀ ≈ 2:1. Sometimes PAN is associated with HBsAg.

Signs and symptoms:
- General features: Fevers, abdominal pain, malaise, weight↓, arthralgia.
- Renal: (75%) Main cause of death. Hypertension, hematuria, proteinuria, renal failure, intrarenal aneurysms, vasculitis.
- Vascular: BP↑; claudication.
- Cardiac: (80%) Coronary arteritis and consequent infarction. ↑BP and heart failure. Pericarditis. In Kawasaki disease (childhood PAN variant), coronary aneurysms occur.
- Pulmonary: Pulmonary infiltrates and asthma occur in vasculitis (some say that lung involvement is incompatible with PAN, calling it then Churg–Strauss syndrome).
- CNS: (70%) Mononeuritis multiplex, sensorimotor polyneuropathy, seizures, hemiplegia, psychoses.
- GI: (70%) Abdominal pain (any viscus may infarct), malabsorption because of chronic ischemia.
- Skin: Urticaria, purpura, infarcts, livedo reticularis, nodules.
- Blood: WBC↑, eosinophilia (in 30%), anemia, ESR↑, CRP↑.

Diagnosis: This is most often made from clinical features in combination with renal or mesenteric angiography. ANCA is classically negative.

Treatment: Treat hypertension aggressively. Refer to rheumatology. Use high-dose prednisone, and then cyclophosphamide.

Polymyalgia rheumatica (PMR)

Common in those over 70yrs who have symmetrical aching and morning stiffness in shoulders and proximal limb muscles for >1 month ± mild polyarthritis, tenosynovitis (eg carpal tunnel syndrome, p350, occurs in 10%), depression, fatigue, fever, weight↓, and anorexia. It may come on suddenly, or over weeks. It overlaps with GCA. ♀:♂ ≈ 2:1 *Tests:* ESR usually >40mm/h; CK usually ↔; alk phos↑; mild anemia *Differential diagnosis:* Recent onset RA; hypothyroidism, primary muscle disease, occult malignancy or infection, neck lesions, bilateral subacromial impingement lesions, spinal stenosis. *Treatment:* prednisone 15–20mg/24h PO; ↓dose slowly after symptoms have been controlled at least one month (in the light of symptoms & ESR). Most need steroids for ≥2yrs. Preventing osteoporosis is essential (p286).

Giant cell (cranial/temporal) arteritis (GCA)

GCA has PMR symptoms in up to 25% of people. Common in the elderly, it is rare under 55yrs. *Symptoms:* Headache, scalp and temporal artery tenderness (eg on combing hair), jaw claudication, amaurosis fugax, or sudden blindness in one eye. *Tests:* ESR↑, CRP↑, platelets↑, alk phos↑, anemia. If you suspect GCA, do an ESR, start prednisone 1mg/kg/24h PO *immediately*. Some advocate higher doses IV (up to 1000mg) if visual symptoms (ask an ophthalmologist). Osteoporosis prophylaxis essential. Get temporal artery biopsy (several cm in length because skip lesions occur) in the next few days. NB: The immediate risk is blindness, but longer term, the main cause of death and morbidity in GCA is steroid treatment! Reduce prednisone after 5–7d in the light of symptoms and ESR; ↑dose if symptoms recur. Typical course: 1–2yrs, though it can reoccur.

Oncology

Daniel Laheru, M.D.

Contents

Introduction

Since Richard Nixon signed the historic National Cancer Act on Decembe 23, 1971 to focus and prioritize federal resources to advance cancer clinic. and basic science research, there have been a number of notable achieve ments particularly in solid tumors such as germ cell tumors and hematolog malignancies including Hodgkins lymphoma and ALL and AML. Such notab breakthroughs have been largely realized by visionary researchers integratir classical methods of drug development with innovative clinical trial desigr

What has impeded systematic progress in achieving similar successes i other cancers has been a lesson in both human psychology as well as th realization that the molecular signaling pathways that control ce proliferation and growth were largely unrecognized. The identification o molecular target-specific therapy would provide the potential of maxima therapeutic benefit while minimizing toxicity to normal cells.

The *tour de force* that led to the sequencing and analysis of the human genom in 2001 provided researchers with the critical tools to begin to identify an differentiate cancer from normal tissue at the genetic level. While the implica tions of this landmark project are still being realized, it has become eviden that the identification of critical genes and proteins involved in cell divisio and growth are just the beginning. The full characterization of the micro environment in which these genes control these molecular switches, and ou ability to understand how to manipulate these complicated non-linear matrice with targeted therapies, are of equal value and have become the new discov ery and treatment paradigm in oncology. The potential has raised expectation for unprecedented progress in the near future. However, even as bette treatments are being developed, the best treatment remains earlier diagnosi and improved screening methods for those at risk. This review will provid only a general overview of the epidemiology, genetics, screening, and trea ment of some select cancers.

Looking after people with cancer

No rules guarantee success, but there is no doubt that getting to know your patient, making an agreed management plan, and seeking out the right expert for each stage of treatment *all* need to be central activities in oncology. These issues center around communication, and the personal attributes of the doctor as a physician. There is nothing unique about oncology here—but in oncology these issues are highly focused. It is never too early to start palliative care (*with* other treatments).

Psychological support Examples include:
- Allowing the patient to express anger, fear—or any negative feeling (anger can anesthetize pain).
- Counseling, eg with a breast cancer nurse (mastectomy preparation).
- Cognitive and behavioral therapy reduces psychological morbidity associated with cancer treatments.
- Group therapy reduces pain, mood disturbance, and the frequency of maladaptive coping strategies.
- Meta-analyses have suggested that psychological support can have some effect on improving outcome measures such as survival.

Advice on breaking bad news
1 Choose a quiet place where you will not be disturbed.
2 Find out what the patient already knows or surmises (often a great deal).
3 Find out how much the person wants to know. You can be surprisingly direct about this. 'Are you the sort of person who, if anything were amiss, would want to know all the details?'
4 Give some warning—eg 'there is some bad news for us to address'.
5 Share information about diagnosis, treatments, and prognosis. Specifically list supporting people (eg nurses) and facilities (eg hospices). Try asking 'Is there anything else you want me to explain?' Don't hesitate to go over the same ground repeatedly. Allow denial: Don't force the conversation.
6 Listen to any concerns raised; encourage the airing of feelings.
7 Summarize and make a plan. Offer availability.
8 Follow through. The most important thing is to leave the patient with the strong impression that you are with them.

Don't imagine that a single blueprint will do for everyone. Be prepared to use *whatever* the patient gives you. This requires close observation of verbal and non-verbal cues. Because humans are very complex, we all frequently fail. Don't be put off: Keep trying.

Epidemiology

It is intuitive that an appreciation of the precise magnitude of cancer cases diagnosed each year in the US is imprecise as complete cancer registration has not yet been achieved in many states. However, data from the Surveillance, Epidemiology, and End Results (SEER) program of the National Cancer Institute (NCI) which covers about 10% to 14% of the US population estimates that approximately 1.4 million new cases of invasive cancer will be identified in 2005.

The incidence of selected most common cancers for men and women are identified in **Fig. 12.1**. These numbers do not include carcinoma in situ of any site except urinary bladder, nor does it include basal and squamous cell cancers of the skin. The incidence reflects a slight ↑ when compared to recent years.

For example, the estimated new cancer cases in the US in 2004 was approximately 1.368 million. The expected deaths for these same selected cancers are identified in **Fig. 12.2**.

Mortality rates have ↓ across all four major cancer sites in men and in women except for female lung cancer in which rates have been stable. The incidence trends are mixed, reflective of the recent initiatives in public policy or awareness and screening. Many cancers including pancreas, breast, and prostate cancer have continued to demonstrate slight ↑ every year. Lung cancer incidence rates are declining in men and leveled off for the first time in women after ↑ for many decades. Colorectal cancer incidence rates have ↓. The incremental ↑ in incidence rates of prostate cancer and female breast cancer may be attributable to ↑ screening through prostate-specific antigen testing (for prostate cancer) and mammography (for breast cancer). Conversely, the slight ↓ in colorectal cancer incidence may represent the fact that screening tests such as colonoscopy are still completed in the minority of eligible individuals. The ↑ in female breast cancer incidence may also reflect ↑ use of hormone replacement therapy and/or ↑ prevalence of obesity. Some additional cancers which have noted a slight ↑ for unclear reasons include hepatocellular cancer.

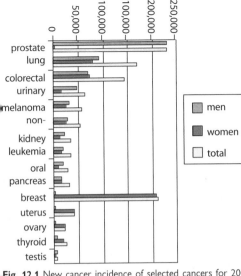

Fig. 12.1 New cancer incidence of selected cancers for 2005 (Data from Jemal *et al.*: Cancer Statistics 2005. CA *Cancer J Clin*. 2005 Jan–Feb; **55**(1): 10–30)

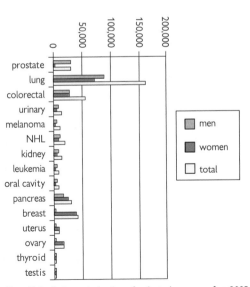

Fig. 12.2 Estimated deaths of selected cancers for 2005 (Data from Jemal *et al.* 2005. Cancer Statistics 2005. CA *Cancer J Clin*. **55**(1): 10–30)

Oncology and genetics

The majority of cancers are believed to be sporadic. However, a number of gene mutations, which predispose to cancer, have been identified. Much progress has been made at understanding a number of cancers at the genetic level although it is beyond the scope of this chapter to provide a comprehensive review of this. However, some of the genetic underpinnings for some of the most common and notable cancers have recently been described.

Familial colorectal cancer ~20% of those with colorectal cancer (CRC) have a family history of the disease. There have been a number of hereditary syndromes identified from this group including familial adenomatous polyposis (FAP), and hereditary nonpolyposis colorectal cancer (HNPCC). The genes responsible for these syndromes have also been identified and characterized. FAP accounts for <1% of hereditary CRC but is the best characterized cancer genetic syndrome. The identified genetic mutation has been mapped to chromosome 5 and is known to be autosomal dominant. FAP is characterized by innumerable colonic adenomas at an early age with the development of overt cancer in 100% of patients by age 40–50. Patients who have a mutation in the locus for FAP [adenomatous polyposis coli (APC) gene] or who have one or more first degree relatives with FAP or an identified APC mutation are at considerable risk and require yearly colonoscopies at an early age. As the incidence of developing CRC is essentially 100% in patients with FAP and because of the elevated risk of developing metachronous (ie with lesions occuring at different times) CRC, these patients are often recommended one of three prophylactic surgeries: 1) total proctocolectomy with ileostomy; 2) total proctocolectomy with ileal pouch-anal anastamosis (IPAA); 3) colectomy with ileorectal anastamosis (IRA).

Of the hereditary syndromes, HNPCC (Lynch syndrome I and II) is the most common, accounting for approximately 2–7% of the total. Patients with HNPCC typically develop CRC later than patients with FAP with age of onset during the fourth and fifth decades. The genetic alterations are more heterogeneous than for FAP, with the majority of individuals linked to chromosomes 2, 3, and 7. The molecular fingerprint of HNPCC is the microsatellite instability (MSI) phenotype which is a germline mutation caused by a number of genes particularly MLH1 and MSH2. MSH2/MLH1 gene testing is the gold standard but for a variety of reasons including cost, this testing is performed in only selected cases. The diagnosis of HNPCC is complex as it is based initially on both clinical evaluation and a careful assessment of family history followed by MSI and MSH2/MLH1 testing only if strict clinical criteria have been met. Despite a complex diagnosis algorithm, such screening is thought to underestimate the true incidence of HNPCC.

Familial breast cancer In breast cancer, numerous studies have shown that the risk of developing breast cancer ↑ if a first degree relative is diagnosed with breast cancer. For example, if a mother or sister has been diagnosed with bilateral breast cancer and the age at diagnosis was premenopause, the absolute risk to other first degree relatives approaches 50%. If the diagnosis in the affected relative was post-menopause, the risk is ↓ to ~10%. ~5% of women with breast cancer report a family history. BRCA1 (mapped to chromosome 17) and BRCA2 (mapped to chromosome 13) mutations account for most cases of breast cancer. Of note, BRCA2 mutations predispose carriers to a number of cancers including pancreas and colorectal, prostate, gastric, oral cavity, hepatobiliary, and ovarian cancer as well as melanoma. The risk of developing male breast cancer is higher in individuals with BRCA2 mutations whereas the risk of developing ovarian cancer is higher in individuals with BRAC1 mutations. Most of the identified mutations within each of these genes are associated with loss of function, suggesting that BRCA1 and BRCA2 are tumor suppressor genes.

Familial prostate cancer ~5% of those with prostate cancer have a family history: The genetic basis is multifactorial. There is a modestly elevated life time risk of prostate cancer for male carriers of BRCA1 and BRCA2 mutations, although the molecular basis of this remains to be elucidated. Mutations in BRCA1/BRCA2 or in the genes on chromosomes 1 and X do not account for all family clusters of prostate cancer and so it is clear that other genes must be involved. In one twin study, 42% of the risk was found to be genetic.

Genetic tests can also tell if chemotherapy is likely to work: Chemotherapy fails in 17% of colon cancer patients—ie those with certain mutations.[1]

Examples of cancers with a familial predisposition

Cancer/syndrome	Gene	Chromosome	
Breast and ovarian cancers	BRCA1	17q	(OPPOSITE)
	BRCA2	13q	
HNPCC	MSH2	2p	(OPPOSITE)
	MLH1	3p	
	PMS2	7p	
Familial polyposis (colorectum)	APC	5q	
von Hippel–Lindau (kidney, CNS)	VHL	3p	
Carney complex	PRKAR1A	17q	
Multiple endocrine neoplasia type I (pituitary, pancreas, thyroid)	MEN1	11q	(p285)
Multiple endocrine neoplasia type 2	RET	10q	(p285)
Basal cell naevus syndrome (CNS, skin)	PTCH	9q	
Retinoblastoma (eye, bone)	Rb	13q	
Li–Fraumeni syndrome (multiple)	TP53	17p	
Neurofibromatosis type I (CNS; rare)	NF1	17q	
Neurofibromatosis type 2 (common) (meningiomas, auditory neuromas)	NF2	22	
Familial melanoma	INK4A	9p	

1 Shown by the microsatellite instability status being 'high-frequency'. Microsatellites are stretches of DNA in which a short section is repeated several times. 5-FU chemotherapy only improves survival in microsatellite stable or low-frequency microsatellite unstable tumors. S Gallinger 2003 *NEJM* **249** 209

Screening: Colorectal and breast cancer

It is intuitive that the earlier any cancer is identified, the higher the likelihood of a curative treatment. The development of a screening test for cervical cancer (the Pap smear) has been the paradigm for an effective screening test. This has proven to be true in a number of cancers but has also proven to be surprisingly elusive or controversial in others. It is again beyond the scope of this general review to comprehensively identify screening guidelines for all cancers. Rather, a few of the most common or deadliest cancers will be highlighted. The results are summarized in the following table.

Screening tests and recommendations for selected cancers

Cancer	Screening test	Recommendations
CRC	Colonoscopy	Starting at age 50 if no risk factors, repeat every 10yrs
Breast cancer	Mammography	Starting at age 40, repeat yearly
Lung cancer	CT scan	No recommendations
Pancreas cancer	EUS	No recommendations, EUS investigational for high risk families
Prostate cancer	PSA	No recommendations

Screening for colorectal cancer

Data from a number of randomized and non-randomized studies would currently support options including fecal occult blood testing (FOBT) in combination with sigmoidoscopy or colonoscopy alone. The test of choice remains controversial.

A recently published study from the Veteran's Administration Medical system performed colonoscopy on 2885 patients at 13 different Veterans Affairs Medical Centers to determine whether or not the patients had invasive cancer, large colon polyps, or colon polyps that had visible or microscopic signs suggesting they were precancerous. These findings were called 'advanced neoplasia' if they were found on the colonoscopic examination. The participants also underwent FOBT before the colonoscopy. The researchers then performed colonoscopy, and made careful observations of their findings in the sigmoid colon and rectum (the regions of the colon that would usually be seen through the sigmoidoscope). Examination of the rectum and sigmoid colon during the colonoscopy was defined as a surrogate for a sigmoidoscopy), and their findings throughout the remainder of the colon (which would usually be seen only with the colonoscope). The researchers then determined what percentage of cases detected by colonoscopy were also detected by the FOBT tests and were seen in the area usually examined with the sigmoidoscope, the two less extensive screening techniques.

Among patients who had advanced neoplasias detected by their colonoscopy, an FOBT detected only 24% of the patients with advanced neoplasias; sigmoidoscopy would have detected 70%; and combined testing would have detected 76%, meaning that about 25% of all the patients with advanced neoplasias detected by colonoscopy would have been missed if a colonoscopy was not performed.

Why, then, do most clinical-practice guidelines provide a number of options and not recommend colonoscopy exclusively? The first reason is that the standard of care evidence required to support screening with colonoscopy without reservation is not all derived from randomized trial data. Evidence-based guidelines frequently restrict their highest recommendations to technology that has been proved in large-scale, randomized trials to reduce the burden of illness. Fecal occult-blood testing has been studied in this way; colonoscopy has not. The second reason relates to adherence to recommendations and patients' preferences. Colonoscopy may be uncomfortable and requires a preparative bowel cleansing schedule. However, if the colonoscopy is negative, it need be performed only once every 10yrs, whereas other tests such as sigmoidoscopy must be performed more frequently. The third reason is risk. An earlier study in this same patient population reported the risk of serious complications including bleeding and perforation was approximately 0.3%.

The fourth reason is economic. A mathematical model of the costs and consequences (measured in terms of life expectancy) of 22 screening strategies for colorectal cancer has been published incorporating not only the cost of the screening test (eg, colonoscopy was assumed to cost $1012) but that of all subsequent events (eg, the treatment of metastatic cancer). They suggest that if the cost of colonoscopy could be reduced by 23%, the expenditure required to achieve one more year of life with screening colonoscopy would be substantially reduced, and such screening would be made more economically attractive.

The fifth reason why colonoscopy is not recommended or covered is availability. The current supply of clinicians trained in colonoscopy may not be adequate to screen everyone who turns 50, let alone the large population between 50 and 75 yrs of age who have not been screened.

The recommendations from The American Cancer Society (ACS) recommends that people without risk factors, such as a family history of the disease or inflammatory bowel disease, begin screening at age 50. The ACS has three preferred options for screening of people at average risk:
• A colonoscopy every 10yrs
• A yearly FOBT combined with flexible sigmoidoscopy every 5yrs
• A double contrast barium enema every 5yrs.

Screening for breast cancer- The current screening guidelines for breast cancer recommend screening mammography for women aged 50–69. Within the US the recommendations include women >40yrs and older. However, there is some recent debate regarding these guidelines with respect to the recommendation of screening at age 40. A number of randomized clinical trials have demonstrated that screening mammography reduces the risk of developing breast cancer by about 20–35% in women aged 50–69yrs with slightly less benefit in women aged 40–49. Women in their 40's have a lower incidence of developing breast cancer as well as denser breast tissue which could lower the sensitivity of the screening mammography. As such, it has been suggested based on statistical modeling that in order to prevent one breast cancer death after 14–20yrs, between 500 and 1800 women who are 40yrs of age would need to undergo regular screening mammography.

Screening: Lung, pancreatic, and prostrate cancer

Screening for lung cancer

The earliest screening methods for lung cancer included sputum for cytology and/or chest radiography and were, on the whole, disappointing. However improved imaging modalities such as high resolution CT have provided new opportunities. Like all screening tests for cancer, the possible benefits must be weighed against the potential risk of the test, harm of false positive tests given the subsequent additional tests that may be required to follow-up suspicious screening evaluations, and additional costs. For example, lung cancers classically appear on CT scans as non-calcified nodules. However, only a small percentage of non-calcified nodules will be actually determined to be lung cancer. In one study, 20% of lung nodules obtained by thoracotomy to follow-up on a suspicious lung nodule was subsequently identified to be benign. A strategy proposed by the Early Lung Cancer Action Project was to determine the rate of growth of nodules.

For non-calcified nodules that were <1cm in diameter, high-resolution CT scanning was repeated at 3 months. Among individuals who were referred for needle biopsy on the basis of lung growth, the positive predictive value was 90%. In addition, the use of PET scanning integrated with traditional CT imaging has been proposed as a useful complement. A recent screening study of 1035 high-risk persons (ie, those with a history of more than 20 pack-years of smoking) combined CT scanning with PET imaging if CT imaging identified a suspicious nodule. PET imaging was subsequently performed in 42 persons with suspicious nodules. Of the 20 PET scans that were classified as positive, 18 were confirmed to be diagnostic of lung cancer. The National Cancer Institute initiated the National Lung Cancer Screening Trial in 2002 to evaluate whether CT screening leads to a significant improvement in mortality associated with lung cancer; full accrual was completed in February 2004. The trial included 50,000 subjects who were randomly assigned to undergo CT screening or chest radiography annually for 3yrs with planned follow-up for mortality through 2009.

Currently, neither the American Cancer Society nor the U.S. Preventive Services Task Force recommend that CT scanning be performed in asymptomatic but at risk individuals.

Screening for pancreas cancer

As has been the story for other cancers, CT scanning has not proven to be sensitive enough in diagnosing early pancreas cancer. Endoscopic ultrasonography is currently used in investigational studies for screening and early detection of familial pancreatic cancer and its precursors. Endoscopic ultrasonography (EUS) is a standard diagnostic predominantly outpatient technique which involves endoscopy plus high frequency ultrasound imaging of the pancreas (parenchyma and ducts, unlike ERCP which images the ducts and adjacent areas from the upper gastrointestinal tract. Tissue sampling can also be readily performed from multiple sites under EUS guidance without accompanying pain or need for local anesthesia (unlike percutaneous fine needle aspiration) with a high diagnostic yield for pancreatic lesions and lymph node metastases. When used for screening high-risk individuals, EUS imaging can be followed by biopsy of pancreatic masses, cystic lesions or evidence of intraductal papillary mucinous neoplasm (IPMN) and collection of pancreatic secretions from the duodenum for molecular marker analysis following secretin stimulation. A recent study for individuals considered high risk for developing pancreas cancer (defined as a study patient having ≥3 first degree family members with pancreas cancer) using EUS as a screening modality identified one early invasive pancreas cancer and one pre-invasive cancer

Screening for prostate cancer

Screening for prostate cancer remains controversial. While there has been ↓a decline in prostate cancer mortality, this is thought to be a function of improved treatment as opposed to improved early screening. The US Preventive Services Task Force does not recommend routine screening for prostate cancer with digital rectal examination (DRE), serum PSA, or transrectal ultrasound of the prostate. The American Cancer Society, the American College of Physicians, and the American Urological Association recommend that clinicians advise patients of the risks and benefits of screening to assist them in deciding whether or not to have these tests performed. In general, men 50yrs and older with a reasonable certainty of a 10-yr life expectancy should be screened annually or biennially. Patients with an elevated risk of disease (eg, African Americans and those with a family history) should be screened beginning at an earlier age (45yrs).

Oncological emergencies

A patient who becomes acutely ill can often be made more comfortable with simple measures, but some problems require specific treatment.

Spinal cord compression Requires urgent and efficient treatment to preserve neurological function. A high index of suspicion is essential. *Causes:* Typically extradural metastases. Others: Extension of tumor from a vertebral body, direct extension of the tumor, or fracture. *Signs & symptoms:* Back pain with a root distribution, weakness and sensory loss (a level may be found), bowel and bladder dysfunction. *Tests:* Urgent MRI. *Management:* Dexamethasone 8–16mg IV then 4mg/6h PO. Discuss with neurosurgeon and clinical oncologist immediately.

Superior vena cava (SVC) obstruction with airway compromise SVC obstruction is not an emergency unless there is tracheal compression with airway compromise: Usually there is time to plan optimal treatment, and this is to be preferred, rather than rushing into therapy which may not be beneficial. *Causes:* Typically lung cancer; rarely from causes of mediastinal enlargement (eg germ cell tumor); lymphadenopathy (lymphoma); thymus malignancy; thrombotic disorders (eg Behçet's or nephrotic syndromes); thrombus around an IV central line; hamartoma; ovarian hyperstimulation; fibrotic bands (lung fibrosis after chemotherapy). *Signs & symptoms:* Dyspnea; orthopnea; swollen face & arm; cough; plethora/cyanosis; headache; engorged veins. *Pemberton's test:* On lifting the arms over the head for >1min, there is ↑facial plethora/cyanosis, JVP↑ (non-pulsatile), and inspiratory stridor. *Tests:* Sputum cytology, CXR, CT, venography. *Management:* Get a tissue diagnosis if possible, but bronchoscopy may be hazardous. Give dexamethasone 4mg/6h PO. Consider balloon venoplasty and SVC stenting, eg prior to radical or palliative chemo- or radiotherapy (depending on tumor type).

Hypercalcemia Affects 10–20% of patients with cancer, and 40% of those with myeloma. *Causes:* Lytic bone metastases, production of osteoclast activating factor or PTH-like hormones by the tumor. *Symptoms:* Lethargy, anorexia, nausea, polydipsia, polyuria, constipation, dehydration, confusion, weakness. Most obvious with serum Ca^{2+} >12.0mg/dL. *Management:* Rehydrate with 3–4L of 0.9% saline IV over 24h. Avoid diuretics. Give bisphosphonate IV (consider maintenance therapy, IV or PO). Best treatment is control of underlying malignancy. In resistant hypercalcemia, consider calcitonin.

Raised intracranial pressure Due to either a primary CNS tumor or metastatic disease. *Signs & symptoms:* Headache (often worse in the morning), nausea, vomiting, papilledema, seizures, focal neurological signs. *Tests:* Urgent CT is important to diagnose an expanding mass, cystic degeneration, hemorrhage within a tumor, cerebral edema, or hydrocephalus due to tumor or blocked shunt since the management of these scenarios can be very different. *Management:* Dexamethasone 4mg/6h PO, radiotherapy, and surgery as appropriate depending on cause.

Tumor lysis syndrome Rapid cell death on starting chemotherapy for rapidly proliferating leukemia, lymphoma, myeloma, and some germ cell tumors can result in a rise in serum urate, K^+, and phosphate, precipitating renal failure. Prevention is with good hydration and *allopurinol* 24h *before* chemotherapy; dose example if renal function OK: 300mg/12h PO. If creatinine >1.2mg/dL: 100mg alternate days.

Inappropriate ADH secretion p618; febrile neutropenic regimen. See p495.

Treating hypercalcemia with bisphosphonates

Ensure adequate hydration (eg with 0.9% saline IVI). Zoledronic acid and pamidronate are 2 options.

Disodium pamidronate

Calcium (mg/dL; corrected)	Single-dose pamidronate (mg)
<12	30
12–14	60
>14	90

Infuse slowly, eg 30mg in 300mL 0.9% saline over 3h via a large vein. Max dose: 90mg. Response starts at ~3–5d, peaking at 1wk.

SE: 'Flu symptoms, bone pain, $PO_4^{3-}\downarrow$, bone pain, myalgia, nausea, vomiting, headache, lymphocytopenia, $Mg^{2+}\downarrow$, seizures (rare).

Zoledronic acid is significantly more effective in reducing serum Ca^{2+} than previously used bisphosphonates. Usually, a single dose of 4mg IVI over 2h will normalize plasma Ca^{2+} within a week. A higher dose should be used if corrected Ca^{2+} is 12mmol/L. *SE:* 'Flu symptoms, bone pain, $PO_4^{3-}\downarrow$, confusion, thirst, taste disturbance, nausea, pulse$\downarrow$, WBC$\downarrow$, creatinine$\uparrow$.

Symptom control in severe cancer

Pain Do not undertreat with analgesia: Aim to *prevent*—or *eliminate* pain.

Types of pain Don't assume that the cancer is the cause (abdominal pain eg, may be from constipation). Seek the mechanism. Pain caused by nerve infiltration and damage via local pressure may respond to amitriptyline (eg 10–50mg at night). Bone pain (eg presenting with back pain) may respond to NSAIDs, radiotherapy, or a nerve block.

Identify each symptom and type of pain.

Management (1) Pain is affected by mood, morale, and meaning. Explain its origin to both the patient and relatives, and plan rehabilitation goals. (2) Use oral analgesics if possible—aim to prevent pain with regular prophylactic doses (eg 4-hourly); do not wait for pain to recur. (3) Modify the pathological process where possible, eg radiotherapy; hormones; chemotherapy; surgery

With analgesia, work up the pain ladder until pain is relieved (see BOX). Monitor response carefully. Laxatives and antiemetics are often needed with analgesics. *Adjuvant analgesics:* NSAIDs, steroids, muscle relaxants, anxiolytic, anti-depressants.

Giving oral morphine: Start with aqueous morphine 5–10mg/4h PO. A double dose at night can be used to promote 8h of sleep. Most patients need no more than 30mg/4h PO. A few need much more. Aim to change to extended-release morphine (eg MS Contin tablets every 12h), when daily morphine needs are known. In morphine-resistant pain (persisting when 60mg/4h is given) consider adjuvant analgesics, methadone, or ketamine (specialist use only).

Vomiting: Prevent from before the 1st dose of chemotherapy, to avoid antici-patory vomiting before the next dose. Give orally if possible, but if severe vomiting prevents this, give rectally or subcutaneously. *Agents to try:* Meto-clopramide 10mg/8h po; ondansetron 4–8mg/8–12h po/IV; haloperidol 0.5–2mg/24h (max 5mg).

Shortness of breath: Consider supplementary O_2 or morphine. Use of relaxa-tion techniques and benzodiazepines can be useful. Assess for pleural or pericardial effusion. If there is significant pleural effusion, consider thoraco-centesis ± pleurodesis. If there is a malignant pericardial effusion, consider pericardiocentesis (p146), pericardiectomy, pleuropericardial windows, external beam radiotherapy, percutaneous balloon pericardiotomy, or peri-cardial instillation of immunomodulators or sclerosing bleomycin.

Venipuncture problems: Repeated venipuncture with the attendant risk of painful extravasation and phlebitis may be avoided by insertion of skin tun-nelled catheter (eg a Hickman line)—a single or multilumen line—into a major central vein (eg subclavian or internal jugular). It is inserted using a strict antiseptic technique. Patients can look after their own lines at home, and give their own drugs. Problems include: Infection, blockage (flush with 0.9% saline or dilute heparin, eg every week), axillary, subclavian, or superior vena cava thrombosis/obstruction, and line slippage. Even more convenient portable delivery devices are available, allowing drugs to be given at a preset time without the patient's intervention.

The analgesic ladder

Rung 1	*Non-opioid*	Aspirin; acetaminophen; NSAID
Rung 2	*Weak opioid*	Codeine; dihydrocodeine; dextropropoxyphene; tramadol; oxycodone (some place this on rung 3)
Rung 3	*Strong opioid*	Morphine; diamorphine; hydromorphine; fentanyl ± adjuvant analgesics.

If 1 drug fails to relieve pain, move up ladder; do not try other drugs at the same level. In new, severe pain, rung 2 may be omitted.

IV delivery of opioids, haloperidol, cyclizine and metoclopramide and hyoscine, giving 24h cover. Or suppositories (below) or *fentanyl transdermal patches:* If not previously exposed to morphine, start with one low-strength patch (25mcg/h). Remove after 72h, and place a new patch at a different site. 25, 50, 75, and 100mcg/h patches are made. $t_{\frac{1}{2}} \approx 17h$.

Suppositories can also be used if unable to tolerate oral route. For pain: Try oxycodone 30mg suppositories (eg 30mg/8h ≈ 30mg morphine). Agitation: Try diazepam 10mg/8h suppositories.

Other agents and procedures to know about (alphabetically listed)
- Bisacodyl tablets (5mg), 1–2 at night, help opioid-induced constipation.
- C(h)olestyramine 4g/6h PO (1h after other drugs) helps itch in jaundice.
- Enemas, eg arachis oil, may help resistant constipation.
- H_2-antagonists (eg cimetidine 400mg/12h PO) help gastric irritation—eg associated with gastric carcinoma.
- Haloperidol 0.5–5mg/24h PO helps agitation, nightmares, hallucinations, and vomiting.
- Hydrogen peroxide 6% cleans an unpleasant-feeling coated tongue.
- Hyoscine hydrobromide 0.4–0.6mg/8h SC or 0.3mg sublingual: Vomiting from upper GI obstruction or bronchial congestion.
- Nerve blocks may lastingly relieve pleural or other resistant pains.
- Low-residue diets may be needed for post-radiotherapy diarrhea.
- Metronidazole 400mg/8h PO mitigates anaerobic odors from tumors; so do charcoal dressings (Actisorb®).
- Polyethylene glycol sachets 2–4/12h for 48h to shift resistant constipation with overflow.
- Naproxen 250mg/8h with food: Fevers caused by malignancy or bone pain from metastases (consider splinting joints if this fails).
- Spironolactone 100mg bd PO + bumetanide 1mg/24h PO for ascites.
- Steroids: Dexamethasone: Give 8mg IV stat to relieve symptoms of superior vena cava or bronchial obstruction—or lymphangitis carcinomatosa. Tablets are 2mg (≈15mg prednisolone). 4mg/12–24h PO may stimulate appetite, or reduce ICP headache, or induce (in some patients) a satisfactory sense of euphoria.
- Supplemental humidified O_2 helps hypoxic dyspnea.
- Thoracocentesis (±bleomycin pleurodesis) in pleural effusion.

Cancer therapy

It is beyond the scope of this chapter to provide a comprehensive review of treatment options for each malignancy. However, as noted earlier, there have been some remarkable achievements in the management of some solid tumors such as germ cell tumors. The sensitivity of germ cell tumors to platinum-based chemotherapy, together with radiation and surgical measures has led to a cure rate of >99% in early stage disease.

Cancer management Management requires a multidisciplinary team and communication is vital. Most patients wish to have some part in decision making at the various stages of their treatment, and to be informed of their options. Patients are becoming better informed through self-help groups and access to the Internet. Most patients undergo a variety of treatments during the treatment of their cancer and your job may be to orchestrate these.

Surgery In many cases a tissue diagnosis of cancer is made with either a biopsy or formal operation to remove the primary tumor. Although it is sometimes the only treatment required in early tumors of the GI tract, soft tissue sarcomas, and gynecological tumors, it is often the case that best results follow the combination of surgery and chemotherapy. Surgery also has a role in palliating advanced disease.

Chemotherapy Cytotoxics should be given under expert guidance by people trained in their administration. Drugs are often given in combination with a variety of intents: *Neoadjuvant*—to shrink tumors to reduce the need for major surgery (eg mastectomy). There is also a rationale which considers early control of micro-metastasis. *Primary therapy*—as the sole treatment for hematological malignancies. *Adjuvant*—to reduce the chance of relapse, eg breast and bowel cancers. *Palliative*—to provide relief from symptomatic metastatic disease and possibly to prolong survival.

Important classes of drugs include:
- Alkylating agents, eg cyclophosphamide, chlorambucil, busulfan.
- Antimetabolites, eg methotrexate, 5-fluorouracil.
- Vinca alkaloids, eg vincristine, vinblastine.
- Antitumor antibiotics, eg actinomycin D, doxorubicin.
- Others, eg etoposide, taxanes, platinum compounds.

Side-effects depend on the types of drugs used. Nausea/vomiting are most feared by patients and are preventable or controllable in most. Alopecia can also have a profound impact on quality of life. Neutropenia is most commonly seen 10–14d after chemotherapy (but can occur within 7d for taxanes) and sepsis requires immediate attention. (p498).

Extravasation of a chemotherapeutic agent: Suspect if there is pain, burning or swelling at infusion site. *Management:* Stop the infusion, attempt to aspirate blood from the cannula, and then remove. Administer steroids and consider antidotes. Elevate the arm and mark site affected. Review regularly and apply steroid cream. Apply cold pack (unless a vinca alkaloid, in which case a heat compress should be applied).

As was also noted earlier, what has impeded systematic progress in achieving similar successes in other cancers has been the realization that the molecular signaling pathways that ultimately lead to cell proliferation and growth were largely unrecognized. The identification of molecular target-specific therapy would provide the potential of maximal therapeutic benefit while minimizing toxicity to normal cells.

Ligand dependent or independent growth factor receptors: Activate downstream signaling pathways via its ability to phosphorylate and thereby activate downstream proteins to effect unregulated cellular proliferation. As such, inhibitors of receptor kinases with high specificity are currently being tested as anticancer drugs. The discovery of the molecular defect associated with the constitutively active tyrosine kinase fusion protein BCR-ABL, which results from the reciprocal DNA exchange between the long arms of chromosomes 9 and 22 [t(9;22) Philadelphia chromosome], has been identified in >90% of patients with CML. The clinical features of CML and the biology of BCR-ABL have recently been elegantly summarized. The variability in the breakpoint on chromosome 22 is well described and has implications for the disease phenotype. As a result, BCR-ABL inhibition represented an ideal target for drug therapy. This strategy has been validated in clinical trials of CML with imatinib that culminated in its approval in May, 2001 by the Food and Drug Administration. In chronic phase, the hematologic response rate is 95% and cytogenetic response rates range from 50–80%, depending on the stage of disease. Moreover, response rates were also high in blast crisis patients, despite the presence of multiple oncogenic abnormalities in addition to BCR-ABL.

The epidermal growth factor receptor (EGFR): Includes a family of receptor tyrosine kinases comprised of 4 related receptors: EGFR (ErbB1/EGFR/Her1), ErbB2 (Her2/neu), ErbB3 (Her3), and ErbB4 (Her4). The formation of receptor homo- or hetero-dimerization through either ligand dependent or independent activation leads to constitutively activated receptor signaling and has been associated with amplification of downstream signals involving a number of non-linear cellular pathways. The end product of this signaling cascade leads to ↑ cellular proliferation, migration, tissue stromal invasion, resistance to apoptotic signals, and angiogenesis. In addition, EGFR is over-expressed in a significant percentage of solid tumors and is believed to be a marker for poor prognosis and ↓ survival. These properties provide the rationale for the development and testing of EGFR inhibitors. Inhibitors to EGFR have already been tested in clinical trials with FDA approval in 2003 of the oral EGFR tyrosine kinase inhibitor gefitinib (Iressa®, Astra-Zeneca) for third line therapy of advanced non-small cell lung cancer. Many important challenges for the use of EGFR small molecule inhibitors remain including identifying appropriate surrogate markers of activity and in best integrating these therapies with other treatment modalities. Cetuximab (Erbitux®, Imclone Systems) is an IgG1 monoclonal antibody against EGFR that has demonstrated activity in patients with Irinotecan-refractory colorectal cancer. Cetuximab has also shown response to treatment and improvement in progression-free progression in patients with locally advanced head and neck cancer refractory to platinum based chemotherapy. The association of an acne-like rash with activity of drug has been suggested.

The formation of new blood vessels to keep pace with growing tumors is an enormously complicated process that occurs in response to a vast array of molecular signals including oxygen tension (hypoxia inducing factor) and growth factors such as fibroblast growth factor (FGF), transforming growth factor alpha and beta (TGF-α and TGF-β), tumor necrosis factor alpha (TNF-α), insulin growth factor and platelet derived growth factor (PDGF). Vascular endothelial growth factor (VEGF) signaling is a critical rate limiting step in angiogenesis.

Inhibitors to VEGF have already been approved in CRC (bevacizumab) and in breast cancer (trastuzumab) and have been examined in lung, renal, pancreas, head and neck, hepatocellular cancer and non-Hodgkin's lymphoma in ongoing trials.

Radiotherapy

Radiotherapy uses ionizing radiation to produce free radicals which damage DNA. Normal cells are better at repairing this damage than cancer cells, so are able to recover before the next dose (or fraction) of treatment.

Radical treatment is given with curative intent. The total doses given range from 40–70Gy (1Gy = 100cGy = 100rads) in 15–35 daily fractions. Some regimens involving giving several smaller fractions a day with a gap of 6–8h. Combined chemoradiation is used in some sites, eg anus and esophagus, to ↑ response rates.

Palliation aims to relieve symptoms. Doses: 8–30Gy, given in 1, 2, 5, or 10 fractions. Bone pain, hemoptysis, cough, dyspnea, and bleeding are helped in >50% of patients. *'Will this patient benefit from radiotherapy?'* is a frequently asked question. For a formal example assessing risks and benefits. When in doubt, ask an expert (or 2).

Early reactions Occur during, or soon after treatment.
- Tiredness: Common after radical treatments; can last weeks to months.
- Skin reactions: These vary from erythema to dry desquamation to moist desquamation to ulceration; on completing treatment, use moisturizers.
- Mucositis: All patients receiving head and neck treatment should have a dental check-up before commencing therapy. Avoid smoking, alcohol and spicy foods. Antiseptic mouthwashes may help. Soluble analgesics are helpful. Treat oral thrush.
- Nausea and vomiting: Occur when stomach, liver, or brain treated. Try a dopamine antagonist first. If unsuccessful, try 5HT$_3$ antagonist, p392.
- Diarrhea: Usually after abdominal or pelvic treatments. Maintain good hydration. Avoid high-fiber bulking agents; try loperamide.
- Dysphagia. Thoracic treatments.
- Cystitis. Pelvic treatments. Drink plenty of fluids. NSAIDs.
- Bone marrow suppression. More likely after chemotherapy or when large areas are being treated. Usually reversible.

Late reactions Occur months, or years after the treatment.
- CNS: Somnolence, 6–12wks after brain radiotherapy. Treat with steroids. Spinal cord myelopathy—progressive weakness. MRI is needed to exclude cord compression. Brachial plexopathy—numb, weak, and painful arm after axillary radiotherapy. Reduced IQ can occur in children receiving brain irradiation if <6yrs old.
- Lung: Pneumonitis may occur 6–12wks after thoracic treatment, eg with dry cough ± dyspnea. Treatment: Prednisolone 40mg reducing over 6wks.
- GI: Xerostomia—reduced saliva. Treat with pilocarpine 5mg/8h or artificial saliva. Care must be taken with all future dental care as healing is reduced. Benign strictures—of esophagus or bowel. Treat with dilatation. Fistulae—need surgical intervention.
- GU: Urinary frequency—small fibrosed bladder after pelvic treatments. Fertility—pelvic radiotherapy (and cytotoxics) may affect fertility, so ova or sperm storage should be considered. This is a complex area: Get expert help. In premature female menopause or reduced testosterone—replace hormones. Vaginal stenosis and dyspareunia. Impotence—can occur several years after pelvic radiotherapy.
- Others: Panhypopituitarism, following radical treatment involving pituitary fossa. Children need hormones checking regularly as growth hormone may be required. Hypothyroidism—neck treatments, eg for Hodgkin's lymphoma. Cataracts. Secondary cancers, eg sarcomas usually 10 or more years later.

Surgery

Susan L. Gearhart, M.D. and Lisa Jacobs, M.D.

Contents

Surgical terms

Incisions have names

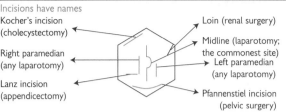

Kocher's incision
(cholecystectomy)

Loin (renal surgery)

Midline (laparotomy;
the commonest site)

Right paramedian
(any laparotomy)

Left paramedian
(any laparotomy)

Lanz incision
(appendicectomy)

Pfannenstiel incision
(pelvic surgery)

Abdominal areas

1	7	2
RUQ		LUQ
3	8	4
RLQ		LLQ
	5	9	6

1, 2: Right & left upper quadrants
3, 4: Right & left flanks
5, 6: Right & left lower quadrants
   7: Epigastrium
   8: Central area (peri-umbilical)
   9: Suprapubic area

Abscess   A cavity containing pus.
Angio-   To do with tubes or blood vessels.
-ectomy   Cutting something out, eg appendectomy.
Chole-   To do with gall or bile.
Cyst   A fluid-filled sac.
Docho-   To do with ducts.

Fistula An abnormal communication between 2 epithelial surfaces, eg enterocutaneous between the bowel and the skin; endothelial in arterio-venous fistulae), eg gastrocolic fistula (stomach/colon). Fistulae commonly close spontaneously but will not do so in the presence of chronic inflammation, distal obstruction, epithelialization of the track, foreign bodies, or malignant tissue.

Ileus Used in this book to mean adynamic bowel (eg no bowel sounds).

Lith Stone, eg nephrolithotomy (cutting kidney open to get to a stone).

Ostomy An artificial opening usually made to create a new connection between 2 conduits or between a conduit and the outside world, eg colostomy: The colon is made to open on to the skin (p424). Stoma means a mouth.

Otomy Cutting something open, eg laparotomy (opening of abdomen).

Plasty A refashioning of something to make it work, eg pyloroplasty relieves pyloric (gastric outlet) obstruction.

Percutaneous Going through the skin (invasive).

Sinus A blind ending tract typically line by epithelium and opens to the skin.

Stent Artificial tube inserted into a biological tube to keep it open.

Trans Going across a structure.

Ulcer An abnormal break in an epithelial surface.

The preoperative evaluation

The purpose of the preoperative evaluation is:
1 To determine the need for surgical intervention
2 To assess the anesthetic risk to the patient
3 To establish a physician/patient relationship.

How to determine if surgical intervention is necessary?

If you can answer yes to any of the following questions, you are heading in the right direction.
1 Is there an emergent life-threatening situation that can be corrected surgically?
2 Is there an eminent life-threatening situation that can be corrected surgically?
3 Is there great probability that a surgical intervention would improve the well-being of an individual?

To determine this, the surgeon may require additional testing to determine if surgery is indicated and to further assess the anesthetic risk to the patient. *For example, a 64yr old man with a newly diagnosed rectal cancer and a history of smoking will need local staging with an ultrasound exam of the tumor, a CT scan of the abdomen and pelvis to evaluate for metastatic disease, a chest X-ray, EKG, and the following laboratory work: CBC, comprehensive panel, PT, PTT. If the patient has cardiac risk factors, an echocardiogram and/or cardiac stress test may need to be performed. For further assessment of any pulmonary conditions, pulmonary function tests may need to be performed.*

More discussion is included with the individual descriptions of the disorders or diseases.

Pre-operative tests

Be guided by the history and examination, and local protocols.

Blood tests

Routine blood tests include CBC, comprehensive panel, and coagulation profile (PT, PTT) in most patients. If Hgb <10g/dL tell anesthesiologist. Investigate/treat as appropriate. A comprehensive panel is particularly important if the patient is starved, diabetic, on diuretics, has significant burns, has hepatic or renal diseases, has an ileus, or is parenterally fed.

In healthy adults less than 40yrs of age,

Cross-matching: Type and cross is recommended for most major surgical cases. For major cardiac, vascular and spine cases, up to 6 units should be available for surgery.

Specific blood tests: LFT in jaundice, malignancy, or alcohol abuse.

Urinalysis: Routine prior to prosthetic device insertion as well as routine abdominal surgery.

β-HCG: Mandatory in ALL pre-menopausal women.

Drug levels: As appropriate (eg digoxin, dilatin, lithium).

Coagulations studies: In liver disease, DIC, massive blood loss, patients already on valproic acid, warfarin, or heparin.

HIV, HBSAG In high risk patients—after appropriate counseling.

Sickle test: In those from Africa, West Indies, or Mediterranean—and others whose origins are in malarial areas (including most of India).

Thyroid function tests: In those with thyroid disease.

Additional tests

CXR: If known smoker, evidence of cardiopulmonary disease, pathology or symptoms, possible lung metastases, or ≥50yrs old.

EKG: Patients with prior coronary revascularization or admission to a hospital for cardiac reasons. Asymptomatic males >45yrs of age, females >55yrs of age without significant co-morbidities (diabetes, obesity, hypertension).

Echocardiogram/stress test: Any patient with cardiac symptoms (chest pain, SOB), known cardiac disease (particularly heart failure) that has not been evaluated recently or has progressed in symptoms to assess adequacy of medical therapy.

Pulmonary function test (PFT): Chronic smoker, known pulmonary disease, sleep apnea, esp. before thoracic surgery

Lower or upper extremity venous duplex: Patients with a history of DVT, prolonged hospitalizations, malignancy, Inflammatory bowel disease, etc. (see DVT prophylaxis). If positive test would consider vena cava filter prior to operation.

American Society of Anesthesiologists (ASA) classification

1 Normally healthy.
2 Mild systemic disease.
3 Severe systemic disease that limits activity; not incapacitating.
4 Incapacitating systemic disease which poses a threat to life.
5 Moribund. Not expected to survive 24h even with operation.

You will see a space for an ASA number on most anesthetic charts. It is a health index *at the time of surgery*. The prefix **E** is used in emergencies. This classification is commonly used to assess the risk of anesthetic complication. Patients with an ASA of 1 have virtually less than 1% risk of death while patient with an ASA of 5 run a 50% risk of intraoperative mortality.

Anesthetic risk assessment and the difficult airway

Begin with the medical history of the patient and family and a general review of systems. Assess cardiopulmonary system, exercise tolerance, existing illnesses, drugs, and allergies. Is the neck unstable (eg arthritis complicating intubation)? Assess past history of: Myocardial infarction, diabetes, asthma, hypertension, rheumatic fever, epilepsy, jaundice. Assess any specific risks, eg is the patient pregnant? Is the neck/jaw immobile (intubation risk)? Has there been previous anesthesia? Were there any complications (eg nausea, DVT) Family history may be relevant eg in malignant hyperthermia; myotonic dystrophy; porphyria; cholinesterase problems; sickle-cell disease.

Drugs Any drug/antiseptic allergies? Inform the anesthesiologist about all drugs even if 'over-the-counter'.

Antibiotics: Tetracycline and neomycin *et al.* may ↑neuromuscular blockade.

Anticoagulants: Tell the surgeon. Avoid epidural, spinal, and regional blocks.

Anticonvulsants: Give as usual pre-op. Post-op, give drugs IV (or by NGT) until able to take orally. Valproate: Give usual dose IV. Phenytoin: Give IV slowly (<50mg/min; monitor ECG). IM phenytoin absorption is unreliable.

Beta-blockers: Continue up to and including the day of surgery as this precludes a labile cardiovascular response.

Estrogen replacement or oral contraceptives: Stop 4wks before major surgery because of the risk of thromboembolic event, and ensure alternative contraception is used.

Digoxin: Continue up to and including morning of surgery. Check for toxicity (ECG; plasma level); do plasma K^+ and Ca^{2+} (succinylcholine ↑K^+ and can lead to ventricular arrhythmias in the fully digitalized).

Diuretics: Beware hypokalemia, dehydration.

Levodopa: Possible arrhythmias when patient under GA.

Lithium: Get expert help; it may potentiate neuromuscular blockade and cause arrhythmias.

MAOI: Get expert help as interaction with opiates and anesthetics may cause hypotensive/hypertensive crises.

Eye-drops: Many get absorbed; anticholinesterases ↑[succinylcholine].

Tricyclics: These enhance epinephrine and arrhythmias.

Predictors of difficult intubation

I do not know of any area of medicine where proper preparation is more important in preventing complications. The overall incidence of difficult intubation is reportedly 5.8%. The incidence for obese patients is 15.8%. Currently the best method of determining the potential for a difficult airway includes the patient's history and physical exam. Any patient who has had a difficult intubation in the past is given an alert bracelet indicating this. Furthermore, a history of maxillofacial trauma, reconstructive surgery, radiation should alert the anesthetist of potential difficulties. Other assessment tools include the following:

Mallampati classification: Estimates the size of the tongue relative to the oral cavity—alone this test is marginally helpful.

Thymomental distance: Distance from thyroid notch to mentum (<4–6cm) is an indication of mouth opening capability

Sternomental distance: Distance from sternum to mentum (<12.5–13.5cm) is an indication of mouth opening capability

Mouth opening: Ability to visualize the glottis on mouth opening—inconsistent

Wilson risk score: Simple summation of risk factor—somewhat reliable score is ≤2.

Cardiac risk assessment and management

The American College of Cardiology and the American Heart Association have published an eight-step guideline regarding cardiac risk assessment in non-cardiac surgery in 1996 which were updated in 2002. Some of these guidelines have been summarized here.

Non-invasive preoperative testing: Should occur if 2 of the 3 following factors are true in any patient:

1 Intermediate clinical predictors are present (Canadian class 1 or 2 angina, prior MI, compensated or prior heart failure, diabetes, renal insufficiency).
2 Poor functional capacity (<4 metabolic equivalent levels on Duke Activity Status Index AJC 1989)
3 High surgical risk procedure (emergency major operation, aortic or PVD surgery, prolonged surgery with large fluid shifts).

Several studies have demonstrated that a LVEF below 35% is associated with an ↑ risk of a coronary event in patients undergoing non-cardiac surgery.

Invasive peri-operative evaluation: Recommended for the following patients prior to undergoing surgery:

1 Patients with suspected or known CAD that have demonstrated a high risk of adverse outcome based on non-invasive testing.
2 Unstable angina or angina not responsive to medical therapy.
3 Equivocal non-invasive test results in patients undergoing high risk surgery.
4 Urgent non-cardiac surgery while convalescing from an acute MI.
5 Peri-operative MI.
6 Candidate for liver, lung, or renal transplant 40yrs old or more, as part of evaluation for transplantation, unless noninvasive testing reveals high risk for adverse outcome.
7 Patients should undergo preoperative coronary bypass grafting before high risk surgery if their long-term outcome would be improved.

Other factors:

1 Prior to surgical intervention, severe hypertension (diastolic >110 mmHg) should be controlled.
2 Symptomatic stenotic lesions (mitral or aortic) are associated with risk of peri-operative severe heart failure and should be treated with intense medical therapy or surgical correction when possible.
3 Arrhythmias and conduction abnormalities—management is identical to non-operative setting, however, pacemakers and ICDs will need to be pro-gramd off prior to surgery because of the concern of electrocautery use.
4 Medical therapy, particularly beta blockade, should be started days prior to planned surgery and continued postoperatively with a dose titrated to achieve a resting heart rate around 50–60bpm. Patients who have a contra-indication to beta-blockade (COPD) may be started on alpha adrenergic agonists.
5 Some studies indicate that maintenance of normothermia and adequate analgesia prevents cardiac events.
6 Because 95% of coronary events may be silent, postoperative EKG monitor-ing should be performed in high risk patients.

All patients who smoke should be encouraged to discontinue smoking prior to surgery.

Prophylactic antibiotics and bowel preparation

The rate of wound infection following surgery ranges from <5% for clean cases without entry into the GI tract to >50% for intra-abdominal perforation. Successful prevention has been demonstrated with the use of intravenous antibiotics only.

Preoperative mechanical bowel preparation especially in the era of routine intravenous antibiotics prior to surgery, has not shown to be beneficial in the prevention of anastomotic complications or wound infections. However, most surgeons find it more aesthetically pleasing and facilitates bowel anastomosis and the identification of intraluminal lesions. The two mechanical bowel preparations utilized are the following:

1 Polyethylene glycol 4L—does not cause electrolyte abnormalities and therefore is commonly used in patients with cardiac disease, renal insufficiency, and the elderly.

2 Sodium phosphate solutions—hypertonic solution leading to dehydration in the elderly and patients already on diuretics, significant electrolyte abnormalities can occur (↑ Na, ↑ Phos, ↓ K, ↓ Ca).

Preoperative oral antibiotics have not shown to be beneficial in the era of intravenous antibiotics in the prevention of wound infections. That being said the most commonly used regimen is neomycin and erythromycin.

Preoperative intravenous antibiotics the surgical literature supports the routine use of intravenous antibiotics in the prevention of wound infections. To be effective, the dose should be given one hour prior to incision. Meta-analysis has demonstrated that a single dose is all that is necessary although frequently three doses are given.

1 1st generation cephalosporin is given in non- contaminated surgery without entry into the GI tract. (eg ancef 1g 1–3 doses q8)

2 2nd generation cephalosporin is given in cases that limited contamination is expected including entry into the GI tract. This antibiotic covers aerobic and anaerobic bacteria. (eg cefotetan 2g 1–2 doses q12)

3 For penicillin allergic patients, penicillins as well as cephalosporins should be avoided (5% cross reactivity). Alternative include clindamycin or vancomycin and gentamicin,

4 For intra-abdominal perforation, coverage with a third generation cephalosporin and metronidazole, a broad spectrum penicillin, or fluoroquinolone is acceptable (eg cefuroxime 1.5g and metronidazole 500mg).

Thomboembolic risk assessment and prevention

Below is the current method of risk assessment for venous thromboembolic disease.

Risk factors for venous thromboembolic disease

Serious risk factors
- Age >60
- Cancer undergoing treatment
- Previous DVT and PE
- Stroke
- Trauma
- Heart and respiratory failure
- Pregnancy and post-partum
- Inherited or acquired hypercoagulability

Other risk factors
- Immobility
- Central venous catheterization
- Acute medical illness or sepsis
- Myeloproliferative disorder
- Inflammatory bowel disease
- Nephrotic syndrome
- Obesity (BMI >30kg/m^2)
- Smoking
- Estrogen use
- Varicose veins

Contraindications to prophylaxis for venous thromboembolic disease include:
- Active, uncontrolled bleeding or high risk of bleeding
- Systemic anticoagulation
- Bacterial endocarditis or pericarditis
- Severe head trauma
- Malignant hypertension
- Threatened abortion
- Severe thrombocytopenia
- Heparin or enoxaparin: Heparin-induced-thrombocytopenia
- Enoxaparin: Spinal tap, epidural instrumentation
- Sequential compression device (SCD): Open wound or extremity with DVT.

Risk categories and management

Risk categories → Prophylaxis

Low risk → **Early mobilization**
- Minor/vascular/laparoscopic/urologic procedures
- Age <40yrs
- NO additional risk factors

Moderate risk → **Heparin 5000U SC bid ± TEDS and SCDs**
- Minor/laparoscopic/gynecological surgery
- Age <40yrs
- With additional risk factors
                    or
- Minor surgery
- Age 40–60yrs
- No additional risk factors
                    or
- Major surgery
- Age <40yrs
- NO additional risk factors

High risk → **Heparin 5000U SC tid or enoxaparin 40mg SC qd**
± TEDs and SCDs
- Any surgery
- Any age >60yrs
- NO additional risk factors
                    or
- Minor surgery
- Age 40–60yrs
- With additional risk factors

Very high risk → **Heparin 5000U SQ tid or enoxaparin 40mg SC qd AND**
TEDs and SCDs
- Major surgery
- Serious risk factors (2 or more)
                    or
- Major surgery
- Age >60yrs
- With any additional risk factor

Informed consent

The purpose of the informed consent is to document that a discussion was undertaken between the surgeon and the patient with regards to the planned procedure. This discussion is paramount with regards to the patient and physician relationship. During this discussion, the physician should feel confident that the patient has a reasonable expectation of what is going to be done at the time of surgery. The patient should be informed of the known foreseeable complications. The patient should also be informed of the alternatives to surgery. All questions should be answered. It is mandatory in many institutions that one-sided surgeries be marked with the surgeon's initials and the agreement of the patient prior to incision (ie nephrectomy).

IV fluid and electrolyte management

The goal of fluid therapy is the normalization of hemodynamic parameters and the body fluid electrolyte composition.

Intraoperative fluids

With the exception of major hemorrhage, avoid taking patient to surgery without adequate resuscitation. Anesthesia compounds shock by inhibiting normal baroreceptor function causing vasodilatation and depressing cardiac contractility.

Most patients can tolerate a 500mL blood loss; however, loss in excess of this may require transfusion.

For third space losses as a result of tissue trauma, isotonic solution such as lactated ringers should be used for replacement. Colloids are expensive and provide no added benefit.

Post-operative fluids

A normal requirement is 2–3L/24h which allows for urinary, fecal, and insensible loss. This maintenance therapy should be supplemented by replacement of the additional fluids needed to replace ongoing third space losses.

Monitor fluid status is best accomplished through close following of vital signs, urinary output, and CVP monitoring.

Urine output: Should be maintained at a level greater than 0.5mL/kg/h.

The first 24 hours: Isotonic solutions (0.9% saline) should be given initially because of ongoing third space losses.

A standard postoperative regimen: (One of many) 2L 5% dextrose with 0.45% saline/24h. Add K^+ post-op (20mEq/L). More K^+ is needed if losses are from the gut (eg diarrhea, vomiting or high NG tube output, intestinal fistula, high output stoma). More saline is appropriate for those at risk of hyponatremia: See BOX.

When to ↑ the above regimen

- Dehydration: This may be by ≥5L if severe. Replace this slowly.
- Shock (all causes, except for cardiogenic shock).
- Operative losses: Check operation notes for extent of bleeding.
- Losses from gut: Replace NGT aspirate volume with 0.45% saline with 20mEq/L potassium.
- Insensible losses: Feverish patients and burns.
- Pancreatitis: There are large pools of sequestered fluid which should be allowed for.
- Losses from surgical drains: check fluid charts and replace significant losses.
- Low urine output (the night after surgery) is commonly due to inadequate infusion of fluids, however, the possibility of bleeding must always be considered. Check JVP, operative drains, proper Foley function and review for signs of cardiac failure. Check urine specific gravity. A sp gravity of >1.012 (more concentrated than plasma) indicates volume depletion or cardiac failure, a urine sp gravity of <1.010 indicates adequate volume resuscitation or renal failure. Treatment is to ↑ IV rate unless patient is in cardiac or renal failure, or bleeding (when blood should be transfused). If in doubt, a fluid challenge may be indicated: 500mL of 0.9% saline over 30min, or 200mL of colloid (Hespan® or albumin) over 30–60min, with monitoring of urine output. Then you may ↑ IV rate (eg to 1L/h of 0.9% saline for 2–3h).
- Patients with evidence or new onset cardiac or renal failure are best managed with CVP monitoring or the insertion of a Swan–Ganz catheter where serial measurements can be made.

Guidelines for success (p616)

- Be simple. Chart losses and replace them. Know the urine output. Aim for 60mL/h; 30mL/h is the minimum in adults ($\frac{1}{2}$mL/kg/h).
- Measure plasma electrolytes if the patient is ill. Regular electrolytes are not needed on young, people with good kidneys unless patient has ongoing losses (vomiting, diarrhea).
- Start oral fluids as soon as possible, the kidney is smarter than the best doctor.

What fluids to use

Hemorrhagic/hypovolemic shock (p686): Insert 2 large IV cannulas (14 or 16 gauge), for fast fluid infusion. Start with crystalloid (eg 0.9% saline) or colloid until blood is available. The advantage of crystalloids is that they are cheap—but they do not stay as long in the intravascular compartment as colloids, as they equilibrate with the total extracellular volume (dextrose is useless for resuscitation as it rapidly equilibrates with the enormous intracellular volume). In practice, the best results are achieved by combining crystalloids and colloids. Aim to keep the hemoglobin above 8mg/dL, and urine flowing at >30mL/h. Monitor pulse and BP often.

Septicemic shock: Infuse isotonic (0.9% saline) fluids to replace third space losses.

Heart or liver failure: Avoid sodium loads.

Excessive vomiting, diarrhea: Use 0.9% saline and replace losses, including K^+. See chart below:

Urine output↓ (oliguria): Aim for output of >30mL/h in adults ($\frac{1}{2}$mL/kg/h). Anuria means a blocked catheter. Flush or replace catheter. Oliguria is usually due to inadequate replacement of lost fluid. Treat by ↑ fluid input. Acute renal failure may follow shock, nephrotoxic drugs, transfusion, or trauma.

- Review fluid chart and examine for signs of volume depletion.
- Urinary retention is also common, so examine for a palpable bladder.
- Establish normovolemia (a CVP line may help here, normal is 0–5cm H_2O relative to sternal angle); you may need 1L/h IVI for 2–3h.
- Catheterize bladder (for accurate monitoring).

If intrinsic renal failure is suspected, refer to a nephrologist early.

Electrolyte concentrations (mEq/L)

Location	Na^+	K^+	Cl^-	HCO_3^-	H^+	Rate (mL/d)
Salivary	50	20	40	30	–	Up to 1L
Gastric	100	10	140	–	100	Up to 4L
Bile	140	5	100	60	–	Up to 1L
Pancreatic	140	5	75	100	–	Up to 1L
Duodenal	140	5	80	–	–	Up to 2L
Ileum	140	5	70	50	–	Up to 2L
Colon	100	70	15	30	–	–

Electrolyte management in the surgical patient

Hypo- and hypernatremia

Hyponatremia: The most common cause is excess free fluid. Symptoms related to hyponatremia include: Nausea, headaches, weakness, cognition↓, coma, death. Hyponatremia results from infusion of 5% dextrose in H_2O, thiazide diuretics, inappropriate adh secretion.

Treatment: (p618) 0.9% saline IVI; check electrolytes every 2h; aim to bring Na^+ up to 130mmol/L by 1–2mmol/L per hour. Diuretics may be useful in acute hyponatremia, or if the patient is symptomatic.

Hypernatremia: The most common cause is excess free water loss. Less common in surgical patients. Diabetes insipidus (depressed ADH secretion) can result from head trauma. Symptoms occur when Na^+ exceeds 160mEq/mL. include irritability, restlessness, fever, seizures.

Treatment: Free water is administered to correct Na^+ at a rate of 0.7mEq/L/h.

Hypo- and hyperkalemia

Potassium is the major intracellular cation and is the major determinant of intracellular osmolality.

Hypokalemia: A result of total body depletion (diarrhea, hyperaldoteronism) or intracellular redistribution (acute alkolosis, glucose and insulin administration, catecholamine excess). Symptoms include muscle weakness, ileus, arrhythmias; ECG may demonstrate flattened *t*-waves, depressed ST segments, prolonged QT, U waves.

Treatment: Replace K^+ 10mEq/h. A drop of 1mEq/mL in the serum K^+ level represents a total body loss of ~100mEq. Correct acid/base abnormalities.

Hyperkalemia: In the postop patient, usually the result of diminished renal function. Also seen in crush and reperfusion injuries after vascular surgery. Acute elevation in K^+ can result from depolarizing muscle relaxants (eg succinylcholine)

Treatment: ECG changes (peaked T waves) paresthesia, and weakness should be treated with a rapid infusion of calcium gluconate, 1 ampule of sodium bicarbonate, and 50g glucose along with 10U or regular insulin which will temporize for 30min. Need ICU monitoring. Definite treatment includes K^+ wasting diuretics or K^+–Na^+ exchange resin (Kayexalate) 40g in 100mL of sorbitol. Alternatively, hemodialysis should be performed.

Hypo- and hypercalcemia

Hypocalcemia: In the post-op patient is usually secondary to inadvertent or planned total parathyroidectomy. After the resection of a parathyroid adenoma, hypocalcemia may be secondary to temporary non-function of existing glands as a result of atrophy. Other causes include acute pancreatitis and pancreatic fistulas, vitamin D deficiency, renal failure. Symptoms occur with serum level below 8mg/dL and include muscle cramps, perioral tingling, paresthesia, laryngeal stridor, tetany, seizures, psychotic behavior. Check for hyperactive deep tendon reflexes: Chvostek sign and Trousseau sign. ECG changes include prolonged QT interval caused by prolongation of the ST segment.

Treatment: Verify not secondary to a low albumin (check ionized calcium). Intravenous calcium gluconate or calcium chloride (can burn in the IV). Should not be administered at a rate >50mg/min (2.5mEq/min). Oral replacement with calcium gluconate, citrate, or carbonate or TUMs as well as Vitamin D supplementation to ↑ GI absorption.

Hypercalcemia: Primary hyperparathyroidism as a result of a parathyroid adenoma is the most common cause of hypercalcemia. Other causes include chief cell hyperplasia, renal failure, paraneoplastic syndrome, familial hypercalemia. Symptoms include muscle fatigue, weakness, personality disorders, psychoses, coma, hypertension, shortening of QT interval on ECG, nausea, vomiting, abdominal pain, nephrocalcinosis and lithiasis ('bones, stones, and abdominal groans').

Treatment: Serum Ca^+ >14mg/dL must be dealt with immediately. Hydration with 0.9% or 0.45% saline with 20mEq of K^+ intravenously at 200–300mL/h to promote diuresis. Furosemide will enhance Ca^+ excretion. Long-term treatment requires resection of the parathyroid adenoma or the tumor. Metastatic bone disease resulting in hypercalcemia may respond to mithramycin or calcitonin. Metastatic breast disease or hematogenous disease may respond to steroids. ESRD patients on dialysis may respond to a low-calcium dialysate.

Hypo- and hypermagnesemia

Hypomagnesemia: Prolonged period of intravenous fluid without Mg^{2+} replacement is the most common cause in the postoperative period. Symptoms are similar to hypocalcemia. Hypokalemia may develop.

Treatment: Large deficits are best managed by intravenous doses infusion with up to 4g. For mild deficits, magnesium can be given orally.

Hypermagnesemia: Renal failure is the primary reason. Symptoms include depressed neuromuscular function.

Treatment: Calcium antagonizes the effects of magnesium so a slow IV of 5–10mEq of calcium is used in acute cases.

The control of pain

The control of postoperative pain is essential and must be individualized. Numerous studies have indicated that patients recover more quickly, have less complications, and a better experience if their pain is well controlled.

Guidelines for success Review and chart each pain carefully and individually
- Identify and treat the underlying pathology wherever possible.
- Give regular doses rather than on an *as required* basis.
- Choose the best route: Oral, PR, IM, epidural, SC, inhalation, or IV.
- Explanation and reassurance contribute greatly to analgesia.
- Allow the patient to be in charge. This promotes well-being, and does not lead to overuse. Patient-controlled continuous parenteral morphine delivery systems are useful.

Non-narcotic analgesia Tylenol: 650mg/6h PO. Caution in liver impairment NSAIDs, eg ibuprofen 400mg/8h PO or Toradol® 15–30mgIV/6–8h; these are good for musculoskeletal pain and work well as an adjunct to the more potent narcotics. CI: Peptic ulcer, clotting disorder, anticoagulants, renal insufficiency (toradol). Cautions: Asthma, renal or hepatic impairment, pregnancy, and the elderly. Aspirin is contraindicated in children due to the risk of Reye's syndrome.

Opioid drugs for severe pain Morphine (eg 2–4mg/2–4h IV push) or oxycodone (5–10mg/4h PO) or derivatives of these medications are best. Meperidine (Demerol®) is also useful on a short-term basis. Long –term use of meperidine can result in CNS hyper-excitability. These are 'controlled' drugs.

Side-effects of opioids: These include nausea, respiratory depression, constipation, cough suppression, urinary retention, BP↓, and sedation (do not use in hepatic failure or head injury). Dependency is a problem especially with longer acting drugs such as oxycontin. Naloxone may be needed to reverse the effects of excess opioids (p736).

Patient controlled analgesia Morphine or fentanyl is given through an intravenous pump which is controlled by the patient. Intravenous infusion allows the patient to receive the pain medication within 2–5min. The patient is allowed just so much medication every hour. Side effects are nausea, purities, and ileus. The PCA is only effective if the patient is properly educated on its use. Family members must be discouraged not to administer the drug for the patient.

Epidural analgesia Opioids and anesthetics are given into the epidural space by infusion or as boluses. Ask the advice of the Pain Service (if available). Side effects: Thought to be more localized: Watch for respiratory depression, neuromuscular weakness, difficulty voiding, local anaesthetic-induced autonomic blockade (BP↓).

Adjuvant treatments Eg radiotherapy for bone cancer pain; anticonvulsants, antidepressants or steroids for nerve pain, antispasmodics, eg hyoscine (Buscopan® 10–20mg/8h) for intestinal, renal, or bladder colic. Transcutaneous electrical nerve stimulation (TENS), local heat, local or regional anesthesia, and neurosurgical procedures (eg excision of neuroma) may be tried but can prove disappointing. Treat conditions that exacerbate pain (eg constipation, depression, anxiety).

Why is controlling post-operative pain so important?

- Psychological reasons: Pain control is a humanitarian undertaking.
- Social reasons: Pain relief makes surgery less feared by society.
- Biological reasons: There is evidence for the following sequence: Pain → autonomic activation → ↑ adrenergic activity → arteriolar vasoconstriction → reduced wound perfusion → ↓ tissue oxygenation → delayed wound healing → serious or mortal consequences.

Deep vein thrombosis (DVT) and swollen legs

DVTs occur in ~20% of surgical patients, and many non-surgical patients. 65% of below-knee DVTs are asymptomatic; these rarely embolize to the lung.

Risks Age, pregnancy, synthetic estrogen, surgery (especially pelvic/ orthopedic), past DVT, malignancy, obesity, immobility, thrombophilia (p590).

Signs Calf warmth/tenderness/swelling, mild fever, pitting edema.

Differential diagnoses Cellulitis (may coexist); ruptured Baker's cyst (both may coexist).

Tests *D-dimer blood tests* are sensitive but not specific for DVT. They are also raised in infection, pregnancy, malignancy and post-op. A −ve result, combined with a low pre-test clinical probability score is sufficient to exclude (see below). DVT. If d-dimer ↑, or the patient has a high/intermediate pre-test clinical probability score, do compression ultrasound. If this is−ve, a repeat ultrasound may be performed at 1wk to catch early but propagating DVTs. Venography is rarely necessary. Do thrombophilia tests if there are no predisposing factors, in recurrent DVT, or if there is a family history of DVT.

Prevention Stop the OCPs 4wks pre-op. Mobilize early. See above.

Treatment Meta-analyses have shown LMWH (eg enoxaparin 1.5mg/kg/24h SC) to be superior to unfractionated heparin (dose guided by APTT, p574), but extensive ileofemoral thrombi may still require unfractionated heparin as such patients were excluded from the trials. Start warfarin simultaneously, stopping heparin when INR is 2–3; treat for 3 months if post-op (6 months if no cause is found; lifelong in recurrent DVT or thrombophilia). Inferior vena caval filters may be used in active bleeding, or when anticoagulants fail, to minimize risk of pulmonary embolus. Preventing post-phlebotic change: Thrombolytic therapy (to reduce damage to venous valves) and graduated compression stockings have both been tried, but neither has been conclusively shown to be beneficial.

Swollen legs

Bilateral edema implies systemic disease with ↑ venous pressure (right heart failure) or intravascular oncotic pressure (any cause of albumin↓, so test the urine for protein). It is dependent (distributed by gravity), which is why legs are affected early, but severe edema extends above the legs. The exception is the local ↑ in venous pressure occurring in IVC obstruction: The swelling neither extends above the legs nor redistributes. *Causes:* Right heart failure (p126). Low albumin. Venous insufficiency: Acute, eg prolonged sitting, or chronic, with hemosiderin pigmented, itchy, eczematous skin ± ulcers. Vasodilators, eg nifedipine. Pelvic mass. Pregnancy—if BP↑ + proteinuria, diagnose pre-eclampsia: Find an obstetrician urgently. In all the above, both legs need not be affected to the same extent.

Unilateral edema: Pain ± redness implies DVT or inflammation, eg cellulitis or insect bites (any blisters?). Bone or muscle may be to blame, eg trauma (check sensation and pulses: A compartment syndrome with ischemic necrosis needs prompt fasciotomy); tumors; or necrotizing fasciitis.

Impaired mobility suggests trauma, arthritis, or a Baker's cyst.

Non-pitting edema is edema you cannot indent.

Treatment Treat the cause. Giving diuretics to everyone is not an answer. Ameliorate dependent edema by elevating the legs (ankles higher than hips— do not just use foot stools); raise the foot of the bed. Graduated support stockings may help (CI: Ischemia).

Pre-test clinical probability scoring for DVT

In patients with symptoms in both legs, the more symptomatic leg is used.

Clinical feature	Score
Active cancer (treatment within last 6 months or palliative)	1 point
Paralysis, paresis, or recent cast immobilization of leg	1 point
Major surgery or recently bedridden for >3d in last 4wks	1 point
Local tenderness along distribution of deep venous system	1 point
Entire leg swollen	1 point
Calf swelling >3cm compared to asymptomatic leg (measured 10cm below tibial tuberosity)	1 point
Pitting edema (greater in the symptomatic leg)	1 point
Collateral superficial veins (non-varicose)	1 point
Alternative diagnosis as likely or more likely than that of DVT	−2 points

3 or more points: High probability; 1–2 points: Intermediate probability; 0 or fewer points: Low pre-test probability of DVT.

Air travel and DVT

In 1954, Homans first reported an association between air travel and venous thromboembolism. Recently, the supposed risk of DVT and subsequent pulmonary emboli associated with air travel (the so-called 'economy-class syndrome') has been the subject of much public scrutiny. Factors such as dehydration, immobilization, ↓ oxygen tension, and prolonged pressure on the popliteal veins resulting from long periods in confined aircraft seats have all been suggested to be contributory factors. While the evidence linking air travel to an ↑ risk of DVT is still largely circumstantial, the following facts may help answer questions from your patients, family, and friends:

- The risk of developing a DVT from a long distance flight has been estimated at 0.1–0.4/1000 for the general population.
- There is an ↑ risk of pulmonary embolus associated with long distance air travel.
- Compression stockings may ↓ the risk of DVT, though they may also cause superficial thrombophlebitis.
- The role of prophylactic aspirin is still under investigation.
- Measures to minimize risk of DVT include leg exercises, ↑ water intake, and refraining from alcohol or caffeine during the flight.

Glucose management and the diabetic patient

Hyperglycemia results from surgical trauma. Although insulin levels are appropriately elevated, the tolerance of insulin sensitive tissues is ↓. The importance of good glucose regulation (<130mg/dL) in the postoperative period has lead to a significant ↓ in wound infection rates.

Insulin-dependent diabetes mellitus (eg type 1 diabetes mellitus)
- Patients are often well informed about their diabetes; involve them fully when managing their diabetic care.
- Stress or concurrent illness ↑ basal insulin needs.
- Always try to put the patient first on the list (surgery, endoscopy, bronchoscopy, etc.). Inform the surgeon and anesthetist early.
- Stop all long–acting insulin the night before. Get IV access before you need it urgently. If surgery is in the morning, stop all SC morning insulin. If surgery is in the afternoon, have the usual short-acting insulin in the morning at breakfast. No medium- or long-acting insulin.
- Check blood glucose hourly. Aim for 100mg/dL during surgery.
- Check electrolytes and glucose pre-op. Start an IV of 1L of 5% dextrose with 20mmol KCL/8h. Dextrose saline can be given if Na⁺ low, but do not give only saline; dextrose may need constant infusion to maintain blood glucose.
- Start an infusion pump with 50U short-acting insulin in 50mL 0.9% saline. Give according to sliding scale below adjusted in the light of blood glucose.
- Post-op, continue IV insulin and dextrose until patient tolerating food. Finger stick glucose every 2h. Switch to usual SC regimen.

Practical hints:
- Some prefer to control blood sugar with a glucose-potassium-insulin (GKI) infusion.
- If the patient is having minor surgery, and thus will definitely be able to eat post-op, IV insulin may not be necessary. Some advocate giving the patient a small glucose drink early on the morning of surgery, and delaying their morning insulin dose and breakfast till after the procedure.
- If in doubt, check with the anesthesiologist.

Non-insulin-dependent diabetes mellitus (type 2 diabetes)
- These patients are usually controlled on oral hypoglycemics (p271). If diabetes poorly controlled, treat as for type 1 diabetes.
- Do not give long-acting sulphonylureas 24h prior to surgery, as they can cause prolonged hypoglycemia on fasting.
- Beware lactic acidosis in patients on biguanides (eg metformin).
- If the patient can eat post-operatively, simply omit tablets on the morning of surgery and give post-op with a meal.
- If the patient is having major surgery with restrictions to eating post-op, check fasting glucose on the morning of surgery and start IV or SC insulin given according to sliding scale. Post-op, consult the diabetic team as the patient may need a phase of insulin to supplement their oral hypoglycemics.

Diet-controlled diabetes usually no problem, though patient may temporarily become insulin dependent post-op. Monitor finger stick glucose before meals and bedtime. Avoid giving 5% dextrose IVI as a fluid replacement as blood glucose will rise.

IV insulin sliding scale (This is only a guide; values are in mg/dL)

Finger stick glucose (mg/dL)	IV soluble insulin	Alternative SC insulin
<60	None (50% glucose IV)	None (50% glucose IV)
60–130	No insulin	No insulin
131–180	1 U/h	2 U SC
181–250	2 U/h	4 U SC
251–350	3 U/h	6 U SC
>351	6 U/h	8 U SC

Blood transfusion and blood products

Blood should only be given if strictly necessary.
- Know *and use* local procedures to ensure that the right blood gets to the right patient at the right time.
- Take blood for cross-matching from only 1 patient at a time. Label immediately. This minimizes risk of wrong labelling of samples.
- When giving blood, monitor temperature and BP every ½h.

Type and screen requests Find out your local guidelines for elective surgery. Obtaining cross-matched blood quickly is easier if the patient has already been typed and screened. No units are set up for the patient when only a type and screen is requested.

Whole blood (rarely used) *Indications:* Exchange transfusion; grave exsanguination—use cross-matched blood if possible, but if not, use 'universal donor' group O Rh−ve blood, changing to cross-matched blood as soon as possible. Blood >2d old has no effective platelets.

Red cells (packed to make hematocrit ~70%) Use to correct anemia or blood loss. 1U ↑Hb by 1–1.5g/dL. In anemia, transfuse until Hb ~8g/dL.

Platelet transfusion (p584) not usually needed if not bleeding or count is >20 × 10⁹/L. If surgery is planned, get advice if <60 × 10⁹/L.

Fresh frozen plasma (FFP) Use to correct clotting defects: Eg DIC (p576) warfarin over dosage, liver disease. It is expensive and carries all the risks of blood transfusion. Do not use as a simple volume expander.

Human albumin solution (Plasma protein fraction) is produced as 4.5% or 20% protein solution and is basically albumin to use for protein replacement. Both the solutions have much the same Na⁺ content and 20% albumin can be used temporarily in the hypoproteinemic (eg liver disease; nephrotic) who is fluid overloaded, without giving an excessive salt load.

Others Cryoprecipitate (a source of fibrinogen); coagulation concentrates (self-injected in hemophilia); immunoglobulin (anti-D).

Complications of transfusion Management of acute reactions: See BOX
- Early (within 24h): Acute hemolytic reactions (eg ABO or Rhesus incompatibility), anaphylaxis, bacterial contamination, febrile reactions (eg from HLA antibodies), allergic reactions (eg itch, urticaria, mild fever), fluid overload, transfusion-related acute lung injury (TRALI)—basically ARDS due to anti-leukocyte antibodies in donor plasma.
- Delayed (after 24h): Infections (eg viruses: Hepatitis B/C, HIV; bacteria; protozoa; prions), iron overload (treatable with desferrioxamine), graft-versus-host disease, post-transfusion purpura—potentially lethal fall in platelet count 5–7d post-transfusion requiring specialist treatment with IV immuno-globulin and platelet transfusions.

Massive blood transfusion This is defined as replacement of an individual's entire blood volume (>10U) within 24h. Complications: Platelets↓, Ca²⁺↓ clotting factors↓, K⁺↑, hypothermia.

Transfusing patients with heart failure If Hb≤5g/dL with heart failure transfusion with packed red cells is vital to restore Hb to safe level, eg 6–8g/dL, but must be done with great care. Give each unit over 4h with (furosemide, eg 40mg slow IV/PO; do not mix with blood) with alternate units. Check for ↑JVP and basal lung crackles; consider CVP line.

There is a role for patients having their own blood stored pre-op for later use (autologous transfusion). Erythropoietin (EPO) can be used to ↑ the yield of autologous blood in normal individuals.

Transfusion reactions

A rapid spike of temperature (>40°C) at the start of a bag indicates that the transfusion should be stopped (suggests intravascular hemolysis or bacterial contamination). For a slowly rising temperature (<40°C), slow the IVI—this is most frequently due to antibodies against white cells.

Acute transfusion reactions	Action
Acute hemolytic reaction (eg ABO incompatibility) Agitation, T°↑ (rapid onset), ↓BP, flushing, abdominal/chest pain, oozing venopuncture sites, DIC.	STOP transfusion. Check identity and name on unit; tell hematologist; send unit + CBC and electrolytes, PT, PTT, cultures and urine (hemoglobinuria) to lab. Keep IV line open with 0.9% saline. Treat DIC.
Anaphylaxis Bronchospasm, cyanosis,↓BP, soft tissue swelling.	SLOW or STOP the transfusion. Maintain airway and give oxygen. Transfer to ICU and contact code team for intubation.
Bacterial contamination T°↑ (rapid onset), ↓BP, and rigors.	STOP the transfusion. Check identity against name on unit; tell hematologist and send unit +CBC, electrolytes, clotting, cultures & urine to lab. Start broad-spectrum antibiotics.
TRALI (See OPPOSITE) Dyspnea, cough; cxr 'white out'	STOP the transfusion. Give 100% O_2. Treat as ARDS. p174. Donor should be removed from donor panel.
Non-hemolytic febrile transfusion reaction Shivering and fever usually 30–60min after starting transfusion.	SLOW or STOP the transfusion. Give an antipyretic, eg Tylenol® 1g. Monitor closely. If recurrent, use leukocyte-depleted blood or WBC filter.
Allergic reactions Urticaria and itch.	SLOW or STOP the transfusion; give diphenhydramine 25–50mg IV/PO q6–8h. Monitor closely.
Fluid overload Dyspnea, hypoxia, tachycardia, ↑JVP, and basal crepitations.	SLOW or STOP the transfusion. Give oxygen and a diuretic, eg (furosemide) 40mg IV initially. Consider CVP line and exchange transfusion.

Blood transfusion and Jehovah's witnesses

These patients are likely to refuse even vital transfusions on religious grounds. These views must be respected, but complex issues can arise especially if the patient is a child. Alternative methods of hemoconcentration should be offered to these patients. These methods include preoperative erythropoietin and iron and intraoperative normovolemic hemodilution. Consultation with hematology and anesthesiology preoperatively is recommended.

Nutritional support

Over 25% of hospital inpatients may be malnourished. Weight loss of more than 10% of normal body mass may compromise the host by altering the ability to heal wounds or develop an immune response to infection. Operative mortality is ↑ in patients with weight loss of more than 20–25% of total body weight. In contrast, patients with normal body composition who are not hypermetabolic do not require nutritional intervention for up to a period of 5–7 days of inadequate intake.

Why are so many hospital patients malnourished?

1 ↑ nutritional requirements (eg sepsis, burns, surgery).
2 ↑ nutritional losses (eg malabsorption, output from stoma).
3 ↓ intake (eg dysphagia, sedation, coma).
4 Effect of treatment (eg nausea, diarrhea).
5 Enforced starvation (eg prolonged periods *nothing by mouth*).

Identifying the malnourished patient

History: Recent weight change; recent reduced intake; diet change (eg recent change in consistency of food); nausea, vomiting, pain, diarrhea which might have led to reduced intake.

Examination: Examine for state of hydration; dehydration can go hand-in-hand with malnutrition, and over hydration can mask the appearance of malnutrition. Evidence of malnutrition: Poor skin turgor (eg over biceps); no fat between fold of skin; hair rough and wiry; pressure sores; sores at corner of mouth. BMI<19kg/m² suggests malnourishment.

Investigations: Low albumin, prealbumin, and transferring levels are suggestive of poor nutritional status.

Calculations of needs: To estimate caloric needs, the basal metabolic rate is estimated based on height, weight, age, and gender. A stress factor is added to account for the ↑ demands in hospitalized patients and 1000kcal should be added per day when weight gain is desired.

Protein requirements: Approximately 1–2g/kg/d will maintain a positive nitrogen (N) balance. The optimal N/calorie ratio is 1:150. Divide total kcal necessary by 150 to get grams of N. Then multiply the grams of N by 6.25 to calculate grams of protein needed per day.

The remainder of requirements are based on the kcals needed.

Remember: Carbohydrates 3.4kcal/g

Protein 4kcal/g

Fat 9kcal/g

Most patients are well-nourished with 2000–2500kcal (20–40kcal/kg) and 7–14g nitrogen every 24h. Even catabolic patients rarely need more than 2500kcal. Very high calorie diets (eg 4000kcal/24h) can lead to fatty liver. If patient requires nutritional support, seek help from dietician.

Prevention of malnutrition Assess nutrition state and weight on admission, and eg weekly thereafter. Identify those at risk (see above). Nutritional supplements high in caloric count will assist with improving nutritional status.

Enteral nutrition (ie nutrition given into gastrointestinal tract) If at all possible, give nutrition by mouth. An all-fluid diet can meet requirements (but get advice from dietitian). If a patient has a limited capacity to swallow but has passed a swallowing study (eg after stroke), consider puree diet before abandoning food by mouth.

Tube feeding: This is giving liquid nutrition via a tube, eg placed endoscopically, radiologically, or surgically (directly into stomach, ie gastrostomy or into the jejunum). Use nutritionally complete, commercially prepared feeds. Standard feeds (eg Nutrison standard®, Osmolite®) normally contain

1kcal/mL and 4–6g protein per 100mL. Most people's requirements are met in 2L/24h. Specialist advice from dietitian is essential. Nausea and vomiting is less of a problem if feed given continuously with pump, but may have disadvantages compared with intermittent nutrition.

Guidelines for success
- Use jejunal tube feeding when possible.
- Keep height of bed at 30 degrees to avoid aspiration risk.
- Build up feeds gradually to avoid diarrhea and distension.
- Weigh weekly, check blood glucose and plasma electrolytes (including phosphate, zinc, and magnesium, if previously malnourished).
- Working closely with a dietitian is essential.

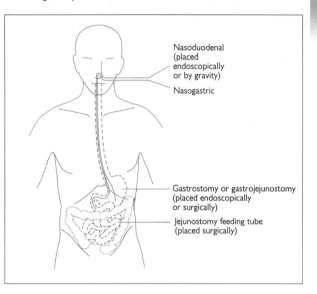

Nasoduodenal (placed endoscopically or by gravity)

Nasogastric

Gastrostomy or gastrojejunostomy (placed endoscopically or surgically)

Jejunostomy feeding tube (placed surgically)

Parenteral (IV) nutrition

Do not undertake parenteral feeding lightly: It has risks. Specialist advice is vital. Only consider it if the patient is likely to become malnourished without it. This normally means that the gastrointestinal tract is not functioning or is not available (eg bowel obstruction or fistula), and is unlikely to function for at least 7d. Parenteral feeding may supplement other forms of nutrition (eg active Crohn's disease when insufficient nutrition can be absorbed in the gut) or be used alone (total parenteral nutrition—TPN). Even if there is GI disease (eg pancreatitis), studies show that enteral nutrition is safer, cheaper, and at least as efficacious.

Administration Nutrition is normally given through a central venous line as this usually lasts longer than if given into a peripheral vein. A peripherally inserted central catheter (PICC line) is another option. Insert under strictly sterile conditions and check its position on x-ray. This line is then dedicated for the use of the administration of nutrition only.

Requirements There are many different regimens for parenteral feeding. Most provide ~2000kcal and 10–14g nitrogen in 2–3L; this usually meets a patient's daily requirements of 20–40kcal/kg and 0.2g nitrogen/kg. ~50% of calories are provided by fat and 50% by carbohydrate. Regimens comprise vitamins, minerals, trace elements, and electrolytes; these will normally be included by the pharmacist.

Complications

Sepsis: (Eg *Staphylococcus epidermidis* and *Staphylococcus aureus*; *Candida*; *Pseudomonas*; infective endocarditis.) Look for spiking pyrexia and examine wound at tube insertion point. If central venous line related sepsis is suspected, the safest course of action is always to remove the line. Do not attempt to salvage a line when *S. aureus* or *Candida* infection has been identified.

Thrombosis: Central vein thrombosis may occur, resulting in pulmonary embolus or superior vena caval obstruction. Heparin in the nutrient solution may be useful for prophylaxis in high-risk patients.

Metabolic imbalance: Electrolyte abnormalities (including K^+, calcium, phosphate, zinc, magnesium); plasma glucose; deficiency syndromes.

Mechanical: Pneumothorax; embolism from CVP tip.

Guidelines for success

• Work closely with nutrition team and pharmacist.
• Practice meticulous sterility. Do not use central venous lines for uses other than nutrition. Remove the line if you suspect infection. Culture the line upon removal.
• Review fluid balance at least twice daily, and requirements for energy and electrolytes daily.
• Check weight, fluid balance, and urine glucose daily throughout period of parenteral nutrition. Check plasma glucose, creatinine and electrolytes (including calcium and phosphate), and full blood count daily until stable and then 3 times a week. Check LFT and lipid clearance 3 times a week until stable and then weekly. Check zinc and magnesium weekly throughout.
• Do not rush. Achieve the maintenance regimen in small steps.

Drains, wounds, and stoma care

Drains

Surgical drains: Abdominal drains placed in surgery are usually closed suction drains (Jackson–Pratt). These drains can also be open drains such as a penrose. Open drains are more commonly associated with infection. Surgical drains should always be brought out a separate incision than the primary incision because of the risk of infection to the primary incision. The purpose of an abdominal drain is to collect fluid that may accumulate after surgery. Common sites to drain include the pelvis, the lateral gutters, and any surgery performed around the pancreas. Drains are also placed above the fascia to drain the subcutaneous tissue especially if skin flaps have been mobilized. Drains are usually removed when the output has dropped. Routine drain care includes drain site care and drain stripping. To strip a drain, the fluid in the drain is stripped through the tubing. Several studies have been performed looking at the benefit of drains in the abdomen and very few have demonstrated a benefit, however, individual surgeons continue to use drains. Another important point about drain management, when cracking or advancing a drain, the drain is removed from the body in increments of 1 to 2 inches a day. The drain must then be re-secured.

External drains: Drainage tubes may also be placed radiographically to drain collection. In general, these drains are not closed suction drains. Care of these drains includes flushing these drains with sterile saline 2–3 times a day.

Tube thoracostomy: Performed to evacuate an ongoing production of air/fluid into the pleural space or fluid that is too viscous to be aspirated by thoracentesis.

If there is a question of a tension pneumothorax, a 14 or 16 gauge angiocatheter should immediately be placed in the second or 3rd intercostals space in the mid-clavicular line on the affected side.

Posterior thoracostomy: To drain hemothorax, pneumothorax (also anterior thoracostomy), persistent pleural effusion, and empyema. After application of local anesthesia, the incision is placed in the 6 intercostals space along the anterior axillary line. Placement of the tube occurs by entering the pleural in the 5th intercostals space and directing the tip posteriorly.

Anterior thoracostomy: For an anterior approach the tube is placed over the 4th rib along the mid-clavicular line. Avoid injury to the intercostals artery and vein by entering the pleural space above the rib.

The tube thoracostomy is then connected to a Pleuravac®.

Tube thoracostomy removal: When the drainage is low and there is no longer a pneumothorax or air leak the chest tube can be removed. The patient is asked to take a deep breath and perform a Valsalva. An airtight dressing is placed over the site once the tube has been removed.

Wounds

All surgical procedures involve the creation of a wound. Factors that prevent wounds from healing include: Lack of good blood supply (smoking and microvascular damage), infection, malnutrition, immunosuppression (diabetes, HIV), radiation, and age.

Clean wounds: Created at the time of elective surgery can be closed primarily. Suture used for wound closure should be placed in tissue with tensile strength such as the dermis or the fascia.

Contaminated wounds: Emergent surgery with free intra-abdominal contamination is best closed by secondary intention. Healing by secondary intention involves closure of a wound by the natural biologic forces of wound contraction. These wounds are dressed with antiseptic gauze moist with saline. Once the wound has granulated with pink healthy tissue other forms of dressing can applied to accelerate healing.

Stomas

A stoma is an artificial union made between 2 conduits (eg a choledocho-jejunostomy) or, more commonly, between a conduit and the outside—eg a colostomy, in which feces are made to pass through a hole in the abdominal wall into an adherent plastic pouch. When choosing the site for a colostomy, avoid areas in scars, the area around the waistline, and creases. The patient should be sitting at the time of stoma marking.

The *stoma nurse* is expert in fitting secure, odorless devices. Ensure patients have their phone number for use before and after surgery. Their visits are more useful than any doctor's in explaining what is going to happen, and what the colostomy will be like, and in troubleshooting post-op problems.

1 *Loop colostomy:* A loop of colon is exteriorized, opened, and sewn to the skin. A rod under the loop prevents retraction and may be removed after 5–7d. This is often called a defunctioning colostomy but this is not strictly true as feces may pass beyond the loop. A loop colostomy is used to protect a distal anastomosis or to relieve distal obstruction. It is often temporary, and more prone to complications than end colostomies. A colostomy does not need to protrude much from the skin because the efflux is not as much as an irritant as in more proximal stomas such as in ileostomy.

2 *End colostomy:* The bowel is divided; the proximal end brought out as a stoma. The distal end may be: Resected (eg abdominoperineal excision of the rectum) left in the abdomen (Hartman's procedure), or exteriorized, forming a 'mucous fistula'.

3 *Double-barrelled (Paul-Mikulicz) colostomy:* The colon is brought out as two openings (similar to a mucus fistula).

Ileostomies protrude from the skin and emit fluid motions which contain active enzymes (so skin needs protecting). These stoma are made to protrude (Brooke) more than a colostomy because of the risk of skin irritation. Furthermore, because the colon is not in continuity, the risk of dehydration is great. Patients must be instructed on careful fluid management. End ileostomy usually follows proctocolectomy, typically for UC. Loop ileostomy can be used to temporarily protect distal anastomoses.

Complications of stomas

Work closely with the stoma nurse, starting pre-operatively.

Early:
- Hemorrhage at stoma site
- Stoma ischemia
- High output (especially ileostomies—can lead to ↑ K^+ and dehydration)
- Obstruction secondary to adhesions
- Stoma retraction.

Delayed:
- Obstruction (failure at operation to close lateral space around stoma)
- Dermatitis around stoma site
- Stoma prolapse
- Parastomal hernia
- Fistula
- Psychological problems.

Thyroid disease, hepatic failure, steroids, anticoagulation, and surgery

Thyroid hormone exerts primary influences on growth and metabolism. It is not a primary mediator of the host response to injury and infection. Frequently, thyroid hormones levels are low in severe illness.

Thyroid surgery for hyperthyroidism: Life-threatening thyrotoxicosis may be precipitated by any operation but especially after thyroidectomy for hyperthyroidism. It is best to bring hyperthyroid patients into a euthyroid state before surgery. If severe, give propylthiouracil 50–200mg q4h for 1wk followed by 200–400mg/d for an additional 5wks prior to surgery or until euthyroid. Aqueous iodine oral solution (Lugol's solution), 0.1–0.3mL/8h PO well diluted with milk or water can also be started prior to surgery.

Mild hyperthyroidism: Start propranolol 80mg/8h po and Lugol's solution as above at the 1st consultation. Stop Lugol's solution on the day of surgery but continue propranolol for 5d post-op.

Thyroid Storm: Severe thyrotoxicosis may result of surgical stress or trauma. The patient may be tachycardia, febrile, and have an altered mental status. Supplemental oxygen should be given to the patient as well as propanolol and hydrocortisone. There is a 10–20% mortality rate associated with thyroid storm.

Hepatic failure and surgery: Patients with hepatic failure are particularly prone to developing oliguria after surgery. The cause of this can be multifactorial and includes pre-renal azotemia, acute renal failure, and the hepatorenal syndrome. The cause of the hepatorenal syndrome is unknown but may be related to intra-hepatic blood flow redistribution and cortical ischemia and inappropriate activation of the rennin-angiotensin system. Development of this syndrome is suggestive of a grim outcome.

Pre-operative preparation:
• Consider arterial line and CVP line to ensure an adequate intravascular volume intra-operatively and post-operatively.
• Insert a urinary catheter.
• Check clotting, and give prophylactic vitamin K (p570).

During surgery:
• Measure urine output
• Alert anesthesiolgist to the removal of large quantities of ascites which may lead to hypovolemia. Consider giving 0.9% saline IV to match the urine output.
• Measure urine output and urine and serum electrolytes and follow closely. Low urine sodium concentration (<10mEq/L) with normal urine osmolality may suggest pre-renal azotemia or the hepatorenal syndrome.
• Give 0.9% saline at rate to match fluid lost through NGT; as well as maintenance fluid.
• Intraoperative ascites drains may be placed to help with anastomotic healing and wound closure. Drain output should be matched ½ cc per CC output with 0.9% normal saline. Spironolactone (50–100mg every 6–8h) may be used to assist in treating ascites.
• Give furosemide if urine output is poor despite adequate intravascular volume.

Surgery in those on steroids or anticoagulants:

Steroids Patients with a history of steroid use in the 6 months prior to surgery may need extra exogenous steroids to cope with the added stress of surgery and the potential for adrenal insufficiency. The amount needed depends on the extent of the surgery and the pre-op dose of steroids. *Major surgery:* Typically give hydrocortisone 50–100mg IV with the pre-med and then every 8h IV/IM for 2d. Then return to previous medication. *Minor surgery:* Prepare as for major surgery except that hydrocortisone is given for 24h only. Adrenal insufficiency results in hypotension. If this is encountered without an obvious cause, it may be worthwhile giving a dose of 50mg hydrocortisone IV.

Those on stable long-term anticoagulants (warfarin and aspirin): All long-term anticoagulants should be stopped 5–7d prior to surgery. Presently, there are enough alternatives that no patient should be on a long-term anticoagulant at the time of surgery. Discuss these issues when arranging consent. Vitamin K or FFP may be needed in emergency surgery. Patients with artificial valves requiring anticoagulation (particularly mitral) and newly placed cardiac stents should be placed on an alternative shorter-acting anticoagulant prior to surgery such as SQ fractionated heparin (lovenox) or, IV unfractionated heparin.

Postoperative care

Postoperative complications and management

Fever Mild fever in the first 24h is typically from atelectasis (needs prompt respiratory therapy, not antibiotics), or tissue damage or necrosis but an ↑ in temperature more than 24h post-op should stimulate an infection evaluation. Check the chest x-ray for pneumonia, the wound, the urine, and the abdomen for signs of peritonitis (eg anastomotic leakage). Examine sites of IV cannula and central venous access for signs of infection. Check the legs for DVT. Send blood for CBC, electrolytes, and culture. Send the urine for analysis. Consider chest x-ray, abdominal CT, and lower extremity duplex depending on the clinical findings.

Confusion This may manifest as agitation, disorientation, and attempts to leave hospital especially at night. Gently reassure the patient in well-lit surroundings, p323. The common causes are:

- Hypoxia (pneumonia, atelectasis, CHF, PE)
- Infection (see above)
- Drugs (opiates, sedatives, and many others)
- Alcohol withdrawal
- Urinary retention; MI or stroke
- Liver/renal failure.

Occasionally, sedation is necessary to examine the patient; consider midazolam (antidote: Flumazenil) or haloperidol 0.5–2mg IM. Reassure relatives that post-op confusion is common and reversible.

Shortness of breath or hypoxia Any previous lung disease?

Sit up and give oxygen, monitoring peripheral O_2 saturation by pulse oximetry. Examine for evidence of:

- Pneumonia/pulmonary collapse/aspiration
- Pulmonary edema (MI or fluid overload)
- Pulmonary embolism (p178)
- Pneumothorax (p179; due to CVP line or intercostal anaesthetic block).

Do CBC, arterial blood gases, CXR, and ECG. Manage according to findings.

BP↓ If severe, tilt bed head down and give O_2. Check pulse rate and measure BP yourself; compare it with that prior to surgery. Post-op ↓BP is commonly due to hypovolemia resulting from inadequate fluid input so check fluid chart and replace losses, usually with colloid initially. Monitor urine output; consider catheterization. A CVP line may be useful to monitor fluid resuscitation. Hypovolemia may also be caused by hemorrhage so review wounds and abdomen. If severe, return to operating room for hemostasis. Beware cardiogenic causes and look for evidence of MI and PE. Consider sepsis and anaphylaxis.

Urine output↓ (oliguria) Aim for output of >30mL/h in adults (½mL/kg/h). Anuria frequently means a blocked or obstructed catheter. Flush or replace catheter. Oliguria is usually due to inadequate replacement of lost fluid. Treat by ↑ fluid input. Acute renal failure may follow shock, nephrotoxic drugs, transfusion, or trauma.

- Review fluid chart and examine for signs of volume depletion.
- Urinary retention is also common, so examine for a palpable bladder.
- Establish normovolemia (a CVP line may help here, normal is 0–5cm H_2O relative to sternal angle); you may need 1L/h IV for 2–3h.
- If intrinsic renal failure is suspected, refer to a nephrologist early.

Nausea/vomiting Any mechanical obstruction, paralytic ileus, or emetic drugs (opiates, digoxin, anesthetics)? Consider AXR, NGT, and anti-emetic.

Other post-op complications Pain (p412), DVT (p414), pulmonary embolus (p178), wound dehiscence.

Follow-up for surgical patients

1 Prior to discharge all patient should be given instructions for follow-up. Determine what further care is needed for the patient.
2 If patients have skin staples, these are usually removed 10–14d after surgery.
3 If a patient has a stoma, this should be attended to by a stoma therapist by at least 4wks after surgery because often the size of the stoma will change.
4 If patient is being treated for a cancer and requires further adjuvant therapy, often the oncologist appreciates a check from the surgeon prior to initiating therapy.

Post-operative bleeding

- Primary hemorrhage: le continuous bleeding, starting during surgery. Replace blood loss. If severe, return to the operating room for adequate hemostasis. Treat shock vigorously (p686).
- Reactive hemorrhage: Hemostasis appears secure until BP rises and bleeding starts. Replace blood and re-explore wound.
- Secondary hemorrhage occurs 1 or 2wks post-op and is the result of infection.

Discharging patients after day-case surgery

After day-case surgery, don't discharge until 'LEAP-FROG' is established:

Lucid, not vomiting, and cough reflex established.
Easy breathing; easy urination.
Ambulating.
Pain relief + post-op drugs dispensed + given. Do they understand doses?
Follow-up arranged.
Rhythm, pulse rate, and bp checked one last time. Is trend satisfactory?
Operation site checked and explained to patient.
Give the primary care provider a call.

The acute abdomen

Any sudden manifestation of a non-traumatic disorder involving pain in the abdominal area for which urgent surgical exploration may be necessary and repeated examination is essential.

Begin by obtaining a careful history of the pain: Ask about the location of the pain, any spreading or shifting, duration, mode of onset, progression, character (dull, sharp, crampy) and any other associated symptoms including: Nausea, vomiting, diarrhea, obstipation, constipation, hematuria, etc.

Types of pain

Visceral pain is mediated by the afferent C fiber and usually is felt in the midline. It is slow in onset and dull. It can be elicited by distension, inflammation, or ischemia.

Parietal pain is mediated by both C fibers and A delta nerve fibers. Abdominal parietal pain is more focused as a result of direct irritation of the somatically innervated parietal peritoneum by pus, bile, GI secretions etc. It is conventional described as occurring in 4 abdominal quadrants (see diagram p433).

Other relevant aspects of history include:
1 Medical and surgical history
2 Menstrual history
3 Drug history
4 Family history
5 Travel history.

Physical exam Observe patient—lying still or writhing, pallor, sweating, feverish. Inspect the abdomen for distension, bruising—grey-turners sign for hemorrhagic pancreatits. Auscultate for bowel sound—hypoactive indicated intra-abdominal infection, hyperactive sounds are noted in bowel obstruction. Palpate in a sequential pattern with the most tender area being touched last. Specific signs on palpation include:
1 Guarding—peritoneal inflammation causing rectus muscle rigidity.
2 Rebound tenderness—discomfort is felt upon releasing your hands from gentle pressure—acute appendicitis.
3 Murphy's sign—palpation in the right subcostal area while inspiring causes abrupt arrest of inspiration secondary to pain—acute cholecystitis.
4 Iliopsoas sign—active flexion or passive extension of the hip illicit pain—psoas abscess in Crohn's disease.
5 Obturators sign—internal or external rotation of the flexed thigh may cause discomfort in the groin area—incarcerated obturator hernia.
6 Costovertebral angle tenderness—punch tenderness of the costovertebral angle—renal colic.

Tests CBC, electrolytes; amylase; LFT; β-HCG; urinalysis; laparoscopy may avert open surgery. CT can be helpful provided it is readily available and causes no delay;

Pre-op care Anesthesia compounds shock, so resuscitate properly first (p686) unless blood is being lost faster than it can be replaced in ruptured ectopic pregnancy, or a leaking abdominal aneurysm, p438. Also do the following:
1 Establish good IV access (two 18 gauge IVs) and begin resuscitation with 0.9% saline
2 Insert Foley and NGT
3 Type and cross-match
4 EKG, AXR, CXR
5 Begin broad spectrum antibiotics if infection is suspected
6 Consent and manage pain.

Clinical syndromes that usually require urgent surgical exploration

■ *Rupture of an organ* (Spleen, aorta, ectopic pregnancy). Shock secondary to cardiovascular collapse (eg faints or orthostatic BP↓ by ≥20mmHg on standing) is a leading sign. Abdominal swelling may be seen. Delayed rupture of the spleen may occur weeks after trauma.

■ *Peritonitis* (Perforation of peptic ulcer, diverticulum, appendix, bowel, or gall bladder). Signs: Prostration, shock, lying still, tenderness (± rebound/percussion pain), board-like abdominal rigidity, guarding, and no bowel sounds. Erect CXR may show gas under the diaphragm on the right side usually—or free intraperitoneal air. NB: Acute pancreatitis (p452) may cause these signs, but does not require a laparotomy—so always check serum amylase.

■ Syndromes that may not require urgent exploration

■ *Local peritonitis:* Eg diverticulitis, cholecystitis, salpingitis, and appendicitis. If abscess formation is suspected (palpable mass, fever, and WBC↑), arrange a diagnostic ultrasound or CT. Drainage can be percutaneous (ultrasound or CT guided), or by laparotomy. Look for 'a sentinel loop' on the plain AXR.

■ *Colic* is a regularly waxing and waning pain, caused by muscular spasm in a hollow viscus, eg gut, ureter, uterus, or gall bladder (in the latter, pain is often dull and constant). Colic causes restlessness, unlike peritonitis.

Other causes of abdominal pain that may masquerade as an acute surgical abdomen in which surgery is not indicated include:

Myocardial infarction	Pneumonia (p158)	Sickle-cell crisis (p566)
Gastroenteritis or UTI	Tabes (p539)	Pheochromocytoma (p295)
Diabetes mellitus (p268)	Zoster (p510)	Malaria (p504)
Pneumococcal peritonitis	Tuberculosis (p506)	Typhoid fever (p543)
Henoch–Schönlein	Porphyria (p628)	Cholera (p535)
Narcotic addiction	Thyroid storm	*Yersinia enterocolitica* (p533)
	PAN (p378)	Lead colic

Accuracy in diagnosing acute abdomen is ~45% so always keep a high index of suspicion. It is better to have a negative surgical exploration than to miss a surgical emergency. With newer minimally invasive techniques in surgery, patient recover and get well quickly. These diagrams go over the causes of an acute abdomen manifested as free intra-abdominal air or peritonitis.

Intestinal ischemia

Acute onset of severe abdominal pain should always suggest the idea of bowel ischemia. Etiology can be classified as the following:

1 Occlusive: Strangulated bowel, large vessel embolic or thrombotic event, ligation of the IMA during aortic surgery
2 Vasospastic: Small vessel non-occlusive intestinal ischemia, ischemic hepatitis, pancreatitis, acalculous cholecystitis
3 Inflammatory: Lupus. Beçhet's disease, angioedema

Acute intestinal ischemia: The most common cause is arterial embolism. Emboli originate from the heart in over 75% of cases and lodge preferentially just distal to the origin of the SMA (see diagram OPPOSITE). Low flow states usually reflect poor cardiac output but there may be other factors such as DIC. Venous thrombosis is uncommon and tends to affect smaller lengths of bowel. The incidence of acute colonic ischemia after aortic surgery is 5–9%. Other risk factors include: Atrial fibrillation, recent myocardial infarction, valvular heart disease, recent cardiac or vascular catheterization, atherosclerotic disease, hypercoaguable state.

A classical clinical triad of occlusive ischemia: Acute severe abdominal pain; no abdominal signs; and rapid hypovolemia (causing shock). Pain tends to be constant and central, or in the right lower quadrant. The degree of pain is often out of proportion to the clinical signs.

Non-occlusive ischemia: (ischemic colitis) Usually presents with generalized abdominal pain, anorexia, bloody stools, and abdominal distension.

Tests: There may be Hb↑ (due to plasma loss), WBC↑, modestly raised plasma amylase, elevated lactate, elevated CPK, and a persistent metabolic acidosis. Early on the AXR shows a 'gasless' abdomen. Arteriography helps but many diagnoses are made at laparotomy. CT/MR angiography may provide a non-invasive alternative to conventional arteriography.

Treatment: Fluid replacement, antibiotics (broad spectrum) secondary to the risk of translocation and, usually, heparin. If arteriography is performed, thrombolytics may be infused locally via the catheter. At surgery dead bowel must be removed. What needs to be removed can be a difficult surgical decision and often the Woods lamp can help. Revascularization of potentially viable bowel should be attempted but is difficult. A second-look laparotomy may be required.

Chronic intestinal ischemia Small bowel chronic ischemia and is typically due to SMA disease. Less common causes of ischemia include vasculitis, trauma, radiotherapy, and strangulation, eg hernias. It presents quite a different picture from acute ischemia, with severe, colicky post-prandial abdominal pain ('gut claudication') with weight loss (food hurts). Auscultation may reveal abdominal bruits. Diagnosis can be made by duplex ultrasound scan of the aorta or on angiography. Treatment requires revascularization with either endovascular or open surgical techniques.

Colonic ischemia usually follows low flow in the watershed areas between the inferior mesenteric artery and the superior mesenteric branches. Griffiths (splenic flexure) and Sudecks (rectosigmoid) points (see diagram OPPOSITE). Patients present with left-sided abdominal pain and bloody diarrhea. There may be fever, tachycardia, blood per rectum, and a leukocytosis. Usually this 'ischemic colitis' resolves, but it may progress to gangrenous ischemic colitis. Colonoscopy will demonstrate a spectrum of findings beginning with hyperemia and ending with frankly dead mucosa. Barium enema may show 'thumbprinting' indentation of the barium due to submucosal swelling. CT will demonstrate diffuse colonic thickening. Symptoms may be mild and result in stricture formation. Treatment may be supportive with fluid replacement and antibiotics or involve surgical removal of the colon with formation of an ileostomy in severe cases.

Gangrenous ischemic colitis This may follow ischemic colitis and is signalled by more severe pain, peritonitis, and hypovolemic shock. After resuscitation, necrotic bowel should be resected and a colostomy or ileostomy formed.

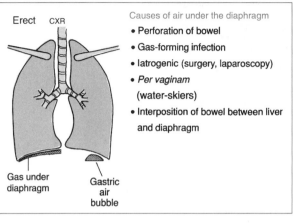

Erect   CXR

Causes of air under the diaphragm

- Perforation of bowel
- Gas-forming infection
- Iatrogenic (surgery, laparoscopy)
- *Per vaginam*
  (water-skiers)
- Interposition of bowel between liver
  and diaphragm

Gas under
diaphragm

Gastric
air
bubble

The causes of parietal pain in the 4 quadrants of the abdomen.

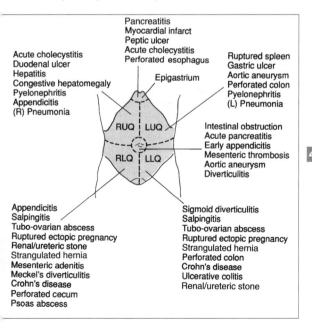

Pancreatitis
Myocardial infarct
Peptic ulcer
Acute cholecystitis
Perforated esophagus

Acute cholecystitis
Duodenal ulcer
Hepatitis
Congestive hepatomegaly
Pyelonephritis
Appendicitis
(R) Pneumonia

Epigastrium

Ruptured spleen
Gastric ulcer
Aortic aneurysm
Perforated colon
Pyelonephritis
(L) Pneumonia

RUQ   LUQ

RLQ   LLQ

Intestinal obstruction
Acute pancreatitis
Early appendicitis
Mesenteric thrombosis
Aortic aneurysm
Diverticulitis

Appendicitis
Salpingitis
Tubo-ovarian abscess
Ruptured ectopic pregnancy
Renal/ureteric stone
Strangulated hernia
Mesenteric adenitis
Meckel's diverticulitis
Crohn's disease
Perforated cecum
Psoas abscess

Sigmoid diverticulitis
Salpingitis
Tubo-ovarian abscess
Ruptured ectopic pregnancy
Strangulated hernia
Perforated colon
Crohn's disease
Ulcerative colitis
Renal/ureteric stone

Gastrointestinal bleeding

Gastrointestinal bleeding is manifested as hematemesis, melena, or hemato
chezia. Melena can be from a gastroduodenal source as well as from the
colon. Small bowel bleeding is rare (<5%). The most common causes of
gastrointestinal bleeding are listed below:

Upper gastrointestinal tract:
• Peptic ulcer disease
• Gastritis
• Gastric neoplasia
• Mallory–Weiss syndrome (see below)
• Delafore lesion
• Varices.

Small intestinal bleeding:
• Angiodysplasia
• Meckel's diverticulum
• Crohn's enteritis
• Neoplasia
• NSAID abuse.

Large intestinal bleeding:
• Diverticulosis (30–50%)
• Colitis—inflammatory, infectious, or ischemic (20%)
• Angiodysplasia (10%)
• AV malformations
• Anorectal disease
• Neoplasia.

Initial management: Directed toward resuscitation and include the following
1 Establish IV access with two large bore IVs (16 gauge).
2 Draw blood for type and cross-match, CBC, PT,PTT, and electrolytes.
3 NGT aspirate to rule out upper GI source although can be inaccurate.
4 Foley catheterization and O_2 administration is based on the severity of
   the bleed.
5 Obtain history regarding the use of warfarin, plavix, aspirin, or NSAIDs.

Diagnostic tests: For bleeding <1cc/min: EGD and colonoscopy

For bleeding ≥1cc/min: Angiography for localization and possible treatment
radionucleotide bleeding scan, endoscopic evaluation, surgery

Therapeutic interventions: Most causes of upper gastrointestinal bleeding
are now managed endoscopically with either electrocautery, heater probe
banding, or injection of epinephrine, Similar, lower tract bleeding can also be
managed endoscopically but more frequently will require surgery.

Arterial embolization or coiling is routinely performed for gastroduodenal
bleeding because of the low risk of end organ ischemia. However, only highly
selective embolization can be performed for colonic bleeding secondary to
the risk of ischemia following embolization (20%).

Surgical intervention for colonic bleeding from a source that has NOT been
identified either colonoscopically or angiographically is a subtotal colectomy.
If the bleeding source has been identified, a colonic segmentectomy can be
performed. The decision whether or not to re-anastomose the bowel is
based on the overall health of the patient and the amount of bleeding that
has occurred. A transfusion requirement of greater than 10 units is associated with a higher anastomotic leak rate.

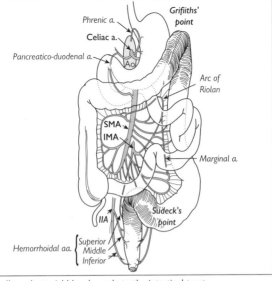

Phrenic a.

Grifiiths' point

Celiac a.

Pancreatico-duodenal a.

Ao

Arc of Riolan

SMA

IMA

Marginal a.

IIA

Sudeck's point

Hemorrhoidal aa. { Superior / Middle / Inferior }

The collateral arterial blood supply to the intestinal tract

Mallory–Weiss syndrome

A 1–4cm submucosal tear occurring at the gastroesophageal junction usually following forceful retching. The lesion is diagnosed on EGD. Brisk bleeding will require surgical repair by the creation of an open high gastrotomy and oversewing the bleeding ends. Alternatively, with less brisk bleeding the lesion can be controlled with endoscopic electrocautery.

Trauma

Trauma is the leading cause of death in the US for individuals <45yrs of ag
Death as a result of trauma can occur immediately as a result of hemorrhag
severe head injury, loss of airway, pneumothorax, and fatal heart injury. Oth
causes of death can be less immediate and include sepsis and multiple orga
system failure. Surgical training under the auspices of Advanced Trauma Li
Support (ATLS) has devised an algorithm for maximizing the care of th
trauma patient. The basics of this algorithm are the ABCDE of primary surve
in trauma care and are the following:

A. **Airway and cervical spine protection**—an airway can be maintaine
with a simple jaw thrust and bagging. A definitive airway can be estab
lished either by orotracheal, nasotracheal, or surgical airway and is ind
cated in: Apnea, inability to maintain airway or oxygenation by othe
means, and airway protection in inhalation injuries, head injuries etc.
   i. Spinal cord injuries must be assumed in all patients and therefor
   inline manual cervical traction should be used during intubation
   ii. A surgical airway should be performed through use of the cricothy
   roid membrane when oral or nasotracheal intubation can not b
   successfully performed.

B. **Breathing and ventilation**—expose the chest to assess breathing
Keep an eye out for the following disorders that will inhibit adequat
breathing.
   i. Tension pneumothorax—hypotension with distended neck veins-
   treat initially with large-bore IV placed in the second intercostal
   space in the mid-clavicular line.
   ii. Flail chest—multiple rib fractures often associated with pneumothora
   and pulmonary contusion.
   iii. Massive hemorrhage and hemothorax—requires thoracostomy an
   possibly thoracotomy if >1000cc drain immediately or patient be
   comes hemodynamically unstable.
   iv. Open pneumothorax—initial treatment is the placement of a steril
   occlusive dressing taped on three sides with a flutter valve. Definit
   treatment is a chest tube.

C. **Circulation**
   i. Shock—recognize and resuscitate with 0.9% NS or LR. Assume hemor
   rhage and be prepared to give O neg blood. Other causes of shock i
   trauma include tamponade, tension pneumothorax, air embolus
   myocardial contusion, and spinal cord injury resulting in neurogeni
   shock. Cardiac tamponade—can be diagnosed on bedside ultrasoun
   (focused assessment with sonography for trauma—FAST). Manage
   ment usually requires pericardial window.
   ii. interventions:
      1. Apply direct pressure to external bleeding.
      2. Two large-caliber IVs and possibly cordis for large volume rapi
      infusion.
      3. Infusion of crystalloid using 3:1 rule and give type specific c
      O neg blood for class III or IV shock (see OPPOSITE).
      4. Send patients blood for type and cross-match, hemoglobir
      chemistries, β-HCG in female patients.

Classes of shock

Class I. Blood volume loss <15% associated with mild tachycardia

Class II. Blood volume loss 15–30%. Signs include tachycardia, tachypnea, ↓ pulse pressure.

Class III. Blood volume loss of 30–40%. Marked tachycardia and tachypnea, hypotension and confusion

Class IV. Blood volume loss of >40%. Severe tachycardia, hypotension, narrow pulse pressure, obtundation.

D. **Disability**—refers to a brief neurologic assesment. This assessed via a measurement for the level or consciousness also known as the Glasgow coma scale (see below). Altered mental status may be the result of hypoxia, shock, drugs, alcohol, but consider injury to the central nervous system until proven otherwise.

Glasgow coma scale

Assessment of eye opening (1–4)

Assessment of verbal response (1–5)

Assessment of motor response (1–6)

If total is ≤8, high potential for severe CNS injury.

E. **Exposure**—undress the patient to evaluate every area to make sure no injury is missed. Broken bones are commonly missed in the intoxicated trauma patient. Once this is done, the patient should be covered to prevent hypothermia.

Following the primary survey for trauma, a secondary survey is undertaken. This begins with an AMPLE history—Allergies, Medicines, Past medical and surgical history, Last meal, Exposures (tetanus). A complete head-to-toe examination is performed and vital signs are reassessed. Any further interventions are arranged.

Aortic aneurysm and dissection

Aortic aneurysm True aneurysms are abnormal dilatations of arteries. They should be distinguished from 'false' aneurysms, which are collections of blood around a vessel wall eg following trauma. Aneurysms may be fusiform or sac-like (eg Berry aneurysms in the circle of Willis). Common sites: Aorta, iliac, femoral, and popliteal arteries. Atheroma is the usual cause; also connective tissue disorders (eg Marfan's, Ehlers–Danlos), and infections (eg endocarditis, or tertiary syphilis). Complications from aneurysms: Rupture; thrombosis; embolism; pressure on other structures; infection.

Symptomatic and ruptured abdominal aortic aneurysm (AAA)

Signs & symptoms: Intermittent or continuous abdominal pain (radiates to back, lower abdomen, or groins), collapse, an expansile abdominal mass (ie the mass expands and contracts: Swellings that are pulsatile merely transmit the pulse, eg nodes overlying arteries), and mottling over the lower extremities. Other associated findings in patients with AAA include hypertension ~ 40%, peripheral aneurysms ~ 20%. The main differential diagnoses are myocardial infarction and pancreatitis. If in doubt, assume a ruptured aneurysm.

Management

1 Start two large bore IVs
2 Send type and cross-match for 12 units, CBC, electrolytes, EKG, and if in doubt, cross table lateral plain film of the abdomen which will demonstrate aortic calcification
3 Take the patient to the operating room. Do not order other investigations. You will waste precious time.
4 The patient is prepped and draped while awake and only put to sleep when the surgeon is ready to cut. Surgery involves clamping the aorta above the leak (usually at the diaphragmatic hiatus. Alternatively, a large bore foley can be placed in the proximal end of the aorta and inflated to temporary tamponade the bleeding. A Dacron® graft (eg 'tube graft' or, if significant iliac aneurysm also, a 'trouser graft' with each 'leg' attached to an iliac artery). Presently, the role of endoluminal placement of stent grafts for ruptured AAA is being investigated (see below).

Outcomes: Mortality—treated: 21–70%; untreated: 100%.

Asymptomatic AAA

Prevalence: 3% of those >50yrs. Trials suggest that aneurysms <5.5cm across might safely be monitored by regular examination and ultrasound/CT. Risk of rupture below this size is <1%/yr, compared with ~25%/yr for aneurysms >6cm across. Aneurysms larger than this, rapidly expanding (>1cm/yr) or symptomatic should be considered for elective surgery. It should be noted that ~75% of aneurysms monitored in this way will eventually need repair. Elective operative mortality is ~5%. Studies show that age >80yrs is not a reason to decline surgery

Open operations can sometimes be avoided by the placement of an endoluminal stent graft via the femoral artery. When successfully positioned, such stents can lead to shorter hospital stays and fewer transfusions than with conventional surgery. Many patients are not suitable for such stents, however, because of the anatomy of their aneurysms. There is also a risk that the stent will leak.

Preparation for surgery is similar to the above preparation with the addition of a preoperative cardiac and pulmonary evaluation. A mechanical bowel prep is preferred. Urinalysis should be performed and antibiotics given prior to incision

Postoperative care and complications Patients will usually spend time in the intensive care unit postoperatively. Peripheral pulses are monitored. The most common complications following aortic surgery include:

1 Renal insufficiency: Usually hypovolemic but you must be concerned about injury from aortic cross-clamping leading to embolization.

438

2 Ischemic colitis: Secondary to IMA ligation. Can start as early as 12h after surgery.

3 Spinal cord ischemia: Occurs when the blood supply to the distal spinal cord is compromised and results in paraplegia. The injured artery is known as the artery of Adamkiewicz and can arise anywhere from T8 to L4.

Aorta dissection

Blood splits aortic media with sudden tearing chest pain (± radiation to back). As dissection unfolds, branches of the aorta occlude leading sequentially to hemiplegia (carotid), unequal arm pulses and bp, paraplegia (anterior spinal artery), and anuria (renal arteries). Aortic incompetence and inferior mi may develop if dissection moves proximally. Aortic dissection is classified according to the Stanford classification.

Stanford classification

Type A. Primary intimal tear located in the ascending aorta
   2/3rd of all dissections
   Ehler–Danlos syndrome, Marfan's

Type B. Dissection limited to the descending thoracic aorta with the intimal tear located near the subclavian artery
   1/3rd of all dissections
   Ruptured atherosclerotic plaque

Management:

Type A dissections Because the risk of intrapericardial rupture and left ventricular failure, all patients with type A dissections should be considered for surgery. Cross-match 10U blood; do ECG & CXR (expanded mediastinum is rare). • CT/MRI or transesophageal echocardiography (TEE). Take to ICU; hypertensive: Keep systolic at ~100–110mmHg: Labetolol (p132) or esmolol (p119; t½ is ultra-short) by IVI is helpful here. Peri-operative mortality: ≤12%.

Type B dissections May extend and cause symptoms as a result of poor flow to peripheral vessels. Symptomatic extension is treated surgically or by endovascular techniques with fenestration, stenting, or bypass. To prevent extension, anti-hypertensive therapy is started.

Limb ischemia

Chronic ischemia This is due to atherosclerosis. Its chief feature is intermittent claudication (from the Latin, meaning to limp). Cramping pain is felt in the calf, thigh, or buttock after walking for a fairly fixed distance (the claudication distance). Ulceration, gangrene, and foot pain at rest, eg burning pain at night relieved by hanging legs over side of bed are cardinal features of critical ischemia.

Signs: Absent pulses; cold, white leg(s); atrophic skin; punched out ulcers (often painful); postural color change.

Tests: Exclude DM, arteritis (ESR/CRP). Do CBC (anemia, infection); electrolytes (renal disease); lipids (dyslipidemia); syphilis serology; ECG (cardiac ischemia). Do coagulation profile and type and cross-match if planning arteriography. *Ankle—brachial pressure index (Doppler):* Normal ≈ 1. Claudication ≈ 0.9–0.6. Rest pain ≈ 0.3–0.6. Impending gangrene ≤0.3 or ankle systolic pressure <50mmHg. Do *arteriography, digital subtraction arteriography or color duplex imaging* to assess the extent and location of stenoses and the quality of distal vessels ('run off'). If only distal obliterative disease is seen, and little proximal atheroma, suspect arteritis, previous embolus, or diabetes mellitus.

Management: Many claudicants improve with conservative treatment, ie quit smoking, ↓weight, more exercise—ideally a supervised exercise program. Treat diabetes, hypertension (avoid β-blockers), and hyperlipidemia. Aspirin has a role. Vasodilators rarely help.

Percutaneous transluminal angioplasty is good for short stenoses in big arteries (a balloon is inflated in the narrowed segment). Stents maintain artery patency after angioplasty, and are beneficial for iliac artery disease. If atheromatous disease is extensive but distal run off is good (ie distal arteries filled by collateral vessels), they may be a candidate for arterial reconstruction by a bypass graft. Vein grafts are often used but prosthetic grafts are an option. Aspirin helps prosthetic grafts to remain patent; warfarin may be better after vein grafts and in high-risk patients.

Sympathectomy (chemical or surgical) may help relieve rest pain. It may not be appropriate in diabetic patients with peripheral neuropathy.

Amputation may relieve intractable pain and death from sepsis and gangrene. The decision to amputate must be made by the patient, usually against a background of failed alternative strategies. The level of amputation must be high enough to ensure healing of the stump. Rehabilitation should be started early with a view to limb fitting.

Acute ischemia This may be due to thrombosis in situ (in ~41%), emboli (38%), graft/angioplasty occlusion (15%), or trauma. There is little difference in presenting signs. Mortality: 22%. Amputation rate: 16%.

Signs/symptoms: 5 Ps—the part is pulseless, painful, pallor, paraesthetic, and paralysed. Onset of fixed mottling implies irreversibility. Emboli commonly arise from the heart (infarcts, AF) or an aneurysm (aorta, femoral, or popliteal). ►The limb may be red, but only when dependent, leading to disastrous misdiagnosis of gout or cellulitis.

Management: ►This is an emergency and may require urgent surgery or angioplasty. Ischemia <12h is associated with 93% limb salvage rate, whereas, ischemic time >12h is associated with only a 78% limb salvage rate and a 30% mortality. If diagnosis is in doubt, do urgent arteriography. If the occlusion is embolic, the options are surgical embolectomy (Fogarty catheter) or local thrombolysis, eg t-PA (p571). Anticoagulate with heparin before and after either procedure. Later, look for the embolic source: Echocardiogram; ultrasound of aorta, popliteal and femoral arteries. Ischemia following trauma and acute thrombosis may require urgent reconstruction.

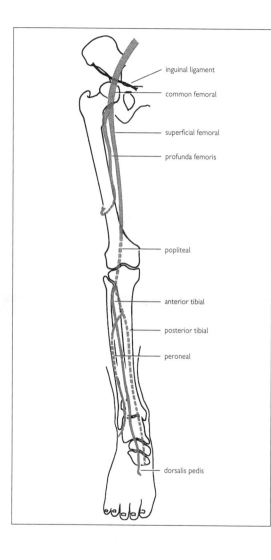

inguinal ligament

common femoral

superficial femoral

profunda femoris

popliteal

anterior tibial

posterior tibial

peroneal

dorsalis pedis

Acute appendicitis

Appendicitis is primarily a disease of adolescents and young adults and is uncommon in individuals over the age of 55yrs. The female/male ratio is 1.2:1.5. Although the incidence of acute appendicitis approaches 20% in some reports, there has been a notable decline in the incidence for all age groups over the past 30yrs.

Pathogenesis Epidemiologists have demonstrated that genetic, dietary, and infectious factors are associated with development of acute appendicitis. Appendiceal inflammation results from luminal obstruction of the appendiceal orifice lymphoid hyperplasia, fecolith, or filarial worms. This inflammation allows for invasion of GI organisms through the appendix wall. There may also be impaired ability to prevent invasion.

Symptoms: Often referred to as the 'great masquerader', the diagnosis of acute appendicitis is not always straight forward. A careful review of symptoms is essential.

Pain is the most important symptom; In general, as inflammation begins, there is central abdominal colic as a result of stimulation of the visceral pain fibers. Once the peritoneum becomes inflamed, the pain shifts to the right lower quadrant (RLQ) and becomes more constant. On examination, RLQ point tenderness (↑ pain on palpation) or rebound tenderness (↑ pain on release) may be present. Rovsing's sign (pain more in the RLQ than the LLQ when the LLQ is pressed. RLQ pain may also be elicited on rectal exam. In women, do a vaginal examination: Does she have cervical motion tenderness or discharge? RE-EXAMINE frequently if unsure of diagnosis.

Other signs and symptoms

- Tachycardia
- Lying still
- Flushing
- Low-grade fever
- Leukocytosis
- Anorexia
- Rare vomiting, diarrhea, or constipation

Essential studies:

cbc—to evaluate for a leukocytosis

Urinalysis—evaluate for WBC's and bacteria indicating bladder infection (can be misleading); RBCs which may suggest kidney stone.

βHCG—R/O pregnancy (ectopic).

Additional studies:

Abdominal x-rays—usually demonstrates a paucity of gas in the RLQ. May also see fecolith.

Abdominal CT scan—highly sensitive for appendiceal inflammation (thickening of appendiceal wall) but can not always separate acute and chronic inflammation

Abdominal ultrasound—sensitive for evaluation of ovarian cyst or abscess, hydrosalpinx.

Differential diagnosis	Cholecystitis	Crohn's disease
Ectopic pregnancy	Diverticulitis	Ovarian cyst or abscess
Mesenteric adenitis	Salpingitis	Kidney stone
Cystitis	Menstral cramps	Meckel's diverticulitis

Complications of acute appendicitis: Perforation (does not appear to cause later infertility in girls); appendix mass; appendix abscess.

An appendix mass may result when an inflamed appendix becomes covered with omentum or loops of small bowel. The mass is palpable on exam and easily seen on abdominal CT scan. Some advocate early surgery, but initial management is usually conservative—NPO and antibiotics (eg cefuroxime 1.5g/8h IV and metronidazole 500mg/8h IV). Mark out the size of the mass and proceed to drainage if the mass develops into an abscess (see below). If the mass resolves some perform an interval (ie delayed) appendicectomy.

An appendix abscess may result if an appendix mass fails to resolve. Signs of abscess formation include enlargement of the mass or if the patient gets more toxic (pain↑; temperature↑; pulse↑; WBC↑). Treatment usually involves drainage, either surgical or percutaneous (under radiological guidance). Antibiotics alone may bring about resolution, eg in >90% of children.

Surgical treatment

Once decision is made to operate, make patient NPO and hydrate with NS. Metronidazole 1g/8h + cefuroxime 1.5g/8h, 1 to 3 doses IV starting 1h pre-op, reduces wound infections. Appendectomy performed laporascopically or through a RLQ incision at McBurney's Point (one-third the distance between the anterior superior iliac crest and the umbilicus). Metronidazole 1g/8h + cefuroxime 1.5g/8h, 1 to 3 doses IV starting 1h pre-op, reduces wound infections. Some surgical hints include:

- Laparoscopic appendectomy ↓ recovery time and incidence of wound infections, but ↑ risk of intra-abdominal abscesses.
- If the appendix is perforated, most advocate closing the fascia but leaving the wound open for closure by secondary intention.
- If the appendiceal stump is difficult to locate and close and the appendix has ruptured, leave a drain because patient is at risk to develop GI leak and fistula.
- If the appendix is associated with an unusual mass, always think of carcinoid or cystadenoma of the appendix. These tumors may cause luminal obstruction and lead to appendicitis. Larger tumors (>2cm) will require formal R hemicolectomy which should be performed at the time of surgery or once pathology is confirmed.

443

Appendicitis in pregnancy

Appendicitis occurs in ~1/1000 pregnancies. Mortality is higher, especially from 20wks gestation. Perforation (15-20%), and ↑ fetal mortality from ~1.5% (for simple appendicitis) to ~30%. As pregnancy progresses, the appendix migrates, so pain is often less well localized. Prompt assessment is vital; laparotomy should be performed by an experienced surgeon.

Diverticular disease

A *diverticulum* is an out-pouching of the wall of the gut. The term *diverticulosis* means that diverticula are present, whereas *diverticular disease* implies they are symptomatic. *Diverticulitis* refers to inflammation within a diverticulum. Although diverticula may be congenital or acquired and can occur in any part of the gut, by far the most important type is acquired colonic diverticula, to which this page refers.

Pathogenesis: Most occur in the sigmoid colon with 95% of complications at this site but right-sided, as well as small bowel diverticula do occur. Lack of dietary fiber is thought to lead to high intraluminal pressures which force the mucosa to herniate through the muscular bowel wall near where vessels penetrate the wall. Nearly 50% of the population in the Western world over the age of 50 have diverticulosis.

Symptoms: 15–30% of patients with diverticulosis have symptomatic diverticular disease. The most common symptoms is left lower quadrant (LLQ) pain. Pain usually occurs after eating and persists. Associated symptoms include low grade fever, diarrhea or obstipation, and anorexia. Rarely do patients experience nausea or vomiting. On exam, LLQ point and rebound tenderness may be present,

Complications of diverticular disease

Free perforation: A free communication exists between the colon and the peritioneal cavity. There is ileus, peritonitis, ± shock. Free fluid in air is noted on imaging studies.

Hemorrhage: Is usually sudden and painless. It is a common cause of big rectal bleeds. Bleeding usually stops with bed rest.

Fistula: Colovesical—complaints of pneumoturia (air in urine stream) or fecaluria (feces in urine stream):
• Colovaginal—complaints of fecal vaginal discharge
• Coloenteric—complaints of persistent diarrhea.

Abscess: Eg with swinging fever, leukocytosis, and localizing signs eg boggy rectal mass.

Post-infective strictures may form in the sigmoid colon and present with large bowel obstruction.

Studies: CBC, urine analysis & culture.

Uncomplicated diverticulitis:
• ABD and pelvic CT scan initially
• Colonoscopy or barium enema once symptoms resolve to R/O cancer.

Complicated diverticular disease:
• Abdominal x-ray to R/O free air
• CT cystogram to R/O colovesical fistula
• Barium enema to R/O colovaginal fistula
• Small bowel series to R/O coloenteric fistula
• Colonoscopy to R/O cancer.

Treatment:

Uncomplicated diverticular disease:
• A 7–14d course of IV or oral antibiotics (ciprofloxacin 500mg bid and Flagyl 250–500mg PO tid).
• Keep NPO till pain resolves.
• Avoid narcotics which may constipate.
• Encourage a *high-fiber diet* with dietary supplements (Metamucil®) Antspasmodics such as Bentyl® 10mg PO 4x a day.
• Repetitive attacks requiring hospitalization of documented diverticular disease should be treated with either laparoscopic or open surgical resection of the diseased colon.

- Recurrence of LLQ pain after surgery is more common in patients who have not had a complete resection of the distal sigmoid and in patients with irritable bowel syndrome (IBS) as well as diverticular disease

Complicated diverticular disease:

Free perforation: Laparotomy, a Hartman's procedure may be used (temporary end colostomy + partial colectomy or perforectomy). It is sometimes possible to do on table colon lavage via the appendix stump, then immediate anastomosis (so avoiding repeat surgery to close the colostomy).

Hemorrhage: Transfusion may be needed. Highly selective embolization or colonic resection may be necessary after locating bleeding points by angiography or colonoscopy (cautery ± local epinephrine injections may obviate the need for surgery). If bleeding site identified and surgery is necessary for bleeding a limited resection can be performed. Otherwise, a total abdominal colectomy with either an ileostomy or ileorectal anastomosis is performed.

Fistula: Treatment is surgical, eg laparoscopic or open colonic resection as well as removal of the fistula. Successful laparoscopic resection is less likely when a fistula is present. Colovesical fistula to the dome of the bladder >> trigone. Consider urology consult for stents and reconstruction.

Abscess: Antibiotics ± CT or ultrasound-guided drainage may be needed. This should be followed by definitive resection in 6wks or sooner if no clinical improvement (<25%).

Post-infective strictures: Stent colon if necessary and prep if possible to perform a primary anastomosis

Hernias

Definition Any congenital or acquired defect in a musculoaponeurotic structure through which an epithelialized or peritonealized sac protrudes through. Hernias involving bowel are said to be irreducible if they cannot be pushed back into the right place. This does not mean that they are either necessarily obstructed or strangulated. Gastrointestinal hernias are obstructed if bowel contents cannot pass through them—the classical features of intestinal obstruction soon appear. Strangulated hernias are a result of ischemia to the bowel which requires urgent surgery.

Sites of hernias

Inguinal hernia See p488.

Pantaloon hernia Both indirect and direct inguinal hernias occurring in the same patient.

Femoral hernia Bowel enters the femoral canal, presenting as a mass in the upper medial thigh or above the inguinal ligament where it points down the leg, unlike an inguinal hernia which points to the groin. They occur more often in women than men and are likely to be irreducible and to strangulate. *Anatomy*: The neck of the hernia is felt below and lateral to the pubic tubercle (inguinal hernias are above and medial to this point). The boundaries of the femoral canal are anteriorly and medially the inguinal ligament; laterally the femoral vein and posteriorly the pectineal ligament. The canal contains fat and Cloquet's node. *Treatment*: Surgical repair is recommended.

Para-umbilical hernias These occur just above or below the umbilicus. Risk factors are obesity and ascites. Omentum or bowel herniates through the defect. Surgery involves repair of the rectus sheath.

Epigastric hernias These pass through linea alba above the umbilicus.

Incisional hernias These follow breakdown of muscle closure after previous surgery (seen in 11–20%). If obese, repair is not easy. A randomized trial of repairs favoured mesh over suture techniques.

Spighelian hernias These occur at the lateral edge of the rectus sheath, below and lateral to the umbilicus.

Lumbar hernias These occur through 1 of the lumbar triangles.

Richter's hernia This involves bowel wall only—not lumen.

Obturator hernias These occur through the obturator canal. Typically there is pain along the medial side of the thigh in a thin woman.

Levator hernias These occur when fat or rectum balloons out the levator muscles of the pelvic floor

Other examples of hernias
- Of the nucleus pulposus into the spinal canal (slipped disc).
- Of the uncus and hippocampal gyrus through the tentorium (tentorial hernia) in space-occupying lesions.
- Of the brainstem and cerebellum through the foramen magnum (Arnold-Chiari malformation).
- Of the stomach through the diaphragm (hiatal hernia, p197).
- Of the terminal (intravesical) portion of the ureter into the bladder, with cystic ballooning between the mucosa and muscle layers. This is a uretero-cele and results from stenosis of the ureteral meatus.

Symptoms
- Reducible hernias are associated with a dull ache and a bulge that go away with recumbency and worsening with physical activity. A neuralgia can occur from injury to a sensory nerve lying at the site of the hernia. ie ilioinguinal nerve and the inguinal hernia or obturator nerve and the obturator canal.
- Incarcerated or strangulated hernias (5%) will be associated with more severe pain, nausea, and vomiting

Treatment

- Symptomatic hernias should be considered for operative repair. Patients should be encouraged to lose weight and to stop smoking to improve the outcome of hernia repair. Several trials of laparoscopic repair for large incarcerated hernias using in-lay vs. on-lay mesh have demonstrated improved outcomes.
- If incarcerated, a gently trial of reduction with manual pressure can be attempted.
- Strangulated hernias should be operatively repaired immediately.

Some examples of hernias

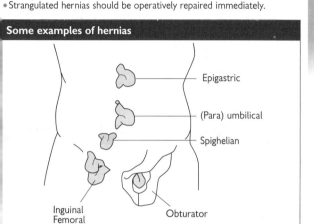

Epigastric

(Para) umbilical

Spighelian

Inguinal
Femoral

Obturator

Reproduced with permission from PA Grace & N Borley
2002, 'Surgery at a Glance', Blackwell Science

Inguinal hernias

Indirect hernias pass through the internal inguinal ring as a result of incomplete closure of the processus vaginalis at birth. Direct hernias enter through the posterior wall of the inguinal canal through an acquired defect in the transverses abdominus aponeurosis and transversalis fascia. Overall, indirect hernias are more common than direct hernias. However, direct hernias are more common in adults and indirect are more common in children. The anatomic landmark distinguishing these hernias is the inferior epigastric artery; indirect is lateral, direct is medial through *Hesselbach's triangle*: Medial edge of rectus abdominis, lateral edge of inferior epigastric artery and inferior edge of inguinal ligament. Predisposing conditions include: Chronic cough, constipation, urinary obstruction, heavy lifting, ascites, previous abdominal surgery, prematurity. Relations of the inguinal canal are:

Floor: Inguinal ligament.

Roof: Fibers of transversalis and internal oblique.

Front: External oblique aponeurosis + internal oblique for the lateral ⅓.

Back: Laterally, transversalis fascia; medially, conjoined tendon

Contents of the inguinal canal

- Spermatic cord in men
- Round ligament in women
- Testicular artery
- Deferential vessel
- Pampiniform plexus of veins
- Ilioinguinal nerve
- Genital branch of the genitofemoral nerve
- Cremasteric artery and muscle
- Internal spermatic fascia

Examining the patient Always look for previous scars, feel the other side and examine the external genitalia. Then ask: Is the lump visible? If so, ask the patient to reduce it—if they cannot, make sure that it is not a scrotal lump. Ask them to cough. Inguinal hernias appear inferomedial to the external ring. If no lump is visible, feel for a cough impulse. If there is no lump, ask the patient to stand and repeat the cough.

Irreducible hernias You may be called because a long-standing hernia is now irreducible and painful. It is always worth trying to reduce these yourself—to prevent strangulation and bowel necrosis (a grave event, demanding prompt laparotomy). Use the flat of the hand, directing the hernia from below, up towards the contralateral shoulder. Sometimes, as the hernia obstructs, reduction requires perseverance, which may be rewarded by a gurgle from the retreating bowel, and can thus spare unnecessary surgery.

Surgical repairs Advise patients to diet and stop smoking pre-op. Laparoscopic and open mesh techniques (eg Lichtenstein repair) have replaced other methods briefly described below:

'Shouldice' repair with its multilayered suture involving both anterior and posterior walls of the inguinal canal.

Bassini repair floor of inguinal canal to the rectus sheath and to the shelving edge of the inguinal ligament (poupart ligament)

McVay repair 'Cooper's ligament repair' approximates the floor of the inguinal canal to cooper's ligament between the pubic tubercle to the femoral vein.

In mesh repairs, a polypropylene mesh reinforces the posterior wall. Recurrence rate is less (<2% mesh vs. 10% no mesh). Local anaesthetic techniques have lead to day-case 'ambulatory' surgery. Laparoscopic repair is also possible, and gives similar recurrence rates. This can be done through the peritoneal cavity or through a pre-peritoneal approach. There is less post-operative pain and an earlier return to work after a laparoscopic repair, and undiagnosed contralateral hernias can be identified. Care must be taken to avoid injury to the iliohypogastric nerve which may occur by placing a holding tack too far laterally along the abdominal wall. This results in severe chronic pain.

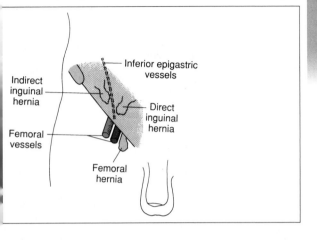

Benign diseases of the biliary tract

Bile contains cholesterol, bile pigments (from broken down Hb), and phospholipids. If the concentrations of these vary, different kinds of stones may be formed. Stones cause chronic inflammation ± colic.

Pigment stones: Most common type of stone worldwide. Small, friable, and irregular. Causes: Hemolysis.

Cholesterol stones: Most common type of stone in the US. Large, often solitary. Causes: Female sex, age, obesity.

Mixed stones: Faceted (calcium salts, pigment, & cholesterol).

Gallstone prevalence: 8% of those over 40yrs. 90% remain asymptomatic for which no treatment is commonly offered.

Biliary colic: Follows stone impaction in the neck of the gall bladder (GB), which may cause epigastric or RUQ pain after eating fatty foods.

Acute cholecystitis: Pain, fevers, and WBC↑ with +ve US findings is suggestive of cholecystitis. Other symptoms include nausea and vomiting. If the stone moves to the CBD, jaundice may occur.

Murphy's sign: Press over the RUQ. Ask the patient to breathe in. This causes pain and arrest of inspiration as an inflamed GB is impinged. It is only +ve if the same test in the LUQ does not cause pain.

Acalculus cholecystitis: Pain, fever, and WBC↑ with biliary stasis and delayed GB emptying on HIDA without evidence of stones. Commonly seen in critically ill, immunosuppressed patients and in patients on TPN.

Chronic cholecystitis: Vague abdominal discomfort, distension, nausea, flatulence, and intolerance of fats may also be caused by reflux, ulcers, irritable bowel syndrome, relapsing pancreatitis, or tumor (stomach, pancreas, colon, GB). Ultrasound is used to image stones, and to assess common bile duct (CBD) diameter. MRCP (p208) is increasingly being used to check for stones in the CBD.

Complications of gallstones:

Obstructive jaundice with CBD stones: RUQ pain and jaundice—unusual to have a total bilirubin >10mg/dL.

Cholangitis—Bile duct infection usually resulting from a blocked duct. Charcot's triad RUQ pain, jaundice, and fevers; Reynold's pentad with the addition of hypotension and mental status changes—worse prognosis.

Gallstone ileus: A stone perforates the GB entering the duodenum; it may then obstruct the terminal ileum. X-ray: Air in CBD, small bowel fluid levels, and a stone. Duodenal obstruction is rarer (Bouveret's syndrome).

Pancreatitis (see p452)

Empyema of the gallbladder: The obstructed gb fills with pus.

Mirizzi syndrome: Impaction of the cystic duct with a large stone causing obstruction of the CBD.

Tests: WBC, RUQ ultrasound (thickened GB wall, pericholecystic fluid, and stones), hida cholescintigraphy to check for GB emptying (useful if diagnosis uncertain after ultrasound).

Magnetic resonance cholangio-pancreaticogram (MRCP) images the bile duct for the presence of stones. Gallstones are only radio-opaque on plain abdominal films in ~10% of cases.

Medical management: NPO, pain relief (avoid morphine which may cause sphincter of oddi dysfunction), IV fluids, and antibiotics if evidence of inflammation/infection; common organisms include *E. coli*, Enterococci, and *Klebsiella* (eg cefuroxime 1.5g/8h IV and metronidazole 500mg/8h IV, or zosyn 3.375mg/6h IV).

Surgical treatment: Cholecystectomy (eg laparoscopic). If ultrasound or MRCP shows a dilated CBD with stones, ERCP with sphincterotomy is used to remove stones, usually prior to surgery or at the time of surgery with CBD exploration (if there is no obstruction/cholangitis), a stone-trapping basket on the end of a choledochoscope introduced through the cystic duct at laparoscopy can be done. In suitable candidates, do laparocopic cholecystectomy within 72h; early surgery is associated with fewer complications and lower conversion rates to open cholecystectomy. Mortality: <1%. If delayed, relapse occurs in 18%. Otherwise, operate after 6–12wks. In elderly or high-risk patients unsuitable for surgery, percutaneous cholecystostomy may be useful; cholecystostomy can still be performed at a later date.

Complications of laparoscopic cholecystectomy:

Injury to the right hepatic duct, accessory duct, or common bile duct: All will require drainage of biloma and possible intrahepatic biliary drain. Depending on the site of injury, reconstruction with a Roux-en-Y choledochojejunostomy may have to be performed.

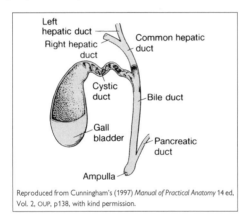

Reproduced from Cunningham's (1997) *Manual of Practical Anatomy* 14 ed, Vol. 2, OUP, p138, with kind permission.

Pancreatitis

Pancreatic inflammation resulting in injury to the gland and the surrounding retroperitoneal tissues. Most common in adults over the age of 30yrs. Overall mortality 6–20%. There may be rapid progress from a phase of mild edema of the pancreas associated with fluid sequestration to one of necrotizing pancreatitis. In fulminating cases, the pancreas is replaced by gray-black necrotic material. Death may be from shock, renal failure, sepsis, or respiratory failure, with contributory factors being protease-induced activation of complement, kinin, and the fibrinolytic and coagulation cascades. May be acute or chronic.

Causes 'GET SMASHED': *G*allstones, *E*thanol, *T*rauma, *S*teroids, *M*umps, *A*uto-immune (PAN), *S*corpion venom, *H*yperlipidemia (↑Ca^{2+}, hypothermia), *E*RCP, (also emboli), *D*rugs (eg azathioprine, asparaginase, mercaptopurine, pentamidine, didanosine, diuretics); also pregnancy. Often none found.

Symptoms Gradual or sudden severe epigastric or central abdominal pain (radiates to back); vomiting with signs of gastric outlet obstruction are prominent.

Signs Tachycardia, fever, jaundice, shock, ileus, rigid abdomen ± local/generalized tenderness and periumbilical discoloration '*Cullen's sign*' or, at the flanks '*Grey Turner's sign*'.

Tests No test is pathognomonic. Serum amylase elevation (amylase may be normal even in severe pancreatitis as amylase starts to fall within the 1st 24–48h, may be abnormally elevated secondary to renal failure or alternative source—salivary gland, fallopian tube). Serum lipase is derived from pancreatic acinar cells and elevation may indicate acinar cell injury. Blood gases. Biochemical analysis. Abdominal films: No psoas shadow (retroperitoneal fluid↑), 'sentinel loop' of proximal jejunum (solitary air-filled dilatation). CT helps assess severity. Ultrasound (if gallstones). ERCP. Differential diagnosis: Any acute abdomen (p430), myocardial infarct.

Management
- NPO (may need NGT).
- IV fluid resuscitation with 0.9% saline until vital signs are satisfactory and urine flows at >30mL/h. If shocked or elderly, consider CVP. Insert a urinary catheter.
- Analgesia: Demerol 75–100mg/4h IM, or morphine (a better analgesic, but *may* cause Oddi's sphincter to contract more) + prochlorperazine.
- Hourly pulse, BP, and urine flow; daily CBC, *Comprehensive panel:* Glucose, amylase, lipase, blood gas—about 1/3 of patient will have respiratory compromise. Supplemental O_2 if P_aO_2↓ is low.
- In suspected abscess formation or pancreatic necrosis (on contrast-enhanced CT), consider parenteral nutrition ± laparotomy & debridement. Antibiotics may help in *severe* disease.
- ERCP + gallstone removal may be needed if there is progressive jaundice.

Prognosis (See BOX) Several grading systems exist. Presently APACHE II score is used to assess likelihood of mortality. Some patients suffer recurrent pancreatitis so often that near-total pancreatectomy is contemplated. Evidence is accumulating that 'oxidant' stress is important here, but initial clinical trials of free radical scavengers have been disappointing.

Complications—*Early: Shock, ARDs* (p174), renal failure, DIC, Ca^{2+}↓, (10mL of 10% calcium gluconate IV slowly is, rarely, necessary; albumin replacement has also been tried), glucose↑ (transient; 5% need insulin). Later (>1wk): Pancreatic necrosis, pseudocyst (fluid in lesser sac, eg at ≥6wks), with fever, a mass, and persistent ↑amylase/LFTs. It may resolve or need drainage, externally, or into the stomach (may be laparoscopically). Abscesses need draining. Bleeding is from elastase eroding a major vessel (eg splenic artery); embolization of the artery may be life-saving. Thrombosis may occur in the splenic and gastroduodenal arteries, or in the colic branches of the superior mesenteric artery (SMA), causing bowel necrosis.

Ransom criteria

On admission
- Age >55yrs
- WBC >16,000/uL
- Glucose >200mg/dL
- LDH >350IU/L
- SGOT >250IU/L

After 48h
- Hct ↓ 10%
- BUN ↑ 5mg/dL
- Ca^{2+} <8mg/dL
- P_aO_2 <60mmHg
- Base deficit >4mEq/L
- Fluid sequestration >6L
- Mortality is 30% if 3 criteria met, 40% for 5–6 criteria, 100% for 7–8.

Intestinal obstruction

This disorder is the result of inability of normal secretions and waste to pass through the GI tract. It is best to separate intestinal obstruction into two major sites, small intestine and large intestinal obstruction.

Symptoms: Both large and small intestinal obstruction is associated with anorexia and colicky abdominal pain with distension. In small bowel obstruction, vomiting occurs earlier, distension may be less. In large bowel obstruction, the pain is more constant. Obstipation is common but constipation need not be absolute (ie no feces or flatus passed). Fever is an ominous sign and when associated with localized peritonitis, always worry about strangulation.

Causes: *Small bowel:* Adhesions are the number one cause in the US, hernias external/internal of the most common worldwide, intussusception, Crohn's disease, radiation enteritis, gallstone ileus, tumor, foreign body.

Large bowel: Tumor, sigmoid or cecal volvulus, feces, diverticular or ischemic stricture.

Physical exam: Examine for distension and borborygmie, auscultate for bowel sounds—no bowel sounds may indicate ileus without obstruction, high-pitched bowel sounds are the hallmark of obstruction

Tests:
- CBC, electrolytes (K^+ and Mg^{2+})
- Urine analysis and culture—may cause ileus.
- AXR (plain abdominal x-ray) look for abnormal gas patterns (gas in the fundus of stomach and throughout the large bowel is normal).
- On erect AXR look for horizontal fluid levels within the small bowel as well as central gas shadows and no gas in the large bowel. Small bowel is identified by valvulae conniventes that completely cross the lumen (large bowel haustral folds do *not* cross all the lumen's width). In large bowel obstruction, AXR shows gas proximal to the block (eg in cecum) but not in the rectum.
- Abdominal and pelvic CT scan with oral contrast may demonstrate dilated loops of bowel to a transition point followed by compressed loops of bowel. Be careful immediately administering IV contrast because often these patients are dehydrated and may have renal insufficiency.

Management

General principles: The site, speed of onset, and completeness of obstruction determine therapy. Strangulation and large bowel obstruction require surgery soon. Paralytic ileus and incomplete small bowel obstruction can be managed conservatively, at least initially.

- *Conservative options:* Pass NGT and give IV fluids to rehydrate and correct electrolyte imbalance, (p616). Recurrent small bowel obstruction requiring hospitalization may be better served with exploratory laparotomy.
- *Surgery:* Strangulation requires emergency surgery, as does 'closed loop obstruction'—large bowel obstruction with tenderness over a grossly distended cecum (>8cm), which occurs when the ileocecal valve remains competent despite bowel distension. Usually large volumes of iv fluid must be given. For less urgent large bowel obstruction, there is time for an enema to determine if a complete or partial obstruction exists and to try to clear the obstruction and to correct fluid imbalance.

Sigmoid volvulus occurs when the bowel twists on the mesentery and can produce a severe, rapid strangulated obstruction. There is a characteristic axr with an 'inverted u' loop of bowel. It tends to occur in the elderly, constipated patient, and is often managed by sigmoidoscopy and insertion of a flatus tube, but sigmoid colectomy is sometimes required. If sigmoid volvulus is able to be decompressed, it is recommended that the colon be prepped and removed during the same hospitalization.

Cecal volvulus similar but less common than sigmoid volvulus, this is found in patients with a mobile cecum. Treatment is surgical resection or cecal pexy.

Pseudo-obstruction is like mechanical GI obstruction but no cause for obstruction is found. *Predisposing factors:* Malignancy, electrolyte disturbances (eg ↓K⁺), recent surgery. *Presentation:* There is nausea and post-prandial bloating. Acute colonic pseudo-obstruction is called Ogilvie's syndrome. This is common in the elderly, institutionalized patient. *Treatment:* Manage conservatively. Neostigmine or colonoscopic decompression is sometimes useful in acute cases. Weight loss is a problem in chronic pseudo-obstruction. There is a case for investigating the cause by colonoscopy or water-soluble contrast enema in most instances of suspected mechanical obstruction.

Rectal prolapse (procidentia)

Full-thickness concentric prolapse of the rectum through the anus; in contrast to mucosal prolapse seen with hemorrhoidal disease. True incidence is unknown but seen in F>M with ratio of 6:1 over 60yrs. In children be concerned about cystic fibrosis.

Symptoms: Prolapse of the rectum usually with defecation; often have constipation, fecal incontinence, uterine and bladder prolapse.

Exam: Have patient do enema while in clinic and observe prolapse. Assess strength of sphincter muscles and evaluate for anterior compartment prolapse. Perform colonoscopy to look for possible lead point and for possible solitary rectal ulcer.

Management: Stool bulking agents (fiber). Surgery is mainstay. Two approaches either transperineal or transabdominal. Best result with transabdominal but depends on health of patient. Colonic resection recommended if constipation is present. Incontinence improves in 80% of patients with repair of prolapse alone.

Transperineal procedures:
- Delorme—rectal mucosectomy
- Altmeier—full-thickness rectal resection transanally
- Tirsch wire—suture around the anus.

Transabdominal approaches:
- Ripstein rectopexy—anterior mesh rectopexy
- Open suture rectopexy or Laparoscopic Wells procedure—presacral suture rectopexy
- Frykman-Goldberg—sigmoid resection with presacral suture rectopexy
- Anterior resection.

Fecal incontinence Inability to control the loss of gas or stool per anus. Majority in females from obstetrical injury (forceps, vacuum, 3rd and 4th degree tears). Prevalence is 0.5–11%. Requires frequent pad usage.

Anatomy: Internal sphincter innervated by intestinal myenteric plexus and is under involuntary control—provides a large portion of anal tone which is further ↑ by the external sphincters innervated by the pudendal nerve and under voluntary control.

Exam: Patulous anus and anal excoriation.

Tests:
- Pudendal nerve terminal motor latency—document functioning nerves
- Transrectal ultrasound—demonstrate sphincter defects
- Anorectal manometery—records resting and squeeze tone.

Management: Imodium will ↑ internal sphincter tone.

Surgical correction with overlapping sphincteroplasty has a 50% 5-yr success rate. Can be repeated. Newer options include sacral stimulation and the artificial bowel sphincter.

Hemorrhoids

The anus is lined by mainly discontinuous areas of spongy vascular tissue—the anal cushions, which contribute to anal closure. Viewed from the lithotomy position, their positions are at 3, 7, and 11 o'clock or right anterior and posterior and left lateral. Hemorrhoids are attached by smooth muscle and elastic tissue to the supporting structure of the anal canal, but are prone to displacement and disruption, either singly or together. The effects of gravity (our erect posture), ↑ anal tone, straining at stool may make them become both bulky and loose, and so to protrude. They are vulnerable to trauma and bleed readily from the capillaries of the underlying lamina propria, hence their name—hemorrhoids (meaning *running blood* in Greek). Because the bleeding is from capillaries, it is bright red. (Hemorrhoids are *not* varicose veins.)

Symptoms: The patient notices bright red rectal bleeding, often coating stools or dripping into the pan after defecation. There may be mucous discharge and pruritis ani. Severe anemia may occur. Often patients complain of mass that needs to be pushed back into the anus. If patient complains of pain, either fissure or thrombosed hemorrhoid* is present. As there are no sensory fibers above the dentate line (squamomucosal junction), hemorrhoids are not painful unless they thrombose when protruded. Fissures and hemorrhoids commonly occur together.

Exam: • An abdominal examination to rule out other diseases. • A rectal examination: Prolapsing hemorrhoids are obvious. • Proctoscopy to see the internal hemorrhoids. • Sigmoidoscopy to identify rectal pathology higher up (you can get no higher up than the rectosigmoid junction).

Classification and treatment: All patients should be instructed on the use of a high-fiber diet and refraining from straining and long trips to the bathroom.

Infra-red coagulation: Applied for 1.5–2s, 3–8 times to localized areas works by coagulating vessels, and tethering mucosa to subcutaneous tissue.

Sclerosants: (2mL of 5% phenol in oil injected above the dentate line; Side effects: Impotence; prostatitis)

Rubber band ligation: Do <3 band-treatments per session; a cheap treatment, but needs skill. Banding produces an ulcer to anchor the mucosa (see: Pain, bleeding, infection).

Conventional hemorrhoidectomy: Excision and ligation of vascular pedicles, as day-case surgery, needing ~2wks off work. Side effects: Hemorrhage or stenosis.

Stapled hemorrhoidectomy: Results in quicker return to normal activity than conventional surgery because of less pain. Will not remove large protruding anal tags (4th degree).

Hemorrhoidal classification and treatment		
Stage	**Definition**	**Treatment**
I	Enlarged with bleeding	Fiber Suppositories Sclerotherapy
II	Protrusion with spontaneous reduction	Fiber Suppositories Banding
III	Protrusion requiring manual reduction	Fiber Banding Conventional or stapled hemorrhoidectomy
IV	Irreducible protrusion	Fiber Stapled hemorrhodectomy in selected cases Conventional hemorrhoidectomy

457

Treatment of prolapsed, thrombosed hemorrhoid is with excision if <72h, otherwise analgesia, sitzbaths, and bed rest. Pain usually resolves in 2wks.

Anal fissure

Anal fissure is a midline longitudinal split in the squamous lining of the lower anus—often, if chronic, with a mucosal tag at the external aspect—the 'sentinel pile'. 90% are posterior (anterior ones follow parturition), and are perpetuated by internal sphincter spasm. Defecation is very painful—and spasm may constrict the rectal artery, making healing difficult.

Primary cause: Diarrhea or hard stools, acquired disorder.

Rare causes: Syphilis, herpes, trauma, Crohn's, anal cancer, psoriasis, more common in the lateral location.

Examine with a bright light. Do a digital rectal exam ± sigmoidoscopy. Groin nodes suggest a complicating factor (eg immunosuppression from HIV).

Treatment: Try 2% lidocaine ointment, extra dietary roughage + good anal toilet, sitz baths. Glyceryl trinitrate ointment (0.2–0.3%) or 0.2% nifedipine ointment relieves pain and ischemia caused by chronic fissures and spasm, and can prevent need for surgery, but may cause headache. If conservative measures fail, consider day-case lateral partial internal, *sphincterotomy.* Manual anal dilatation (under GA) is also used, but has fallen out of favor due to ↑risk of post-op anal incontinence (24.3% vs. 4.8% for lateral sphincterotomy).

Pilonidal sinus/cyst: Obstruction of natal cleft hair follicles ~6cm above the anus, with ingrowing hair, excites a foreign body reaction, and may cause secondary tracks which open laterally ± abscesses, with foul-smelling discharge.

Treatment is excision of the sinus tract ± primary closure, but is unsatisfactory in 10% of patients. Complex tracks can be laid open and packed individually, or skin flaps can be used to cover the defect.

Anal ulcers are rare: Consider Crohn's disease, anal cancer, TB, syphilis.

Skin tags seldom cause trouble but are easily excised.

Anorectal abscess/fistula is usually caused by enteric organisms (rarely *s. aures* or TB). Location: Perianal (~45%), ischiorectal (≤30%), intersphincteric (>20%), supralevator (~5%). Redness and swelling may spread well into the buttock. Do incision & drainage, eg under GA unless small perianal (+ fistulotomy if needed, eg in Crohn's disease). Associations: DM, Crohn's, malignancy. Don't rely on antibiotics.

Anal cancer: *Risk↑:* Syphilis, anal warts (HPV 16, 6, 11, & 18 implicated), anoreceptive homosexuals (often young). Histology: Squamous cell (80%): rarely basaloid, melanoma, or adenocarcinoma. The patient may present with bleeding, pain, bowel habit change, pruritis ani, masses, and stricture. Differential diagnosis: Condyloma acuminata, leucoplakia, lichen sclerosus, Bowen's, Pagets, or Crohn's disease. Treatment: Radiotherapy + 5-FU + mitomycin/cisplatin is usually preferred to anorectal excision and colostomy, and 75% of patients retain normal anal function.

Gastric and duodenal ulcer disease

Ulcerative disease of the stomach and duodenum has declined in incidence sharply from 1960 until now. Risk factors include smoking, NSAID use, *Helicobacter pylori*, and ↑ acid production or a defect in mucosal defense.

Symptoms: Cardinal feature is epigastric pain described as burning, stabbing, or gnawing relieved by eating or antacids. Other associated symptoms include nausea, vomiting, bleeding, weight loss. Differential diagnosis includes cholelithiasis, pancreatitis, pancreatic cancer, MI, and gastric neoplasia.

Evaluation:
• Barium swallow and UGI
• EGD—biopsy for neoplasia and *H. pylori*
• Recurrent peptic ulceration in unusual places think of Zollinger–Ellison syndrome (gastrinoma). Do secretin stimulation test.

Medical management
• Treat *H. pylori*
• Anti-histamines
• Proton pump inhibitors
• Prostaglandin analogues
• Sucralfate
• Antacids.

Surgical management

Operative intervention is reserved for the treatment of complicated ulcer disease (intractability, hemorrhage, perforation, obstruction).

Operations for benign gastric ulceration

Elective operation for gastric fundus ulceration is rarely needed as ulcers respond well to medical treatment, stopping smoking, and avoidance of NSAIDs. Emergency surgery is sometimes needed for hemorrhage or perforation. Hemorrhage is usually treated by under running the bleeding ulcer base or excision of the ulcer. If the former is done, then a biopsy should be taken to exclude malignancy. Perforation is usually managed by excision of the hole for histology, then closure.

Gastric carcinoma Curative surgical options include D_1 resection (removal of tumor and perigastric lymph nodes) and D_2 resection (removal of the D_1 tier of lymph nodes and the next tier out, along the celiac axis). There is considerable controversy as to which should be performed, as some studies have shown worse morbidity and mortality for D_2 resections performed in Western countries. It is likely that the results reflect the lack of dedicated specialists such as those in Japan, where gastric carcinoma is particularly common. D_2 resections should therefore only be performed in specialist centers.

Pre-pyloric ulceration is considered peptic disease and an anti-acid procedure must be performed.

Partial gastrectomy (the Billroth operations)

Billroth I: Partial gastrectomy with simple re-anastomosis (rejoining).

Billroth II (Polya gastrectomy): Partial gastrectomy. The duodenal stump is oversewn (leaving a blind loop), and anastomosis is achieved by a longitudinal incision further down (into the proximal jejunum).

Physical complications of gastrectomy and peptic ulcer surgery

Recurrent ulceration: Symptoms are similar to those experienced pre-operatively but complications are more common and response to medical treatment is poor. Further surgery is difficult.

Abdominal fullness: Feeling of early satiety (perhaps with discomfort and distension) improving with time. Advise to take small, frequent meals.

Dumping syndrome: Fainting and sweating after eating due to food of high osmotic potential being dumped in the jejunum, causes rapid fluid shifts. 'Late dumping' is due to rebound hypoglycemia and occurs 1–3h after meals. Both tend to improve with time but may be helped by eating less sugar, and more guar and pectin (slows glucose absorption). Acarbose may also help to reduce the early hyperglycemic stimulus to insulin secretion.

Bilious vomiting: This is difficult to treat—but often improves with time.

Diarrhea: May be disabling after vagotomy. Codeine phosphate may help.

Gastric tumor: A rare complication of any surgery which affects acid production.

Amylase ↑: If abdominal pain too, this may indicate afferent loop obstruction after Billroth II surgery (needs emergency surgery).

Metabolic complications *Weight loss:* Often due to poor calorie intake.

Bacterial overgrowth ± malabsorption (the blind loop syndrome) may occur.

Anemia: Usually from lack of iron hypochlorhydria and stomach resection. B_{12} levels are frequently low but megaloblastic anemia is rare.

Osteomalacia: There may be pseudofractures which look like metastases.

Complications of peptic ulcer surgery

	Recurrence	Dumping	Diarrhea	Metabolic
Partialgastrectomy	2%	20%	1%	++++
Vagotomy & pyloroplasty	7%	14%	4%	++
Highly selectivevagotomy	>7%	6%	<1%	0

(These values are approximate and depend on the skill of the surgeon.)

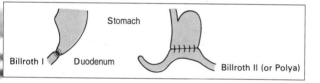

Stomach

Billroth I   Duodenum   Billroth II (or Polya)

Surgery for duodenal ulcer

Peptic ulcers usually present as epigastric pain and dyspepsia (p196). There is no reliable method of distinguishing clinically between gastric and duodenal ulcers. Although management of both is usually medical in the 1st instance (with *H. pylori* eradication, p196) surgery still has a role.

Surgery is usually only required for complications such as *hemorrhage, perforation*, and *pyloric stenosis*, though may be considered for the few patients who are not responsive/tolerant to medical therapy.

Several types of operation have been tried but, as whenever considering an operation, one must consider efficacy, side-effects, and mortality.

Elective surgery may be undertaken for patients who are intolerant to or who fail to respond to medical treatment:
- Highly selective vagotomy: May be useful in patients unable to tolerate medical treatment. The vagus supply is denervated only where it supplies the lower esophagus and stomach. The nerve of Laterget to the pylorus is left intact; thus, gastric emptying is unaffected. The results of surgery are greatly dependent on the skill of the surgeon.
- Vagotomy and pyloroplasty: A vagotomy reduces acid production from the stomach body and fundus, and reduces gastrin production from the antrum. However, it interferes with emptying of the pyloric sphincter and so a drainage procedure (eg pyloroplasty) must be added. This operation is now almost obsolete, and is only performed in exceptional circumstances.
- Gastrectomy is rarely required in the modern management of peptic ulcer disease.

Emergency surgery may be required for the following complications:
- Hemorrhage may be controlled endoscopically by adrenaline injection, cautery, laser coagulation, or heat probe. Operation should be considered for severe hemorrhage or rebleeding, especially in the elderly. At surgery, the bleeding ulcer base is under run or oversewn. Occasionally, the gastro-duodenal artery must be ligated.
- Perforation: Most patients undergo surgery, though some advocate an initial conservative approach (NPO, ng tube, iv antibiotics) in patients without generalized peritonitis—this can prevent surgery in up to 50% of such cases. If emergency surgery is required, laparoscopic repair of the hole will usually suffice. *H. pylori* eradication should be commenced post-op.
- Pyloric stenosis: This is a late complication, presenting with vomiting of large amounts of food some hours after meals. (Adult pyloric stenosis is a complication of duodenal ulcers, and has nothing to do with congenital hypertrophic pyloric stenosis.)

Treatment: Endoscopic balloon dilatation, followed by maximal acid suppression, may be tried in the 1st instance (NB: 5% risk of perforation). If this is unsuccessful, a drainage procedure (eg gastro-enterostomy or pyloroplasty) ± highly selective vagotomy may be performed, often laparoscopically. The operation should be done after correction of the metabolic defect—hypochloremic, hypokalemic metabolic alkalosis.

Surgery for gastroesophageal reflux disease (GERD)

Fundoplication for GERD

The goal of surgery for GERD is to re-establish lower esophageal sphincter tone and prevent continued esophageal inflammation.

Indications:
• Failure of medical therapy
• Barrett's esophagus without dysplasia
• Recurrent pneumonia secondary to aspiration
• Mechanically defective sphincter.

Evaluations:
• Videoesophagram
• Upper GI endoscopy
• Esophageal manometry and 24h pH monitoring.

Multivariant analysis has shown that three factors are significant predictors of an excellent to good outcome for antireflux surgery: 1) an abnormal 24h pH score, 2) the presence of symptoms of heartburn and regurgitation, 3) a clinical response to acid suppression therapy. Large hiatal hernias and long-term chronic disease maybe associated with a shortened esophagus. Failure of laparoscopic fundiplication is higher in patients with a shortened esophagus.

Procedure: Gastric fundoplication involves wrapping the gastric fundus around the lower esophagus, closing the hiatus, and securing the wrap in the abdomen. There are various types of procedure eg Nissen (360° wrap), Toupe (270° posterior wrap), Watson (anterior hemifundoplication). Now usually performed laparoscopically which, when performed in specialist centers, is at least as effective at controlling reflux as open surgery but with a lower morbidity. Wound infections and respiratory complications are also more common in open surgery, and the incidence of dysphagia is similar for the two procedures.

Obesity surgery

Patients are eligible for surgical management of morbid obesity if their body mass index (BMI) is over 40 without a co-morbidity and $\geq$ 35 with the addition of co-morbidity. Surgical treatment can result in ½ to 1/3 of weight being lost within the first 1 to 1.5 years following surgery. This requires a great deal of patient education and cooperation. Many co-morbidities will reverse.

Co-morbidity of obesity:
- Cardiovascular dysfunction
- Non-insulin dependent diabetes
- Respiratory insufficiency
- ↑ intra-abdominal pressure leading to GERD, urinary incontinence, venous stasis
- Nephrotic syndrome
- Pseudotumor cerebri
- Degenerative osteoarthritis
- Cholelithiasis
- Infectious complications
- Sexual hormone dysfunction
- Colon cancer
- Psychosocial impairment.

Surgical procedures include:
- Gastric procedures—restrictive
- Gastroplasty—horizontal stapling, vertical banded gastroplasty (VBGP)
- Gastric bypass—formation of a small gastric pouch which is drained via a gastrojejunostomy
- Small bowel bypass—malabsorptive
  - Jejunoileal bypass—obligatory malabsorption associated with numerous complications (cirrhosis) and now avoided.
  - Partial biliopancreatic bypass—both restrictive and malabsorptive with small gastric pouch emptying into small bowel without pancreatic and biliary secretions because this is emptying into terminal ileum thus minimizing absorption.

Breast lumps and breast cancer

History: The presenting complaint: Mass, nipple discharge, pain, change in the skin of the breast, or abnormal mammogram; how the complaint changes over time and with the menstrual cycle. Previous breast problem. or surgery.

Risk factors: Menstrual history; parity; age of first childbirth; use of hormon replacement therapy, birth control pills, or tamoxifen; family history of breas or ovarian cancer

Examination: Inspect the breast (arms both up and down) noting; contou of the breast, nipple/areolar complex, skin overlying the breast (specifical for redness or dimpling), and symmetry. For abnormalities identified not symmetry, fixation to the skin or chest wall, and characteristics of the lum Nodal evaluation of the axillary, supraclavicular, and cervical basins.

Investigations: Clinical examination is crucial and all suspicious of abnor malities, whether suspicious by imaging or physical examination, must underg biopsy preferably by core needle biopsy

Imaging includes: • Mammography • Ultrasound • Magnetic resonance imag ing • For nipple discharge investigations also include ductogram.

Many breast cancers are identified by breast imaging and have no symptom

Abnormalities of the breast: *Causes of lumps:* Fibroadenoma, cyst, cance fibroadenosis, mastitis, galactocele, abscess, fibrocystic change; non-breas lumps; lipoma, fat necrosis, and sebaceous cyst. *Abnormal mammogram find ings:* Micro-calcification, architectural distortion or density, asymmetric den sity. *Causes of abnormal mammogram:* Fibroadenoma, cyst, cancer, duct carcinoma in-situ, atypical hyperplasia, radial scar, columnar cell hyperplasi *Causes of nipple discharge:* Duct ectasia (green/red, often multiple ducts an bilateral), intraductal papilloma/adenoma/carcinoma (bloody/brown, ofte single duct and unilateral), lactation.

Management: Core needle biopsy is used to diagnose most abnormalitie identified on either mammogram or physical examination. If there are disco dance between the abnormal finding and the pathology, excisional biopsy performed. If there is concordance and the pathology is benign, no furthe investigation is necessary with the following exceptions. For mastitis, con tinue breast feeding if lactating, and treat with antibiotics. Abscesses must b drained and wound care initiated. If the finding is atypical hyperplasia, exc sional biopsy is recommended and consider of the use of tamoxifen fo prevention. For nipple discharge, microdochectomy/total duct excision

Breast cancer

Risk factors: Nulliparity, first pregnancy after age 30, early menarche, lat menopause, HRT >5yrs, BRCA mutation (p385), family history of first degre relative with breast cancer at a pre-menopausal age or ovarian cancer, pe sonal history of breast cancer.

TNM Staging: TIS *in situ;* T1 <2cm; T2 2–5cm; T3 >5cm; T4 fixed to che wall or skin or/and inflammatory breast cancer.

N0 negative nodes; N1 1–3 positive nodes; N2 4–10 positive nodes; N3 >1 positive nodes.

M0 no metastases; M1 metastases present.

Early breast cancer: Wide local excision (WLE) with radiation therapy (RT) C mastectomy plus or minus reconstruction, with sentinel lymph node biops or axillary lymph node dissection. WLE plus RT has equal survival but high local recurrence rates compared to mastectomy.

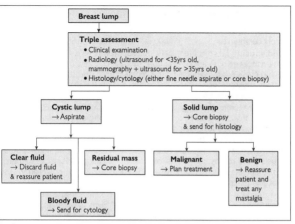

Staging

Assess liver function test and calcium levels; CT scan of the chest and abdomen; and bone scan. A PET scan may be used. Staging reserved for high risk patients or those with symptoms.

Adjuvant therapy: *Radiation Therapy* for all patients with WLE; post-mastectomy RT to the chest wall for T3 or T4 and N2 or N3 tumors. RT results in ↓ local regional recurrence. *Chemotherapy* improves survival with the most common combination being doxorubicin based with taxanes added for high risk patients. Herceptin is used for *HER-2 neu* positive disease. *Endocrine therapy* for those patients that are estrogen or progesterone receptor positive. Tamoxifen is most commonly used for 5yrs post-operatively. Aromatase inhibitors may also be used in post-menopausal women with possibly lower side affects. In pre-menopausal women with estrogen receptor positive tumors, ovarian ablation/suppression can be considered.

Treatment of metastatic disease: RT can be used for metastatic lesions at high risk for functional deficit; hormonal therapy is effective in many patients with estrogen receptor positive disease; after failure of one hormonal therapy, switching to another may be effective.

Preventing breast cancer deaths

Promoting 'breast awareness': Mammography: The detection rates of mammography are 6.4 cancers per 1000 healthy women over age 50. Breast cancer screening with mammography ↓ deaths in women over 50 by 25%. Prevention with the use of tamoxifen is possible for high risk women (equal to a risk of a women age 60) resulting in a 50% risk reduction.

Sentinel lymph node biopsy:

Sentinel lymph node biopsy is used in staging breast cancer patients. For those patients that are sentinel lymph node negative, no addition surgery is completed in the axilla, for those that are positive a completion axillary dissection is performed. Sentinel lymph node biopsy has a risk of lymphedema of 2% with minimal risk of functional deficit of the arm. Axillary lymph node dissection has a risk of lymphedema of 10–20% with 20% of patients having functional deficit of the arm. The sentinel lymph node procedure is completed as follows: A vital blue dye and/or radiocolloid is injected either peritumorally or in the retroareolar area; an incision is made in the axilla and gamma probe or visual inspection is used to identify and remove the sentinel lymph node for pathologic assessment. Multi-center trials report identification rates >90% and false negative rates <12%.

Colorectal adenocarcinoma

This is the 3rd most common cancer diagnosed and 2nd most common cause cancer deaths in the US with 156,000 estimated cases and 56,000 deaths this yea

Predisposing factors Neoplastic polyps, UC, Crohn's, familial adenomato polyposis, previous cancer, low-fiber diet. NSAIDs may be protective. Gene ics: No close relative affected: Colorectal cancer risk is 1:50. One 1st degre relative affected: Risk = 1:17; if 2 affected, 1:10 (refer when 10yrs young than the youngest affected relative).

Polyps are lumps that appear above the mucosa. There are 3 types:
1 *Inflammatory:* Ulcerative colitis, Crohn's, lymphoid hyperplasia.
2 *Hamartomatous:* Juvenile polyps, Peutz-Jeghers' syndrome.
3 *Neoplastic:* Tubular or villous adenomas: Malignant potential, esp. if >2c
Symptoms of polyps: Passage of blood/mucus per rectum. They should k biopsied and removed if they show malignant change. Most can be reache by the flexible colonoscope to avoid the morbidity of colectomy. Che resection margins are clear of tumor.

Presentation of cancer: Depends on site: *Left-sided:* Bleeding per rectum; altere bowel habit; tenesmus; mass (60%). *Right:* Weight loss; anemia; abdomin pain. *Either:* Abdominal mass; obstruction; perforation; hemorrhage; fistula

Tests CBC (microcytic anemia); fecal occult blood (FOB); proctoscop sigmoidoscopy, barium enema or colonoscopy (can be done 'virtually' k CT); LFT, CT/MRI; liver ultrasound. CEA may be used to monitor disease a effectiveness of treatment (p626). If polyposis in family, refer for DNA testi once a patient is >15yrs old. Genetic testing may also help determine wt will benefit from chemotherapy—p384.

Spread Local, lymphatic, or by blood (liver, lung, bone) or transcoelom
Surgical treatment Surgery is considered curative for Stage I and II diseas Attention to technique may ↓ local recurrence rates.

Hemicolectomies: Right is for cecal tumors, ascending or proximal transver colon (Extended right including the middle colic artery). Left is for tumors the distal transverse colon, descending colon, and proximal sigmoid colo *Anterior resection* is for distal sigmoid or high rectal tumors. *Abdomin perineal (A-P) resection* is for tumors low in the rectum that are abutting invading the sphincter muscles: Permanent colostomy and removal of rectu and anus. *Low anterior resection* tumors of the mid & low rectum. Stapli devices are helpful. *Radiotherapy* may be used pre-op or post-op in stage a III rectal cancer to ↓ local recurrence. Pre-op radiotherapy + 5-FU is al used to downstage tumor to ↑ sphincter preservation rates. *Adjuvant thera* Reserved generally for stage III and IV disease, except in rectal cancer whe T3N0 disease is treated with adjuvant therapy to ↓ local recurrence. *Chem therapy:* Usually 5-FU based chemotherapy ± folinic acid and newer ager (eg irinotecan, oxaliplatin) for 6 months post-op ↑ survival in patients wi stage III or IV colorectal cancer. The role of chemotherapy in Stage II (T3N tumors is under investigation.

Patients with resectable hepatic metastases (<4), >1yr disease free interv and no extrahepatic spread will have improved survival following hepat metastectomy

Stage	TNM classification	Treated 5yr survival (%) AJCC 1988
I	T1–2 N0	~90
II	T3–4 N0	~75
IIIA	T1–2 N1	~80
IIIB	T3–4 N1	~65
IIIC	Tx N2	~45
IV	TxNxM1	<10

Location of cancers of the large bowel

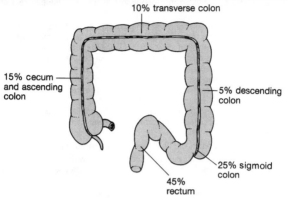

10% transverse colon

15% cecum and ascending colon

5% descending colon

25% sigmoid colon

45% rectum

NB: These are averages: Black females tend to have more proximal neoplasms, while White men tend to have more distal neoplasms.

Signs and symptoms of colorectal cancer

- Rectal bleeding and/or a persistent change in bowel habit for >6wks.
- Persistent rectal bleeding without anal symptoms any age, with no obvious external evidence of benign anal disease.
- Recent onset of looser stools and/or ↑ frequency of defecation, persisting for >6wks.
- Iron-deficiency anemia without an obvious cause and Hb <10g/dL.
- An easily palpable abdominal or rectal mass.

Universal adult screening for colorectal cancer

A number of screening methods have been proposed. Evidence from randomized trials is currently only available for FOB screening, however.

- FOB screening every 2yrs with home tests reduces mortality by 15–33%, but false +ve rates are high (up to 10% of those screened) and there are problems with acceptability. The patient has to be on a special diet while 2 out of 3 consecutive stool samples are tested. Sample rehydration improves sensitivity but ↑ false +ves.
- Sigmoidoscopy can be used to screen for left-sided lesions with 90% sensitivity and 99% specificity within the region of the scope. Case–control studies suggest ~60% reduction in risk of death from colorectal cancer by the finding of a lesion within the reach of the scope. Limitations include acceptability, cost, and not picking up right-sided lesions.
- Colonoscopy examines *all* the colon and is the most accurate test. It is already used in those at ↑risk of colorectal cancer due to personal or family history, adenoma, or UC/Crohn's. Limitations include perforation problems (2/1000 vs. 1/10,000 for sigmoidoscopy), cost, need for sedation, acceptability to patients, and the availability of trained endoscopists.

Pancreatic cancer

Pancreatic cancer is divided into neoplasms of the exocrine pancreas and endocrine pancreas.

Neoplasms of the exocrine pancreas: Pancreatic ductal adenocarcinoma is the 10th leading new cancer diagnosis and the 4th leading cause of cancer death in the US with the number of new cases (32,000) equaling the number of deaths. This cancer is more common in men, African Americans, and individuals over 70 yrs of age. The only known risk factor is smoking. Other factors that suggest an association is family history, chronic pancreatitis, and previous gastric surgery. 70% of pancreatic ductal cancers occur in the head (periampullary), 15% occur in the body, 10% occur in the tail, and 5% are diffuse. The most common presentation for periampullary tumors is painless jaundice. Other associated symptoms include weight loss, epigastric pain, nausea, and vomiting.

Tests: Bilirubin, ALK phos, CA 19–9. Contrast enhanced spiral CT ± ERCP.

Palliation for periampullary cancer can be achieved with gastrojejunostomy and hepaticojejunostomy at the time or attempted resection or with transhepatic stents.

Treatment: Surgical resection, when possible, provides the greatest survival benefit. For tumors of the head, a pancreaticoduodenctomy (*Whipple procedure*) is done. Small respectable tumors of the head of the pancreas result in a 20% 5-yr survival. For tumors of the tail, a distal pancreatectomy ± splenectomy is performed. These tumors tend to be much larger at the time of diagnosis because patients are largely asymptomatic. Adjuvant chemotherapy and radiation has been shown to ↑ survival following curative resection for pancreatic cancer.

Neoplasms of the endocrine pancreas

Islet cell type	Hormone	Syndrome	Clinical features	Diagnostic test	% Malignant
α cell	Glucagon	Glucagonoma	Migratory rash, diabetes, diarrhea	↑ Glucagon after tolbutamide	Nearly 100%
β cell	Insulin	Insulinoma	Hypoglycemia, mental confusion	↑insulin	10%
δ cell	Somatostatin	Somatostatinoma	Dyspepsia, diabetes, gallstones, steatorrhea	↑glucose without ↑ketones	Nearly 100%
δ₂ cell	VIP	VIPoma	Diarrhea?	—	40%
G cell	Gastrin	Gastrinoma	(Zollinger–Ellison) Severe PUD, diarrhea	↑gastrin after secretin 70%	

The primary treatment of endocrine tumors of the pancreas is excision. If disease is unresectable, systemically active therapy can be directed at the products of the tumors (eg H2 receptor blockers in ZES, diazoxide in insulinomas, somatostatin analogues).

Thyroid nodules and cancer

The *single thyroid lump* is a common problem; ~10% will be malignant.

Causes: Cyst, adenoma, discrete nodule in multi-nodular goiter, malignancy

Examination: Watch the neck during swallowing water. Stand behind and feel thyroid for size, shape, tenderness, and mobility. Percuss for retrosternal extension. Any nodes? Bruits? If the thyroid is enlarged (goiter), ask these 3 question.
- Is the thyroid smooth or nodular?
- Is the patient euthyroid, thyrotoxic (p280), or hypothyroid (p282)? Do TSH,T3 & T4
    - *Smooth, non-toxic goiter:* Endemic (iodine deficiency); congenital; goitrogens; thyroiditis; physiological; Hashimoto's thyroiditis (an autoimmune disease thought to be due to apoptosis induced by lymphocytes bearing Fas ligands combining with thyrocytes bearing Fas).
    - *Smooth, toxic goiter:* Graves' disease.
- *Any nodules? Many or one?* If >4cm across, malignancy is more likely. *Multinodular goiter:* Usually euthyroid but hyperthyroidism may develop. Hypothyroidism and malignancy are rare.

Tests: Ultrasound, to see if the lump is solid or cystic or part of a group of lumps

Radionucleotide scans may show malignant lesions as hypofunctioning or 'cold', whereas a hyperfunctioning 'hot' lesion suggests adenoma

Fine needle apirate (FNA) and do cytology on the fluid. No clinical/lab test is good enough to tell for sure if follicular neoplasms found on FNA are benign, so such patients are referred for surgery.

What should you do if high-resolution ultrasound shows non-palpable nodules?

Such thyroid nodules can usually just be observed provided they are:
- <1cm across (most are; ultrasound can detect lumps <2mm; such 'incidentalomas' occur in 46% of routine autopsies) and asymptomatic.
- There is no past history of thyroid cancer or radiation.
- No family history of medullary cancer. (If any present, do ultrasound-guided FNA; excise if cytology is malignant.)

Thyroid neoplasia 5 types: • Follicular: 25%. Middle-aged, spreads early via blood (bone, lungs). Well-differentiated. Treat by total thyroidectomy and T4 suppression and radioiodine (^{131}I) ablation. • *Anaplastic:* Rare. ♀:♂ ≈ 3:1. Elderly, poor response to any treatment. In the absence of unresectable disease, excision + radiotherapy may be tried. • *Medullary:* 5%. Sporadic (80%) or part of MEN syndrome (p285). May produce calcitonin. They do not concentrate iodine. Do thyroidectomy + node clearance (do pheochromocytoma screen pre-op). External beam radiotherapy should be considered to prevent regional recurrence.
- *Papillary:* 60%. Often in young; spread to nodes and lung. Treatment: Total thyroidectomy (to remove non-obvious tumor) ± node excision + radioiodine to ablate residual cells may all be needed. Give T4 to suppress TSH. Prognosis is better if young and female.
- *Lymphoma:* 5%. ♀:♂ ≈ 3:1. May present with stridor or dysphagia. Do full staging pre-treatment (chemoradiotherapy). Assess histology for mucosa-associated lymphoid tissue (MALT) origin (associated with a good prognosis).

Thyroid surgery indications: Pressure symptoms, hyperthyroidism, carcinoma, cosmetic reasons. Render euthyroid pre-op, by antithyroid drugs and/or propranolol. Check vocal cords by indirect laryngoscopy pre- and post-op.

Early complications: Recurrent laryngeal nerve palsy, hemorrhage (▶if compresses airway, instantly remove sutures for evacuation of clot), hypo-parathyroidism (check plasma Ca^{2+} daily, usually transient), thyroid storm (symptoms of severe hyperthyroidism—treat by propranolol PO or IV, antithyroid drugs, and iodine, p726). *Late complications:* Hypothyroidism.

Esophageal cancer

Benign tumors make up 1%—most common Leiomyoma or GIST. The incidence of esophageal cancer is on the rise, especially in Western countries. The types of esophageal cancer include squamous cell, adenocarcinoma, small cell cancer. The most common presenting symptoms are dysphagia and weight loss.

Squamous cell cancer of the esophagus
- More common world wide
- Associated with cigarette use and alcohol
- More common in the proximal 1/3 of the esophagus.

Adenocarcinoma
- More common in the US
- Associated with Plummer–Vinson syndrome, obesity, reflux esophagitis ± Barrett's esophagus (there is a 44-fold ↑risk of adenocarcinoma if severe reflux for >10 yrs).

Evaluation
- Barium swallow
- EGD with biopsy
- Endoscopic ultrasound
- CT scan
- Staging laparoscopy

Staging for esophageal cancer and 5-year survival		
TNM	Stage	5-year survival
TisN0M0	0	100
T1N0M0	I	85
T2N0M0, T3N0M0	IIA	45
T1N1M0, T2N1M0	IIB	20
T3-T4N1–2M0	III	10
AnyTAnyN M1	IV	<4

Treatment
Resection
- Transthoracic (radical) resection with en-bloc lymphadenectomy—3 incision
- Transhiatal resection—easier to perform.

Reconstruction
- Gastric pull-up with pyloroplasty based upon the right gastric artery
- Colonic interposition.

Adjuvant therapy
- Given preoperatively (neoadjuvant) or postoperatively for Stage II or III tumors.
- Cisplantin, 5-FU
- Radiation
- Palliation with metal stents for stage IV disease.

Gastric cancer

The incidence of gastric cancer, unlike esophageal, has dropped dramatically in the last 70 years (approximately 70%). Risk factors include: Lower economic status, smoking, consumption of salted, smoked food, atrophic gastritis, genetic factors (HNPCC), *H. pylori*.

Adenocarcinoma accounts for >90%, others include squamous cell, carcinoid, GIST, lymphoma.

Pathology The adenocarcinoma may be polypoid, ulcerating, or leather bottle type (linitis plastica). Some are confined to mucosa and submucosa—so-called 'early' gastric carcinoma.

Presentation symptoms: Often non-specific. Dyspepsia (p196) lasting >1 month in patients aged ≥40–50yrs demands GI investigation. Others: Weight loss, vomiting, dysphagia, anemia. Signs suggesting incurable disease: Epigastric mass, hepatomegaly, jaundice, ascites (p212), large left supraclavicular (Virchow's) node (Troissier's sign), acanthosis nigricans. Spread is local, lymphatic, blood-borne, and transcoelomic eg to ovaries (Krukenberg tumor).

4 *Evaluation*
* EGD with multiple biopsies—always biopsy ulcers
* Endoscopic ultrasound
* CT scan/MRI to evaluate for metastatic disease.

Staging for gastric cancer

TNM	Stage
TisN0M0	0
T1N0M0	IA
T1N1M0, T2N0M0	IB
T1N2M0, T2N1M0, T3N0M0	II
T2N2M0, T3N1M0, T4N0M0	IIIA
T3N2M0	IIIB
T4N1–3M0, T1–3N3M0, or M1	IV

Treatment
* Endoscopic mucosal resection may remove early cancers limited to the mucosa.
* Surgical—resection with gross negative margins of 6cm.
* Need at least 15 lymph nodes harvested to determine the nodal status of the disease.
* Adjacent organs should be resected en-bloc only if involved with tumor AND only one organ is involved.
* Stage II and IIIA may benefit from a more extensive nodal dissection D_2 (12 lymph node stations) vs. D_1 (6 lymph node stations) with an improved 5-yr survival 80% vs. 55% respectively.
* Reconstruction is performed with a Roux-en-Y end-to-side esophagojejunostomy.
* Adjuvant therapy includes radiation and 5-FU-based chemotherapy.

473

Cutaneous neoplasms

Cutaneous neoplasms are the most commonly diagnosed tumor in the U
with 600,000 new cases annually. The most common cutaneous neoplasm
include:
- Basal cell cancer
- Squamous cell cancer
- Melanoma:
  - 5th most common malignancy in the US
  - only accounts for 3% of all skin cancers but leads to 65% of all skin cancer related deaths.

The evaluation and treatment of cutaneous neoplasms is based upon
whether the lesion is melanoma or non-melanoma skin cancers.

Melanoma

Risk factors:
- Fair complexion
- Sun exposure
- Previous history of melanoma
- Dysplastic nevi syndrome
- Large congenital nevi—have a 5–20% lifetime risk of developing.

Types of melanoma
- Lentigno maligna ~ 10–15%, least aggressive
- Superficial spreading ~70%
- Nodular melanoma ~15–30%, most aggressive
- Acryl letiginous melanoma ~2–8%, seen in greater percentage or darker skinned individuals (African Americans, Asians, Hispanics).

Most common sites
- Women: Legs
- Men: Back of body.

Depths of invasion	Staging: JCC	~5-yr survival*
<0.75mm	Stage IA	99%
0.76–1.5 mm	Stage IB	90%
1.5–4 mm	Stage IIA	75%
>4 mm	Stage IIB	65%
Any depth + 1 nodal station	Stage III	40%
Any depth + >1 nodal station	Stage IV	0%
Or disseminated disease		

*Dependent on site as well

Treatment

Wide local excision is the primary method of local control of the lesion. Th
margin of excision is based upon the thickness of the lesion.

Appropriate margins for wide local excision of primary melanoma	
Thickness of primary lesion	Margin
Melanoma in situ	5mm
<1mm	1cm
1–4mm	2cm
>4mm	≥2cm

entinel lymph node dissection indications: 1) Primary melanoma ≥1 mm because 10% chance of lymph node spread, 2) Clinically negative nodal basin, 3) No *v*idence of distant disease.

rocedure: Should be performed concurrently with wide local excision because *n*proves accuracy. An intradermal injection with technetium-sulfur-colloid is *e*rformed around the lesion.

*h*e sentinel node is located by use of a gamma probe to identify the site of a *o*t focus (≥10x background counts), the use of isosulfan blue dye will also *l*low for easier identification of the sentinel node.

ymphadenectomy Indications and procedure: 1) Patients with known nodal *s*ease determined clinically or on sentinel node dissection. Intermediate *h*ickness melanoma and sentinel node can not be performed. 2) Nodal *i*ssections should be complete. 3) The risk of upper or lower extremity *m*phadema associated with a axillary or inguinal dissection is ~10%.

ites of spread or recurrence Local, distant cutaneous sites (in transit), distant *o*dal sites, lung, liver, brain, bone, gastrointestinal tract, thyroid.

djuvant therapy Interferon α—very toxic and therapy lasts for 1yr, Radiation *o*r palliation.

Non-melanoma skin cancer
isk factors
- Chemical carcinogens
- HPV
- Previous skin radiation.

Basal cell carcinoma
- Most common
- Little or no aggressive potential.

Squamous cell carcinoma (SCC)
- Contain keratin pearls
- Bowen's disease—in situ cancer that occurs around the anus
- Queyrat erythoplasia—in situ cancer that occurs around the penis
- Marjolin's ulcer—aggressive SCC in old scar.

Treatment
- Moh surgery—for basal cell and SCC in certain hard to reconstruct areas
- Layered excision of tumor to limit the amount of tissue removed
- SCC requires 1cm margin
- Adjuvant therapy
- Chemotherapy—mitomycin, 5-FU, cisplatin (anal)
- Radiation.

Common urological disorders

Torsion of the testis

The aim is to recognize this condition early on so that prompt surgical intervention can be undertaken and preserve both the fertility and hormone function of the involved testis.

If in any clinical doubt, and timely color Doppler ultrasound is not available, surgical exploration is mandatory. A missed torsion is one of the most common reasons for medical malpractice claims!

Symptoms: Sudden onset of pain in one testis, which makes walking uncomfortable. (Pain in the abdomen, nausea, and vomiting are common.)

Signs: Inflammation of one testis—it is tender, hot, and swollen. The testis may lie high and transversely. Torsion may occur at any age but is most common at 11–30yrs.

Tests: Doppler US (may demonstrate lack of blood flow to testis). Isotope scanning was used but its use has declined with the widespread availability of color Doppler ultrasound.

Treatment: ▶Ask consent for possible orchiectomy + *bilateral* fixation (orchidopexy). At surgery expose and untwist the spermatic cord. If the color of the testis returns and it pinks up, return it to the scrotum and fix *both* testes to the scrotum. If you are unsure of the status of the testis, incise the tunica albuginea and if you see bright red blood then the blood supply has been reconstituted.

Differential diagnosis: The main one is epididymitis but here the patient tends to be older, there may be symptoms of urinary infection and more gradual onset of pain. Also consider testis tumor, trauma, and an acute hydrocoele. NB: *Torsion of the hydatid of Morgagni*—remnants of the Müllerian ducts—occurs a little earlier, and causes less pain (the patient can often walk with no pain, unlike in testicular torsion)—and its tiny blue nodule may be discernible through the scrotal skin. It is thought to be due to the surge in gonadotrophins which signal the onset of puberty. *Idiopathic scrotal edema* a benign condition, and is differentiated from torsion by the absence of pain and tenderness.

Urinary retention & benign prostatic hyperplasia

Retention means not emptying the bladder (∵ *obstruction* or ↓*detrusor power*).

Acute retention The bladder is usually tender, containing ~600mL of urine. The cause in men is usually prostatic obstruction, eg precipitated by anticholinergics, 'holding on', constipation, pain, anaesthetics, alcohol, infection (p240). *Examine:* Abdomen, PR, perineal sensation (cauda equina compression).

Investigations: Midstream urine, analysis and culture, CBC, and prostate-specific antigen (PSA) (p627). Renal ultrasound and bladder ultrasound.

Tricks to aid voiding: Analgesia, privacy on hospital wards, ambulation, standing to void, voiding to the sound of running taps—or in a hot bath.

If the tricks fail: Catheterize (p657) and drain bladder. After eg 7d, trial without catheter may work (esp. if <75yrs old and <1L drained or retention was triggered by a passing event, eg general anaesthesia).

Prevention: Finasteride reduces prostate size and retention risk.

Chronic retention is more insidious. Bladder capacity may be >1.5L. Presentation: Overflow incontinence, acute on chronic retention, a lower abdominal mass, UTI, or renal failure. Prostatic enlargement is the common cause. Others: Pelvic malignancy, rectal surgery; DM; CNS disease eg transverse myelitis/MS; zoster (S2–S4). ▶Only catheterize the patient if there is pain, urinary infection, or renal impairment (eg urea >12mmol/L). Institute definitive treatment promptly. Intermittent self-catheterization is sometimes required. Both bladder and renal ultrasound may be informative.

Catheters and catheterization (p657).

Prostate cancer (p478).

Benign prostatic hypertrophy (BPH) is common (24% if aged 40–64; if older, 40%). ↓ urine flow (eg <15mL/s) is associated with frequency, urgency and voiding difficulty.

Managing BPH:

History: Severity of symptoms and impact on life. Rectal examination.
Effect on bladder/kidneys: Ultrasound (residual volume↑, hydronephrosis).
Electrolytes: Renal function.
MSU: Rule out infection.
Rule out cancer: PSA[1], transrectal ultrasound ± biopsy. Then consider:

1 *Transurethral resection of the prostate* (TURP, a common operation; ≤14% become impotent). Cross-match 2U. Consider perioperative antibiotics, eg cefuroxime 1.5g/8h IV, 3 doses. Beware excessive bleeding post-op and clot retention. ~20% of TURPs need redoing within 10yrs.

2 *Transurethral incision of the prostate* (TUIP) involves less destruction than TURP, and less risk to sexual function, while achieving similar clinical improvement in symptoms. It achieves its effect by relieving pressure on the urethra. It is perhaps the best surgical option for those with small glands <30g—ie ~50% of those operated on in some areas.

3 *Retropubic prostatectomy* is an open operation.

4 *Transurethral laser-induced prostatectomy* (TULIP).

5 *Drugs* may be useful in mild disease, and while awaiting TURP, eg:
- α-blockers: Eg *tamsulosin* 400mcg/24h PO; alternatives: Alfuzosin, doxazosin, terazosin. These ↓smooth muscle tone (prostate *and* bladder). SE: Drowsiness, depression; dizziness; BP↓; dry mouth; ejaculatory failure; extra-pyramidal signs; nasal congestion; weight↑. They are the drugs of choice.
- 5α-reductase inhibitors: *Finasteride* (5mg/d PO ↓testosterone's conversion to dihydrotestosterone). It is excreted in semen, so warn to use condoms; ♀: Avoid handling crushed pills. SE: Impotence; libido↓. Effects on prostate size are limited and slow, so, if α-blockers fail, many try surgery next.

6 *Wait and see* is an option, but risks incontinence, retention, and renal failure.

Advice for patients concerning transurethral prostatectomy

Pre-op consent issues may center on risks of the procedure, eg:
- Hematuria/hemorrhage
- Infection; prostatitis
- Hematospermia
- Impotence ~10%
- Hypothermia
- Incontinence ≤10%
- Urethral trauma/stricture
- Clot retention near strictures
- Post TURP syndrome ($T°$↓; Na^+↓)
- Retrograde ejaculation (common)

Post-operative advice:
- Avoid driving for 2wks after the operation.
- Avoid sex for 2wks after surgery. Then get back to normal. The amount ejaculated may be reduced (as it flows backwards into the bladder—harmless, but may cloud the urine. It means you may be infertile. Impotence may be a problem after TURP, but do not expect this: In some men, erections improve. Rarely, orgasmic sensations are reduced.
- Expect to pass blood in the urine for the first 2wks. A small amount of blood colors the urine bright red. Do not be alarmed.
- At first you may need to urinate *more* frequently than before. In 6wks things should be much better—but the operation cannot be guaranteed to work (8% fail, and lasting incontinence is problem in 6%; 12% may need repeat TURPs within 8yrs, compared with 1.8% of men undergoing open prostatectomy).
- If feverish, or if urination hurts, take a sample of urine to your doctor.

Urinary tract malignancies

Renal cell carcinoma (hypernephroma, Grawitz tumor) arises from the proximal renal tubular epithelium.

Epidemiology: 90% of renal cancers; mean age 55yrs; ♂:♀=2:1.

Clinical features: 50% are incidental findings during abdominal imaging for other symptoms. Hematuria, flank pain, abdominal mass, anorexia, malaise, weight loss, PUO may occur. Rarely, invasion of left renal vein compresses the left testicular vein causing a left varicocele. Spread may be direct (renal vein), via lymph nodes, or hematogenous (bone, liver, lung).

Tests: Blood: CBC (polycythemia from erythropoeitin secretion); ESR; electrolytes, alk phos. *Urine:* RBCs; cytology. *Imaging:* Ultrasound; CT/MRI; renal angiography (if partial nephrectomy or palliative embolization are being considered; angiography can be done by CT); IVP (filling defect in kidney ± calcification); CXR ('cannon ball' metastases).

Treatment: Radical nephrectomy either open or laparoscopic. Metastatic disease is reason to consider immunotherapy with interferon-α or interleukin-2. *Prognosis:* 5yr survival: 45%.

Transitional cell carcinoma (TCC) may arise in the bladder (50%), ureter, or renal pelvis. *Epidemiology:* Age >40yrs; ♂:♀=4. *Risk factors:* Smoking; drugs (cyclophosphamide, phenacetin); industrial carcinogens (azo-dyes, β-naphthalene). Schistosomiasis is a risk factor for squamous cell carcinoma of the bladder. *Presentation:* Painless hematuria; frequency, urgency, dysuria, or urinary tract obstruction. *Diagnosis:* Urine cytology; IVP; cystoscopy + biopsy; CT/MRI scan. *Treatment:* See *Bladder tumors* p482. *Prognosis:* Varies with clinical stage/histological grade: 10–80% 5yr survival.

Wilms' tumor (nephroblastoma) is a childhood tumor of primitive renal tubules and mesenchymal cells. It presents most commonly with an abdominal mass and hematuria. *Investigations:* Ultrasound with careful examination of the renal vein; CT/MRI scan. May biopsy only if tumor is massive and preoperative chemotherapy will be given. *Treatment:* Nephrectomy; with adjunctive radiotherapy and chemotherapy depending on pathological stage. *Prognosis:* 90% 5yr survival.

Prostate cancer is the 2nd commonest malignancy of men. *Incidence:* Rises with age: 80% in men >80yrs (in autopsy studies). *Associations:* ↑testosterone, +ve family history. Most are adenocarcinomas arising in the peripheral prostate. Spread may be local (seminal vesicles, bladder, rectum) via nodes, or hematogenous (sclerotic bony lesions). *Symptoms:* May be asymptomatic or nocturia, hesitancy, poor stream, terminal dribbling, or urinary obstruction. Weight↓ ± bone pain suggests metastases. *Digital rectal exam:* May show a hard, irregular prostate. *Diagnosis:* ↑PSA (p627; normal in 30% of small cancers); transrectal ultrasound and biopsy; bone scan; CT/MRI. .

478

Treatment: *Local disease:* Which is better: *Radical prostatectomy, radiotherapy* or *watchful waiting* with serial PSA monitoring? One trial (N=695) found radical prostatectomy improved disease-specific mortality, but not overall survival, when compared with watchful waiting. Radical surgery does risk erectile dysfunction and incontinence. Some centers recommend. Brachytherapy for local disease. *Metastatic disease:* Hormonal drugs may give benefit for 1–2yrs. Gonadotrophin-releasing analogues, eg 12-weekly goserelin (10.8mg SC as Zoladex LA®) first stimulate, and then inhibit pituitary gonadotrophin output. Alternatives: Cyproterone acetate; flutamide; diethylstilboestrol. *Symptomatic treatment:* Analgesia; treat hypercalcemia; radiotherapy for bone metastases or spinal cord compression.

Prognosis: 10% die in 6 months, but 10% live >10yrs. *Screening:* Rectal examination; PSA; transrectal ultrasound. There are problems with all (p627).

Advice to asymptomatic men asking for a PSA test

The prostate lies below the bladder, and surrounds the tube taking urine out. Prostate cancer is common in older men. Many men over 50 (to whom this advice applies) consider a PSA test on their blood to detect prostatic cancer. *Is this a good idea?*

The test itself has no side effects, provided you don't mind giving blood and time. There is indirect evidence of benefit of screening from the US where fewer radical prostatectomies reveal cancer-affected lymph nodes than those done before widespread PSA-based screening. Intensive screening and treatment for prostate cancer does not, however, appear to be associated with lower prostate-specific mortality in retrospective studies.

Prognostic factors in prostate cancer

A number of prognostic factors are used to help determine whether watchful waiting or aggressive therapy should be undertaken in prostate cancer. These include age, overall general health and risk factors, pre-treatment PSA level, tumor stage (as measured by the TNM system), and tumor grade—as measured by its Gleason score. Gleason grading is from 1 to 5, with 5 being the highest grade, and carrying the poorest prognosis. A pathologist determines the Gleason grade by analysing histology from two separate areas of tumor specimen, and adds them to get the total Gleason score for the tumor, from 2 to 10. Scores from 8 to 10 suggest an aggressive tumor, from 5 to 7 suggest intermediate grade, whereas from 2 to 4 suggest indolent tumor. Patients with high Gleason scores (6–7) are more likely to be treated aggressively, especially if they are young and/or have higher stage disease.

Urinary incontinence

Think twice before inserting a urinary catheter.

Carry out rectal examination to exclude fecal impaction.

Is the bladder palpable after voiding (retention with overflow)? Do not think of people as either dry or incontinent but as incontinent in certain circumstances, ie stress-cough, laughing. Attending to these circumstances is as important as focusing on the physiology.

Incontinence in men Enlargement of the prostate is the major cause of incontinence: Urge incontinence (see below) or dribbling may result from the partial retention of urine. TURP may weaken the bladder sphincter and cause incontinence. Troublesome incontinence needs specialist assessment.

Incontinence in women

1 *Functional incontinence,* ie when physiological factors are relatively unimportant. The patient is 'caught short' and too slow in finding the toilet because of eg immobility or unfamiliar surroundings.

2 *Stress incontinence:* Leakage of urine due to incompetent sphincter. Leakage typically occurs when intra-abdominal pressure rises (eg coughing, laughing). The key to diagnosis is the loss of small (but often frequent) amounts of urine when coughing, etc. Examine for pelvic floor prolapse. Look for cough leak with the patient standing and with full bladder. Stress incontinence is common during pregnancy and following childbirth. It occurs to some degree in about 50% of post-menopausal women. In elderly women, pelvic floor weakness, eg with uterine prolapse or urethrocele is the commonest cause.

3 *Urge incontinence* is the most common type seen in hospital practice. The urge to pass urine is quickly followed by uncontrollable complete emptying of the bladder as the detrusor muscle contracts. Large amounts of urine flow down the patient's legs. In the elderly it is usually related to detrusor instability (a urodynamic diagnosis) or organic brain damage. Look for evidence of: Stroke; Parkinson's; dementia. Other causes: Urinary infection; diabetes; diuretics; 'senile' vaginitis; urethritis.

In both sexes incontinence may result from diminished awareness due to confusion or sedation. Occasionally incontinence may be purposeful (eg preventing admission to an old people's home) or due to anger.

Management *Check for:* UTI; diabetes mellitus; diuretic use; fecal impaction. Do urine analysis and culture. *Stress incontinence:* Pelvic floor exercises may help. Intravaginal electrical stimulation may also be effective, but is not acceptable to many women. A ring pessary may help uterine prolapse, eg while awaiting surgical repair (this must be preceded by cystometry and urine flow rate measurement to exclude detrusor instability or sphincter dyssynergia). Surgical options for stress incontinence include Burch colposuspension and sling procedures; a variety of minimal access techniques (eg involving tension-free vaginal tape) have also been tried but remain unproven.

If urge incontinence: Examine for spinal cord and CNS signs (including cognitive test); and for vaginitis—treat with estriol 0.1% cream (eg Ovestin®, one applicator dose twice weekly for a few months)—consider cyclical progesterone if prolonged use, if no hysterectomy, to avoid risk of uterine cancer. The patient (or carer) should complete an 'incontinence' chart for 3d to obtain the pattern of incontinence. Maximize access to toilet; advise on toileting regimen (eg every 4h). The aim is to keep bladder volume below that which triggers emptying. Drugs may help reduce night-time incontinence but are generally disappointing. Consider aids (absorbent pad; bedside commode).

Do urodynamic assessment before any surgical intervention.

Bladder tumors

What appear as benign papillomata rarely behave in a purely benign way. They are almost certainly indolent transitional cell (urothelial) malignancies. Adenocarcinomas and squamous cell carcinomas are rare in the West (the latter may follow schistosomiasis). Histology is important for prognosis: Grade 1—differentiated; Grade 2—intermediate; Grade 3—poorly differentiated. 80% are confined to bladder mucosa, and only ~20% penetrate muscle (↑ mortality to 50% at 5yrs).

Presentation Painless hematuria; recurrent UTIs; voiding irritability.

Associations Smoking; aromatic amines (rubber industry); chronic cystitis; schistosomiasis (↑risk of squamous cell carcinoma); pelvic irradiation, and history of cytoxan exposure.

Tests *Urine:* Microscopy/cytology (cancers may cause sterile pyuria).
• IVP may show filling defects ± ureteric involvement.
• Cystoscopy with biopsy is diagnostic.
• Bimanual EUA helps assess spread.
• CT/MRI or lymphangiography may show involved pelvic nodes.

Staging Complex and changing (EUA = examination under anaesthesia)

Tis	Carcinoma-*in-situ*	Not felt at EUA
Ta	Tumor confined to epithelium	Not felt at EUA
T1	Tumor in mucosa or submucosa	Not felt at EUA
T2	Superficial muscle involved	Rubbery thickening at EUA
T3	Deep muscle involved	EUA: Mobile mass
T4	Invasion beyond bladder	EUA: Fixed mass

Treatment of transitional cell carcinoma (TCC)
Tis/Ta/T1: (80% of all patients.) Electrocautery via cystoscope. Consider intravesical chemotherapeutic agents (eg mitomycin C) for multiple small tumors or high-grade tumors. Immunotherapy with intravesical BCG is useful in high-grade tumors and carcinoma-*in-situ*.

T2–3: Radical cystectomy is the 'gold standard'. Radiotherapy gives worse 5yr survival rates than surgery, but preserves the bladder. 'Salvage' cystectomy can be performed if radiotherapy fails, but yields worse results than primary surgery. Post-op chemotherapy (eg M-VAC: Methotrexate, vinblastine, adriomycin, and cisplatin) is toxic but effective. Methods to preserve the bladder with transurethral resection/partial cystectomy + systemic chemotherapy have been tried, but long-term results are disappointing. The patient should have all these options explained by a urologist *and* an oncologist.

T4: Usually palliative chemo/radiotherapy. Chronic catheterization and urinary diversions may help to relieve pain.

Cystectomy complications include sexual and urinary malfunction. To avoid a urostoma, a continent urinary reservoir may be made from the patient's ileum.

Follow up History, examination, and regular cystoscopy: *High-risk tumors:* Every 3 months for 2yrs, then every 6 months; *low-risk tumors:* First follow-up cystoscopy after 9 months, then yearly.

Tumor spread Local—to pelvic structures; lymphatic—to iliac and para-aortic nodes; hematogenous—to liver and lungs.

Survival This depends on age at surgery. For example, the 3yr survival after cystectomy for T2 and T3 tumors is 60% if 65–75yrs old, falling to 40% if 75–82yrs old (in whom the operative mortality is 4%). With unilateral pelvic node involvement, only 6% of patients survive 5yrs. The 3yr survival with bilateral or para-aortic node involvement is nil.

Massive bladder hemorrhage may complicate treatment; consider alum solution bladder irrigation (safer than formalin): It is an in-patient procedure.

s asymptomatic microscopic hematuria significant?

Dipstick tests are often done routinely as part of a new admission. If microscopic hematuria is found, but the patient has no related symptoms, what does this mean? Before rushing into a barrage on investigations, consider:

- A meta-analysis found incidence of urogenital disease (eg bladder cancer) was no higher in those with asymptomatic microhematuria than those without[1].
- Asymptomatic microscopic hematuria is the sole presenting feature in only 4% of bladder cancers, and there is no evidence that these are less advanced than malignancies presenting with macroscopic hematuria.
- When monitoring those with treated bladder cancer for recurrence, microscopic hematuria tests have a sensitivity of only 31% in those with superficial bladder malignancy, in whom detection would be most useful.
- Although 80% of those with flank pain due to a renal stone have microscopic hematuria, so will >50% of those with flank pain but no stone.

The conclusion is not that urine dipstick testing is useless, but that results need should not be interpreted *in isolation*. Smokers and those with a +ve family history for urothelial malignancy may be investigated differently from those with no risk factors (eg ultrasound, cystoscopy ± referral to a renal physician in some patients), but in a young fit athlete, the diagnosis is more likely to be exercise-induced hematuria.

JAMA 1989, Sep 1; 262(9): 1214–9.

Gynecology

Disorders of the vulva The area surrounding the vagina that is loosely cover[ed] by skin and is affected by pathologic processes that affect squamous epithelium

Benign disorders include:

Bartholins gland cyst or abscess: Obstruction of the mucus secreting gland su[r]rounding the vagina leads to super infection, polymicrobial, needs marsupializati[on] and antibiotics. Undrained abscess of either bartholins gland or perianal may le[ad] to necrotizing fasciitis. More common in diabetics, immuno-compromised, and history of atherosclerotic disease.

Pre-malignant and malignant conditions:

Vulvar intraepithelial neoplasia (VIN): Presents either asymptomatic or wi[th] pruritis. Appearance is white and red papular or macular rash. 5% acetic acid m[ay] help visualize. Document lesions and biopsy. Often associated with human pap[il]loma virus (HPV). Look for peri-anal lesions as well.

Histological grade: VIN I (mild dysplasia), VIN II (moderate), VIN III (severe dyspl[asia] or carcinoma in situ).

Treatment: Local excision, CO_2 laser

Vulvar cancer: 5% of female genital malignancies, look for vaginal and anorect[al] involvement. VIN is usually precursor lesion. 90% squamous cell, also melanom[a]. Inguinal and pelvic lymph nodes involved 20% of cases if lesion is <2cm, 40% [of] cases if lesion is >2cm. Treatment: Unilateral lesions <2cm can be treated wi[th] wide local excision (WLE). All others are treated with WLE and bilateral inguina[l] femoral lymphadenectomy. If node negative 5-yr survival approaches 90%; inguin[al] node mets ~40%, pelvic nodes ~20%.

Disorder of the vagina

Benign disorders:

Pelvic organ prolapse: Results 2° to weakness in pelvic support. Risk factor[s] include: Pregnancy and childbirth, ↑ in intra-abdominal pressure (respirator[y] disease, obesity), postmenopausal atrophy, and connective tissue disorder.

Presentation: Pelvic pressure, coital difficulty, backache, protrusion from th[e] vagina, vaginal spotting, urinary incontinence, fecal incontinence or obstructe[d] defecation.

Evaluation: Clinical exam, urodynamics, radiographic studies include cystocolp[o] proctography, dymamic pelvic MRI.

Treatment: Pessary if unfit for surgery. Abdominal suspension procedures inclu[d]ing sacrocolpopexy or sacrocolpoperineopexy.

Premalignant or malignant conditions

Vaginal cancer: Rare, most are extensions from either vulvar or cervical cancer[s]. Usually squamous cell (90%), adenocarcinoma, sarcoma (DES exposure), mela[no]noma in 10%. Surgery has a limited role. Radiation therapy is the mainstay. Poo[r] survival rates.

Disorders of the uterus

Benign disorders:

Hyperplasia or uterine polyps: Presentation is abnormal uterine bleeding. Laser o[r] cauterization of the endometrium is the method of treatment.

Leiomyoma (fibroids): 25% of women in reproductive years have fibroids. Risk o[f] malignant degeneration is <0.5%. GnRH analogs, myomectomy, embolization hysterectomy are all methods of treatment.

Cervicitis: Common organisms include *Trichomonas vaginalis, Chlamydia trachom[a]tis, N. gonnorrheae, Herpes simplex virus.* Presentation: Vaginal discharge, pruritis. Clinical findings: Yellow discharge and erythematous cervix on inspection. Cervic[al] motion tenderness on bimanual exam. Treatment is antibiotics and education.

Pelvic inflammatory disease (PID): Spread of organisms in the endocervix throug[h] the endometrium to the fallopian tubes and beyond. Common organisms include

Chlamydia trachomatis, N. gonnorrheae, Hemophilus influenzae. Criteria for diagnosis include lower abdominal pain, mucopurulent cervical discharge on exam, bilateral adnexal tenderness. Associated findings include fever, leukocytosis,

Treatment: For questionable diagnosis laparoscopy is helpful. There are usually erythematous tubes and with a sticky exudate. Antibiotics are the mainstay treatment. Outpatient treatment is ceftriaxone 250 mg intramuscular and doxycycline 100 mg bid for 10–14d. Re-examine outpatients within 48h. A tubo-ovarian abscess is the most severe form of PID. Inpatient antibiotics will resolve abscess in 75%, drainage is necessary either operatively or via interventional radiology in 25%.

Malignant disorders:
Cervical cancer
Approximately 20% of female genital cancers. Adenocarcinoma (90%) or Squamous cell cancer (10%). Spreads primarily through direct extension and into the regional pelvic lymph nodes. Treatment is either radiotherapy or surgery with similar 5-yr survival rates. Localized disease has a 5-yr survival rate of 80–90%, metastatic disease to the lymph nodes ~40% 5-yr survival.

Endometrial cancer: Most common female genital cancer. Risk factors include nulliparity, obesity, delayed menopause, chronic anovulation, and unopposed postmenopausal estrogens. Presenting symptom is bleeding. Types include adenocarcinoma (90%)

Evaluation incudes transvaginal ultrasound and endometrial sampling. Treatment of localized disease is surgical and includes extrafascial abdominal hysterectomy and bilateral salpingo-oophorectomy. Poorly differentiated endometrial cancer and extension into the cervix of beyond the superficial myometrium should undergo selective pelvic and periaortic lymph node sampling. Additional radiotherapy is commonly employed in these patients. 5-yr survival for superficial stage I disease is 80%; stage II disease is 60%, and 30% for advanced disease.

Disorders of the ovary
Benign disorders:
Benign follicular, corpus luteal and theca lutein cysts are the most common. Usually disappear with new menstral cycle or oral contraception. Cysts >10cm are unlikely to disappear.

Teratoma: Commonly seen in women of reproductive age. Often bilateral. Ovarian cystectomy is recommended treatment.

Serous or mucinous cystadenoma: Benign epithelial tumors. Treated with cystectomy or oophorectomy. Intraoperative frozen section may be important to determine whether or not these cysts contain malignant cells. If so, and the patient is postmenopausal, bilateral oophorectomy and hysterectomy is recommended.

Ectopic pregnancy: Risk factors include: History of PID, use of infertility drugs, intrauterine contraceptive device. Any women of childbearing age with lower abdominal pain should have a βHCG drawn. Small ectopic pregnancies may be treated with methotrexate. Laparoscopy or laparotomy is otherwise performed.

Malignant disorders:
Ovarian cancer: 25% of all female genital cancers. Risk factors include ↑ age, ↓ fertility, family history, Peutz–Jeghers' syndrome, Turner syndrome. Presentation is often late and consists of abdominal pain and swelling, gastrointestinal symptoms, adnexal mass.

Evaluation: CBC, chemistry, CA-125, α –fetoprotein, CT, IVP,

Treatment: Abdominal hysterectomy with bilaterally salpingo-oophorectomy, lymphadenectomy, and tumor cytoreduction. Adjuvant chemotherapy (taxol) and/or radiation are given for advanced disease. 5yr survival from epithelial ovarian cancer is 70% for stage I, 30% for stage II, and <15% for stage III and IV.

Infectious diseases (ID)

John G. Bartlett, M.D.

Contents

Relevant pages in other sections

Prophylactic antibiotics in surgery (p404); infective endocarditis (p140); pneumonia (p158); atypical pneumonia (p160); lung abscess (p161); bronchiectasis (p163); fungi and the lung (p164); UTI (p240); encephalitis (p337); ▸▸meningitis (p336); septic arthritis (p365).

US notifiable diseases

AIDs
Anthrax
Legionellosis
Listeriosis
Lyme disease
Malaria
Rubella
Salmonellosis
SARS
Botulism
Brucellosis
Chanchroid
Chlamydia trachomatis, genital
Cholera
Coccidioidomycosis
Cryptosporidiosis
Cyclosporiasis
Measles
Shigellosis

Streptococcal disease, invasive, group A
Streptococcal toxic shock
Streptococcal pneumoniae, drug-resistant
Diphtheria
Ehrlichiosis
Syphillis
Tetanus
Toxic shock
Trichinellosis
Meningococcal disease
Tuberculosis
Tularemia
Mumps
Pertussis
Typhoid fever
Varicella

Yellow fever
Encephalitis, arboviral (Califonia, Eastern equine, Powassan, St. Louis, Western equine, West Nile)
E. coli (EHEC)
Giardiasis
Gonorrhea
Haemophilus influenzae
Plague
Poliomyelitis, paralytic
Psittacosis
Q fever
Hansen disease (leprosy)
Hantavirus, pulmonary
Hemolytic uremic syndrome
Hepatitis, acute viral
Rabies, animal and human
Rocky Mountain spotted fever
Leptospirosis

MMWR **52**(54);1–85, 2005.

488

Examples of pathogens from various types of bacteria

This table is not exhaustive.

Gram positive cocci
Staphylococci (p530):
  coagulase +ve, eg *Staphylococcus aureus*
  coagulase –ve, eg *Staph. epidermidis*
Streptococci[1] (p530):
  β-hemolytic streptococci
  Streptococcus pyogenes (Lancefield group A)
α-hemolytic streptococci
  Strep. Mitior
  Strep. pneumoniae (pneumococcus)
  Strep. Sanguis
Enterococci (non-hemolytic)[2]:
  Enterococcus mutans
  E. Faecalis
Anaerobic streptococcus

Gram positive bacilli (rods)
Aerobes
Bacillus anthracis (anthrax: p530)
Corynebacterium diphtheriae (p531)
Listeria monocytogenes (p531)
Nocardia species

Anaerobes:
Clostridium
Cl. botulinum (botulism: p531)
Cl. perfringens (gas gangrene: p531)
Cl. tetani (tetanus: p534)
Cl. difficile (antibiotic-associated colitis)
Actinomyces:
Actinomyces israeli (p531), *A. naeslundii*
A. odontolyticus, A. viscosus

Obligate intracellular bacteria:
Chlamydia (p526)
  Chlamydia trachomatis
  C. psittaci
  C. pneumoniae
Coxiella burnetii (p542)
Bartonella (p542)
Ehrlichia (p542)
Listeria
Rickettsia (typhus, p543)
Legionella pneumophilia (p160)
Mycoplasma pneumoniae (p160)

Gram negative cocci
Neisseria:
  Neisseria meningitidis (meningitis, septicemia)
  N. Gonorrheae (gonorrhea, p528)
Moraxella:
  Moraxella catarrhalis (pneumonia, p533)

Gram negative bacilli (rods)
Enterobacteriaceae (p532):
  Escherichia coli
  Shigella species (p535)
  Salmonella species (p535)
  Citrobacter freundii, C. koseri
  Klebsiella pneumoniae, K. oxytoca
  Enterobacter aerogenes, E. cloacae
  Serratia marascens;
  Proteus mirabilis/vulgaris
  Morganella morganii
  Providencia species
  Yersinia enterocolitica, Y. pestis
  Y. Paratuberculosis
Pseudomonas aeruginosa (p532)
Hemophilus influenzae (p532)
Brucella species (p532)
Bordetella pertussis (p532)
Pasteurella multocida (p533)
Vibrio cholerae (p535)
Campylobacter jejuni (p501)
Anaerobes:
  Bacteroides (wound infections)
  fusobacterium
  Helicobacter pylori (p196)
Mycobacteria:
  mycobacterium tuberculosis (TB, p506)
  M. Bovis
  M. leprae (leprosy, p536)
'Atypical' mycobacteria:
  M. avium intracellulare (p520)
  M. scrofulaceum, M. kansasii
  M. marinum, M. malmoense
  M. ulcerans, M. xenopi, M gordonae
  M. fortuitum, M. chelonae, M. flavescens
  M. Smegmatis-phlei
Spirochetes (p538):
  Treponema (syphilis; yaws; pinta)
  Leptospira (Weil's disease)
  Borrelia (relapsing fever; Lyme disease)

1 Streps are classified according to hemolytic pattern (α, β-, or non-hemolytic) or by Lancefield antigen (A–G), or by species (eg *Strep. pyogenes*). There is much crossover among these groups; the above is a generalization for the chief pathogens.
2 Clinically, epidemiologically and in terms of treatment, enterococci behave unlike other streps.

Viruses (classification)

DNA viruses

A *Double-stranded DNA*

Papova virus	Papilloma virus: Human warts
	JC virus: Progressive multifocal leukoencephalopathy, PML
Adenovirus	>30 serotypes
	10% viral respiratory disease
	7% viral meningitis

Herpes viruses

    Herpes simplex virus (HSV) 1 & HSV 2 (p510)
    Herpes (varicella) zoster virus
    Cytomegalovirus—CMV, also called HHV-5, (p515)
    Herpes virus 6 & 7 (HHV-6 & 7): Roseola infantum;
    also post-transplant, like CMV
    Epstein–Barr virus (EBV) (p511)
    –Infectious mononucleosis (glandular fever)
    –Burkitt's lymphoma; nasopharyngeal carcinoma
    HHV-8: Kaposi's sarcoma

Pox viruses	(1) Variola: Smallpox (now officially eradicated)[1]
	(2) Vaccinia, cowpox
	(3) Orf, cutaneous pustules, caught from sheep
	(4) Molluscum contagiosum, pearly umbilicated papules, typically seen in children or with HIV.

Hepatitis B virus (p516)

B *Single-stranded DNA*

Erythrovirus	Erythema infectiosum (fifth disease) 'slapped cheek'
formerly parvovirus	appearance ± aplastic crises

RNA viruses

A *Double-stranded RNA*

Reovirus	eg rotavirus, infantile gastroenteritis

B *Positive single-stranded RNA*

Picornavirus	(1) Rhinovirus, common cold, >90 serotypes
	(2) Enterovirus
	(i) Coxsackie A (meningitis, gastroenteritis)
	Coxsackie B (pericarditis, Bornholm disease)
	(ii) Polio virus
	(iii) Echovirus (30% viral meningitis)
	(iv) Hepatitis A virus
Togavirus	(1) Rubella
	(2) Alphavirus
	(3) Flavivirus (yellow fever, dengue, hepatitis C)
Coronavirus	eg Urbani SARS-associated coronavirus

C *Negative single-stranded RNA*

Orthomyxovirus	Influenza A, B, C
Paramyxovirus	Parainfluenza, mumps, measles, respiratory syncitial virus (RSV)
Arenavirus	Lassa fever, some viral hemorrhagic fevers, lymphocytic-choriomeningitis virus (LCM)
Rhabdovirus	Rabies
Bunyavirus	Some viral hemorrhagic fevers

D *Retrovirus*

HIV-1, HIV-2, (p518)
HTLV-1, HTLV-2

---

1 Although officially declared eradicated by WHO in 1979, there have been some recent concerns that the virus may fall into the hands of those who would use it as a biological weapon.

Travel advice

The majority of travel-related illnesses are not infections but due to other events such as accidents, indiscretions (alcohol ± promiscuous sexual contact), and other illnesses. Most infections are due to ignorance or indiscretions. *Advice to travelers is more important than vaccination*: Eg simple hygiene, malaria prophylaxis, and protective measures. Take time to advise travellers on the benefits of safe sex and the risks of HIV and other STDs. *Malaria* is a large concern in endemic areas as is *cholera* and *traveller's diarrhea, p535.*

Vaccinations: [L = live vaccine]	Doses needed	Gap between doses: 1st & 2nd	2nd & 3rd	Booster interval
Yellow fever	1			10yrs
Typhoid SC (Typhim VI®)	1			3yrs
Tetanus	3	4wks	4wks	10yrs
Polio	3	>4wks	>4wks	10yrs
Rabies pre-exposure	3	7–28d	6–12 months	2–3yrs
Meningococci	1			3yrs
Japanese encephalitis	3	1–2wks	2–4wks	2yrs
Tick encephalitis	3	1–3 months	9–12 months	3yrs
Hepatitis A (Havrix monodose®)	1	6–12 months		10yrs
If 1–15yrs use Havrix Junior®	1	6–12 months		
Hepatitis B	3	1 month	5 months	5yrs
if travelling soon:		1wk	3wks	1yr

Suggested vaccines: *Africa:* Meningitis, typhoid, diphtheria, tetanus, polio, hepatitis A ± yellow fever. *Asia:* Meningitis (quadrivalent vaccine against meningitis A, C, W135, and Y for Saudi Arabia), typhoid, diphtheria, tetanus, polio, hepatitis A. Consider rabies and encephalitis. *S America:* Typhoid, diphtheria, tetanus, polio, hepatitis A ± yellow fever. *Travel if immunocompromised:* Avoid live vaccines. Hepatitis B vaccine p223.

Preventing traveler's diarrhea

Water: If in doubt, boil all water. Chlorination is an alternative but does not kill amebic cysts. Tablets are available from pharmacies. Filter water before purifying. It is important to distinguish between simple gravity filters and water purifiers (which also attempt to sterilize chemically). Make sure that all containers are disinfected. Try to avoid surface water and intermittent tap supplies. In Africa assume that all unbottled water is unsafe. With bottled water, ensure the rim is clean and dry. Avoid ice.

Food: Hot, well-cooked food is safest. Avoid salads and peel your own fruit. If you cannot wash your hands, discard the part of the food which you are holding. In those in whom traveler's diarrhea might be most serious, consider a standby course of ciprofloxacin.

491

Susceptibility of some bacteria to certain antibiotics

	Penicillin V & G	Flucloxacillin	Ampicillin & Amoxicillin, Azlocillin, Ticarcillin, piperacillin	Cefradine & Cefaclor	Cefuroxine & Cefotaxime	Ceftazidime	Imipenem & Meropenem	Erythromycin & Clarithromycin	Clindamycin	Tetracyclines	Chloramphenicol	Trimethoprim	Aminoglycosides eg Gentamicin	Vancomycin & Teicoplanin	Metronidazole	Ciprofloxacin	Co-amoxiclav
Staph. aureus (penicillin-sensitive)	1	2	2	2	2	0	2	2R	2R	2R	2	2	2	2	0	2	2
Staph. aureus (penicillin-resistant)	R	1	R	2	2	0	2	2R	2R	2R	2	2	2	2	0	2	2
Strep. (group A)	1	2	2	2	2	0	2	2	2	2R	2	2	R	2	0	2	2
Strep. pneumoniae	1ᵃ	2	2	2	2	0	2	2	2	2R	2	2	R	2	0	2	2
Enterococcus faecalis	R	R	1	R	R	R	2	R	R	R	R	R	2R	2	0	1	R
N. meningitidis	1	2	2	2	2	2	2	R	R	2	2	2	R	R	0	2	2
Listeria monocytogenes	1	2	1	0	0	0	2	2	2	2	2	2	2	R	0	R	2
H. influenzae	0	R	1R	1R	2	2	2	2	R	2	2	2	2	R	0	2	2
E. coli	R	R	2R	1R	2	2	2	R	R	2R	2	1R*	2	R	0	2	2
Klebsiella species	R	R	R	1R	2	2	2	R	R	2R	2	1R*	2	R	0	2	2
Serratia/Enterobacter species	R	R	2R	2R	2	2	2	R	R	2R	2	1R*	2	R	0	2	2R
Proteus species	R	R	2R	1R	2	2	2	R	R	R	2	1R*	2	R	0	2	2
Pseudomonas aeruginosa	R	R	R	R	R	1R	2	R	R	R	R	1R*	2	R	0	2	R
Bacteroides fragilis	R	R	2	R	R	R	2	R	2R	R	2R	R	R	R	1	R	2
Other Bacteroides species	2	R	2	R	R	R	2	R	2R	R	2R	R	R	R	1	R	2
Clostridium difficile	0	0	0	0	0	0	0	0	0	0	0	0	0	1	1	0	0

NOTE: 1 = susceptible, 1st choice. 2 = 2nd choice. R = resistance likely. 0 = usually inappropriate. R* = resistance is rare in most areas.

Antibiotics: Penicillins

General advice The most common error is to give antibiotics without knowing the infectious organism and then to stop them before the infection is controlled. This may promote the spread of antibiotic resistance. In general, avoid giving antibiotics until the lab has cultured the organism unless the patient is very ill and in need of immediate treatment. In which case, culture blood, urine, sputum, and any other relevant samples before treating with empiric antibiotics.

Antibiotic (and its uses):	Usual adult dose:	In renal failure:
Amoxicillin As ampicillin but better absorbed PO. For IV therapy, use ampicillin.	250–500mg/8h PO 3g/ 12h in recurrent or severe pneumonia	↓Dose if CC <10
Ampicillin Broader spectrum than penicillin; more active against Gram –ve rods, but β-lactamase sensitive. Amoxicillin is better absorbed PO.	1–2g/4–6h IM/IV	↓Dose dose if CC<10
Ampicillin/sulbactam C(Unasyn®)used in abdominal sepsis and severe respiratory infection	1–2g q 6h IV	CC<10, Q 12h
Clavulanate-Amoxicillin Augmentin® = clavulanic acid 125mg + amoxicillin 250mg; use as for ampicillin but β-lactamase inhibitor confers a much broader spectrum. May cause LFT↑.	1–2 tab/8–12h PO; Avoid clavulanic acid toxicity (LFT↑) by giving 2nd tab as amoxicillin. I	If CC 10–50, give 1–2 tab/12h; if CC <10, 1–2 tab/24h
Oxacillin For Gram +ve coagulase producer+	0.5–3g IV q4–6h up to to 12g/d. 0.5–1g PO q6h	No change
Penicillin G Most streptococci, meningococcus, gonococcus, syphilis, gas gangrene, anthrax, actinomycosis, and many anaerobes.	300–600mg/6h IV, 2.4g/ 4h in meningitis. If dose >1.2g, inject at rate <300mg/min	Massive doses may cause Na+↑ & K+↓, and, in renal failure, seizures
Penicillin V As for penicillin G but less active. Used as prophylaxis or to complete an IV course.	250–500mg/6h PO; take ½h before food	In severe renal failure, give doses every 12h
Piperacillin Very broad spectrum incl. anaerobes & *Pseudomonas*. Inactive against *Staphs*. Reserve only for those with severe infections. May be used with aminoglycosides (but not in the same IV).	3–4g/4–6h slowly IV if severe infection. Tazocin®= tazobactam 500mg + piperacillin 4g: Dose: 4.5g/8h IV over 3–5min	↓Dose if CC↓: CC 10–50: 4g/6h CC <10: 3–4g/8h
Procaine penicillin Depot injection; good for syphilis and gonorrhea.	Syphilis: 600mg/24h IM for 14d, gonorrhea: Start dose 3.6g if male 2.5g if female	Dose unaltered
Ticarcillin Very broad spectrum, eg *Pseudomonas, Proteus*. Use with an aminoglycoside. More active than azlocillin or piperacillin.	Timentin® contains 3g ticarcillin + 200mg clavulanic acid; dose: 3.2g/8h IV (/4h in severe infections)	If CC 10–50 dose is 2g/4–8h If CC <10, dose is 2g/12h

493

(CC=creatinine clearance, mL/min)

Penicillin side-effects • Hypersensitivity: Rash (ampicillin rashes need not indicate penicillin allergy but 'penicillin-allergic' implies allergy to *all* penicillins); serum sickness (2%); anaphylaxis (<1:100,000). • In huge overdose or intrathecal injection: Seizures and coma. • Diarrhea (pseudomembranous colitis is rare). • Electrolyte imbalance if given IV.

Antibiotics: Cephalosporins

Spectrum Most cephalosporins are active against methicillin-sensitive staphylococci (including β-lactamase producers), streptococci (except group D, *Enterococcus faecalis & faecium*), pneumococci, *E. coli*, some *Proteus*, *Klebsiella*, *Hemophilus*, *Salmonella*, and *Shigella*. 2nd generation drugs (cefuroxime, cefamandole) are active against *Neisseria* and *Hemophilus*. 3rd generation drugs (cefotaxime, cefta-zidime, ceftriaxone) have better activity against Gram –ve organisms. Ceftazidime has less Gram +ve activity, especially against *Staph. aureus*, and is used in the treatment of *Pseudomonas* infections. Cefepime is 4th generation and has activity vs. both Gram +ve and Gram –ve aerobic bacteria.

Uses Cephalosporins (cefaclor, cefadroxil, cefradine, cefalexin, cefuroxime axetil) may be used in pneumonias, otitis media, skin and soft tissue lesions, and UTIs, but they are not 1st-line agents. They may be used as 2nd-line agents, or to complete a course that was started with an IV cephalosporin. The major use of cephalosporins is parenteral, eg as prophylaxis in surgery (p404) and in post-operative infection. Suspected life-threatening infections, eg severe pneumonia, meningitis, or Gram –ve septicemia may be treated empirically with a 3rd generation drug. Cephalosporins may also become the drugs of 1st choice in certain situations, such as penicillin sensitivity (NB: 10% cross-sensitivity) or where aminoglycosides are better avoided.

The principal **adverse effect** of the cephalosporins is hypersensitivity. This is seen in <10% of penicillin-sensitive patients. There may be GI upset, reversible changes in liver function tests, eosinophilia, rarely neutropenia, nephrotoxicity, and colitis. There are reports of clotting abnormalities, and there may be false +ve results for glycosuria or the Coombs' test. Most broad-spectrum cephalosporins potentiate warfarin.

Antibiotic	Adult dose	Notes
		Cc = creatnine clearance /mL/min. RF = Renal failure, CC^M = cc/1.73m body area
Cefaclor	250–500mg/8h PO Max: 4g/24h	No dose change in RF
Cefadroxil	500mg–1g/12h PO	In RF give 1g loading dose, then: if CC^M 26–50: 1g/12h if CC^M 11–25: 1g/24h if CC^M 0–10: 1g/36h
Cefazolin	Mild infection 0.5–2g q6–8h IV Severe infection 1–2g q8h	Cc 35–54: 250–1000mg q12h Cc 11–34: 125–500mg q12h Cc <10: 125–500 q12h
Cefepime	1–2g/12h IVI	Good activity against *Pseudomonas*, enterobacter, other resistant Gram –ve organisms, and *S. aureus*. if CC 10–50: 1–2g/12h if CC ≤10: 1g/24h

Antibiotic	Adult dose	Notes
Cefixime	Syrup = 100mg/5mL ½–1yr: 3.75mL/d 1–4yrs: 5mL/d 5–10yrs: 10mL/d Adult dose: 400mg q 12–24h	Active against streptococci, coliforms, *Hemophilus*, *Proteus* and anaerobes, staphylococci, *E. faecalis*, and Pseudo-monas are resistant. In RF: Normal dose if CC >20mL/min
Cefotaxime	1–2g/12h IV/IM Max 4g/8h (gonorrhea: 500mg stat)	Broad spectrum. For serious infections only (severe pneumonia, meningitis). Unreliable activity against Pseudomonas. If CC <10, give 2g/24h max.
Cefoxitin	0.5–2g q4–6h IV/IM Max 12g/24h Gonorrhea: 2g stat (deep IM) with probenecid 1g PO	Active against Bacteroides, so useful in bowel surgery and pre-operatively. In RF load with 1–2g, then: if CC 10–50: 1–2g/8–12h if CC <10: 2g/24–48h
Ceftazidime	UTI: 1–3g q8–12h IV	Broad spectrum, incl. most Pseudomonas
	Other: 1–2g/8h Max: 1g/8h if elderly	For serious infections only. Used in empiric treatment of neutropenic sepsis.
	Route: IV/IM but avoid IM if dose >1g	In RF load with 1g, then: if CC 31–50: 1g/12h if CC 16–30: 1g/24h if CC 6–15: 500mg/24h if CC ≤5: 500mg/48h
Ceftriaxone	1–4g daily IM/IV give ≤1g at each IM site with 3.5mL 1% lidocaine	Many Gram +ve and –ve infections. Used in meningitis (p336), pre-colonic surgery, and gonorrhea. No activity against Listeria, enterococci, and Pseudomonas. Can be used in RF unless CC <10, then limit dose to 2g/d and check levels
Cefuroxime	250–500mg/12h PO 750mg–1.5g/8h IV/IM; Max IV: 3g/8h In RF ↓dose	Broad spectrum & good Gram –ve activity. Used in: Surgical prophylaxis; post-op infections; severe pneumonia. if CC 10–20: 750mg/12h if CC <10: 750mg/24h

Antibiotics: Others

496

Antibiotic (and uses)	Adult dose	Notes (CC=creatinine clearance, mL/min)
Amikacin See gentamicin.	15mg/kg × 1/d or 7.5mg/kg/12h IV; (lower dose in renal failure)	Resistance is less common than with gentamicin.
Azithromycin See clarithromycin, also good against *N. gonorrhoae*.	500mg PO for 3d.	SE: See erythromycin.
Chloramphenicol Rarely used 1ˢᵗ-line. May be used in typhoid fever & *Haemophilus* infection. Also in blind ℞ of meningitis if patient allergic to both penicillins and cephalosporins. Avoid late in lactation & pregnancy.	12.5mg/kg/6h PO or IV; 25mg/kg/6h may be used in septicemia or meningitis	SE (rare): Marrow aplasia (check CBC often), neuritis, GI upset. Avoid long or repeated courses and in liver impairment or if CC <10mL/min. *Interactions:* Warfarin, rifampicin, phenytoin, sulfonylureas, phenobarbital.
Ciprofloxacin Used in adult cystic fibrosis, typhoid, *Salmonella*, *Campylobacter*, prostatitis, and serious or resistant infections. Avoid overuse.	250–750mg/12h PO 200–400mg/12h IVI over ≥½h (over 1h, if 400mg used)	A good oral anti-pseudomonal agent. β-lactamase-resistant. Halve dose if CC <10. SE: Rashes, D&V, LFT ↑; potentiates theophylline.
Clarithromycin A macrolide, like erythromycin, used for: *S. aureus*, streptococci, *Mycoplasma*, *H. pylori*, *Chlamydia*, MAI (p520).	250–500mg/12h PO for 7–14d. *H. pylori:* 500mg/12h PO for 1wk as triple therapy. MAI may need 12wks	Halve dose if CC <10. *Interactions:* Ergot, warfarin, carbamazepine, theophyllines, zidovudine; never use with terfenadine or pimozide.
Clindamycin Active against Gram+ve cocci including penicillin resistant staph, and anaerobes.	150–300mg/6h PO; max 450mg/6h PO. 0.2–0.9g/8h IV or IM (by IVI only, if >600mg used)	Stop if diarrhea occurs (pseudomembranous colitis, p199). Used in *Staph.* bone/joint infection.
Doxycycline Used in travellers' diarrhea, *Chlamydia*, leptospirosis, syphilis, & brucellosis.	200mg PO on 1ˢᵗ day then 100–200mg/24h; max 200mg/d in severe infections	As for tetracycline, but may be used in renal failure.
Erythromycin Macrolide, used in penicillin allergy. Used 1ˢᵗ line in atypical pneumonia, p160.	250–500mg/6h PO (≤4g/d in *Legionella*). 6.25–12.5mg/kg/6h IVI (adult and child)	SE: D&V; phlebitis in IV use. Potentiates warfarin, theophylline, terfenadine, ergotamine, carbamazepine.
Gentamicin Spectrum-wide but poor against streps & anaerobes, so use with a penicillin and/or metronidazole. Synergy with ampicillin against Enterococcus. For potentially serious Gram –ve infections or prophylaxis in IE.	1.5–2mg/kg/8h or 5mg/kg × 1/d IV ↓Dose in renal failure. Typical once daily dose: 160mg/d in uncomplicated infection. Single stat dose for 'simple' infections: 5mg/kg then no more or review.	In uremia, give usual loading dose then ↓ frequency. Avoid: • Prolonged use • Concurrent furosemide • In pregnancy or myasthenia gravis. SE: Oto- & nephrotoxicity.

Antibiotic (and uses):	Adult dose	Notes
Imipenem (+cilastatin) Very broad spectrum: Gram +ve & –ve organisms, anaerobes & aerobes. β-lactam stable.	0.25–1mg/6h IVI; dose if CC 6–20: 250mg/12h or 3.5mg/kg/d, whichever is less; high doses risks seizure. CC <5, dialyse	Avoid in pregnancy and lactation. SE: Seizures; diarrhea, N&V; myoclonus, eosinophilia, WCC↓, Coombs' +ve; LFTs abnormal.
Levofloxacin UTIs, skin infections ,and community acquired pneumonia	250–750mg q 24h IV or PO	CC <50: 250MG IV Q24–48H
Linezolid Oxazolidinone used for MRSA, & VRE	600mg/12h PO/IV	May cause reversible pancytopenia if Rx >2wks
Meropenem See imipenem.	0.5–1g/8h IVI, max 2g/8h	Causes fewer seizures than imipenem.
Metronidazole Drug of choice vs anaerobes, *Gardnerella, Entameba histolytica,* & *Giardia lamblia;* use PO in pseudo-membranous colitis.	250–500mg tid PO or 0.5–1g q12h IV. PR dose: 1g/8h for 3d then 1g/12h. IVI dose: 500mg/8h for ≤7d	Disulfiram reaction with alcohol, interacts warfarin, phenytoin, cimetidine; care in liver failure.
		Breast-feeding and pregnancy: Avoid high-dose regimens.
Minocycline Spectrum > tetracycline.	100mg/12h PO	As tetracycline, but more SE (hepatitis, pneumonitis).
Nitrofurantoin UTI.	50mg/6h PO with food	CI: CC <50. SE: Fibrosis.
Rifampin Mycobacteria, prophylaxis in meningitis contacts.	Dose example: 600mg/24h PO before breakfast.	↓Dose in liver disease. Interferes with birth control pill.
Tetracycline Used in chronic bronchitis; 1st line in *Chlamydia,* Lyme disease, mycoplasma, brucellosis, rickettsia.	250–500mg/6h PO ac 500–1000mg/12h IVI (not if liver disease). IV preparation not available in UK.	Avoid if <12yrs old, in pregnancy, and if CC <50. Absorption ↓by iron, milk, and antacids. SE: Photosensitivity, D&V.
Tobramycin As gentamicin; better against *Pseudomonas.*	1.5–2mg/kg q 8h or 5mg/kg × 1/d IV Dose↓ in renal failure	Less toxic than gentamicin. Once daily dose: 5.1mg/kg/d.
Trimethoprim/sulfamethoxazole TMP/SMZ(Bactrim) Sulfamethoxazole 400mg + trimethoprim 80mg. 1st choice in *Pneumocystis carinii,* toxoplasmosis and nocardia. **NB:** Can act against *S. aureus*	0.2–20mg/kg/d (TMP) PO or IV 1–3 DS TAB PO bid	SE (mostly ∵ sulfonamide, elderly at ↑risk): Jaundice; Stevens–Johnson syn; marrow depression; folate↓. If CC 15–30, halve dose frequency after 3d. Avoid if CC <15. CI: G6PD deficiency.
Vancomycin PO: pseudomembranous colitis if metronidazole is contraindicated; IV: MRSA & other Gram +ve organisms (not *Erysipelothrix* species).	125mg/6h PO; 500mg/6h IVI over 1h or 1g/12h IVI over 100min; do peak level 2h post-IVI, eg after dose 3; aim for <30mg/L, & <10mg/L before dose 4	In renal failure, get help; nomograms are available. SE: Renal and ototoxicity. Do not overuse (↑risk of multiple resistance.

Empiric treatment

History: A detailed history may reveal the source of infection: Ask about respiratory, GI and GU symptoms; any travel or possible immunocompromised state? If acquired in the hospital, then follow local guidelines for nosocomial infection. *Examination:* Evalute the fever curve and examine for localizing signs. *Investigations:* If possible, culture all possible sources before treating (blood, sputum, urine, feces, skin/wound swabs, CSF, aspirates). Also check CBC, ESR, CRP, electrolytes, LFT, clotting, malaria film, save acute phase serum, serum for virology, CXR, ABG (as clinically indicated). Dipstick the urine. *Treatment:* Follow local guidelines. Change to the most appropriate drug once sensitivities are known. Treatment of most infections should not exceed 7d. Intravenous antibiotic therapy should preferably not exceed 48h–72h; review the need and change to PO if possible. If in doubt, ask for Infectious Disease consultation.

Infection	Treatment
Urinary tract infection	TMP/SMZ 160/800mg/12h PO
Cellulitis	Oxacillin
Wound infection	Await swab results
	Otherwise, oxacillin 1g/6h IV
Pneumonia	
Mild community-acquired	Amoxicillin 500mg/8h PO
	Azithromycin 500mg/d × 3d
Possible atypical pneumonia	Erythromycin 500mg/6h PO
Severe community-acquired	Cefuroxime 1.5g/8h IV
	+ erythromycin 1g/6h IV
	Levofloxacin 750mg PO or IV qd.
	ceftriaxone 2g IV qd + Azithromycin
	500mg PO or IV qd × 3d
Hospital-acquired	Cefuroxime 1.5g/8h IV or Zosyn® 4.5g/8h IV
Meningococcus	Penicillin G
Pneumococcus	and ceftriaxone 2g/12h IV
Hemophilus	
Listeria	Add ampicillin 2g/4h IVI
If HSV encephalitis possible	Add acyclovir 10mg/kg/8h IV
Endocarditis	
Empirical therapy	Oxacillin[2] + gentamicin IV
Strep. viridans	Oxacillin + gentamicin IV
Enterococcus faecalis	Amoxicillin + gentamicin IV
Staph. aureus, Staph. epidermidis	Oxacillin + gentamicin IV
Prosthetic valve	Vancomycin + gentamicin + rifampicin
Osteomyelitis/septic arthritis	Oxacillin 1g/6h IV then clindamycin PO
Septicemia	
Urinary tract sepsis	Cefuroxime 1.5g/8h IV + gentamicin IV
Intra-abdominal sepsis	Cefuroxime 1.5g/8h IV
	+ metronidazole 500mg/8h IV
Meningococcal sepsis	Ceftriaxone 2g/12h IV
Neutropenic sepsis	Zosyn® 4.5g/8h IV[1] over 3–5min + gentamicin
Skin or bone source	Oxacillin 1g/6h IV
Unknown cause	Cefuroxime 1.5g/8h IV + gentamicin 5mg/kg IV once daily + metronidazole 500mg/8h IV

Zosyn = piperacillin + tazobactam
Use vancomycin if penicillin allergic or resistant
All IV does should be given slowly, eg over 5mins.

Prognosis: Poor if very old or young, BP↓, WBC↓, P_aO_2↓, DIC, hypothermia.

---

1 Tazocin = piperacillin 4g (p493) + tazobactam 500mg.
2 Use vancomycin if penicillin-allergic, or suspected penicillin resistance eg MRSA.

Drug abuse and infectious diseases

Always consider this when there are evasive answers or unexplained findings. Ask direct questions: 'Do you use any drugs? Have you ever injected drugs? Does your partner use any drugs? Do you share needles? Have you ever had an HIV test?

Behavioral clues:

Temporary resident. 'Just passing through your area and need some pain medicine'.

Demands analgesia/antiemetics. Knows formulary well: 'I just need some Percocet for my renal colic'.

Erratic behavior on the ward; unexplained absences; mood swings.

Unrousable in the mornings; agitation from day 2.

Heavy smoking; strange smoke smells (cannabis, cocaine, heroin).

Physical clues:

Acetone or glue smell on breath (solvent abuse).

Small pupils (opiates), reversed by naloxone.

Needle tracks on arms, groin, legs; between toes; difficuly IV access.

Abscesses and lymphadenopathy in nodes draining injection sites.

Signs of drug-associated illnesses (eg endocarditis, p140; AIDS, p518, chronic viral hepatitis).

Common and possible presentations in drug abusers

Unconscious (p682)	Narcotics (consider nalaxone, p736), barbiturates, solvents, benzodiazepines.
Psychosis or agitation	Ecstasy (p737), LSD, amphetamine, anabolic steroids, benzodiazepines. Haloperidol may help.
Asthma or dyspnea	Is there opiate-induced pulmonary edema? Asthma may follow the smoking of heroin.
Lung abscess	Right-sided endocarditis (*Staph*) until proved otherwise.
Fever/FUO	Is it endocarditis?
Shivering & headache	After a 'bad hit' (chemical/organism contamination). Beware of myoglobinuria, DIC, renal failure. Do blood cultures and consider empiric antibiotics
Abscesses	If over injection site, then often of mixed organisms.
DVT	Eg on injecting suspended tablets into groin. Is there compression damage (compartment syndrome)? Do CPK.
Pneumonia	Pneumococcus, hemophilus, TB, pneumocystis (p520).
Tachyarrhythmia	(If young); cocaine, amphetamines, endocarditis.
Jaundice	Hepatitis B, C, or D; anabolic steroids (cholestasis).
'Lymphadenopathy with fever'	May be presentation of HIV seroconversion illness.
Osteomyelitis	Including spinal. *Staph. aureus*/Gram –ve organisms.
Constipation	If severe, opiate abuse may be the cause.
Blindness	Consider fungal ophthalmitis ± endocarditis.
Runny nose	Opiate withdrawal (+colic/diarrhea, yawns, lacrimation, dilated pupils, insomnia, myalgia, mood↓; can occur in neonates if mother is an opiate abuser); cocaine use.
Neuropathies	Consider solvent abuse.
Infarctions	(eg of spinal cord, brain, heart): Suspect cocaine use.

499

General management A non-judgemental approach will produce better cooperation and may avoid the patient leaving against medical advice. Establish firm rules, and if necessary a written contract, of acceptable behavior. NSAIDs are useful for pain relief. Do not prescribe benzodiazepines.

Commercial sex workers need STD screen and cervical cytology as carcinoma-*in-situ* is common. Screen for hepatitis B (provide vaccination when indicated); safe sex and safe injection advice. HIV testing and work with community teams.

Fever of unknown origin (FUO)

Most fevers are caused by self-limiting viral infections. Here fever may be caused by the body's immune response to infection resulting in the production of cytokines. A FUO is defined as a prolonged fever (>3wks), temperature ≥38.5°, undiagnosed despite 3d in the hospital, or 2 outpatient visits. Bacteremia is not a common cause of FUO.

Causes Infections: TB, culture-negative endocarditis, mononucleosis syndromes. Remainder of infections are *rare* and evaluation for their presence may lead to unnecessary and useless tests. Infection (23%); multisystem diseases, eg connective tissue diseases (22%); tumors (20%); drug fever (3%); miscellaneous diseases (14%). It is often impossible to reach a diagnosis (25% in one series).

Infections TB, culture neg endocarditis, mononucleosis syndromes, remainder are rare, abscesses are easily detected with CT scan (*Salmonella*, *Brucella*, *Borrelia*, leptospirosis). Rheumatic fever is rare; endocarditis may be culture-negative (eg Q fever); TB (CXR may be normal, culture sputum, urine ± gastric aspirate); other granulomas (eg toxoplasmosis); parasites (eg amebic liver abscess, malaria, schistosomiasis, trypanosomiasis); fungi and HIV. Asking '*Where have you been*' is vital: Find an expert on that area, or else you will miss diagnoses you may have never heard of.

Neoplasms Especially lymphomas (any pattern: Pel–Ebstein fever, p582, is rare)—myeloma, hypernephroma. Occasionally solid tumors (especially with hepatic metastasis—breast, lung GI). Fever with leukemia is usually due to infection.

Connective tissue disease Rheumatoid arthritis, polymyalgia rheumatica, Still's disease, giant cell arteritis, granulomatous hepatitis, SLE, PAN, Kawasaki disease.

Others Drugs (T°↑ may occur months after starting but remits within days of stopping; eosinophilia is a inconsistent clue); pulmonary embolism; stroke; Crohn's; ulcerative colitis; sarcoid; amyloid; familial Mediterranean fever—recurrent polyserositis (peritonitis, pleurisy) + fevers, abdominal pain, and arthritis; treat with colchicines.

Examples of intermittent fevers SBE; TB; filarial fever; amyloid; *Brucella*. *Daily fever spikes:* Abscess; malaria; schistosomiasis; *Saddleback fever (eg fever for 7d, then ↔ for 3d):* Colorado tick fever; Borrelia; Leptospira; dengue; Ehrlichia (p542). *Longer periodicity:* Pel–Ebstein. *Remitting* (diurnal variation, not dipping to normal): Amebiasis; malaria; Salmonella; Kawasaki disease; CMV.

History Note especially sexual history, IV drug abuse, immunosuppressive illness, foreign or distant travel (p502), animal (or people) contacts, bites, cuts, surgery, rashes, mild diarrhea, drugs (including non-prescription), immunization, sweats, weight↓, and itching.

Examination Remember teeth, rectal/vaginal exams, skin lesions, lymphadenopathy, hepatosplenomegaly, nails, joints, temporal arteries.

Tests Stage 1(the first days): CBC, ESR, electrolytes, LFT, CRP, WBC differential, save acute phase serum, blood cultures (several, from different veins, at various times of day; prolonged culture may be needed for *Brucella*); baseline serum for virology, sputum microscopy and culture (specify for TB), urine dipstick, microscopy, and culture stool for microscopy (ova, cysts, and parasites), CXR. Serology is rarely useful in developed countries.

Stage 2: Repeat history and examination every day. Protein electrophoresis, CT (chest, abdomen). Rheumatoid factor, ANA, antistreptolysin titer, Mantoux, ECG, bone marrow, lumbar puncture. Consider PSA, carcionembryonic antigen, and withholding drugs, one at a time for 48h each. Consider temporal artery biopsy (p379). HIV test counseling.

Stage 3: Follow any leads uncovered. Consider echocardiography, CT, liver biopsy. Bronchoscopy.

Stage 4: Treat for TB, endocarditis, vasculitis, or trial of aspirin/steroids.

Gastroenteritis

Ingestion of certain bacteria, viruses, and toxins (bacterial and chemical) is a common cause of diarrhea and vomiting (p198). Contaminated food and water are common sources, but often no specific cause is found. Ask about details of food and water taken, cooking method, time for onset of symptoms, and whether other diners were affected. Ask about swimming, canoeing, etc.

Organism/Source	Incubation	Clinical features	Food
Staph. aureus	1–6h	D&V, P, hypotension	Meat
Bacillus cereus	1–5h	D&V	Rice
Red beans	1–3h	D&V	
Scrombotoxin	10–60min	D, flushing, sweating erythema, hot mouth	Fish
Salmonella	12–48h	D&V, P, fever, septicemia	Meat, eggs, poultry
Cl. perfringens	8–24h	D, P afebrile	Meat
Cl. botulinum	12–36h	V, paralysis	Home canned food
Cl. difficile		Colitis (p199)	
Vibrio parahemolyticus	12–24h	Profuse D; P, V	Seafood
Vibrio cholerae	2h–5d	See p535	Water*
Campylobacter	2–5d	P, fever	Milk, poultry, water*
Listeria		meningoencephalitis; 'I've got 'flu'; miscarriages	Cheese, pâtés
Small round-structured viruses (SRSV)	36–72h	D&V, fever malaise	Any food
Norovirus	1–5d	Vomiting and diarrhea	Food or water
E. coli type 0157	12–72h	Bloody D *hemolytic-uremic syndrome	Hamburger
Y. enterocolitica	24–36h	D, P, fever, appendicitis symptoms	Milk*
Cryptosporidium[1]	4–12d	D	Cow→water→man
Giardia lamblia	1–4wks	P544	Water*
Entameba histolytica	1–4wks	Bloody D p544	*
Rotavirus	1–7d	D&V, fever, malaise	*
Shigella	2–3d	Bloody D, P, fever	Any food

V=vomiting; **D**=diarrhea; **P**=abdominal pain. *May be food- or water-borne.

Tests *Stool microscopy and culture,* if patient has been travelling and fails to respond to empiric therapy, is from an institution or at day care, an outbreak is suspected, has bloody diarrhea or persistent fever. Perform *C. difficile* toxin assay if diarrhea is associated with antibiotic exposure.

Prevention Basic hygiene. When abroad, avoid unboiled/unbottled water, ice cubes, salads, and unpeeled fruit. Eat only freshly prepared hot food. Beverages should be purified water, alcohol or carbonated.

501

Management Usually symptomatic. Maintain *oral fluid intake* (± oral rehydration solution). For severe symptoms (but not in dysentery), give *antiemetic* (eg prochlorperazine 12.5mg/6h IM) and an *antidiarrheal* (eg codeine 30mg PO/IM or loperamide 4mg initially then 2mg after each loose stool). *Antibiotics are only indicated if systemically unwell, immunosupressed or elderly:*
• Cholera: Tetracycline ↓ transmission. • Salmonella: Ciprofloxacin 500mg/12h PO, 200–400mg/12h IV × 5–7d • Shigella: Ciprofloxacin 500mg/12h PO × 1–3d • C. jejuni: Erythromycin 500mg PO bid × 5d × 5d • C. difficile: Stop implicated drug; start metronidazole 500mg PO tid or oral vancomycin 125mg qid • Cyclospora: TMP-SMZ 1 DS PO bid × 7–10d • Giardia: Metronidazole 250–750mg PO tid × 7–10d • E. histolytica: Metronidazole 750mg PO tid × 5–10d • Isospora TMP-SMZ 1 DS bid × 7d

1 Cryptosporidium is a fungus prevalent in HIV infection, eg related to drinking unboiled water. Self-limiting if CD4 count is ≥100. Quantify oocyst excretion. If Rx is needed, ask a microbiologist. Various treatments are tried, eg azithromycin with paromomycin 1g/12h PO, but none is of proven value.

Evaluating the tropical traveler

In every ill traveler, consider:

1 *Malaria* (p504): Presentation: Fever, rigors, headaches, dizziness, flu-like symptoms, diarrhea, thrombocytopenia. Complications: Anemia, hyperparasitemia (>5%), renal failure, pulmonary edema, cerebral edema. Diagnosis Serial thick and thin blood films. **NB**: Mosquitoes may stowaway in luggage causing malaria in non-tropical areas.

Typhoid (p543): Presents with fever, relative bradycardia, abdominal pain, dry cough, constipation, lymphadenopathy, headache, splenomegaly ± rose spots (rare). *Complication*: GI perforation. *Diagnosis*: Blood or BM culture.

Dengue fever (p541): Presents with fever, headache, myalgia, rash (flushing or petechial), thrombocytopenia, and leukopenia. Diagnosis: Serology.

Amebic liver abscess (p544): Presents with fever, jaundice, RUQ pain. Do serology and ultrasound. Blood cultures to rule out septicemia.

NB: A visit to the tropics does not preclude the mundane fevers—eg flu.

Jaundice Think of viral hepatitis, cholangitis, liver abscess, leptospirosis, typhoid, malaria, dengue fever, yellow fever, hemoglobinopathies.

Hepatosplenomegaly Viral hepatitis, malaria, *Brucella*, typhoid, leishmaniasis, schistosomiasis, toxoplasmosis.

Gross splenomegaly Malaria, visceral leishmaniasis (kala-azar).

Diarrhea & vomiting: Enterotoxigenic *E. coli* (Travelers' diarrhea) is most common. Consider *Salmonella, Shigella, Campylobacter, Giardia lamblia, Vibrio cholerae, Yersinia, Cryptosporidia, Isospora, E. coli 0157, Enteroinvasive E. coli, Aeromonas, Rotavirus, Norovirus*, etc. If diarrhea prolonged, consider protozoal infection of small bowel or tropical sprue (p232). In HIV: MAC, CMV, cryptosporidia, microsporidia, and *Isospora belli*.

Respiratory symptoms Common respiratory pathogens (p160), typhoid, *Legionella*, TB, Q fever, histoplasmosis, Löffler's syndrome.

Arthritis Gonococcus; septicemia; viruses (Ross river, Chikungunya et al p365).

Erythema nodosum *Causes*: Strep, TB, leprosy, fungi, Crohn's, ulcerative colitis, sarcoidosis, pregnancy, drugs (sulfonamides).

Anemia hookworm, malaria, kala-azar, hemolysis, malabsorption.

Skin lesions scabies (itchy allergic rash + burrows, eg in finger web-spaces, p326), orf (pustules), molluscum contagiosum (pearly, punctate, papules), leprosy (p336, anesthetic, hypopigmented areas), tropical ulcers, typhus ('eschar' = scab), leishmaniasis (ulcers/nodules), myiasis (nodules—larvae of various insects); drug reactions.

Acute abdomen Perforation of a typhoid ulcer, toxic megacolon in amebic or bacillary dysentery, sickle-cell crisis, ruptured spleen.

502

Rarities to consider Use local emergency isolation policy.

Rabies (p340) and other CNS viral infections, eg encephalitis (p337).

Yellow fever (p541) Suspect in travelers from Africa.

Lassa fever: Occurs in Nigeria, Sierra Leone, or Liberia. *Signs*: Fever; exudative sore throat; face edema; shock. Δ: PCR/EM; serology. R: ISOLATE & refer.

Marburg and Ebola virus: Seen in Sudan, Zaire, Kenya. *Signs*: Fever, myalgia, diarrhea, N&V, pleuritic pain, hepatitis, shock, and bleeding tendency. A maculopapular rash appears on day 5–7 and desquamates in <5d. Patients may bleed from all orifices and gums. Δ: PCR/EM; serology. R: Isolate & refer.

Viruses causing hemorrhage: Dengue, Marburg, Lassa, Ebola, Crimea-Congo fever, hemorrhagic fever with renal syndrome, yellow fever.

The details of the travel history (eg areas visited, immunization and prophylaxis taken, any exposure to disease) are very important, even if you cannot interpret them yourself. Seek expert opinion early.

Incubation times for fever in the tropical traveller[1]

The incubation times below are typical, but considerable variation occurs.

<14d	14d to 6wks	>6wks
Undifferentiated fever		
Malaria	Malaria	Malaria
Typhoid	Typhoid	Hepatitis B or E
Leptospirosis	Leptospirosis	Kala-azar
Dengue fever	Hepatitis A or E	Lymphatic filariasis
Rickettsiae	Acute schistosomiasis	Schistosomiasis
Acute HIV infection		Amebic liver abscess
Fever with CNS signs		
Viral and bacterial meningitis and encephalitis	East African trypanosomiasis	Rabies
East African trypanosomiasis	Rabies	
Poliomyelitis		
Fever with chest signs		
Influenza	Tuberculosis	Tuberculosis
Legionellosis	Q fever	
Q fever		
Acute histoplasmosis		
SARS		

Immunization

Active immunization usually stimulates the immune system (humoral and cellular immunity). *Passive immunization* provides pre-formed antibody (non-specific or antigen-specific).

Immunizations

At birth	Hepatitis B vaccine #1: If mother is HBsAg +ve give HBIG	
2 months	DPT-HiB (diphtheria, pertussis, tetanus)	
	Hemophilus influenzae Type b)	
	Oral polio #1	
	Hepatitis B #2	
3 months	Repeat DPT, HiB and Polio #2	
4 months	Repeat DPT-HiB and polio #3	Hepatitis B #3
12–18 months	Measles/mumps/rubella (MMR® vaccine)#1	
4–5yrs	DPT-HiB #4 Polio booster #4. MMR® #2.	
10–14yrs	Hepatitis B #4. Meningococcal vaccine.	
15–18yrs	Polio #5 + tetanus + low-dose diphtheria (=Td) booster.	
Any age	Consider yearly flu vaccine (if in 'at risk' category, p512).	
Adults	Boosters of tetanus every 10yrs and Polio. Pneumococcal vaccine every 5yrs, if at risk.	

An acute febrile illness is a contraindication to any vaccine. Give live vaccines either together, or separated by ≥3wks. Caution with live vaccines in patients who are immunodeficient (transplants, cancer chemotherapy, steroids, HIV infection)—seek expert advice.

Immunization in special situations If *splenectomized/hyposplenic (eg sickle cell):* Polyvalent pneumococcal; Hib; annual flu vaccine. *Chronic lung, heart, liver or kidney disease, diabetes:* Pneumococcal; annual flu vaccine.
►Always check for malaria in any sick patient from an endemic area.

503

1 ET Ryan 2002 *NEJM* **347** 505

Malaria^ND: Clinical features and diagnosis

Plasmodium protozoa, injected by the female *Anopheles* mosquito (~12 sporozoites/bite), multiply in RBCs (>10^8–10^{12} trophozoites per infection) so causing hemolysis, RBC sequestration, and cytokine release. Malaria is one of the most common causes of fever and illness in the tropics. *P. falciparum* is estimated to kill 1 million people each year.

P. falciparum malaria Incubation: 12d. Most travellers present within 2 months. *Symptoms:* Non-specific flu-like prodrome: Headache, malaise, myalgia, and anorexia followed by fever and chills ± syncope. Classic periodic fever (peaking every 3rd day, ie tertian) headache and rigors are unusual initially. *Signs* Anemia, jaundice, and hepatosplenomegaly. No rash or lymphadenopathy. *Complications: Cerebral malaria:* Seizures ± confusion then coma. Focal signs unusual. May have variable tone, extensor posturing; upgoing plantars, dysconjugate gaze. Mortality: ~20%. *Metabolic (lactic) acidosis* giving labored deep (Kussmaul's) breathing also major cause of death. *Anemia* is common due to hemolysis of parasitized RBCs. Elevated transaminase levels, *hyperparasitemia* (>5% of RBCs parasitized), and *hypoglycemia* can occur in severe malaria (8% of adults) or with quinine therapy. *Acute renal failure* from acute tubular necrosis, sometimes with hemoglobinuria ('*blackwater fever*'), and *pulmonary edema* are important causes of death in adults. Shock may develop in severe malaria (*algid malaria*) from bacterial septicemia, dehydration or, rarely, splenic rupture. In pregnancy, the risk of death (mother or fetus) is high. Use chemoprophylaxis in pregnant women in endemic areas of transmission. *Relapse* occurs as parasites lie dormant in the liver (*P. vivax* and *ovale*) or at low levels in the blood (*P. malariae*). Nephrotic syndrome (glomerulonephritis) may occur in chronic *P. malariae* infection.

Diagnosis Serial thin & thick blood films (needs much skill, don't always believe –ve reports, or reports based on thin film examination alone); if *P falciparum*, what is the level of parasitemia? Serology is not useful. Other tests: CBC (anemia, elevated transaminase, thrombocytopenia), clotting (DIC p576), glucose (hypoglycemia), ABG/lactate (lactic acidosis) ELECTROLYTES (renal failure), urinalysis (hemoglobinuria, proteinuria, casts), blood culture.

Poor prognostic signs (Severe *falciparum* malaria) parasite index >5% pregnancy, respiratory distress, seizures, coma, papilledema, pulmonary edema, acidemia (HCO$_3^-$ <15mEq/L), anemia, DIC, renal failure. If ≥20% (or >10^4/mcL) of parasites are mature trophozoites or schizonts, the prognosis is poor, even if few parasites seen (reflects critical mass of sequestered RBCs).

Pitfalls in malaria

- Failure to take a full travel history, including stop-overs in transit and failure to check if the patient has already received treatment which might make the blood smear negative.
- Delay in treatment while seeking lab confirmation.
- Failure to examine enough blood films before excluding the diagnosis.
- Belief that drugs will work, when the parasite is often one step ahead.
- Not having IV quinine available immediately. (Quinidine is an alternative.)
- Not observing *falciparum* patients closely for the first few days.
- Forgetting that malaria is an important cause of coma, deep jaundice, severe anemia, and renal failure in the tropics.

Malaria: Treatment and prophylaxis

Treatment If species unknown or mixed infection, treat as *P. falciparum*. Nearly all *P. falciparum* is now resistant to chloroquine and in many areas is also resistant to Fansidar® (pyrimethamine + sulfadoxine). If in doubt consider as resistant. Chloroquine is the drug of choice for benign malarias in most parts of the world, but chloroquine-resistant *P. vivax* occurs in Papua New Guinea, Indonesia, some areas of Brazil, Colombia, and Guyana. Never rely on chloroquine if used alone as prophylaxis.

Falciparum malaria: If the patient can swallow and there are no complications, give 650mg quinine salt/8h PO for 7d, + doxycycline 100mg/12h x 3–7d, or pyrimethamine/sulfacloxin 3 tabs last day of quinine. *Alternatives:* Atovaquone + proguanil (Malarone®) 4 tabs once daily (both for 3d with food). If seriously ill, take to ICU, and give quinidine IV with telemetry. Observe for QT prolongation, ventricular arrhythmias, hypotension and hypoglycemia. Artesunate or artemether have also been used IV.

Benign malarias: Give chloroquine PO as 600mg initially, 300mg 6h later, then 300mg/24h at 24h and 48h. If *P. vivax/ovale*, give primaquine 15mg/24h for 14–21d (22.5mg if Chesson strain from SE Asia/west Pacific) after chloroquine to treat liver stage and prevent relapse. Screen for G6PD deficiency first.

Other treatments: Acetaminophen for fever. Transfuse if severe anemia. Consider exchange transfusion if patient severely ill. Monitor BP, urine output, blood glucose frequently. Daily parasite count, platelets, electrolytes, LFT.

Examples of prophylaxis *Prophylaxis does not give full protection.* Risks are very variable; get local advice. Avoid mosquito bites between dusk and dawn: Wear long-sleeved clothes, use repellents (DEET), insecticide-treated bed nets. Except for Malarone®, take drugs from 1wk before travel (to reveal any SE) and continue for 4wks after return. None are required if just visiting cities of East Asia. There is no good protection for parts of SE Asia.

Recommended prophylaxis: Caribbean, North Africa, and Middle East: Chloroquine ± proguanil. *Latin America, sub-Saharan Africa, SE Asia, and Oceania:* Mefloquine 250mg (1 tab) weekly starting 1wk prior to travel and continue until 4wks post travel or doxycycline 100mg/d from 1wk before travel to 4wks post travel. *Central America north of Panama Canal:* Chloraquine 300mg/wk starting 1wk before travel to 4wks post travel.

If area has poor medical care and traveller not pregnant, also carry standby treatment course (eg Riamet®, Malarone®).

Adult prophylactic doses: Chloroquine (base[1]): 300mg/wk PO. *Proguanil:* 200mg/24h PO. *Doxycycline:* 100mg/24h PO starting 1wk before and continue to 4wks after returning. *Mefloquine:* 250mg/wk PO for adults if no risk of pregnancy starting 1wk before and continue to 4wks after returning. *Malarone®:* 1 tablet/24h PO starting 1d before travel, and continuing till 7d after return from malarious area.

Antimalarial SE: Chloroquine: Headache, psychosis, retinopathy (chronic use). *Fansidar®:* Stevens–Johnson, erythema multiforme, LFT↑, blood dyscrasias. *Primaquine:* Epigastric pain, hemolysis if G6PD-deficient, methemoglobinemia. *Mefloquine:* Nausea, dizziness, dysphoria, sleep disturbance, neuropsychiatric symptoms, long $t_{1/2}$. Ideally start prophylaxis 3wks prior to travel to reveal any SE. Avoid mefloquine if: • Low risk of chloroquine-resistant malaria, eg 1wk trip to East African coastal resort. • Past or family history of epilepsy, psychosis need to perform complicated jobs (eg pilots) • Risk of pregnancy within 3 months of last dose. Interactions: Quinidine, halofantrine. *Malarone®:* Abdominal pain, nausea, headache, dizziness.

---

1 150mg chloroquine base ≈ 250mg chloroquine phosphate (PO) ≈ 200mg chloroquine sulfate (IV).

Mycobacterium tuberculosis: Clinical features

TB kills nearly 3 million/yr worldwide. If one includes HIV-related TB, then T is the leading infectious cause of death worldwide, despite being treatable for the past 50yrs. Worldwide prevalence: 2 billion people.

Primary TB Initial infection is usually pulmonary (by droplet spread). A lesion forms and its draining nodes are infected. There is early distant spread of the bacilli, then an immune response suspends further multiplication at all site. Primary TB is often asymptomatic, or there is fever, anorexia, productive cough or conjunctivitis (small, multiple, yellow-grey nodules near the limbus). Acid-fast bacilli (AFBs) may be found in sputum. CXR may be abnormal. The commonest non-pulmonary *primary* infection is GI, typically affecting the ileocaecal junction and associated lymph nodes.

Post-primary TB Any form of immunocompromise may allow reactivation eg malignancy; diabetes; steroids; debilitation (esp. HIV or old age). The lung lesions (usually upper lobe) progress and fibrose. Any other site may become the main clinical problem. Tuberculomas contain few AFB, unless they erode into a bronchus, where the favorable environment ensures rapid multiplication, rendering the patient highly contagious. In the elderly or immunocompromised, dissemination of multiple tiny foci throughout the body (including back to the lungs) results in miliary TB.

In third world 40–50% of active TB patients have HIV infection and 40–50% of AIDS patients have active TB.

Pulmonary TB: This may be silent or present with cough, sputum, malaise, weight loss, night sweats, pleurisy, hemoptysis (may be massive), pleural effusion, or superimposed pulmonary infection. *Investigation and treatment* p508. An aspergilloma/mycetoma (p164) may form in the cavities.

Miliary TB: Occurs following hematogenous dissemination. Clinical features may be non-specific. CXR shows characteristic reticulonodular shadowing. Look for retinal TB. Biopsy of lung, liver, lymph nodes, or marrow may yield AFB or granulomas.

Meningeal TB: Subacute onset of meningitic symptoms: Fever, headache, nausea, vomiting, neck stiffness, and photophobia.

Genitourinary TB: May cause frequency, dysuria, flank/back pain, hematuria, and, classically, sterile pyuria. Take 3 early morning urine samples (EMU) for AFB. Renal ultrasound may help. Renal TB may spread to bladder, seminal vesicles, epididymis, or fallopian tubes.

Bone TB: Look for vertebral collapse adjacent to a paravertebral abscess (Pott's vertebra). Do biopsies for AFB stains and culture.

Skin TB (lupus vulgaris): Jelly-like nodules, eg on face or neck.

Peritoneal TB: This causes abdominal pain. Look for AFB in ascites (send *large* volume to lab); laparotomy may be needed.

Acute TB pericarditis: Think of this as a primary exudative lesion.

Chronic pericardial effusion and constrictive pericarditis: These reflect chronic granulomata. Fibrosis and calcification may be prominent with spread to myocardium.

Additional points in all those with TB:
- Advise HIV testing.
- Notify local health department to arrange contact tracing and screening.
- Explain that prolonged treatment will be necessary.
- All patients should receive directly observed therapy (DOT). Monitoring of blood tests will be needed (LFTs).
- Explain the need for respiratory isolation procedures while infectious until 3 neg sputa for AFB or 1 neg induced sputum for AFB.

TB with AIDs and multi-drug resistant (MDR) TB

Directly observed treatment strategy (DOTS) prevents MDR-TB. In areas where MDR-TB is common, DOTS-plus (involving the rational use of second-line drugs) may be a solution.

TB is a common, serious, but treatable complication of HIV infection. It is estimated that 30–50% of those with AIDS in the developing world also have TB. TB is probably no more infectious when occurring in the context of HIV. Interactions of HIV and TB are as follows:
• Mantoux tests may be negative with CD4 <200.
• ↑ reactivation of latent TB from the early stage of HIV.
• Presentation may be atypical.
• Previous BCG vaccination does not prevent development of TB.
• Smears may be negative for AFB in 50% of patients with pulmonary TB with or without HIV. Smears that are positive tend to contain few AFB. This makes culture all the more important and is vital to characterize drug resistance.
• Atypical CXR: Lobar or bibasal pneumonia, hilar lymphadenopathy.
• Extrapulmonary and disseminated disease is much more common.
• More toxicity from highly-active antiretroviral therapy (HAART, p524) and anti-TB therapy due to drug interactions with rifampin.
• Antiretroviral therapy reconstitutes CD4 count and immune function, which may lead to a paradoxical worsening of TB symptoms.
• Isoniazid prophylaxis in HIV is standard: 300mg qd x 9 month. With HIV infection add pyridoxine (vitamin B6) 50mg qd.

Respiratory isolation is essential when TB patients are near other patients including those HIV +ve. Nosocomial (hospital-acquired) and MDR-TB are now major problems worldwide, affecting both HIV +ve and HIV –ve people. Mortality is ~80%. Test TB cultures against 1st and 2nd line chemotherapeutic agents; 5+ drugs may be needed in MDR-TB.

First line antitubercular agents: *Second line antitubercular agents:*

Isoniazid	Ofloxacin	Aminosalicylic acid
Rifampicin	Ciprofloxacin	Cycloserine
Ethambutol	Moxifloxacin	Capreomycin
Pyrazinamide		Streptomycin
		Amikacin
		Kanamycin
		Ethionamide

Stopping the spread of MDR-TB Chief goals: *Early identification; full treatment; isolation.* Control may be linked to:
• Early isolation of suspected patients. A suspicious CXR or a past history of MDR-TB is enough. Don't wait to prove the diagnosis. Isolate if cough >2wks and abnormal chest X-ray.
• The ability to obtain 3 expectorated sputum or on sample obtain by bronchoscopy or sputum induction Ziehl–Nielsen (ZN)/auramine stains in a timely fashion.
• Directly observing & confirming that patients take all prescribed drugs.
• Wearing of special masks by staff.
• Sputum induction/expectoration being confined to isolation rooms.
• Providing negative air pressure in isolation rooms.
• Only stop isolation after ≥3 sputum samples are AFB –ve on culture for MDR-TB.
• Frequent tuberculin skin surveillance tests for workers and contacts.
• Contact evaluation.

507

TuberculosisND: Diagnosis and treatment

Diagnosis In all suspected cases, it is important to obtain the relevant clinical samples (sputum, pleural fluid, pleura, urine, pus, ascites, peritoneum, or CSF) for culture to establish the diagnosis. Get advice on testing contacts from health department.

Microbiology: Send 3 expectorated sputum samples for AFB stain and culture. If no expectorations, one bronchoscopy sample or one induced sputum sample should be used. Biopsy any suspicious lesions in liver, lymph nodes or bone marrow. AFB are bacilli that resist acid–alcohol decolorization under auramine or Ziehl–Neelsen (ZN) staining. Cultures undergo prolonged incubation (up to 12wks).

TB PCR: Allows rapid identification of rifampicin (and likely multi-drug) resistance. Occasionally useful for diagnosis in sterile specimens.

Histology: The hallmark is the presence of *caseating granulomata*.

Radiological features: CXR may show *consolidation, cavitation, fibrosis, and calcification* in pulmonary TB.

Immunological evidence of TB may be helpful:
- *Tuberculin skin test:* Test only if there is risk
- Test is positive if >5mm with HIV, close contact of TB case, fibrosis on X-ray, or immunosuppressed (prednisone >15mg/d × >1 month, etc)
- >10mm if recent immigrant, IVDU, resident or employee of prison or jail, nursing home, shelter, diabetes, renal failure, leukemia, lymphoma, weight loss, gastrectomy, child <4yrs.
- Recent converter defined as >10mm ↑ in induration within 2yrs

All above categories should be treated for latent TB regardless of age

Treatment of pulmonary TB *Before treatment:* Stress importance of compliance (helps the patient and prevents the spread of resistance). Check CBC, liver, and renal function. Test color vision (Ishihara chart) and acuity before and during treatment if ethambutol dose is ≥25mg/kg/d as ethambutol may cause (reversible) ocular toxicity. Patients often forget to take pills, so consider DOT, as follows:

Initial phase (8wks on 4 drugs):
1 Rifampicin (RIF) 600mg PO 3 times/wk.
2 Isoniazid (INH) 15mg/kg PO 3 times/wk + pyridoxine 10mg/24h.
3 Pyrazinamide (PZA) 2.5g PO 3 times/wk. 56–75kg: 2.5g 76–90kg: 3g
4 Ethambutol (EMB) 30mg/kg PO 3 times a week.

Monitor LFT at baseline and with symptoms on monthly review.

Continuation phase (4 months on 2 drugs) rifampicin and isoniazid at same doses. (2 Rifinah 300® tablets = rifampicin 600mg + isoniazid 300mg). If resistance is a problem: Resistance: INH, drug: RIF/PZA/ETH ± FQ; Resistance: RIF, drug: INH/PZA/ETH/± fluoroquinolone (FQ); Resistance: INH/RIF, drug: FQ/PZA/ETH/aminoglycoside.

Phase 1 (8wks)	Phase 2 (18wks)
INH/RIF/PZA/EMB	INH/RIF
7d/wk × 8wks	7d/wk × 18wks
5d/wk × 8wks	5d/wk × 18wks
7d/wk × 2wks, then 2×/wk × 6wks	2d/wk × 18wks
3d/wk × 8wks	3×/wk × 18wks
INH/RIF/EMB	INH/RIF
7d/wk × 8wks	7d/wk × 31wks
5d/wk × 8wks	2d/wk × 31wks

Give pyridoxine throughout treatment.

Steroids *may* be indicated in meningeal and pericardial disease.

Main side-effects Seek help in renal or hepatic failure, or pregnancy.

Rifampicin: Hepatitis (a small rise of AST is acceptable, stop if ALT is 5 × ULN bilirubin rises), orange discoloration of urine and tears (contact lens staining), inactivation of birth control pills, flu-like syndrome with intermittent use.

Isoniazid: Hepatitis, neuropathy, pyridoxine deficit, agranulocytosis.

Ethambutol: Optic neuritis (color vision is the first to deteriorate).

Pyrazinamide: Hepatitis, non-gout polyarthritis arthralgia (gout is a contrain-dication).

Chemoprophylaxis for asymptomatic tuberculous infection

Immigrant or contact screening may identify patients with TB without symptoms or radiographic changes. In such patients, chemoprophylaxis may be useful to kill the infective organisms and prevent possible disease progression at a later date. This involves administration of INH 600mg/d x 9mo.

In all cases, standard anti-TB therapy should be initiated once any evidence of active disease (clinical or radiographic) is found.

Preventing TB in HIV +ve people

Primary prophylaxis against TB is indicated in some HIV +ve patients. In Africa, about 50% of those with HIV develop TB, and 80% of those with TB are HIV +ve. Isoniazid (eg 300mg/d PO; give with pyridoxine) is the most common agent used. If there is a known contact with a person infected with isoniazid-resistant TB, rifampicin is an alternative. The duration of prophylaxis has been the subject of debate.

Indications for primary prophylaxis:
• If the patient has not had BCG and the Mantoux test is >5mm.
• If BCG vaccinated (>10yrs ago), consider prophylaxis if Mantoux >10mm.
• If there is recent exposure to someone with active TB.

Herpes infections

Varicella zoster Chickenpox is the primary infection; after infection virus remains dormant in dorsal root ganglia. Reactivation causes shingles. Shingles affects 20% at some time. High-risk groups: Elderly or immunosuppressed. *Clinical features:* Pain in a dermatomal distribution precedes malaise and fever by a few days. Some days later macules, papules, and vesicles develop in the same dermatome. Thoracic dermatomes and the ophthalmic division of trigeminal nerve are most vulnerable. If the sacral nerves are affected, urinary retention may occur. Motor nerves are rarely affected. *Ramsay-Hunt syndrome* (zoster of the ear + VIIth nerve palsy). Recurrence suggests immunosuppression. *Investigations* are rarely necessary. Culture or electron microscopy of vesicle fluid confirm the diagnosis. *Indications for treatment:* Most patients will want treatment (to ↓risk of post-herpetic neuralgia); if seen early, give Valacyclovir 1g PO tid x 7–10d or famciclovir 500mg PO tid. If immunocompromised give acyclovir 10mg/kg/8h IV for 10d. Control pain with oral analgesic ± gabapentin, tricyclics, carbamazepine lidocaine patch and/or narcotics (underutilized). There is evidence to support a 4wk course of prednisolone to reduce post-herpetic neuralgia. If the conjunctiva is affected, apply 3% acyclovir ointment 5 times a day. Beware iritis. Measure visual acuity often. Advise patient to report *any* visual loss at once. SE of acyclovir: Renal impairment (check electrolytes) vomiting, urticaria, encephalopathy. *Complications:* Post-herpetic neuralgia in the affected dermatome can persist for years, and be very hard to treat. Try carbamazepine, phenytoin, amitriptyline, gabapentin, or capsaicin cream and narcotics. As a last resort, ablation of the appropriate ganglion may be tried. Refer to a pain clinic.

Herpes simplex virus (HSV) Manifestations of primary infection:

1 *Systemic infection*, eg fever, sore throat, and lymphadenopathy may pass unnoticed. If immunocompromised, it may be life-threatening with fever, lymphadenopathy, pneumonitis, and hepatitis.

2 *Gingivostomatitis:* Ulcers filled with yellow slough appear in the mouth.

3 *Herpetic whitlow:* A breach in the skin allows the virus to enter the finger, causing a vesicle to form. Often affects childrens' nurses.

4 *Traumatic herpes (herpes gladiatorum):* Vesicles develop at any site where HSV is ground into the skin by brute force.

5 *Eczema herpeticum:* HSV infection of eczematous skin; usually children.

6 *Herpes simplex meningitis:* This is uncommon and usually self-limiting (typically HSV II in women during a primary attack).

7 *Genital herpes:* Usually HSV II. ♂: Grouped vesicles and papules develop around anus and penis (with pain, fever, and dysuria) ± palms, feet, or throat. Give analgesia and one of the regimens below for acute, or recurrent presentations. Suppressive therapy can be provided if there are frequent (≥6/yr) or severe recurrences.

	Acute	Recurrent	Suppression
Acyclovir	400mg PO tid x 7–10d	400mg PO tid x 2–3d	400mg bid
Famciclovir	500mg PO tid x 7–10d	125mg PO bid x 3–5d	250mg bid
Valacyclovir	1g PO bid x 7–10d	500mg PO qd x 3d	0.5–1g qd

8 *Severe disease:* Acyclovir 10mg/kg q8h IV

9 *Acyclovir resistance:* Foscarnet 120–200mg/d IV or topical cidofovir get 1% applied qd x 5d

10 *Encephalitis:* Acyclovir 10–15mg/kg q8h IV x 14–21d

11 *Keratitis:* Trifluridine eyedrops, 1 drop q2h up to 9x/d x 21d

12 *HSV keratitis:* Corneal dendritic ulcers. *Avoid steroids.*

13 *Herpes simplex encephalitis:* Usually HSV I. Spreads centripetally, eg from cranial nerve ganglia, to frontal and temporal lobes. *Suspect if* fever, seizures, headaches, odd behavior, dysphasia, hemiparesis, or coma or subacute brainstem encephalitis, meningitis, or myelitis. *Diagnosis:* Urgent PCR on CSF sample (CT/MRI and EEG may show temporal lobe changes but are non-specific and unreliable; brain biopsy rarely required). Seek expert help: Adm

to ICU; careful fluid balance to minimize cerebral edema (consider mannitol, p722); *prompt* acyclovir, eg 10mg/kg/8h IV for 10d, saves lives. Mortality: 19% if treated with acyclovir, 70% if untreated.

4 *Tests:* Rising antibody titers in 1° infection; culture; PCR for fast diagnosis.

5 *Recurrent HSV:* HSV lying dormant in ganglion cells may be reactivated by illness, immunosuppression, menstruation, or even sunlight. Cold sores (perioral vesicles) are one manifestation. Acyclovir cream is not recommended.

Infectious mononucleosis

This is a common disease of young adults which may pass unnoticed or cause acute illness. Spread is thought to be by saliva or droplet. The incubation period is uncertain, but may be 4–5wks. The disease is caused by the Epstein–Barr virus (EBV), which preferentially infects B-lymphocytes. There follows a proliferation of T-cells (the 'atypical' mononuclear cells) which are cytotoxic to EBV-infected cells. The latter are 'immortalized' by EBV infection and can, very rarely, proliferate to form a picture indistinguishable from immunoblastic lymphoma in immunodeficient individuals (whose suppressor T-cells fail to check multiplication of these B-cells).

Symptoms and signs Sore throat, fever, anorexia, malaise, lymphadenopathy, palatal petechiae, splenomegaly, hepatitis, and hemolytic anemia. Occasionally encephalitis, myocarditis, pericarditis, neuropathy. Rashes may occur, particularly if the patient is given ampicillin.

Investigations *Blood film* shows a lymphocytosis (up to 20% of WBC) and atypical lymphocytes (large, irregular nuclei). Such cells may be seen in many viral infections (eg CMV, HIV, parvovirus, dengue fever), toxoplasmosis, leukemias, lymphomas, drug hypersensitivity, and lead poisoning.

Heterophil antibody tests (eg Monospot®): Heterophil antibodies develop early and disappear after ~3 months. These antibodies agglutinate sheep red blood cells. They can be absorbed (and thus agglutination is prevented) by ox red cells, but not guinea-pig kidney cells. This pattern distinguishes them from other heterophil antibodies. These antibodies do not react with EBV or its antigens. *False +ve* Monospot® tests may occur in hepatitis, parvovirus infections, lymphoma, leukemia, rubella, malaria, carcinoma of pancreas, and SLE.

Immunology: EBV-specific IgM implies current infection. IgG shows that the patient has been previously infected.

Differential diagnosis Streptococcal sore throat (may coexist), CMV, viral hepatitis, HIV seroconversion illness, toxoplasmosis, leukemia, diphtheria.

Treatment Avoid alcohol and trauma to LUQ. Steroids are rarely recommended for severe symptoms. *Ampicillin and amoxicillin should not be given for sore throats as they may cause a severe rash in those with acute EBV infection.*

Complications Depression, fatigue, and lethargy which may persist for months. Also, thrombocytopenia, ruptured spleen, splenic hemorrhage, upper airways obstruction (may need observation on ICU), secondary infection, pneumonitis, aseptic meningitis, Guillain–Barré syndrome, renal failure, lymphoma, and autoimmune hemolytic anemia. All are rare.

Other EBV-associated diseases EBV is associated with Burkitt's lymphoma in Africa, and nasopharyngeal carcinoma in Asia. EBV+ve large cell (B-cell) lymphomas occasionally appear in the immunocompromised, eg post-transplantation lymphoproliferative disorder. The EBV genome has also been found in the Reed–Sternberg cell of Hodgkin's lymphoma. Oral hairy leukoplakia is caused by EBV and may respond to antivirals such as acyclovir and valaciclovir.

511

Influenza

This is the most important viral respiratory infection because of its frequency and complication rate, particularly in the elderly. In pandemics, millions may die, particularly when new strains evolve. The virus (RNA orthomyxovirus) has three types (A, B, C). Only types A and B cause significant morbidity in humans. Subtyping (for type A) is by hemagglutinin (H) and neuraminidase (N) characteristics. Frequent mutations give strains with new antigenic properties. Minor changes (antigenic drift) and especially major changes (antigenic shift) place whole areas at risk. WHO classification specifies: Type/host origin/geographic origin/strain no./year of isolation/subtype, eg A/Swine/Taiwan/ 2/87/ (H3, N2).

Spread is by droplets or hands. *Incubation period:* 1–4d. *Infectivity:* 1d before to 7d after symptoms start. *Immunity:* Those attacked by one strain are immune to that strain only. *Convalescence:* May be slow.

Symptoms Fever, headache, malaise, myalgia, nausea, vomiting, conjunctivitis/eye pain (even photophobia).

Tests Rapid flu test (70% sensitive) is the standard for hospitalized patients. *Serology* (paired sera; takes >2wks). *Culture* (1wk, from nasopharyngeal swabs). *PCR:* (eg 36h; sensitivity 94.2%; specificity ~100%).

Complications Bronchitis 20%, pneumonia (esp. *S. pneumoniae Staph. aureus*), sinusitis, otitis media, encephalitis, pericarditis, Reye's syndrome (coma, LFT↑).

Treatment Bed rest ± aspirin. If severe pneumonia and, most authorities recommend rapid transfer to ICU as sepsis and hypoxia may rapidly progress to circulatory collapse and death.

Antivirals: Oseltamivir 75mg PO bid, all for 5d eases symptoms in H2,N2; H3,N2; & H1,N1 outbreaks if started within 48h of onset of symptoms. Amantadine and rimantadine are only effective against type A virus. *Zanamivir* (an inhaled neuramindase inhibitor) and oseltamivir are active against influenza types A and B **NB:** Inhalation is not an ideal route, eg if elderly. SE: Bronchospasm; oropharyngeal edema.

Medication	Zanamivir	Oseltamivir A + B
Activity	A + B	
Dose Treatment	100mg inhaled bid x 5d	75mg PO bid x 5d
Prophylaxis	Not FDA approved	75mg PO qd
Side effects	Cough, asthma	GI intoler.
Price	+++	+++

Prevention • Use whole *trivalent vaccine* (from inactivated viruses). It is prepared from current serotypes and takes <2wks to work. *Indications:* All healthcare workers with patient contact, all persons >50yrs, all pregnant women (2nd & 3rd trimester) and patients with high risk comorbidities: Neurologic disorders, diabetes; chronic lung, heart or renal disease; immunosuppression; hemoglobinopathies. *Dose:* 0.5mL SC (once). SE: Mild pain or swelling (17%). Fever, headaches, and malaise are reported in 10%. *Flumist:* Live attenuated flu vaccine for immunocompetent persons aged 5–49yrs. Patients should be isolated and on respiratory precautions. Outpatients should be >3 feet from other patients and wear a surgical mask.

Advice on antivirals for preventing and treating influenza

Individuals 'at risk' are those with any of the following: Chronic respiratory diease (asthma, COPD), significant cardiovasular disease (excluding patients with hypertension alone), chronic renal impairment, diabetes mellitus, age >65yrs, or patients who are immunocompromised.

Oseltamivir (Tamiflu®): Recommended for *treatment* (eg 75mg/12h PO for 5d) of adults if given within 48h of onset of influenza symptoms. Effectiveness for influenza pneumonia is not known.

Used for *prophylaxis* (eg 75mg/24h PO for 14d (until vaccine is effective)) in 'at risk' adults who have *both* not been effectively protected by vaccination, *and* have been exposed within 4d to someone with an influenza-like illness. This includes those vaccinated less than 2–3wks previously.

The common cold (coryza)

Rhinoviruses are the main culprits (>80 strains), and cause a self-limiting nasal discharge (which becomes mucopurulent over a few days). *Incubation:* 2–4d. *Complications:* (6% in children) Otitis media, pneumonia, febrile convulsions. *Treatment:* None is usually needed. If nasal obstruction in infants hampers feeding, 0.9% saline nose drops may help. In adults, a careful study has shown that zinc gluconate trihydrate 13.3mg in a candy lozenge, 5 × daily, reduced duration by ~50%; SE: Nausea, metallic taste.

Toxoplasmosis

The protozoan *Toxoplasma gondii* infects via gut, lung, or broken skin. Cat (the primary host) excrete oocysts, but the ingestion of poorly cooked infected meat by humans may be as important as contact with cat feces. In humans, the oocysts release trophozoites, which migrate widely, with a predeliction for eye, brain, and muscle. Toxoplasmosis occurs worldwide, but is common in the tropics. Infection is lifelong. HIV may reactivate it. NB: Rat are also sources of infection.

The patient *In any granulomatous uveitis or necrotizing retinitis, think of toxoplasmosis.* Most infections are asymptomatic. Symptomatic acquired toxoplasmosis resembles infectious mononucleosis, and is usually self limiting. Eye infection, usually congenital, presents with posterior uveitis often in the 2nd decade of life, and may cause cataract. In the immunocompromised (eg AIDS), encephalitis with CD4 <100, ring enhancing lesion(s) on MRI and positive IgG serology, clinical symptoms include focal neurological signs, stroke or seizures.

Tests Acute infection is confirmed by a 4-fold rise in antibody titer over 4wks or specific IgM. Parasite isolation is difficult but easily seen on histopathology; lymph node or CNS biopsy may be diagnostic. Cerebral CT may show characteristic multiple ring-shaped contrast-enhancing lesions in compromised hosts, especially those with AIDS.

Treatment Often none is needed: Seek expert advice. If the eye is involved or in the immunocompromised pyrimethamine 200mg PO ×1, then 50mg (<60kg) or 75mg (>60kg) PO qd plus sulfadiazine 1mg (<60kg) PO q6h plus leukovorin 10-20mg PO qd x ≥6wks, then pyrimethamine 25-50mg PO qd, + sulfadiazine 500-1000mg PO qid + leucovorin 10-25mg PO qd. If pregnant, get expert help. Alternatives: Pyrimethamine + leukovorin + either clindamycin or atovaquone or TMP-SMZ x 6wks, then half dose.

Congenital toxoplasmosis May cause abortion, neonatal seizures, chorio doretinitis, hydrocephalus, microcephaly, or cerebral calcification. Worse prognosis if early infection.

Cytomegalovirus (CMV)

CMV may be acquired by direct contact, blood transfusion, or organ transplantation. After acute infection, CMV becomes latent but the infection may reactivate at times of stress or immunocompromise. If immunocompetent, primary infection is usually asymptomatic, but acute hepatitis may occur. In transplant recipients or post bone marrow transplantation: Fever > pneumonitis > colitis > hepatitis > retinitis. In AIDS: Retinitis > colitis > esophagitis > CNS disease. (Here '>' means 'is more common than'.)

Diagnosis of acute CMV infection is occasionally difficult; growth of the virus is slow and there may be prolonged CMV excretion from a distant source of infection. CMV PCR (including quantitative tests) of blood/CSF/bronchoalveolar lavage are becoming widely available but utility is unclear. CMV retinitis is diagnosed by fundus exam in atypical host; no lab tests are necessary. Histopathology (lung, gut, etc) shows typical inclusions.

Treat only if serious infection (eg immunocompromised), with valganciclovir 900mg PO bid x 21d, then 900mg qd. Alternatives: IV ganciclovir, foscarnet.

Congenital CMV Look for: Jaundice, hepatosplenomegaly, and purpura. Chronic defects include mental retardation, cerebral palsy, epilepsy, deafness, and eye problems. Treatment: None is established.

Viral hepatitis

Hepatitis A virus (HAV) RNA virus *Spread:* Fecal–oral, often in travelers o
institutions. Most infections occur in childhood. *Incubation:* 2–6wks. *Symptoms*
Prodromal symptoms include fever, malaise, anorexia, nausea, arthralgia. Jaundice
develops ± hepatomegaly, splenomegaly, and adenopathy. *Tests:* Serum transami
nases rise 21–42d after exposure. IgM rises from day 25 and signifies recent infec
tion. IgG remains detectable for life. *Treatment:* Supportive. Avoid alcoho
Prevention: Passive immunization with normal human immunoglobulin (0.02mL/k
IM) gives <3 months' immunity to those at risk (travelers, household contacts,
Active immunization is with Havrix Monodose®, an inactivated protein derived
from HAV. *Dose:* If >16yrs old, 1 IM dose (1mL to deltoid) gives immunity for 1y
(10yrs if further booster is given at 6 months). *Prognosis:* Usually self-limiting
Fulminant hepatitis occurs rarely. Chronic liver disease does not occur.

Hepatitis B virus (HBV) DNA virus. *Spread:* Blood products, IV drug abusers
sexual intercourse, vertical transmission. Risk groups: Health workers, hemophili
acs, hemodialysis, sexually promiscuous, homosexuals, and IV drug users (IVDU)
Endemic in the Far East, Africa, and Mediterranean. *Incubation:* 1–6 months. *Clinica
features:* Resemble hepatitis A but extrahepatic manifestations are more common
eg arthralgia, urticaria. *Tests:* HBsAg (surface antigen) is present from 1 to 6 month
after exposure. HBeAg (e antigen) is present for 1½–3 months after the acute
illness and implies high infectivity. The persistence of HBsAg for >6 months define
carrier status and occurs in 5–10% of infections (chronic infection). Antibodies to
HBcAg (anti-HBc) imply past infection; antibodies to HBsAg (anti-HBs) alone implie
vaccination. HBV PCR allows monitoring of response to therapy. *Vaccination* (p223)
may be universal in childhood or just for high-risk groups. Passive immunizatio
(specific anti-HBV immunoglobulin) may be given to non-immune contacts afte
high-risk exposure. *Treatment:* Supportive. Avoid alcohol. About 5–6% with acute
HBV infection develop chronic HBV, define by persistence of HBsAg >6 months
Chronic HBV may respond to interferon-α or antivirals, eg adefovir, tenofovir
lamivudine or entecavir. Unlike HCV, cure is rare so the goal of therapy is conver
sion to eAg negativity (most likely with viral interferon) or reduction in viral loa
and rates of disease progression. Immunize sexual contacts. *Complications:* Fulmi
nant hepatic failure (rare); relapse; prolonged cholestasis; chronic hepatitis (5–10%,
cirrhosis; hepatocellular carcinoma (HCC: 10-fold ↑risk if HBsAg +ve, 60-fold ↑risk
both HBsAg and HBsAg +ve); glomerulonephritis; cryoglobulinemia.

Hepatitis C virus (HCV) RNA flavivirus. *Spread:* Blood, IVDU, sexual, unknow
(40%). Early infection often mild/asymptomatic. ≈70–80% develop chronic infec
tion; 20–30% get cirrhosis within 20yrs; a few also get hepatocellular cancer (HCC
Tests: LFT (typically AST:ALT <1 until cirrhosis develops, p212), anti-HCV antibodies
recombinant immunoblot assay, quantitative HCV-PCR. Liver biopsy if HCV-PC
+ve to assess degree of liver damage and need for R. *Treatment:* Interferon-α +
ribavirin is used in chronic infection; pegylated interferon-α is superior to IFN-α
Treating acute infection with IFN-α may ↓ progression to chronic disease but th
indication is controversial. *Complications:* Cirrhosis, HCC with chronic HCV, th
goal of treatment, unlike HBV, is cure as indicated by sustained viral suppressio
defined as no detectable HCV at 6 months after treatment.

Hepatitis D virus (HDV) Incomplete RNA virus, exists only with HBV. *Spread*
Coinfection or superinfection with HBV. *Clinical features:* ↑ risk of acute hepati
failure and cirrhosis. *Tests:* Anti-HDV antibody. *Treatment:* Interferon-α ha
limited success in treatment of HDV infection.

Hepatitis E virus (HEV) RNA virus. Similar to HAV. Common in India. Hig
mortality in pregnancy. *Diagnosis:* Serology. No effective treatment/vaccine

Hepatitis GB Parenterally transmitted. Causes asymptomatic post-transfusio
hepatitis. One type (HGB-C) can cause fulminant liver failure.

Differential diagnosis *Acute hepatitis:* Alcohol, drugs, toxins, EBV, CM
leptospirosis, malaria, Q fever, syphilis, yellow fever. *Chronic hepatitis:* Alcoho
drugs, autoimmune hepatitis (p217), Wilson's disease (p218).

Serological markers of HBV infection

	Incubation	Acute	Carrier	Recovery	Vaccinated
LFTs		↑↑↑	↑	Normal	Normal
HBsAg	+	+	+		
HBeAg	+	+	±		
Anti-HBs				+	+
Anti-HBe			±		
Anti-HBc IgM		+	±		
Anti-HBc IgG		+	+	+	

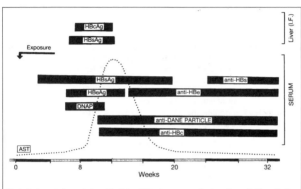

Virological events in acute hepatitis B in relation to serum amino-transferase (AST) peak. IF = immunofluorescence; Ag = antigen; HBs = hepatitis B surface; HBC = hepatitis B core; HBe = hepatitis B e antigen; DNAP = DNA polymerase.

Using ribavirin with pegylated interferon-α in HCV

This combination is indicated in moderate and severe chronic hepatitis C infection if liver biopsy shows necrosis, inflammation and fibrosis. Efficacy is less if: • HCV genotype G1, 4, 5, or 6 is involved • ↑Viral load • Older patients • Excessive delay before R starts • Blacks (vs Caucasians) • Male sex • HIV+ve.

NB: Pegylated interferon has an inert tail retarding its elimination (hence it may be given SC once weekly). Contraindications include: • Autoimmune hepatitis • Severe liver dysfunction or decompensated cirrhosis • Severe, unstable or uncontrolled heart disease in past 6 months • Depression that is not controlled • Pregnancy or pregnancy potential (♂ or ♀) (ribavirin is pregnancy category x) • hemoglobinopathies (a CI to ribavirin). • Unstable HIV infection

Human immunodeficiency virus (HIV)

Over 40 million people are HIV positive; over half are in Africa (WHO 2004). HIV-1 (a retrovirus) is responsible for most cases worldwide. HIV-2, a related virus, produces a similar illness, perhaps with a longer latent period.

More than 3 million have acquired immunodeficiency syndrome (AIDS); most are women and children in sub-Saharan Africa. AIDS is one end of a spectrum of disease caused by HIV, and is defined as the presence of one or more AIDS-defining illnesses ± evidence of HIV infection. New cases in US average 40,000/yr (40% MSM, 24% IVDU, heterosexual 29%, perinatal transmission 0.2%)

Transmission for global experience is primarily by sexual contact (84%), and infected blood or blood products, IV drug abuse or perinatally. In developed countries, the screening of blood donors and sterilizing blood products has greatly reduced the risk. In the developing world, ↑ numbers of infected children being born.

Immunology HIV binds, via its gp120 envelope glycoprotein, to CD4 receptors on helper T-lymphocytes, monocytes, macrophages, and neural cells. CD4 +ve cells migrate to the lymphoid tissue where the virus replicates producing billions of new virions. These are released, and in turn infect new CD4 +ve cells. As the infection progresses depletion or impaired function of CD4 +ve cells predisposes to the development of immune dysfunction.

Virology HIV is a double-stranded RNA retrovirus. After entry into the cell, the viral reverse transcriptase enzyme (hence retrovirus) makes a DNA copy of the RNA genome. The viral integrase enzyme then integrates this into the host DNA. The core viral proteins are initially synthesized as large polypeptides that are cleaved by the viral protease enzyme into the enzymes and building blocks of the virus. The completed virions are then released from the cell by characteristic budding. The number of circulating viruses (viral load) predicts progression to AIDS.

Stages of HIV infection *Acute infection* is often asymptomatic. *Seroconversion* may be accompanied by a 1–2wk illness 2–6wks after HIV infection: Fever, malaise, myalgia, pharyngitis, maculopapular rash or meningoencephalitis (rare). A period of *asymptomatic infection* follows although one-third of patients will have *persistent generalized lymphadenopathy (PGL)*, defined as nodes >1cm diameter at ≥2 extra-inguinal sites, persisting for 3 months or longer. There may be opportunistic infections, prior to AIDS such as tuberculosis, pneumococcal pneumonia oral *Candida*, oral hairy leucoplakia, herpes zoster. *AIDS* is a stage in HIV infection characterized by the presence of an indicator disease (p520) or a CD4 count <200/mm^3.

AIDS prognosis Untreated, death in ~20 months; longer by an average of 15yrs if treated with the 2005 regimen.

Diagnosis is based on detecting anti-HIV antibodies in serum. Acute infection may be detected by the presence of P24 antigen or HIV RNA by PCR and precedes the appearance of IgM and IgG (within 3 months). During the asymptomatic period, there are high titers of IgG to core and envelope proteins. As immunodeficiency develops, IgG titer to core protein falls, and P24 antigenemia recurs. New rapid diagnostic kits for detecting anti-HIV antibodies are point-of-care tests that can be read by the provider at 20min. Positive tests require confirmation; negative tests are definitive.

Prevention About 40% of transmissions occur during early acute infection prior to seroconversion. This makes detection of acute infection for counseling a high priority if prevention is ever going to be successful.

Condoms for *any* sexual contact, or abstinence; blood screening; disposable equipment, IVDU drug rehabilitation, ART for occupational exposure, antiretroviral therapy, and, in the case of infants, perinatal antiretroviral therapy for mother and infant (± Cesarean section), and bottle-feeding (but may not reduce infant mortality, in developing countries where hygiene is poor).

Complications of HIV infection

All patients with a new diagnosis of HIV should have a tuberculin test and be tested for toxoplasma, CMV, hepatitis B/C, and syphilis serology, to identify past or current infections that may develop as immunosuppression progresses. All AIDS-defining diagnoses are seen almost exclusively with a CD4 count <200/mm³ and some (disseminated MAC and CMV) are seen only with a CD4 count of <50.

Pulmonary *Pneumocystis jiroveci* pneumonia is the most common life-threatening opportunistic infection in AIDS (p160). Treatment: High-dose TMP/SMZ IV or PO, trimethoprim-dapsone PO, primaquine-clindamycin PO, atovaquone PO, or pentamidine by slow IVI for 3wks. Steroids are beneficial if severe hypoxemia (pO₂ <70). Primary prophylaxis (eg TMP/SMZ or dapsone PO) is indicated while CD4 count <200. Secondary prophylaxis is the same and continued after 1st attack until CD4 count >200 for >3 months. Other pathogens include *M. tuberculosis* (p508); *M. avium intracellulare (MAI); fungi* (Aspergillus, cryptococcus, histoplasma); parasites (toxoplasmosis, cryptosporidiosis, isospora), viruses (HSV, CMV, JC virus). Also: *Kaposi's sarcoma*, lymphoma, lymphoid interstitial pneumonia, and non-specific pneumonitis.

GI tract Oral pain may be caused by *candidiasis*, HSV or aphthous ulcers, or tumors. *Oral candida* is treated with nystatin suspension/pastilles or clotrimazole lozenges. *Esophageal* involvement causes dysphagia ± retrosternal discomfort. R: Fluconazole, or itraconazole, caspofungin or IV amphotericin for 2wks. Relapse is common. *HSV* and *CMV* also cause esophageal ulceration which may be difficult to differentiate from *Candida* by barium studies. *Anorexia and weight loss* are common in HIV infection. *Elevated lft and hepatomegaly* are common; causes include drugs, viral hepatitis, AIDS sclerosing cholangitis, or *MAI*. *MAI* causes fever, night sweats, malaise, anorexia, weight↓, abdominal pain, diarrhea, hepatomegaly, and anemia. *Diagnosis:* Blood cultures, but requires 7–14d for growth, biopsies (lymph node, liver, colon, bone marrow). R: Ethambutol + clarithromycin ± rifabutin/rifampicin (see BOX). *Primary prophylaxis:* Eg azithromycin 1200mg weekly, while CD4 <100. Acute diarrhea is often caused by *salmonella, C. difficile,* and viruses. *Chronic diarrhea* may be caused by bacteria (MAC), protozoa (*Cryptosporidium, Microsporidium, Isospora belli, cyclospora*), viruses (*CMV, adenovirus*), or meds esp. LPV/r and NFV. *Perianal disease* may be due to recurrent HSV ulceration, perianal warts, squamous cell carcinoma (rare). Kaposi's sarcoma and lymphomas can also affect the gut.

Neurological *Acute HIV* is associated with transient meningoencephalitis, myelopathy, and peripheral neuropathy. *Chronic HIV* is associated with several CNS syndromes: Most common are HIV-associated dementia (HAD) attributed to HIV, toxoplasmosis encephalitis, cryptococcal meningitis and peripheral neuropathy, AIDS-related dementia, HIV-related meningitis, CMV encephalitis, progressive multifocal leukoencephalopathy (PML) (p514), and vacuolar myelopathy. *T. gondii* is the chief CNS pathogen in AIDS, presenting with focal symptoms/signs. CT/MRI shows ring-shaped contrast enhancing lesions. Treat with pyrimethamine (and folinic acid) + sulfadiazine or clindamycin for 6 months. Treat toxo until CD4 >100 x 3–6 months. Primary prophylaxis (eg TMP/SMZ PO) is indicated in patients with serum antitoxoplasma IgG and CD4 <100. *Cryptococcus neoformans* (p548) causes an insidious meningitis, often without neck stiffness. Diagnosis: CSF cryptococcal antigen assay

Treatment: Amphotericin + flucytosine IV; fluconazole in milder cases. 20% mortality despite treatment. Secondary prophylaxis with fluconazole is needed until CD4 is 100–200 x ≥6 months. *Tumors* affecting the CNS include primary cerebral lymphoma, B-cell non-Hodgkin's lymphoma. CSF JC virus PCR is useful in distinguishing lymphoma from PML.

Eye *CMV retinitis* (acuity↓ ± blindness) may affect 45% of those with AIDS. Fundoscopy shows characteristic appearance. Treatment: Ganciclovir intraocular device + valganciclovir PO; Alternative: IV ganciclovir, foscarnet, cidofovir. Treatment has traditionally been lifelong, but trials suggest that therapy may be stopped in some patients when CD4 >150 after HAART (p524).

Treatment of opportunistic infections in HIV

Infection	Treatment/side-effects
Tuberculosis	This is the most lethal opportunistic infection (WHO 2004); p508.
Pneumocystis jiroveci	*TMP/SMZ* (=trimethoprim 1 part + 5 parts sulfamethoxazole) 120mg/kg/d IV OR PO in 3–4 divided doses for 14d. (SE: Nausea, vomiting, fever, rash, myelosuppression) *Prednisolone* 40–60mg PO daily (reducing dose) with taper if severe hypoxemia. *2nd line agents:* Primaquine + clindamycin, dapsone—trimethoprim, pentamidine, atovaquone. *Pentamidine isetionate* 4mg/kg/d by slow IV infusion for 14–21d (SE: Hypotension, hyper- or hypoglycemia, renal failure, hepatitis, myelosuppression, arrhythmias). *Secondary prophylaxis* (eg co-trimoxazole 480mg/24h PO; same dose as primary prophylaxis) essential after 1st attack.
Candidiasis	Local treatment: *Nystatin* suspension/*Clotrimazole* lozenges 4 times/d. Systemic treatment: *Fluconazole* 100–200mg/d PO (SE: Nausea, hepatitis) *or* ketoconazole 200mg/d PO (SE: Nausea, hepatitis, rash, platelets↓) *or* itraconazole (liquid) 200mg/d PO (SE: CHF, nausea, hepatitis). *Amphotericin B* (p164) is used in severe systemic infections. Relapse is common.
Toxoplasmosis	*Sulfadiazine* 1g/6h (or *clindamycin* 600–1200mg/6h) + *pyrimethamine* 25mg/8h PO + folinic acid 15mg/d. *Secondary prophylaxis:* Toxoplasmosis: Pyrimethamine 200mg × 1, then 100mg PO qd + sulfonamide 1–1.5g + folinic acid 15mg qd × 6wks, then half dose of all drugs until CD4 >150 × 3mo.
Cryptococcal meningitis	*Amphotericin B* 0.7mg/kg/d and *flucytosine* 5mg/kg/6h PO eg for 2wks, then fluconazole 400mg qd × 10wks, then fluconazole 200mg/d until CD4 >100–200 × ≥3mo (SE: Nausea, vomiting, rash, myelo-suppression, renal impairment). OR, in milder disease *fluconazole* 800mg on days 1–3, then 400–800mg/d (better tolerated). *Secondary prophylaxis:* Fluconazole 200mg/24h PO.
CMV retinitis	Vitracert implant + valganciclovir 900mg PO bid × 21d then 900mg PO qd or valganciclovir PO alone (peripheral lesions and expected immune reconstitution). Alternatives: Ganciclovir 5mg/kg/12h IV for 14–21d then 5mg/kg qd (SE: Myelosuppression) or *foscarnet* 60mg/kg/8h IV for 2wks, then 90mg/kg qd. SE: Renal impairment, ↑ ulcers. Or *cidofovir:* Start with 5mg/kg IV once weekly for 2wks (given with probenecid and IV fluids), then reduce to weekly doses. Valganciclovir is po and gives levels comparable to IV form. Maintenance therapy may be discontinued in patients with CD4 >150.
MAI	*Clarithromycin* 500mg/12h + *ethambutol* 15mg/kg/24h ± either *rifabutin* or *rifampicin* 450–600mg/d (adjust dose with concurrent PIs) ± *ciprofloxacin* 500mg/12h, all PO. *Secondary prophylaxis* is required eg clarithromycin 500mg/12h + ethambutol 15mg/kg/24h; may be dis-continued when culture –ve, CD4 >200 × ≥6mo and patient is asymptomatic.

521

What every doctor should know about HIV

HIV care should be managed by an expert. HIV in developed countries is primary management of antiretroviral drugs and their toxicities and controlling HIV viral load—not opportunistic infections.

Preventing HIV spread • Promote *lifelong* safer sex, barrier contraception, and reduction in the number of partners. Videos, followed by interactive discussions, is one way to double the use of condoms. Another way is the *100% condom program* involving distribution of condoms to brothels, with enforcement programs enabling monitoring and encouraging condom use at any sex establishment. Such programs are estimated to have prevented 2 million HIV infections in Thailand.
• ↑ testing enhances counseling, partner notification, and early treatment.
• Warn everyone about the dangers of sexual tourism/promiscuity.
• Tell drug users not to share needles. Use needle exchange programs.
• Vigorous control of other STDs can reduce HIV incidence.
• Strengthen awareness of clinics for STDs.
• Encourage pregnant women to have HIV tests. (Caesarean sections and HAART during pregnancy can prevent vertical transmission)
• All HIV infected persons should have partner notification.

Occupational exposure and needle-stick injury

(Seroconversion rate: ~0.4% for HIV; 30% for hepatitis B if HBeAg +ve and recipient is unvaccinated); 1.9% for hepatitis C.
• Wash well; do not suck or immerse in bleach.
• Note name, address, and clinical details of 'donor'.
• Report incident to Occupational Health and fill out an accident form.
• Rapid HIV test on source if HIV status unknown. Also test source for HBV (HBsAg) and HCV (anti-HCV). Immunize (active and passive) against hepatitis B at once, if needed. Counsel (HIV risk <0.5% if 'donor' is HIV +ve) and test recipient at baseline 3, 6, ±12months (seroconversion may take this long).
• Weigh risks which are based on the viral load in the donor and the severity of injury—volume of blood and depth of injury. Informed consent in a donor is sometimes required for HIV serology. (Mucous membrane exposure carries very low risk.) Give 4wks of drugs, if possible within 1h of exposure: (p524) *Higher-risk:* Typically a two drug regimen consisting of (3TC or FTC) plus AZT, TDF or d4T and for more severe injuries a third drug is added—preferably LPV/r, FPV/r, ATV/r, or SQV/r are alternatives. Avoid NVP and ABC. Use EFV with caution due to teratogenicity and CNS complications.

HIV test counseling If in doubt, get help from an AIDS care center. Routine tests in the recipient are HIV serology at baseline, 6wks, 3 months and 6 months. Viral load to detect acute infection should not be done unless symptomatic. Routine tests in the donor are rapid HIV serology, anti-HCV and H BsAg if these data have not been done previously.
• Do post-test counseling (eg to re-emphasize ways to ↓risk exposure).
• *Counseling throughout HIV illness:* A key issue when a person who is dying from HIV is making a will. Legal help may be needed on housing, employment, and guardianship of children. Making advance directives needs special skill.

Acute seroconversion As HIV gets more treatable, recognizing this early phase becomes more important. The clinical features are similar to infectious mononucleosis; perform tests if there are unusual signs, eg oral candidiasis, recurrent shingles, leukopenia, or CNS signs (antibody tests may be negative but viral P24 antigen and HIV RNA levels are ↑ in early infection). As always, the first best 'test' is to take a thorough history. If you *do* identify acute seroconversion illness, get expert help promptly. Counseling to prevent HIV transmission is critical.

Monitoring HIV infection

Baseline tests: CBC, chemistry profile, chest xray, CD4 count, HIV viral load, HIV resistance test (optional), toxoplasmosis serology, PPD, PAP smear, screen for HBV (HBsAg and anti-HBc), screen for HCV (anti-HCV), syphilis serology. Optional tests: Baseline lipids, FBS, CVM IgG, urine NAAT for GC and CT, wet mount for Trichomonas, G6PD.

Monitoring: CBC, CD4 and viral load q3–4months

When to treat HIV infection (US guidelines)[1]

In deciding when to recommend anti-HIV treatment, extensive recent long-term studies involving clinical end points such as death are available and consistently show extraordinary benefit. Mortality, AIDS rates and hospitalization rates are ↓ by 60–80%. It is now estimated that s extends survival by 179months—nearly 15yrs.

Indications to start therapy:

AIDS

CD4 count <200

Consider if CD4 count 200–350 based on viral load, patient preference, slope of CD4 decline

The desired response to HAART is a ↓ in HIV RNA by 1 log in 1–4wks, to <500c/mL at 8–16wks and to <50c/mL at 24wks. The accompanying CD4 ↑ average 30–50mm^3 in the first 3–4months and then 100–150/mm^3/yr.

The major concerns with HAART are:

1 Virologic failure which is usually due to poor adherence and often results in resistance.
2 Adverse effects of the drugs, both short-term and long-term.

1 DHHS Guidelines: www.aidsinfo.nih.gov

Antiretroviral agents

ALL HIV care should be supervised by an HIV expert.

HAART (highly active antiretroviral therapy) generally involves combining two nucleoside analogue reverse transcriptase inhibitors (NRTI) with *either* a protease inhibitor (PI), a boosted PI, *or* a non-nucleoside reverse transcriptase inhibitor (NNRTI).

Nucleoside analogue reverse transcriptase inhibitors (NRTI)
- Zidovudine (Azidothymidine, AZT) was the first anti-hiv drug. Dose: 300mg/12h PO. SE: Anemia, leukopenia, gastrointestinal disturbance, lactic acidosis.
- Didanosine (DDI; Videx ec®) Dose: 250mg/24h PO if wt <60kg; 400mg/24h if >60kg. SE: Pancreatitis, lactic acidosis, peripheral neuropathy, GI disturbance. Stop treatment if significant rise in amylase. Take on empty stomach.
- Lamivudine (3TC) is probably the best tolerated antiretroviral. Dose: 150mg/12h or 300mg QD PO. SE: with HBV co-infection there may be flare in hepatitis with HBV resistance, immune reconstitution or flare if 3TC is stopped.
- Stavudine (D4T) Dose: 40mg/12h PO if wt >60kg; 30mg/12h PO if <60kg. Stop treatment if peripheral neuropathy, lipoatrophy, hypertriglyceridemia, pancreatitis, lactic acidosis.
- Tenofovir (TDF) dose: 300mg/24h PO. SE: Rare causes of renal failure incl. Fanconi syndrome, and ABV flare if TDF stopped.
- Abacavir (ABC) dose: 300mg/12h or 600mg qd PO. SE: Hepatitis, hypersensitivity syndrome (5–8%)—rash, fever, vomiting; may be fatal if rechallenged.
- Emtricitabine (FTC) dose: 200mg/24h PO. SE: Same as lamivudine.

Protease inhibitors (PI) PIS are often given with low dose ritonavir (200–400mg/d PO), which enhance drug levels except with nelfinavir (NFV). All PIS are metabolized by the cytochrome P450 enzyme system. They may therefore ↑ the concentrations of certain drugs by competitive inhibition of their metabolism, if administered concomitantly. PIs associated with body fat redistribution: ↑ abdominal fat, breast enlargement, and a buffalo hump. Other class specific SE: Hyperlipidemia, hyperglycemia, insulin resistance, gastrointestinal disturbance. ATV does not alter lipids or cause insulin resistance.

Indinavir Dose: 1200mg bid PO, 1h before or 2h after a meal. SE: Dry mouth, taste disturbance, pruritis, alopecia, nephrolithiasis, ↑LFT.

Ritonavir (RTV) Dose: 600mg/12h PO. Now used to boost other PIs as indicated by: PI/r.

Saquinavir Dose: SQV/r—1000/100mg bid or 2000/100mg QD PO. SE: GI intolerances, rash, hepatitis, lipodystrophy, paraesthesiae.
- Nelfinavir (NFV) dose: PO. SE: Hepatitis, diarrhea, ↑CK.
- Lopinavir/Ritonavir (LPV) (Kaletra®). Dose: 400mg (+100mg ritonavir)/BID PO. SE: GI intolerances, rash, hepatitis, lipodystrophy.
- Atazanavir (ATV) dose: 400mg QD with food or with RTV 300mg/100mg QD with food SE—hyperbilirubinemia (benign), GI intolerance (Note: Does not cause hyperlipidemia or insulin resistance).
- Tipranavir (TPV) dose: With RTV 400/200mg bid only for salvage; SE hepatotoxicity, rash, GI intolerances, CNS bleed (rare).
- Fosamprenavir (FPV) dose: With RTV 700/100mg bid or 1400/200mg QD.
- Darunivar dose: With RTV 600/100mg bid; salvage only. SE: GI intolerance, hepatitis, lipodystrophy.

Non-nucleoside reverse transcriptase inhibitors (NNRTI) These may interact with drugs metabolized by the cytochrome P450 enzyme system, which they either induce or inhibit depending on the concomitantly administered drug.

Nevirapine (NVP) Dose: 200mg/24h for 2wks, then 200mh/12h PO. Resistant mutants emerge readily. SE: Stevens–Johnson syndrome, toxic epidermal necrolysis, hepatitis incl. fatal hepatic necrosis.

Efavirenz (EFV) Dose 600mg/24h PO. SE: Rash, sleep disturbance, dizziness in first 2–3wks. Avoid in pregnancy due to teratogenicity (category D).

Golden rules in HIV therapy

- Start HAART early, ideally before CD4 count <200.
- Explain to patients that regimens are complex and stress the importance of strict adherence.
- Use three anti-HIV drugs (minimizes replication and resistance).
- Monitor plasma viral load and CD4 count. Aim for undetectable viral loads (<50 copies/mL) within 4–6months of starting HAART. Suspect poor adherence or transmitted resistance if viral load rebounds.
- If virologic goals are not achieved the cause is resistance or failure of drug to reach target (usually due to non-adherence, but possibly due to drug interactions, food effect etc). The usual reasons to change therapy are toxicity or virologic failure.
- If toxicity: Substitute for the implicated drug
- If viral failure: Review adherence and drug interactions etc. Changes in regimen are then made based on genotypic resistance tests.
- For multiple failures consider enfuvirtide, often with TPV, LPVr, or other new agent that targets resistant HIV

Sexually transmitted disease (STD)

Incidence While great progress has been made in the last decade in treating STDs, this still remains a major health problem with over 19 million new cases reported each year (nearly half in ages 15–24). *Chlamydia* remains the most commonly reported infectious disease in the US with nearly 1 million cases reported in 2004, with over 300,000 cases of gonorrhea and nearly 8000 cases of syphilis reported (a rise of 8% from the previous year).

Presentation Vaginal or urethral discharge (p528), genital lesions, or HIV. Herpes (p510). Syphilis (p539). *Chlamydia* (often symptomless but may cause infertility or ectopic pregnancy). Genital warts. Salpingitis. Crab lice.

History Ask about timing of last intercourse; contraceptive method; sexual contacts; duration of relationship; sexual practices and orientation; past STDs, menstrual and medical history; antimicrobial therapy.

Examination Detailed examination of genitalia including inguinal nodes and pubic hair. Scrotum & male urethra. Rectal examination, pelvic & speculum examination.

Tests Refer to STD clinic. Urine: Dipstick and culture for GC and C. trachomatis. Ulcers: Take swabs for HSV culture (viral transport medium) and dark field microscopy for syphilis (*T. pallidum*). *Men:* Urethral smear for Gram stain and culture for *N. gonorrheae* (send quickly to lab in Stuart's medium); urethral swab for *Chlamydia*. *Women:* High vaginal swab in Stuart's medium for microscopy and stain for *Candida, Gardnerella vaginalis*, anaerobes, *Lactobacillus Trichomonas vaginalis*); endocervical swab for *Chlamydia trachomatis*. *Chlamydia* (an obligate intracellular bacteria) is usually asymptomatic, but easy to detect with urinary nucleic acid amplification tests (NAAT) test. *Blood tests:* Syphilis, hepatitis B and C, and HIV serology.

Follow-up Arrange to see patients at 1wk and 3 months, with repeat smears, cultures, and syphilis serology. Patients should avoid sex until treatment is completed. Partners should be referred for screening and treatment. Most effective is to give the treatment course for the partner to the patient since this is more likely to result in treatment.

Scabies *(Sarcoptes scabeii)* Spread is common in families. *Presentation:* Papular rash (on abdomen or medial thigh; itchy at night) + burrows (in digital web spaces and flexor wrist surfaces). *Incubation:* ~6wks (during which time sensitization to the mite's feces and/or saliva occurs). Penile lesions produce red nodules. *Diagnosis:* Tease a mite out of its burrow with a needle for microscopy. This may fail but if a drop of oil is placed on the lesion, a few scrapes with a scalpel may provide feces or eggs. ℞: Treat all the household. Give written advice. Apply malathion 0.5% liquid (Derbac-M®). Include the head in those <2yrs old, elderly, or immunocompromised. Remember to paint *all* parts, including soles (avoid eyes); wash off after 24h.

Lymphogranuloma *Presentation:* Inguinal lymphadenopathy and ulceration *Causes:* Lymphogranuloma venereum, chancroid *(Hemophilus ducreyi)*, or granuloma inguinale *(Calymmatobacterium granulomatis*, ie donovanosis). The latter causes extensive, painless, red genital ulcers and pseudobuboes, ie abscesses near inguinal nodes, with possible elephantiasis ± malignant change. Diagnosis: 'Closed safety-pin' inclusion bodies in cytoplasm of histiocytes. Treatment: Doxycycline 100mg/12h PO until all lesions epithelialized; alternatives include azithromycin, erythromycin, or tetracycline.

Genital Ulcer Disease

Agent	Diagnosis	Treatment
HSV	Culture or antigen assay	Acyclovir, famciclovir or valacoclovir
Syphilis	Dark field exam	Penicillin
Chancroid	Culture of *H. ducreyi*	Azithromycin, fluoroquinolone, ceftriaxone

Chlamydia screening to prevent pelvic inflammatory disease

It has been known for several years that *Chlamydia* infection correlates with involuntary infertility and chronic abdominal pain. Large screening programs are currently in place in countries such as Sweden and the US. Several large scale studies in the US showed screening (using the urine ligase chain reaction) to be both feasible and acceptable to patients[1]. Whether national screening will be as straightforward remains to be seen. Urinary NAAT testing is standard in most STD clinics and some HMO's in the US since 1993[2]

1 M Catchpole 2003 *Sex Transm Infect* **79** 16–27
2 MMWR 2002;51:RR–15

Vaginal discharge and urethritis

Some vaginal discharge may be physiologic. Most discharges which are smelly or itchy are due to infection. A very foul discharge may be due to a foreign body (eg forgotten tampons).

Discharges rarely resemble their classical descriptions.

Vaginal yeast infection *(Candida albicans)* Thrush is the most common cause of discharge and is classically described as white curds. The vulva and vagina may be red, fissured, and sore. This is not an STD so partner treatment is unnecessary. *Risk factors:* Pregnancy; immunodeficiencies, diabetes, birth control pills, antibiotics. *Diagnosis:* Microscopy: Strings of mycelium or oval spores. Culture on Sabouraud's medium is rarely indicated except to test in vitro sensitivity in refractory cases. *Treatment:* A single imidazole pessary, eg clotrimazole 500mg, + cream for the vulva. A single dose of fluconazole 150mg PO is an alternative. Reassure that thrush is not sexually transmitted.

Trichomonas vaginalis (TV) Produces vaginitis and a thin, bubbly, fishy smelling discharge. It is sexually transmitted. Exclude gonorrhea (which may coexist). The motile flagellate may be seen on wet film microscopy, or cultured. *Treatment:* Metronidazole 400mg/12h PO for 5d or 2g PO x 1. Treat the partner. If pregnant, use the 5d regimen.

Bacterial vaginosis presents with fishy smelling discharge. The vagina is not inflamed and itch is common. Vaginal pH is >5.5 resulting in alteration of bacterial flora ± overgrowth, eg of *Gardnerella vaginalis, Mycoplasma hominis, Mobiluncus* and anaerobes, eg *Bacteroides* species with too few lactobacillae. There is ↑risk of pre-term labor and amniotic infection if pregnant. *Diagnosis:* Stippled vaginal epithelial 'clue cells' may be seen on wet microscopy. Culture. *Treatment:* Metronidazole 400mg/12h PO for 5d, or clindamycin cream.

Gonorrhea *neisseria gonorrhea* (gonococcus, GC) can infect any columnar epithelium, eg urethra, cervix, rectum, pharynx, conjunctiva. Incubation: 2–10d. *Symptoms:* ♂: Purulent urethral discharge ± dysuria; or proctitis, tenesmus, ± discharge PR if homosexual. ♀: Usually asymptomatic, but may have vaginal discharge, dysuria, proctitis. Pharyngeal disease is often asymptomatic. *Complications—Local:* Prostatitis, cystitis, epididymitis, salpingitis, Bartholinitis. *Systemic:* Septicemia, eg with petechiae, hand/foot pustules, arthritis; Reiter's syndrome; endocarditis (rare). *Obstetric:* Ophthalmia neonatorum. *Long-term:* Urethral stricture, infertility. *Treatment:* One dose of *ciprofloxacin* 500mg PO. Resistance is a problem in ≥10%. Alternatives: Levofloxacin, eg 250mg PO stat. Treat for chlamydia too (eg doxycycline 100mg/12h PO for 7d, or a single dose of azithromycin 1g PO) as 50% of patients with urethritis or cervicitis will have concomittant *C. trachomatis* infection. Trace contacts. No intercourse or alcohol until cured.

Non-gonococcal urethritis is commoner than GC. Discharge is thinner and signs less acute, but this may not help diagnosis. Women (typically asymptomatic) may have cervicitis, urethritis, or salpingitis (pain, fever, infertility). Rectum and pharynx are not infected. *Organisms:* *C.trachomatis* (special swabs are needed); *Ureaplasma urealyticum; Mycoplasma genitalium; Trichomonas vaginalis; Gardnerella;* Gram –ve and anaerobic bacteria; *Candida. Complications:* Similar to local complications of GC. *Chlamydia* may cause Reiter's syndrome and neonatal conjunctivitis. *Treatment:* 1wk of doxycycline 100mg/12h PO. A single dose of azithromycin 1g PO is an alternative where compliance is likely to be problematic. Trace contacts. Avoid intercourse during treatment and alcohol for 4wks.

Non-infective urethritis Traumatic; chemicals; cancer; foreign body.

Miscellaneous Gram-positive bacteria

Staphylococci When pathogenic, these are usually *Staph. aureus*. Typically, they cause localized infection of skin, lids, or wounds. Severe infections with *Staph. aureus* include: Pneumonia, osteomyelitis, septic arthritis, endocarditis, and septicemia. Production of β-lactamase, which destroys many antibiotics, is the main problem. *Staph. aureus* toxins may cause food poisoning (p501) or the toxic shock syndrome toxin (TSST-1): Shock, confusion, fever, a rash with desquamation of digits, diarrhea, myalgia, CPK↑, platelets↓ (associated with the use of hyperabsorbent tampons that are no longer marketed). *Staph epidermidis (albus)* is increasingly recognized as a pathogen in the immuno-compromised, particularly in connection with IV lines or any prosthesis. When isolated from a culture, *Staph. epidermidis* can usually be assumed to be a contaminant unless recovered ≥2 times from a normally sterile site. It is often enough to remove the infected line. Deep *Staph.* infections need ≥4wks of oxacillin 500mg/6h IV ± removal of foreign bodies, eg prostheses.

Methicillin-resistant Staph. aureus (MRSA) is the big issue in hospital-acquired infection, causing pneumonia, septicemia, wound infections, and deaths. In the US, about 50% of *S. aureus* isolates are in nosocomial infections are MRSA. MRSA is more often spread nosocomially. Community-acquired MRSA (US 300 strain) is a new form of staphylococcal infections which is due to strains that are clonal, global, and harbor genes for the Panton-Valentine leukociden that is associated with virulence. These strains usually harbor the mec IV element that confers resistance to beta-lactams. Sensitivity tests usually show susceptibility to clindamycin, doxycycline, gentamicin and TMP-SMZ. The most common infections are large furuncles that require surgical drainage. Other less common infections are necrotizing fasciitis, necrotizing pneumonia and pyomyositis. *Management:* Furuncles require drainage and antibiotics are optional; if used the usual recommendation is TMP-SMZ or doxycycline. For necrotizing pneumonia due to the US 300 strain the recommendation is vancomycin or linezolid or vancomycin combined with clindamycin and/or rifampin *Nosocomial MRSA:* The usual drug is vancomycin; more recently there has been the introduction of linezolid and daptomycin. All 3 are essentially universally active vs. MRSA.

Preventive measures: • Isolate recently admitted patients with suspected MRSA. • Group MRSA patients together or place in single isolation rooms. • Wash hands and stethoscope! (Use alcohol-based products) • Ask about the need for eradication (with *mupirocin*). • Be meticulous in looking after intravascular catheters. • Surveillance swabs of patients and staff during outbreaks. • Use gowns/gloves when dealing with infected or colonized patients. Masks may be needed during contact with MRSA pneumonia.

Streptococci Group A streptococci (eg *Strep. pyogenes*) are common pathogens, causing wound and skin infections (eg impetigo, erysipelas), tonsillitis, scarlet fever, necrotizing fasciitis, toxic shock, or septicemia. Late complications are rheumatic fever and post-streptococcal glomerulonephritis. *Strep. pneumoniae* (pneumococcus, Gram +ve diplococcus) causes pneumonia, otitis media, meningitis, septicemia, peritonitis (rare). Resistance to penicillin is a problem. *Strep. sanguis, Strep. mutans,* and *Strep. mitior* (of the 'viridans' group), *Strep. bovis,* and *Enterococcus faecalis* all cause SBE. *Enterococcus faecalis* also causes UTI, wound infections, and septicemia. *Strep. mutans* is a very common cause of dental caries. *Strep. milleri* forms abscesses, eg in CNS, lungs, and liver. Most streptococci are sensitive to the penicillins, but *Enterococcus faecalis* and *Enterococcus faecium* may present some difficulties. They usually respond to a combination of ampicillin and an aminoglycoside, eg gentamicin. Vancomycin-resistant enterococci (VRE) have been reported. Some strains of VRE are sensitive to either teicoplanin or Synercid; all appear to be sensitive to linezolid.

Anthrax *(Bacillus anthracis)* Occurs in Africa, Asia, China, Eastern Europe, and Haiti. Spread by handling infected carcasses; well-cooked meat poses *no* risk. Terrorists have attempted to use anthrax as a biological weapon. *Presentation*

Common form: Local cutaneous 'malignant pustule'. Edema may be a striking sign
fever & hepatosplenomegaly. May cause pulmonary or GI anthrax with breath-
essness or massive GI hemorrhage (± meningoencephalitis). *Tests:* CXR may show
widened mediastinum. Gram stain is sometimes diagnostic (Gram +ve rod). *Treatment: Cutaneous disease:* Ciprofloxacin 500mg/12h PO or doxycycline 100mg
bid for 60d. *Pulmonary or GI anthrax:* Ciprofloxacin 400mg/12h or doxycycline
100mg bid IV with clindamycin 900mg/8h IV + rifampicin 300mg/12h IV or Imipenem
g IV q6h. Switch to oral drugs when able; treat for 60d. *Prevention:* Immunization
of animals at risk, and enforcement of sound food-handling and carcass-hygiene
policies. In bioterrorism, doxycycline or ciprofloxacin is highly effective in prevent-
ng disease among those exposed. The mortality for pneumonia treated with
ciprofloxacin and other agents is 40–50%. Must drain bloody pleural effusions.

Diphtheria is caused by the toxin of *Corynebacterium diphtheriae*. Presents with
tonsillitis ± a pseudomembrane over the throat and lymphadenopathy ('bull neck').
℞: Erythromycin 10–12mg/kg/6h IV. *Prevention:* 'Adsorbed Diphtheria Vaccine for
Adults and Adolescents' 0.5mL × 3 at monthly intervals. Give all close contacts
prophylaxis (eg erythromycin 250mg/6h PO for 10d) *before* swab results known.

Listeriosis is caused by *Listeria monocytogenes*, a Gram +ve bacillus with an
unusual ability to multiply at low temperatures. Possible sources of infection
include pâtés, raw vegetables, unpasteurized milk, and soft cheeses (brie,
camembert, and blue-vein types). It may cause a non-specific flu-like illness,
pneumonia, meningoencephalitis, ataxia, rash, or FUO, especially in the immunocompromised, in pregnancy, where it may cause miscarriage or stillbirth, and
in neonates. *Diagnosis:* Culture blood, placenta, amniotic fluid, CSF, and any
expelled products of conception. *Take blood cultures in any pregnant patient with
unexplained fever for 48h.* Serology, vaginal, and rectal swabs don't help (it may
be a commensal here). *Treatment:* Ampicillin IV (erythromycin if allergic) ±
gentamicin. *Prevention in pregnancy:* • Avoid soft cheeses, pâtés, and under-
cooked meat. • Observe 'use by' dates. • Ensure reheated food is piping hot;
observe standing times when using microwaves; throw away any leftovers.

Nocardia species cause subcutaneous infection (eg Madura foot) in warm
climes. If immunocompromised, it may cause abscesses (lung, liver, cerebral).
Microscopy: Branching chains of cocci. *Treatment:* Sulfamethoxazole 3g/12h
PO for 6wks; check blood levels if renal failure. Alternative: Imipenem.

Clostridia *Cl. perfringens* causes wound infections and gas gangrene ± shock or
renal failure after surgery or trauma. *Treatment:* Debridement is essential; benzylpenicillin 1.2–2.4g/6h IV + clindamycin 900mg/8h IV, antitoxin and hyperbaric
oxygen may also be used. Amputation may be necessary. *Clostridia* food poisoning (p501). *Cl. difficile:* Diarrhea (the cause of pseudomembranous colitis following antibiotic treatment, p199). *Cl. botulinum:* (Botulism) *Cl. botulinum* toxin blocks
release of acetycholine causing descending flaccid paralysis. Botulism is not
spread from one person to another. There are 2 adult forms of botulism: Food-
borne and wound botulism. *Risk in IV drug abusers* if heroin is contaminated with
Cl. botulinum. *Signs:* Afebrile, flaccid paralysis, dysarthria, dysphagia, diplopia,
ptosis, weakness, respiratory failure. Autonomic signs: Dry mouth, fixed or
dilated pupils. *Tests:* Find toxin in blood samples or, in the case of wound botulism, by the identification of *Cl. botulinum* in wound specimens by prompt referral
to a reference lab. Samples include: Serum, wound pus, swabs in anaerobic
transport media. *Management:* Get help and transfer to ICU. IM botulinum antitoxin works if given early (eg 50,000U of types A and B with 5000U of type E).
Also give to those who have ingested toxin but who have not yet developed
symptoms. *Cl. botulinum* is sensitive to benzylpenicillin and metronidazole. After
hours, antitoxin can be obtained via CDC @ (404) 639–3670.

Actinomycosis is caused by *Actinomyces israelii*. Usually causes subcutaneous
infections, forming chronic sinuses with sulfur granule-containing pus. It commonly affects the area of the jaw. It may cause abdominal masses (may mimic
appendix mass). *Treatment:* Benzylpenicillin for ≥2wks post-clinical cure, usually
>6 months. Consult with surgeons.

Miscellaneous Gram-negative bacteria

Enterobacteria Some are normal gut commensals, others environmental organisms. They are the commonest cause of UTI and intra-abdominal sepsis especially post-operatively and in the acute abdomen. They are also a common cause of septicemia. Unusually, they may cause nosocomial pneumonia (especially *Klebsiella*) line sepsis and are a rare cause of, meningitis, or endocarditis. These organisms are often sensitive to ampicillin and trimethoprim but in serious infections, use cefuroxime or 3rd or 4th generation cephalosporins, fluoroquinolones, or imperiem ± an aminoglycoside.

Pseudomonas aeruginosa is a serious pathogen, especially in the immunocompromised and in patients with cystic fibrosis. It causes pneumonia, septicemia, UTI, wound infection, osteomyelitis, and cutaneous infections. The main problem is its ↑ antibiotic resistance. *Treatment:* Piperacillin (p593) or mezlocillin + an aminoglycoside. Ciprofloxacin, cefepime ceftazidime, and imipenem are useful against *Pseudomonas*.

Hemophilus influenzae type B typically affects unvaccinated children usually <4yrs old. It causes otitis media, acute epiglottitis, pneumonia, meningitis, osteomyelitis, and septicemia. In adults non-typable strains may cause exacerbations of chronic bronchitis, sinusitis, and pneumonia. *Treatment:* Unreliably sensitive to ampicillin and TMP-SMZ; cefotaxime, fluoroquinolones, azithromycin amox-clavulanate are more reliable. Capsulated types tend to be much more pathogenic than non-capsulated types. *Prevention:* Immunization with HiB vaccine (p503) has resulted in a dramatic fall in incidence.

Plague is caused by *Yersinia pestis*. *Spread:* Fleas of rodents or cats, or droplets from other infected humans. *Incubation:* 1–7d. **Bubonic plague** presents with lymphadenopathy (buboes). **Pneumonic plague** may present with lymphadenopathy or a 'flu-like illness leading to dyspnea, cough, copious, bloody sputum, septicemia, and a hemorrhagic fatal illness. *Diagnosis:* Phage typing o bacterial culture, or a 4-fold rise in antibodies to F antigen. *Treatment:* Isolate suspects. Streptomycin 15mg/kg/12h IV or gentamicin for 10d. If in 1st trimester of pregnancy, amoxicillin 250–500mg/8h PO; if later in pregnancy, co-trimoxazole 480mg/12h PO. Staying at home, quarantine (inspect daily for 1wk), insect sprays to legs and bedding, and avoiding dead animals helps stop spread. *Post-exposure prophylaxis:* Doxycycline 100mg/12h PO for 7d and ciprofloxacin 500mg PO bid x 7 d *Prevention:* Vaccines give no *immediate* protection (multiple doses may be needed).

Brucellosis This zoonosis (carried by domestic animals) is common in the Middle East. Typically affects vets or farmers. *Cause: B. melitensis* (the most virulent), *B. abortus, B. suis,* or *B. canis*. Symptoms may be indolent and last for years—eg fever (FUO), sweats, malaise, anorexia, vomiting, weight loss, hepato-splenomegaly, constipation, diarrhea, myalgia, backache, arthritis, sacro-iliitis, rash, bursitis, orchitis, depression. *Complications:* Osteomyelitis, SBE (culture negative), abscesses (liver, spleen, lung), meningoencephalitis *Diagnosis:* Blood culture (≥6wks but rapid culture systems available, contact lab); serology: If titers equivocal (eg >1:40 in non-endemic zones) do ELISA ± immunoradiometric assays; pancytopenia. *Treatment:* Doxycycline 100mg/12h PO for 6wks + streptomycin 1g/d IM for 2–3wks or gentamicin (↓relapse rate from 2% to 10% *vs* >20%).

Whooping cough is caused by *Bordetella pertussis*. This begins with a prodromal catarrhal phase with fever and cough. After a week or so, the child develops the characteristic paroxysms of coughing and inspiratory whoops. Most children recover without complication, although the illness may last some months. Some, especially the very young, may develop pneumonia (and consequent bronchiectasis) or convulsions and brain damage. *Treatment:* Erythromycin should be given early, if only to limit spread. Azithromycin and TMP-SMZ are also effective.

Pasteurella multocida is acquired via domestic animals, especially cat or dog bites. It can cause cutaneous infections, septicemia, pneumonia, UTI, or meningitis. *Treatment:* Amoxicillin-clavulanate; an IV form is available; the dose, expressed as amoxicillin, is 1g/6–8h IV over 3–4min.

Yersinia enterocolitica In Scandinavia, this is a common cause of a reactive, asymmetrical polyarthritis of the weight-bearing joints, and, in America, of enteritis. It also causes uveitis, appendicitis, mesenteric lymphadenitis, pyomyositis, glomerulonephritis, thyroiditis, colonic dilatation, terminal ileitis and perforation, and septicemia. *Diagnosis:* Serology is often more helpful than culture, as there may be quite a time-lag between infection and the clinical manifestations. Agglutination titers >1:160 indicate recent infection. *Treatment:* None may be needed or ciprofloxacin 500mg/12h PO for 3–5d. TMP–SMX, gentamicin, and 3rd gen cephalosporins are usually effective.

Moraxella catarrhalis (Gram –ve diplococcus) is a rare cause of pneumonia, and occasional cause of exacerbations of COPD, otitis media, sinusitis, and septicemia. *Treatment:* Clarithromycin 500mg/12h PO. Azithromycin, doxycycline, amoxicillin-clavulanate, fluoroquinolones are effective.

Tularemia is caused by *Francisella tularensis* (Gram –ve bacillus), which may be acquired by handling infected animal carcasses. It causes rash, fever, malaise, tonsillitis, headache, hepatosplenomegaly, and lymphadenopathy. There may be papules at sites of inoculation (eg fingers). *Complications:* Meningitis, osteomyelitis, SBE, pericarditis, septicemia. *Diagnosis:* Contact local microbiologist for advice. Only use laboratories with safety cabinets suitable for dangerous pathogens. Swabs and aspirates must be transported in approved containers. *Treatment:* Gentamicin or streptomycin 7.5–10mg/kg/12h IM for 2wks. Oral tetracycline or ciprofloxacin are suitable for chemoprophylaxis. *Prevention:* Find the animal vector; reduce human contact with it as far as possible. Vaccination may be possible for high-risk groups.

Cat scratch disease Mostly due to *Bartonella henselae* (a small, curved, pleomorphic, Gram negative rod) or *Afepilis felis*. Think of this when any three of the following coexist: An inoculating cat scratch; regional lymphadenopathy with –ve lab tests for other causes of lymphadenopathy); establish dx with Warthin-Starry stain of biopsy or serology; skin lesions may resemble Kaposi's sarcoma. *Treatment:* Usually resolves spontaneously within 1–2months. One trial found that azithromycin sped resolution of lymph nodes. Other drugs that have been used include ciprofloxacin, rifampicin and co-trimoxazole. Usually unresponsive *in vivo* despite susceptibility *in vitro*.

Tetanus[ND]

Toxin, *Clostridium tetani*'s exotoxin, tetanospasmin, causes muscle spasm and rigidity, cardinal features of tetanus (='to stretch').

Incidence ~50 people/yr in the US. Mortality: 20%

Pathogenesis Spores of *Cl. tetani* live in feces, soil, dust, and on instruments. A tiny breach in skin or mucosa, eg cuts, burns, ear piercing, banding of hemorrhoids, may allow entry of the spores. (Diabetics are at ↑ risk). Spores may then germinate and make the exotoxin. This then travels up peripheral nerves and interferes with inhibitory synapses.

The patient *15–25% will have no evidence of recent wounds.* Signs appear from 1d to several months from the (often forgotten) injury. There is a prodrome of fever, malaise, and headache before classical features develop. *Trismus* (=lockjaw; difficulty in opening the mouth); *risus sardonicus* (a grin-like posture of hypertonic facial muscles); *opisthotonus* (arched body with hyperextended neck); *spasms* (which at first may be induced by movement, injections, noise, etc., but later are spontaneous; they may cause dysphagia and respiratory arrest); autonomic dysfunction (arrhythmias and wide fluctuations in BP).

Differential diagnosis is dental abscess, rabies, phenothiazine toxicity, and strychnine poisoning. Phenothiazine toxicity usually only affects facial and tongue muscles.

Bad prognostic signs are short incubation, rapid progression from trismus to spasms (<48h), development post-partum or post-infection, and tetanus in neonates and old age.

Treatment Get expert help; use ICU. Monitor ECG + BP. Careful fluid balance.
- Clean/debride wounds, give penicillin or metronidazole 1g/8h for 1wk.
- If tetanus is established, give human tetanus immune globulin (HTIGS) 5000U to neutralize free toxin. Local infiltration of 3000U around a suspicious wound is used in some centers. If only horse antitetanus serum (ATS) is available, give a small SC test dose before giving 10,000U IV + 750U per 24h to the cut for 3d. Some advocate intrathecal administration of antitoxin.
- Early ventilation and sedation if symptoms progress.
- Control spasms with diazepam 0.05–0.2mg/kg/h IV or phenobarbital 1.0mg/kg/h IM or IV + chlorpromazine 0.5mg/kg/6h IM (IV bolus is dangerous) starting 3h after the phenobarbital. If this fails to control the spasms paralyse and ventilate (get anesthetist's help).

Prevention Active immunization with tetanus toxoid is given as part of the 3-stage 'triple' vaccine during the 1st year of life (p503). Boosters are given on starting school and in early adulthood. Once five injections have been given, revaccinate only at the time of significant injury, and consider a final 1-off booster at ~65yrs. *Primary immunization of adults:* 0.5mL tetanus toxoid IM repeated twice at monthly intervals.

Wounds: Any cut merits an extra dose of 0.5mL toxoid IM, unless already fully immune (a full course of toxoid or a booster in last 10yrs). The non-immune will need 2 further injections (0.5mL IM) at monthly intervals. If partially immune (ie has had a toxoid booster or a full course >10yrs previously), single booster is all the toxoid that is needed.

Human tetanus immunoglobulin: This is required for the partially or non-immune patient (defined above) with dirty, old (>6h), infected, devitalized, or soil-contaminated wounds. Give 250–500 units IM, using a separate syringe and site to the toxoid injection.

If immune status is unknown, assume that the patient is nonimmune. Routine infant immunization started in 1961, so many adults are at risk.

Hygiene education and wound debridement are of vital importance.

Enteric fever

Typhoid and paratyphoid are caused by *Salmonella typhi* and *S. paratyphi* (types A, B, and C), respectively. (Other *Salmonella* cause D&V p501.) *Incubation:* 3–21d. *Spread:* Fecal-oral. 1% become chronic carriers. *Presentation:* Usually malaise, headache, high fever with relative bradycardia, cough, and constipation (or diarrhea). CNS signs (coma, delirium, meningism) are serious. Diarrhea is more common after the 1st week. Rose spots occur on the trunk of 40%, but may be very difficult to see. Epistaxis, bruising, abdominal pain, and splenomegaly may occur. *Tests:* First 10d: Blood culture; later: Urine/stool cultures. Bone marrow culture has highest yield (infiltration may cause ↓platelets & WBC). LFT↑. Widal test unreliable. DNA probes and PCR tests have been developed, but are not widely available. *Treatment:* Fluid replacement and good nutrition. There is good evidence that fluoroquinolones (eg ciprofloxacin 500mg/12h PO for 6d) are the best antimicrobial treatment for typhoid. Chloramphenicol is still used in many areas: 1g/8h PO until fever diminishes, then 500mg/8h for a week and 250mg/6h to make up 14d (can be shorter). Other alternatives: Cefotaxime, azithromycin, or amoxicillin (if fully susceptible). In severe disease, give IV ciprofloxacin or IV cefotaxime for 10–14d. In encephalopathy ± shock, give dexamethasone 3mg/kg IV stat, then 1mg/kg/6h for 48h. Drug resistance is a problem, even with ciprofloxacin, eg due to mutations in the DNA gyrase enzyme of *S. typhi*.

Complications: Osteomyelitis (eg in sickle-cell disease); DVT; GI bleed or perforation; cholecystitis; myocarditis; pyelonephritis; meningitis; abscess. Infection is said to have cleared when 6 consecutive cultures of urine and feces are –ve. Chronic carriage is a problem; treat if at risk of spreading disease (eg food handlers). Amoxicillin 4–6g/d + probenecid 2g/d for 6wks may work (alternative: Ciprofloxacin 500mg/12h PO for 6wks) but cholecystectomy may be needed. *Prognosis:* If untreated, 10% die; if treated, 0.1% die.

Bacillary dysentery

Shigella causes abdominal pain and bloody diarrhea ± sudden fever, headache, and occasionally neck stiffness. CSF is sterile. Dysentery may be severe (often *S. flexneri* or *S. dysenteriae*). *Incubation:* 1–7d. *Spread:* Fecal-oral. *Diagnosis:* Stool culture. *Treatment:* Fluids PO. Other active drugs are TMP–SMX and azithromycin. Drugs: Ciprofloxacin 500mg/12h PO for 3–5d. Imported shigellosis is often resistant to several antimicrobials: Sensitivity testing is important. There may be associated spondyloarthritis (p362).

Cholera

Caused by *Vibrio cholerae* (Gram negative comma-shaped rod). Pandemics or epidemics may occur, eg 1990s epidemic in S America and Bangladesh (Bengal *Vibrio cholerae* 0139). *Incubation:* From a few hours to 5d. *Spread:* Fecal-oral. *Presentation:* Profuse (eg 1L/h) watery ('rice water') stools, fever, vomiting, and rapid dehydration (the cause of death). *Diagnosis:* Stool microscopy and culture. *Treatment:* Strict barrier nursing. Replace fluid and salt losses meticulously. Oral rehydration with WHO formula (20g glucose/L) is not so effective as cooked rice powder solution (50–80g/L) in reducing stool volume. Its high osmolarity (310mmol/L vs 200mmol/L) is also unfavorable to water absorption. A single dose of ciprofloxacin 1g PO may reduce fluid loss. *Prevention:* Only drink boiled or treated water. Cook all food well; eat it hot. Avoid shellfish. Peel all vegetables. Heat-killed vaccine (serovar O1) gives limited protection, and is no longer needed for international travel; newer vaccines are non-standard.

LeprosyND

The diagnosis of leprosy (Hansen's disease) must be considered in all who have visited endemic areas who present with painless disorders of skin and nerves. It is not just a tropical disease, and may occur in the US, eg in Texas, Louisiana, and California, as well as Hawaii and Puerto Rico.

Mycobacterium leprae affects millions of people in the Tropics and subtropics. Since the widespread use of dapsone, and WHO elimination campaigns, prevalence has fallen (from 0.5% to 0.4/10,000 in Uganda; from 11% to 4/10,000 in parts of India). Incidence remains stable at about 800,000 new cases/yr worldwide, many of whom are children.

The Patient The incubation period is months to years, and the subsequent course depends on the patient's immune response. If the immune response is ineffective, '*lepromatous*' or '*multibacillary*' disease develops, dominated by foamy histiocytes full of bacilli, but few lymphocytes. If there is a vigorous immune response, the disease is called '*tuberculoid*' or '*paucibacillary*', with granulomata containing epithelioid cells and lymphocytes, but few or no demonstrable bacilli. Between these poles lie those with 'borderline' disease.

Skin lesions: Hypopigmented anesthetic macules, papules, or annular lesions (with raised erythematous rims). Erythema nodosum occurs in 'lepromatous' disease, especially during the 1st year of treatment.

Nerve lesions: Major peripheral nerves may be involved, leading to much disability. Sometimes a thickened sensory nerve may be felt running into the skin lesion (eg ulnar nerve above the elbow, median nerve at the wrist, or the great auricular nerve running up behind the ear).

Eye lesions: Refer promptly to an ophthalmologist. The lower temperature of the anterior chamber favors corneal invasion (so secondary infection and cataract). Inflammatory signs: Chronic iritis, scleritis, episcleritis. There may be reduced corneal sensation (V nerve palsy), and reduced blinking (VII nerve palsy) and lagophthalmos (difficulty in closing the eyes), ± ingrowing eyelashes (trichiasis).

Diagnosis Biopsy a thickened nerve; *in vitro* culture is not possible. Split skin smears for AFB are +ve in borderline or lepromatous disease. Classification matters as it reflects the biomass of bacilli, influencing treatment: The more organisms, the greater the chance that some will be drug resistant.

Other tests: Neutrophilia, ESR↑, IgG↑.

Treatment Ask a local expert about: • Resistance patterns, eg to dapsone when ethionamide may (rarely) be needed • Using prednisolone for severe complications • Is surgery ± physiotherapy needed as well as drug therapy? The administration of some drugs should be supervised (S) whereas others need no supervision (NS). For multibacillary and borderline disease, WHO advises rifampicin 600mg PO monthly (S), dapsone 100mg/24h PO (NS), clofazimine 300mg monthly (S) + 50mg/24h (NS) for 2yrs. In paucibacillary leprosy, rifampicin 600mg monthly (S) and dapsone 100mg/24h (NS) for 6 months. In single skin lesion paucibacillary disease, single-dose therapy (rifampicin 600mg, ofloxacin 400mg, minocycline 100mg, all PO) is advised.

Beware sudden permanent *paralysis* from nerve inflammation caused by dying bacilli (± *orchitis*, *prostration*, or *death*); this 'lepra reaction' may be mollified by thalidomide (**NOT** if pregnant).

Spirochetes

Lyme disease is a tick-borne infection caused by *Borrelia burgdorferi*. Although originally described in Lyme (Connecticut) it is now widespread. Not all will remember being bitten by a tick. *Presentation: Erythema migrans*, ± malaise; cognitive impairment; lymphadenopathy; arthralgia; myocarditis; heart block; meningitis; ataxia; amnesia; cranial nerve palsies (Bell's palsy); neuropathy; lymphocytic meningoradiculitis (Bannwarth's syndrome). *Diagnosis:* Clinical + serology at 4–6wks (if –ve, PCR may help.) *Treatment:* Skin rash: Doxycycline 100mg/12h PO (amoxicillin or penicillin V if <8yrs or pregnant) for 14–21d. Later complications: High-dose IV benzylpenicillin, cefotaxime, or ceftriaxone ×14–28d. *Prevention:* Keep limbs covered; use insect repellent; tick collars for pets; check skin often when in risky areas. Vaccination is no longer available. A single dose of doxycycline 200mg PO given within 72h of a bite is effective prophylaxis; in highly endemic areas, this may be worthwhile (eg if risk is >1%). *Removing ticks:* Suffocate tick with, eg petroleum jelly, then gently remove by grasping close to mouth parts and twisting off; then clean skin.

Endemic treponematoses *Yaws* is caused by *T. pertenue*, which is serologically indistinguishable from *T. pallidum*. It is a chronic granulomatous disease prevalent in children in the rural Tropics. Spread is by direct contact, via skin abrasions, and is promoted by poor hygiene. The primary lesion (an ulcerating papule) appears ~4wks after exposure. Scattered secondary lesions then appear, eg in moist skin, but can be anywhere. These may become exuberant. Tertiary lesions are subcutaneous gummatous ulcerating granulomata, affecting skin and bone. Cardiovascular and CNS complications do not occur. *Pinta* (*T. carateum*) affects only skin; seen in Central and S America. *Endemic non-venereal syphilis* (*bejel; T. pallidum*) is seen in Third World children, when it resembles yaws. In the developed world, *T. pallidum* causes syphilis (p539). *Diagnosis:* Clinical. *Treatment:* Procaine penicillin.

Weil's disease is caused by *Leptospira interrogans* (eg serogroup *L. icterohemorrhagiae*). Spread is by contact with infected rat urine, eg while swimming. *Presentation:* Fever, jaundice, headache, red conjunctivae, tender legs (myositis), purpura, hemoptysis, hematemesis, or any bleeding. Meningitis, myocarditis, and particularly renal failure may develop. AST rise may be small. *Diagnosis:* Rapid serological assays are replacing the old microscopic agglutination test. Also take blood, urine, and CSF culture (take 4–6wks). *Treat* symptomatically; give doxycycline 100mg/12h or, in serious disease, IV benzylpenicillin 600mg/6h for 7d. Prophylaxis (eg doxycycline 200mg/wk PO) may be useful for those at high risk for short periods.

Canicola fever is an aseptic meningitis caused by *Leptospira canicola*.

Relapsing fever This is caused by *Borrelia recurrentis* (louse-borne) or *B. duttoni* (tick-borne). It typically occurs in pandemics following war or disaster, and may kill millions. *Incubation:* 4–18d. *Presentation:* Abrupt onset fever, rigors, and headache. A petechial rash (which may be faint or absent), jaundice, and tender hepatosplenomegaly may develop. Serious complications include myocarditis, hepatic failure, and DIC. Crises of very high fever and tachycardia occur. When the fever abates, hypotension due to vasodilatation may occur and be fatal. Relapses occur, but are milder. *Tests:* Organisms are seen on Leishman-stained thin or thick films. *Treatment:* Tetracycline 500mg PO or 250mg IV as a single dose (but for 10d for *B. duttoni*). Alternative: Doxycycline 100mg/12h PO. The Jarisch–Herxheimer reaction (p539) is fatal in 5%: Meptazinol 100mg IV slowly is given as prophylaxis with the tetracycline, repeated 30min later (with the chill phase) and during the flush phase (if systolic BP <75mmHg). Delouse the patient and their clothes. Doxycycline is useful prophylaxis in high-risk groups.

Syphilis—the archetypal spirochaetal (treponemal) disease

Any anogenital ulcer is syphilis until proven otherwise.

Treponema pallidum enters via an abrasion, during sex. All features are due to an endarteritis obliterans. Previously common in merchant seamen and the armed forces, it is now commonest in homosexuals. *Incubation:* 9–90d.

Four stages

Primary: A macule at site of sexual contact becomes a very infectious, painless hard ulcer (*primary chancre*).

Secondary: Occurs 4–8wks after the chancre. Fever, malaise, lymphadeno-pathy, rash (trunk, face, palms, soles), alopecia, condylomata lata, buccal snail-track ulcers; rarely hepatitis, meningism, nephrosis, uveitis.

Tertiary syphilis follows 2–20yrs latency (when patients are non-infectious): There are *gummas* (granulomas occurring in skin, mucosa, bone, joints, rarely viscera, eg lung, testis).

Quaternary syphilis Cardiovascular: Ascending aortic aneurysm ± aortic regurgitation. *Neurosyphilis: (a) Meningovascular:* Cranial nerve palsies, stroke; *(b) General paresis of insane (GPI):* Dementia, psychoses (fatal untreated; treatment *may* reverse it); *(c) Tabes dorsalis:* Sensory ataxia, numb legs, chest, and bridge of nose, lightning pains, gastric crises, reflex loss, extensor plantars, Charcot's joints. *Argyll Robertson pupil.*

Serology (Two types):

Cardiolipin antibody: Not treponeme-specific. Indicates active disease and becomes negative after treatment. *False +ves* (with negative treponemal antibody): Pregnancy, immunization, pneumonia, malaria, SLE, TB, leprosy, HIV. *Examples:* Venereal disease research laboratory (VDRL) slide test, rapid plasma reagin (RPR), Wassermann reaction (WR).

Treponeme-specific antibody: Positive in 1° disease, remains so despite treatment. *Examples: T. pallidum* hemagglutination assay (TPHA), fluorescent treponemal antibody (FTA–ABS), *T. pallidum* immobilization (TPI) test. Non-specific, also +ve in non-venereal yaws, bejel, or pinta.

Other tests In 1° syphilis, treponemes may be seen by *dark ground microscopy* of chancre fluid; serology at this stage is often –ve. In 2° syphilis, tre-ponemes are seen in the lesions and both types of antibody tests are posi-tive. In late syphilis, organisms may no longer be seen, but both types of antibody test usually remain +ve (cardiolipin antibody tests may wane). In neurosyphilis, CSF antibody tests (particularly FTA and TPHA) are +ve but not standard. PCR may help.

Treatment: Procaine penicillin (=procaine benzylpenicillin) 600mg/24h IM for ~28d (14d in early syphilis). Alternative: Doxycycline 200mg/12h PO for 28d (100mg/12h PO for 14d in early syphilis). Beware *Jarisch-Herxheimer reac-tion:* Fever, pulse↑, and vasodilatation hours after the 1ˢᵗ dose of antibiotic. It is thought to be from sudden release of endotoxin. Commonest in 2° disease; most dangerous in 3°. Consider steroids. If HIV+ve, penicillin may not stop neurosyphilis; consult ID. *Trace contacts.*

PoliomyelitisND

Polio is a highly contagious picornavirus, though only a small proportion of patients develop any illness from the infection. *Spread:* Droplet or fecal–oral; nearly eliminated from globe.

The patient: 7d incubation, then 2d flu-like prodrome, leading to a 'pre-paralytic' stage: Fever, tachycardia, headache, vomiting, neck stiffness, and unilateral tremor. In <50% of patients this progresses to the paralytic stage: Myalgia, lower motor neuron signs, and respiratory failure. *Tests:* CSF: WBC↑, polymorphs then lymphocytes, otherwise normal; paired sera (14d apart); throat swab & stool culture identify virus. *Natural history:* <10% of those with paralysis die. There may be *delayed progression* of paralysis. *Risk factors for severe paralysis:* Adulthood; pregnancy; post-tonsillectomy; muscle fatigue/trauma during incubation period. *Prophylaxis:* Live vaccine PO (p503).

RabiesND

Rabies is a rhabdovirus spread by bites from any infected mammal, eg bats, dogs, cats, foxes, or raccoons (bites may go unnoticed). Nearly all cases in US are from bat bites; nearly all in developing world are dog bites—60,000 cases/yr.

The patient: Usually 9–90d incubation, so give prophylaxis even several months after exposure. Prodromal symptoms include headache, malaise, abnormal behavior, agitation, fever, and itching at the site of the bite. Progresses to 'furious rabies', eg with water-provoking muscle spasms often accompanied by profound terror (hydrophobia). In 20%, 'dumb rabies' starts with flaccid paralysis in the bitten limb and spreads.

Pre-exposure prophylaxis (eg vets, zoo-keepers, customs officials, bat handlers, travellers): Give human diploid cell strain vaccine (1mL IM, deltoid) on days 0, 7, & 28, and again at 2–3yrs if still at risk.

Treatment if bitten where rabies is endemic (if unvaccinated): Seek expert help. Observe the biting animal if possible, to see if it dies (but it is possible that it may not die of rabies before the patient does); asymptomatic carriage occurs but has not (yet) produced rabies in man. Clean the wound. *If previously immunized:* Give vaccine (1mL IM) on days 0 and 3. *If previously unimmunized:* Give vaccine on days 0, 3, 7, 14, and 28 and human rabies immunoglobulin (20U/kg on day 0; half given IM and half locally infiltrated around wound). Rabies is usually fatal once symptoms begin, but survival has occurred (5 reported cases), if there is optimal CNS and cardiorespiratory support. Offer to vaccinate attending staff. Recently reported cure with ketamine + midzolam induced coma + amantadine and avoidance of vaccine. For protocol see www.mcw.edu/rabies

Viral hemorrhagic fevers[ND]

Yellow fever: An epidemic arbovirus disease spread by *Aedes* mosquitoes (Brazil, Bolivia, Peru, and Central and West Africa). *Incubation:* 2–14d. *The Patient:* In mild forms, fever, headache, nausea, albuminuria, myalgia, and relative bradycardia. If severe: 3d of headache, myalgia, anorexia ± nausea, followed by abrupt fever, a brief remission, then prostration, jaundice (± fatty liver), hematemesis and other bleeding, oliguria. *Mortality:* <10% (day 5–10). *Diagnosis:* ELISA. *Treatment:* Symptomatic.

Lassa fever, Ebola virus, Marburg virus, and dengue hemorrhagic fever (DHF) (dengue is the most prevalent arbovirus disease). These diseases may start with sudden-onset headache, pleuritic pain, backache, myalgia, conjunctivitis, prostration, dehydration, facial flushing (dengue), and fever. Bleeding soon supervenes. There may be spontaneous resolution, or renal failure, encephalitis, coma, and death. *Treatment:* Primarily symptomatic; ribavirin is useful in Lassa fever if given early in disease. *Use special infection control measures (Lassa, Ebola, Marburg); get expert help at once.*

Dengue fever (DF) and dengue hemorrhagic fever (DHF)

There is a global pandemic of this RNA flavivirus, related to poor vector control (*Aedes* mosquitoes), urbanization, and rapid migrations bringing new strains (DEN-2) which become more virulent in those who have had mild dengue. Incidence: $50–100×10^6$/yr; 250,000–500,000/yr get DHF.[1]

Infants typically have a simple febrile illness with a maculopapular rash. Older children/adults have flushing of face, neck, and chest or a centrifugal maculopapular rash from day 3—or a late confluent petechiae with round pale areas of normal skin—also headache, arthralgia, jaundice; hepatosplenomegaly; anuria. *Hemorrhagic signs:* (Unlikely if AST normal). Petechiae, GI, gum or nose bleeds, hematuria; hypermenorrhea.

Monitor: Bp; urine flow; WBC↓; platelets↓; PCV; +ve tourniquet test (>20 petechiae inch^2) + PCV↑ by 20% are telling signs (rapid endothelial plasma leak is the key pathophysiology of DHF). ΔΔ: Chikungunya, measles, leptospirosis, typhoid, malaria. *Exclusion:* If symptoms start >2wks after leaving a dengue-endemic area, or if fever lasts >2wks, dengue can be 'ruled out'. *R:* Prompt IV resusc. If in shock (mortality 40%), give a bolus of 15mL/kg; repeat every ½h until BP rises & urine flow >30mL/h.

1 M Guzman 2003 *J Clin Virol* 27
2 Hemorrhagic features in Chikungunya virus infections are rare.

Rickettsia and arthropod-borne bacteria

Rickettsia are intracellular bacteria that are carried by host arthropods and invade human mononuclear cells, neutrophils, or blood vessel endothelium (vasculotropic). All the cataclysmic events of the last century (war, revolution, flood, famine, genocide, and overcrowding) have favored lice infestation. As a result, Rickettsia (in particular typhus) have killed untold millions.

Q fever is caused by *Coxiella burnetii*. It is so named because it was first labelled 'query' fever in workers in an Australian abattoir. *Epidemiology:* Occurs worldwide, and is usually rural, with its reservoir in cattle and sheep. The organism is very resistant to drying and is usually inhaled from infected dust. It can be contracted from unpasteurized milk, directly from carcasses in abattoirs, sometimes by droplet spread, and occasionally by tick bites. *Clinical features* Q fever should be suspected in anyone with a FUO or atypical pneumonia. It may present with fever, myalgia, sweats, headache, cough, and hepatitis. If the disease becomes chronic, suspect endocarditis (typically 'culture-negative'). This usually affects the aortic valve, but clinical signs may be absent. It also causes miscarriages and CNS infection. *Investigations:* CXR may show consolidation, eg multilobar or slowly resolving. Liver function tests may be hepatitic and biopsy may show granulomata. Diagnosis is serologically: Phase I antigens indicate chronic infection; phase II antigens indicate acute infection. PCR may be used on tissue samples. CSF tests may be needed. *Treatment:* Get expert microbiological help. *Acute:* Tetracycline or doxycycline for 2wks. Minocycline, clarithromycin, ciprofloxacin (in pregnancy) and co-trimoxazole have been used. *Chronic:* Ciprofloxacin + rifampicin for 2yrs ± valve replacement. *Prevention:* Vaccination for those whose occupation places them at high risk.

Bartonellosis is caused by *Bartonella bacilliformis*, a Gram negative, motile, bacillus-like organism which parasitizes RBCs. Spread is by sandflies in the Andes, Peru, Equador, Colombia, Thailand, and Niger. Transient immunosuppression leads to associated infections (eg *Salmonella*). *Incubation:* 10–210d (average = 60). *Clinical features:* Fever, rashes, lymphadenopathy, hepatosplenomegaly, jaundice, cerebellar syndromes, dermal nodules (verrugas), retinal hemorrhages, myocarditis, pericardial effusion, edema, and rarely, meningo-encephalomyelitis. *Investigations:* Giemsa-stained blood films. Prolonged incubation of blood cultures. Coomb's negative hemolytic anemia, and hypochromic, macrocytic red cells with a megaloblastic marrow. CSF pleocytosis. Serological tests exist, but are not widely available. *Treatment:* Responds to penicillin, but chloramphenicol or ciprofloxacin (500mg/12h PO for 10d) are often used because of its frequent association with salmonelloses. Steroids may be indicated if there is severe neurological involvement.

Cat scratch disease (p533) is caused by *Bartonella henselae*.

Trench fever is caused by *Bartonella quintana* inoculated from infected louse feces, not only in soldiers, but also in the homeless, and in alcoholics. *Clinical features:* Fever, headache, myalgia, dizziness, back pain, macular rash, eye pain, leg pain, splenomegaly, and rarely, endocarditis. In HIV-infected patients, the skin lesions may resemble Kaposi's sarcoma. *Investigations:* Blood culture, serology, PCR. *Treatment:* Doxycycline 100mg/12h PO for 15d. *Prognosis:* It is not fatal; it may relapse. May cause "culture negative endocarditis" which is difficult to diagnose, requires long therapy.

Ehrlichiosis is caused by *Ehrlichia chaffeensis*, an obligate intracytoplasmic Gram –ve organism, related to Rickettsia. It is spread by ticks. *Symptoms:* Fever, headache, anorexia, malaise, abdominal pain, epigastric pain, conjunctivitis, lymphadenopathy, jaundice, rash, confusion, and cervical lymphadenopathy. *Investigations:* Leukopenia, thrombocytopenia, AST↑. Serology and PCR are used for diagnosis. *Treatment:* May respond to doxycycline 100mg/12h PO for 7–14d.

Typhus: The archetypal rickettsial disease

Typhus rickettsia are transmitted between hosts by arthropods. The incubation period is 2–23d.

Pathology Widespread vasculitis and endothelial proliferation may affect any organ and thrombotic occlusion may lead to gangrene.

Clinical features Infection may be mild and asymptomatic or severe and systemic. There may be sudden onset of fever, frontal headache, confusion, and jaundice. With some species, an *eschar* (black scar at the site of the initial inoculation) may be present. A rickettsial rash may be macular, papular, petechial, or hemorrhagic. Investigations may show hemolysis, neutrophilia, thrombocytopenia, clotting abnormalities, hepatitis, renal impairment. Patients die of shock, renal failure, DIC (p576), or stroke.

Rocky Mountain spotted fever (R. rickettsii) is tick-borne and endemic in the Rocky Mountains and the south-eastern states of the US. The rash begins as macules on the hands and feet and then spreads becoming petechial or hemorrhagic.

Tick typhus (R. conorii) endemic in Africa, the Arabian Gulf, and the Mediterranean. A black eschar may be visible at the site of the infecting bite. The rash starts in the axillae, becoming purpuric as it spreads. *Other features*: Conjunctival suffusion; jaundice, deranged clotting, renal impairment.

Epidemic typhus (R. prowazeki) carried by human lice *(Pediculus humanus)* whose feces are inhaled or pass through skin. It may become latent, and recrudesce later (Brill–Zinsser disease).

Murine (endemic) typhus (R. typhi) is transmitted by fleas from rats to humans. It is more prevalent in warm, coastal ports.

Rickettsialpox (R. akari) Variegate rash: Macular, papular, or vesicular.

Scrub typhus (Orienta tsutsugamushi) Most common in SE Asia.

Diagnosis This is difficult as often the picture is non-specific, the organisms are difficult to grow, and the traditional heterophil antibody Weil–Felix test has low sensitivity and specificity. A rise in antibody titer in paired sera is diagnostic. Latex agglutination, indirect immunofluorescence, and ELISAs are available. An accurate, rapid dotblot immunoassay is available for scrub typhus. Skin biopsy may be diagnostic in Rocky Mountain spotted fever.

Treatment Doxycycline 200mg/d PO or IV or tetracycline 500mg/6h PO for 10–14d. Alternative: Chloramphenicol 500mg/6h PO or IV for 10–14d. Resistance has been reported in northern Thailand.

Poor prognostic factors Older age, male, Black, G6PD deficiency.

Giardiasis

Giardia lamblia is a flagellate protozoon, which lives in the duodenum and jejunum. It is spread by the fecal–oral route. Risk factors for transmission: Travel, immunosuppression, homosexual behavior, achlorhydria, playgroups, and swimming. Drinking water may become contaminated.

Presentation: Often asymptomatic. Lassitude, bloating, flatulence, abdominal discomfort, loose stools ± explosive diarrhea are typical. Malabsorption, weight loss, and lactose intolerance may occur.

Diagnosis: Repeated stool microscopy for cysts or trophozoites may be –ve. Duodenal fluid analysis by aspiration or absorption on to a piece of swallowed string (Enterotest®) may be tried. An ELISA test is available. Finally, a trial of therapy may be needed.

Differential diagnosis: Any cause of diarrhea (p501), tropical sprue (p232), celiac disease (p232).

Treatment: Scrupulous hygiene. Give metronidazole 500mg/12h PO for ~7d, or 2g/24h for 3d. Alternatives: Tinidazole 2g PO once (advise to avoid driving and alcohol). If treatment fails, check for compliance and consider treating the whole family. If diarrhea persists, avoid milk as lactose intolerance may persist for 6wks.

Other GI protozoa *Cryptosporidium* (p501) *Microsporidium* and *Isospora* (occur in AIDS, p520), *Balantidium coli*, and *Sarcocystis*.

Amebiasis

Entameba histolytica occurs worldwide. Spread: Fecal–oral. Boil water and infected food to destroy cysts. Trophozoites may remain in the bowel or invade extra-intestinal tissues, leaving 'flask-shaped' GI ulcers. Presentation may be asymptomatic, with mild diarrhea or with severe amebic dysentery.

Amebic dysentery may occur years after the initial infection. Diarrhea begins slowly, but becomes profuse and bloody. An acute febrile prostrating illness does occur but high fever, colic, and tenesmus are rare. May remit and relapse. *Diagnosis:* Stool microscopy shows trophozoites, blood, and pus cells. Distinguish from *E. dispar* which looks identical, is more common and doesn't cause disease. Fecal antigen detection makes this distinction and is a preferred test. Serology indicates previous or current infection and may be unhelpful in acute infection. H is 99% sensitive for liver abscess *Differential diagnosis:* Bacillary dysentery often has a sudden onset and may cause dehydration. Stools are more watery initially, then bloody. *E. coli* 0157 is a common cause of acute bloody diarrhea without fever *Acute ulcerative colitis* has a more gradual onset and the stools are very bloody. Other causes of bloody diarrhea (p535).

Amebic colonic abscess may perforate causing peritonitis.

Ameboma is an inflammatory mass most often found at the cecum, where it must be distinguished from other RLQ masses.

Amebic liver abscess is usually a single mass in the right lobe, and contains 'anchovy-sauce' pus. There is usually a high swinging fever, sweats, RUQ pain, and tenderness. WBC↑. LFT may be normal or ↑ (cholestatic). 50% have no history of amebic dysentery. *Diagnosis:* Ultrasound/CT ± aspiration; positive serology.

Treatment Metronidazole 500–750mg/8h PO for 7–10d for acute amebic dysentery, then paromomycin 30mg/kg Q 8H PO for 10d to destroy gut cysts. Amebic liver abscess: Metronidazole 400mg/8h IV for 10d; repeat at 2wks as needed; aspirate if no improvement within 72h of starting metronidazole; give diloxanide post-metronidazole.

Trypanosomiasis

African trypanosomiasis (sleeping sickness) In West and Central Africa, *Trypanosoma gambiense* causes a slow, wasting illness with a long latent period. In East Africa, *T. rhodesiense* causes a more rapidly progressive illness. Spread by tsetse flies, entering skin following an insect bite. It spreads via the blood to the lymph nodes, spleen, heart, and brain.

Prevalence: ~500,000, nearly all *T. gambiense*. Wars, famine, and other disasters are contributing to an upsurge in African trypanosomiasis. In these destabilized circumstances, population surveillance and control of wild animal populations is being abandoned.

Presentation: A tender, subcutaneous nodule (*T. chancre*) develops at the site of infection. Two stages follow: *Stage I (hemolymphatic):* Non-specific symptoms including fever, rash, rigors, headaches, hepatosplenomegaly, lymphadenopathy, and joint pains. Winterbottom's sign (enlargement of posterior cervical nodes) is a reliable sign, particularly in *T. gambiense* infections. In *T. rhodesiense* infections, this stage may be particularly severe, with potentially fatal myocarditis. *Stage II (meningoencephalitic):* Occurs weeks (in *T. rhodesiense*) or months (in *T. gambiense*) after initial infection. Patients exhibit CNS features, eg convulsions, agitation, and confusion, with later apathy, depression, ataxia, dyskinesias, dementia, hypersomnolence, and coma.

Diagnosis: Microscopy shows trypomastigotes in blood film, lymph node aspirate, or CSF. Serology is only reliable in *T. gambiense* infections.

Treatment: Seek expert help.
- Treat anemia and other infections first.
- Early (pre-CNS) phase: Pentamidine isethionate 4mg/kg/d IM for 10d. SE: Neutropenia, ↓BP, ↓Ca^{2+}, nephrotoxicity, thrombocytopenia. Alternative: Suramin (SE: Proteinuria, ↑creatinine).
- CNS disease: Melarsoprol[1] eg '3 by 3' regimen IV: 2–3.6mg/kg/d IV for three doses. Repeat at 7d and once more after 10–21d. SE: Pruritus, Jarisch–Herxheimer-like reaction (p539), lethal encephalopathy in up to 10% (abnormal behavior, seizures, coma) — partly preventable with prednisolone (1mg/kg/24h, max 40mg/24h), starting the day before the first injection. Arseno-resistant trypanosomiasis was always fatal until the introduction of difluoromethylornithine (DFMO). Dose example: 100mg/kg/6h IV over 1h for 14d, followed by 75mg/kg/ 6h for 3–4wks. SE: Anemia, diarrhea, seizures, leukopenia, hair loss.

American trypanosomiasis (Chagas' disease) is caused by *T. cruzi*. It occurs in Latin America and is spread by triatomine bugs.

The Patient: Acute disease predominantly affects children. An erythematous, indurated nodule (*chagoma*) forms at the site of infection which may then scar. *Signs:* Fever, myalgia, rash, lymphadenopathy, hepatosplenomegaly. If the eye is infected, unilateral conjunctivitis and periorbital edema may occur (*Romaña's sign*). Occasionally death is from myocarditis or meningoencephalitis. In up to 30% of cases, progression to chronic disease occurs after a latency of eg 20yrs. Multiorgan invasion may cause megaesophagus (dyshagia, aspiration), megacolon (abdominal distension, constipation), or dilated cardiomyopathy (chest pain, heart failure, arrhythmias, syncope, thromboembolism). CNS lesions may occur if HIV +ve.

545

Diagnosis: Acute disease: Trypomastigotes may be seen in or grown from blood, CSF, or lymph node aspirate. Chronic disease: Serology (Chagas' IgG ELISA).

Treatment: Unsatisfactory. Nifurtimox 2mg/kg/6h PO after food, or alternatively benznidazole (3.7mg/kg/12h PO for 60d) are used in acute disease (toxic, and only eliminate the parasite in 50%). Chronic disease can only be treated symptomatically.

1 Melarsoprol is available on a compassionate use protocol through the centers of disease control.

Leishmaniasis

Leishmania protozoa are intracellular organisms that cause granulomata. They are spread by sandflies and occur in Africa, India, Latin America, the Middle East, and the Mediterranean. Clinical effects reflect: (1) The ability of each species to induce or suppress the immune response, to metastasize, and to invade cartilage, and (2) the speed and efficiency of our own immune response. *L. major*, for example, is the most immunogenic and allergenic of cutaneous Old World *Leishmania*, and causes necrosis. *L. tropica* is less immunogenic and causes less inflamed, slow-healing sores with relapsing lesions having tuberculoid histology.

Cutaneous leishmaniasis (oriental sore) A major disease affecting >300,000 people mainly in Africa, India, and S America caused by *L. mexicana*, *L. major*, or *L. tropica*. Lesions develop at the site of the bite, beginning as an itchy papule, from which the crust may fall off to leave an ulcer (*Chiclero's ulcer*). Most heal spontaneously, typically within 3–18 months, with scarring (disfiguring if extensive). *L. mexicana* may cause destruction of the pinna (*Chiclero's ear*).

Diagnosis: Microscopy and culture of aspiration from the edge of the ulcer.

Treatment: Get help. Fluconazole 200mg/d PO for 6wks is effective against *L. major*. Alternatives: Miltefosine 2.25mg/kg/d PO for 4wks; sodium stibogluconate (Sb^V, pentavalent antimony) 10mg/kg/12h IV (max 850mg/d) for 28d; paromomycin, eg 14mg/kg/d IM for 60d with 10mg Sb^V/kg/d IM.

Mucocutaneous leishmaniasis is caused by *L. brasiliensis* and occurs in S. America. Primary skin lesions may spread to the mucosa of the nose, pharynx, palate, larynx, and upper lip and cause severe scarring. Nasopharyngeal lesions are called *espundia*.

Diagnosis: As the parasites may be scanty, a Leishmanin skin test is often necessary to distinguish the condition from leprosy, TB, syphilis, yaws, and carcinoma. Indirect fluorescent antibody tests and PCR tests are available.

Treatment: Sodium stibogluconate (dose as below). Treatment is unsatisfactory once mucosae are involved, so treat all cutaneous lesions early.

Visceral leishmaniasis (kala-azar) Kala-azar means black sickness and is characterized by dry, warty, hyperpigmented skin lesions. It occurs in Asia, Africa, S America, and the Mediterranean. It is caused by *L. donovani*, *L. chagasi*, or *L. infantum* (or rarely, 'visceralizing' of *L. tropica*). Incubation: Months to years. Protozoa spread via lymphatics from minor skin lesions and multiply in macrophages of the reticuloendothelial system (Leishman–Donovan bodies). There are 30 subclinical cases for every clinical case. ♀:♂ ratio >3:1. It is HIV-associated. *Presentation:* See BOX.

Diagnosis: Leishman–Donovan bodies in bone marrow (80%), lymph node or splenic aspirates (95%). Hypersplenism (Hb↓, platelets↓, WBC↓), albumin↓, IgG↑; –ve Leishmanin skin test. Solid-state serology has been developed for field use (K39 antigen). Serology may be –ve if HIV +ve.

Treatment: Seek expert help. WHO regimen: Sodium stibogluconate (Sb^V) 20mg/kg/24h IV or IM, up to 850mg/d, for 30d. SE: Malaise, cough, substernal pain, prolonged Q–T interval, arrhythmias, anemia, uremia, hepatitis. Regimens are changing as 25% fail to respond or relapse—eg 10mg/kg Sb^V/8h for 10d, without the 850mg limit. Alternative: Pentamidine, eg 3–4mg/kg (deep IM) on alternate days, up to 10 doses. SEs may be fatal (BP↓, arrhythmias, glucose↓, diabetes in 4%). Other agents: Paromomycin (amino-sidine), liposomal amphotericin B (AmBisome®). Miltefosine (50mg/12h PO for 21d) is a promising oral alternative.

Post kala-azar dermal leishmaniasis may occur months or years following successful treatment; lesions resemble leprosy.

Clinical features of visceral leishmaniasis

Signs & symptoms:
- Fevers 100%
- Sweats 90%
- Rigors 83%
- Burning feet 52%
- Arthralgia 36%

- Splenomegaly 96%
- Fatigue 88%
- Cough 69%
- Insomnia 42%
- Epistaxis 19%

- Weight↓ 95%
- Appetite↓ 87%
- Hepatomegaly 63%
- Abdominal pain 42%
- Lymphadenopathy

Complications: Over months to years, emaciation and exhaustion occur, with a protuberant abdomen. Intercurrent infections are common, especially pneumococcal otitis, pneumonia and septicemia, tuberculosis, measles. Untreated mortality: >80%.

Fungi

Fungi may cause disease by acting as airborne allergens, by producing toxins or by direct infection. Fungal infection may be superficial or deep, and both are much commoner in the immunocompromised.

Superficial mycoses Dermatophyte infection (*Trichophyton*, *Microsporum*, *Dermatophyton*) causes tinea (ringworm). *Diagnosis:* Skin scraping microscopy. *Treatment:* Topical clotrimazole 1%. Continue for 14d after healing. If intractable, try itraconazole (100–200mg/24h PO for 7d), terbinafine (250mg/24h PO for 4wks) or griseofulvin 0.5–1g/24h (SE: Agranulocytosis; SLE).

Candida albicans causes oral and vaginal infections.

Malassezia furfur causes pityriasis versicolor; a macular rash which appears brown on pale skin and pale on tanned skin. *Diagnosis:* Microscopy of skin scrapings under Wood's light. *Treatment:* Ketoconazole 200mg/24h PO with food for 7d (also available as a cream); alternatively selenium sulfide lotion.

Some superficial mycoses penetrate the epidermis and cause chronic subcutaneous infections such as Madura foot or sporotrichosis. Treatment is complex and may require amputation of the affected limb.

Systemic mycoses *Aspergillus fumigatus* may precipitate asthma, allergic bronchopulmonary aspergillosis (ABPA), or cause aspergilloma (p164). Pneumonia and invasive aspergillosis occur in the immunosuppressed. There is evidence that voriconazole and caspofungin may be superior to amphotericin B in the treatment of invasive aspergillosis.

Systemic *candidiasis* also occurs in the immunocompromised: Consider this *whenever* they get a FUO, line sepsis, endophthalmitis, peritonitis (dialysis pts), eg *Candida* UTI in DM or as a rare cause of prosthetic valve endocarditis. Take repeated blood cultures. Remove line and give amphotericin B or lipid amphoteracin IV (p164), fluconazole 400 IV x 14d or voriconazole 6mg/kg q12h x 2, then 4mg/kg IV q12h. Alternative is caspofungin or amphoteracin plus fluconazole.

Cryptococcus neoformans causes meningitis or pneumonia. It is most common in the immunocompromised, eg AIDS, Hodgkin's, and those on corticosteroids. The history may be long and there may be features suggesting ICP↑, eg confusion, papilledema, cranial nerve lesions. *Diagnosis:* Indian Ink CSF staining; blood culture. Cryptococcal antigen is detected in CSF and blood by latex tests. *Treatment:* Amphotericin B IV over 4h (Fungizone®) 0.7mg/kg/d + flucytosine 25mg/kg/6h PO x 14d, then fluconaole 400mg/dx 10wks, then 200mg/d until CD4 >200 x 6mo. (AIDS patients). If CSF OP is >250mm H$_2$O drain CSF until OP ↓ 50%. Repeat drainage daily until OP is <200. Failure to do this is most common cause of death due to cryptococcal meningitis.

Other fungi, mostly from the Americas and Africa, causing deep infection: *Histoplasma capsulatum*, *Coccidioides immitis*, *Paracoccidioides brasiliensis*, and *Blastomyces dermatitidis* may cause asymptomatic infections, acute or chronic lung disease, or disseminated infection. Acute histoplasma pneumonitis is associated with arthralgia, erythema nodosum, and erythema multiforme. Chronic disease, which is commoner with the other 3 fungi, may cause upper-zone fibrosis or radiographic 'coin lesions'. Diagnosis: CXR, serology, culture, and biopsy. These diseases are treated with itraconazole except coccidioidomycosis which may be treated with fluconazole (especially with cocci meningitis).

Preventing fungal infections This is a goal in the immunocompromised, eg fluconazole 50–400mg/24h after cytotoxics or radiotherapy, preferably started before the onset of neutropenia, and continued for 1wk after WBC returns to normal. Also used as secondary prophylaxis after cryptococcal meningitis in HIV patients.

Candida on ICU: Colonization → invasion → dissemination

Not everyone with a positive yeast culture needs treatment: *Candida* is a common commensal (eg on skin, pharynx, or vagina) but if many sites (urine, sputum, or surgical drains) are colonized, risk of invasion rises, particularly when on ICU with known risk factors:

- Prolonged ventilation   • Urinary catheters   • Intravascular lines
- Broad-spectrum antibiotics • Immunosuppression • IV nutrition

Invasion implies fungus in normally sterile tissues.

Dissemination involves infection of remote organs via the blood (eg endophthalmitis + fungi in lung or kidney). Consider IV amphotericin or fluconazole (itraconazole if unresponsive) in these unequivocal circumstances (especially if your patient is deteriorating):

- A single well-taken +ve blood culture—if risk factors present (above).
- Isolation of *Candida* from any sterile site except urine.
- Yeasts on microscopy on a sterile-site specimen, before culture known.
- Positive histology from normally sterile tissues in those at risk (above).
- Removal/change of IV lines is essential in patients with candidemia.

Consult an ID physician/microbiologist before starting systemic antifungals.

Nematodes (roundworms)

Worldwide, ~1 billion people are hosts to nematodes. Ascariasis can cause GI obstruction, hookworms can stunt growth, necatoriasis can cause debilitating anemia, and trichuriasis causes dysentery and rectal prolapse. Mass population treatment (eg albendazole 400mg/24h PO for 3d) to school children or immigrants from endemic areas *may* be beneficial.

Necator americanus and *Ankylostoma duodenale (hookworms)* Occur in the Indian subcontinent, SE Asia, Central and N Africa, and parts of Europe. Necator is also found in the Americas and sub-Saharan Africa. Numerous small worms attach to upper GI mucosa, causing bleeding and consequent iron-deficiency anemia. Eggs are excreted in the feces and hatch in soil. Larvae penetrate feet, so starting new infections. Oral transmission of *Ankylostoma* may occur. *Diagnosis:* Stool microscopy. *Treatment:* Mebendazole 100mg/12h PO for 3d, and iron.

Strongyloides stercoralis is endemic in the (sub)tropics. Transmitted percutaneously, it causes rapidly migrating urticaria over thighs and trunk (*cutaneous larva migrans*). Pneumonitis, enteritis, and malabsorption may occur. Chronic signs: Diarrhea, abdominal pain, and urticaria. The worms may take bacteria into the bloodstream, causing Gram negative bacterial septicemia ± meningitis. *Diagnosis:* Stool microscopy and culture, serology, or duodenal aspiration. *Treatment:* Tiabendazole 25mg/kg/12h (max 1.5g) for 3d—or albendazole 5mg/kg/12h PO for 3d (recommended doses may not be enough, and 800mg/d PO has been advised for some adults). Ivermectin 0.2mg/kg/24h PO for 72h may be the best for chronic infestations. Hyperinfestation is a problem if immunocompromised (eg on steroids, or, more rarely, in AIDS).

Ascaris lumbricoides occurs worldwide. It looks like (and is named after) the garden worm (*Lumbricus*). An unusual characteristic is that it has 3 finely toothed lips. Transmission is fecal-oral. It migrates through liver and lungs, and settles in the small bowel. It is usually asymptomatic, but death may occur from GI obstruction or perforation. If a worm migrates into the biliary tract, cholangitis or pancreatitis can result. A worm may grow very long (eg 25cm). *Diagnosis:* Stool microscopy shows ova (stained orange by bile); Worms on barium x-rays; eosinophilia (may be absent if immunosuppressed). *Treatment:* Mebendazole 100mg/12h PO for 72h.

Trichinella spiralis occurs worldwide and is transmitted by uncooked pork. It migrates to muscle, causing myalgia, myocarditis, periorbital edema ± fever. *Treatment:* Albendazole 400mg/12h PO for 8–14d, with concomitant prednisolone 40mg/d PO.

Trichuris trichiura (whipworm) may cause non-specific abdominal symptoms. *Diagnosis:* Stool microscopy. *Treatment:* Mebendazole.

Enterobius vermicularis (threadworm) is common in temperate climes. It causes anal itch as it leaves the bowel to lay eggs on the perineum. Apply sticky tape to the perineum and identify eggs microscopically. *Treatment:* Mebendazole 100mg PO. Repeat at 2wks if ≥2yrs. If aged <2yrs, try piperazine 0.3mL/kg/24h for 7d. Treat the whole family. *Hygiene is more important than drugs* as adult worms die after 6wks. Continued symptoms means *reinfection*.

Toxocara canis Commonest cause of *visceral larva migrans*. Presents with eye granulomas (squint, blindness, pigmentary retinopathy) or visceral involvement (fever, myalgia, hepatomegaly, asthma, cough). *Diagnosis:* Ophthalmoscopy, serology, may require histology. *Treatment:* Tiabendazole or diethylcarbamazine is often unsatisfactory. In ocular disease, visible larvae can sometimes be photocoagulated by laser. *Toxocara* is commonly acquired by ingesting soil contaminated by animal feces so de-worm pets regularly, and exclude them from play areas.

Filarial infection

This is common—prevalence of lymphatic filariasis: 120 million worldwide.

1 **Onchocerciasis** is caused by *Onchocerca volvulus* and is transmitted by the black fly. It causes river blindness in 72% of some communities in Africa and S America, affecting 17 million worldwide. A nodule forms at the site of the bite, shedding microfilariae to distant skin sites which develop altered pigmentation, lichenification, loss of elasticity, and poor healing. Disease manifestations are mainly due to the localized host response to dead/dying microfilariae. Eye manifestations include keratitis, uveitis, cataract, fixed pupil, fundal degeneration, or optic neuritis/atrophy. Lymphadenopathy and elephantiasis also occur. *Diagnosis:* Visualization of microfilaria in eye or skin snips. Remove a fine shaving of clean, unanesthetized skin with a scalpel. Put on slide with a drop of 0.9% saline and look for swimming larvae after 30min.

2 **Lymphatic filaria** occur in Asia, Africa, and S America and is transmitted by mosquito vectors. Acute infections cause fever and lymphadenitis. *Wuchereria bancrofti* causes lower limb lymphedema (elephantiasis) and hydrocoeles. *Brugia malaya* causes elephantiasis below the elbow/knee. *Wuchereria* life cycle: A mosquito bites an infected human → ingested microfilariae develop into larvae → Larvae migrate to mosquito's mouth → Biting of another human → Access to bloodstream → Adult filariae lodge in lymphatic system. *Diagnosis:* Blood film, serology. A rapid immuno-chromatographic fingerprick test has been developed for use in the field. *Complications:* Immune hyperreactivity may cause tropical pulmonary eosinophilia (cough, wheeze, lung fibrosis, high eosinophil counts, IgE↑ and IgG↑). It is a major public health problem and is a WHO target for elimination by the year 2020 (starting with Nigeria, Samoa, and Egypt). The current elimination strategy involves mass treatment with a single yearly dose of 2 drugs for 5yrs: Albendazole (400mg) plus *either* ivermectin (200mcg/kg) *or* diethylcarbamazine (6mg/kg). An alternative strategy, involving giving diethylcarbamazine-fortified salt to families for 12 months, has also been found to be effective.

3 **Loiasis** is caused by *Loa loa*. It occurs in Africa and is transmitted by the *Chrysops* fly. It causes painful 'Calabar' swellings of the limbs, eosinophilia, and may migrate across the conjunctiva.

Treatment: Seek expert help. Ivermectin is the drug of choice, eg 1 dose of 150mcg/kg PO repeated, eg every 6 months for *Onchocerca* or 20mcg/kg PO as a single dose for *Wuchereia*. It does not kill adult worms, so repeat treatment may be needed every 6–12 months until adult worms die. Mass treatment campaigns may prevent blindness in some communities, but side-effects may pose problems. Lymphedema responds to compression garments (hard to use) or benzopyrone (coumarin) 400mg/24h PO.

Cestodes (tapeworms)

Taenia solium (pork tapeworm) infection occurs by eating uncooked pork, or from drinking contaminated water. *T. saginata* is contracted from uncooked beef. Both cause vague abdominal symptoms and malabsorption. Contaminated food and water contain cysticerci which adhere to the gut and develop into adult worms. On swallowing the eggs of *T. solium* they may enter the circulation and disseminate throughout the body, becoming cysticerci within the human host (*cysticercosis*). This tapeworm encysts in muscle, skin, heart, eye, and CNS, causing focal signs. *Subcutaneous cysticercosis* causes palpable subcutaneous nodules in the arms, legs, and chest. *Ocular cysticercosis* causes conjunctivitis, uveitis, retinitis, choroidal atrophy, and blindness.

Diagnosis of cysticercosis: This is by fecal microscopy and examination of perianal swabs. • Differentiate *T. solium* from *T. saginata* by examining the scolex or a mature proglottid; the eggs are indistinguishable. • A less technical means of species identification is to ask your patient about *movement* of the worm. If he describes worms vigorously wriggling out of the rectum, they will be *T. saginata*. • An indirect hemagglutination test is available. • The CSF may show eosinophils in neurocysticercosis. A CSF antigen tesct is available. • CT or MRI scan may locate cysts. CXR and X-rays of soft tissues of the thigh may show calcified cysts.

Neurocysticercosis is the commonest cause of seizures in some places, eg Mexico. Other features: Focal CNS signs, eg hemiplegia, odd behavioral, dementia—or no symptoms. Cysticerci may cluster like bunches of grapes ('racemose' form) in the ventricles (causing hydrocephalus) and basal cisterns (causing basal meningitis, cranial nerve lesions, and raised ICP). Spinal cysticerci may cause radicular or compressive spinal symptoms.

Diagnosis: • Stool microscopy and examination of perianal swabs. • Serology: Indirect hemagglutination test. • CSF: May show eosinophils in neurocysticercosis, and a CSF antigen test is available. • CT or MRI scan may locate cysts. • SXR and X-rays of soft tissues may show calcified cysts.

Treatment: Seek expert help. Niclosamide 2g PO in 2 doses, separated by 1h. Neurocysticercosis: Albendazole 7.5mg/kg/12h PO with food, or praziquantel 17mg/kg/8h PO for 30d. An allergic response to the dying larvae should be covered by dexamethasone 12mg/d PO for 21d. Cimetidine (800mg/d PO) is used to ↑ the concentration of praziquantel. The role of steroids in the routine treatment of neurocysticercosis is controversial. NB: If CSF ventricles are involved, you may need to shunt before starting drugs, and drugs may worsen the acute phase of cysticercotic encephalitis.

Diphyllobothrium latum is a fish tapeworm acquired from uncooked fish. It causes similar symptoms to *T. solium*, and is also treated with niclosamide. It is a cause of vitamin B_{12} deficiency.

Hymenolepis nana and *H. diminuta* (dwarf tapeworms) are rarely symptomatic. Treat with niclosamide 2g 1st day, then 1g/24h for 6d. *H. nana* may be treated with a single dose of praziquantel (25mg/kg PO).

Hydatid disease Cystic hydatid disease is a zoonosis caused by ingesting eggs of the dog parasite *Echinococcus granulosus* eg in rural sheep-farming regions. Hydatid is an ↑ public health problem in parts of China, Russia, Alaska, Wales, and Japan. *Presentation:* Most cysts are asymptomatic, but liver cysts may present with hepatomegaly, obstructive jaundice, cholangitis, or FUO. Lung cysts may present with dyspnea, chest pain, hemoptysis, or anaphylaxis. Parasites migrate almost anywhere, eg CNS or it turns up incidentally on CXR. *Diagnosis:* Plain X-ray, ultrasound, and CT of cysts. A reliable serological test has replaced the variably sensitive Casoni intradermal test. *Treatment:* Seek expert help. The drug of choice is albendazole (eg 7.5mg/kg/12h with food; max 800mg/d) for 28d, in 3 cycles. Excise/drain symptomatic cysts. Beware spilling cyst contents (causes anaphylaxis; give praziquantel here). The PAIR approach is commonly used: Puncture → aspirate cyst → inject hypertonic saline → reaspirate. Give albendazole pre- and post-drainage to prevent recurrence. (NB: Alveolar hydatid is caused by *E. multilocularis*.)

Trematodes (flukes)

Schistosomiasis (bilharzia) is the most prevalent disease caused by flukes, affecting 200 million people worldwide. The snail vectors release cercariae which can penetrate the skin, eg during paddling, may cause an itchy papular rash ('swimmer's itch'). The cercariae shed their tails to become schistosomules and migrate via lungs to liver where they grow. ~2wks after initial infestation, there may be fever, urticaria, diarrhea, cough, wheeze, and hepatosplenomegaly ('Katayama fever'). In ~8wks, mature flukes couple and migrate to resting habitats, ie vesical veins (*hematobium*) or mesenteric veins (*mansoni* and *japonicum*). Eggs released from these sites cause granulomata and scarring. Clinical schistosomiasis is an immunological process on the part of the human host which is known to be due to a type IV hypersensitivity (at least for *S. mansoni*) to schistosomal eggs.

The patient is likely to have visited or be from Africa, the Middle East, or Brazil (*S. mansoni*), and present with abdominal pain and stomach upset, and, later, hepatic fibrosis, granulomatous inflammation, and portal hypertension (transformation into true cirrhosis has not been well-documented). *S. japonicum*, often the most serious, occurs in SE Asia, tends to affect the bowel and liver, and may migrate to lung and CNS ('travelers' myelitis'). Urinary schistosomiasis (*S. hematobium*) occurs in Africa, the Middle East, and the Indian Ocean. Signs: Frequency, dysuria, hematuria (± hematospermia), incontinence. It may progress to hydronephrosis and renal failure. There is an ↑risk of squamous cell carcinoma of the bladder.

Diagnosis is based on finding eggs in the urine (*S. hematobium*) or feces (*S. mansoni* and *S. japonicum*) or rectal biopsy (all types). AXR may show bladder calcification in chronic *S. hematobium* infection. Renal ultrasound identifies renal obstruction, hydronephrosis, thickened bladder wall. Schistosoma ELISA is most sensitive.

Treatment Praziquantel: 40mg/kg PO with food divided into 2 doses separated by 4–6h for *S. mansoni* & *S. hematobium*, and 20mg/kg/8h for 1d in *S. japonicum*. Sudden transitory abdominal pain and bloody diarrhea may occur shortly after. Oxamniquine is an alternative for *S. mansoni* infection. Artemether also shows promise, both for prophylaxis in high-risk groups, and as a synergist to praziquantel therapy.

Fasciola hepatica (liver fluke) is spread by sheep, water, and snails. It causes hepatomegaly, then fibrosis. *Presentation:* Fever, abdominal pain, diarrhea, weight↓, jaundice, and eosinophilia. *Tests:* Stool microscopy, serology. *Treatment:* Get help. Triclabendazole 10mg/kg PO, 1 dose (may repeat once), or bithionol 30mg/kg/d, max 2g/d IM (15 doses).

Opisthorchis and **Clonorchis** are liver flukes common in the Far East, where they cause cholangitis, cholecystitis, and cholangiocarcinoma. *Tests:* Stool microscopy. *Treatment:* Praziquantel 25mg/kg/8h PO for 1d.

Fasciolopsis buski is a big intestinal fluke ~7cm long causing ulcers or abscesses at the site of attachment. Treatment: As for opisthorchiasis.

Paragonimus westermani (lung fluke) is contracted by eating raw freshwater crabs or crayfish. Parasites migrate through gut and diaphragm to invade the lungs, causing cough, dyspnea, and hemoptysis. Secondary complications: Lung abscess and bronchiectasis. It occurs in the Far East, S America, and the Congo, where it is commonly mistaken for TB (similar clinical and CXR appearances). *Tests:* Ova in sputum. MRI/CT may disclose CNS/lung lesions. *Treatment:* Praziquantel (25mg/kg/8h PO for 2d) or bithionol (30–50mg/kg on alternate days PO for 10d).

Exotic infections

Exotic infections may be *community-acquired* or *nosocomial*, ie acquired in hospital. The ↑ prevalence of immunosuppression, both drug induced and innate, and the widespread use of broad-spectrum antibiotics have resulted in an ↑ in exotic infections. New techniques such as PCR have enabled the identification of more putative infective agents.

History When an infection is suspected (fever, sweats, inflammation, D&V, WBC↑, or *any* unexplained symptom), ask the patient about:
- Any recent foreign travel?
- Previous travel history?
- Any foreign bodies, eg hip prosthesis, prosthetic heart valves?
- Immunosuppression or risk factors for HIV?
- Any necrotic tissues?
- Any pets at home?
- Any animal or insect bites or scratches?
- Any exposure to illness at work?

Diagnosis Take appropriate cultures (blood, urine, stool, CSF) or swabs as clinically indicated. Consult early with an infectious diseases physician. Consider CXR, ultrasound, or CT as clinically indicated. If the infection appears to be localized, consider surgical debridement ± drainage. Do not give up if you cannot culture an organism; tests may need to be repeated. Perhaps the organism is 'fastidious' in its nutritional requirement or requires prolonged incubation. Even if culture *is* achieved, it may be that the organism is pathogenic or it could be a commensal (ie part of the normal flora for that patient). If culture is not possible, look for antibodies or antigen in the serum or other body fluids. It is generally agreed that a 4-fold ↑ in antibody titers in convalescence (compared with the acute sera) is indicative of recent infection although not diagnostic. PCR is increasingly being used to make identifications; however, it is far from infallible, and contamination with DNA from the lab or elsewhere is a frequent problem.

Treatment Empiric therapy (p498) may be needed if the patient is ill. *The table opposite is for reference purposes only:* No one can remember *all* the details about even the common infectious diseases, let alone the rare ones. Check with a microbiologist for local patterns of disease and antibiotic sensitivity/resistance. *Antibiotic doses:* Penicillins (p493); cephalosporins (p494); other agents (p496).

Organism	Site or type of infection	Treatment example
Acanthameba	Corneal ulcers	Propamidine + neomycin
Acinetobacter calcoaceticus	UTI; CSF; lung; bone; conjunctiva	Gentamicin
Actinobacillus actinomycetemcomitans	IE; CNS; UTI; bone; thyroid; lung Periodontitis; abscesses	Penicillin ± gentamicin
Actinobacillus lignieresii	CSF; IE; wounds; bone; lymph nodes	Ampicillin ± gentamicin
Actinobacillus ureae	Bronchus; CSF post-trauma; hepatitis	Ampicillin ± gentamicin
Aerococcus viridans	Empyema; UTI; CSF; bone	Penicillin ± gentamicin
Aeromonas hydrophila	IE; CSF; cornea; bone; D&V; liver abscess	Gentamicin
Afipia broomeae	Marrow; synovium	Imipenem or ceftriaxone
Alcaligenes species	Dialysis peritonitis; ear; lung	Co-amoxiclav or cetazidime
Arachnia propionica	Actinomycosis; tear ducts; CNS	Penicillin
Arcanobacterium	Throat; cellulitis; leg ulcer	Penicillin
Babesia microti (protozoa)	FUO ± hemolysis if old/splenectomized	Clindamycin + quinine
Bacillus cereus	Wounds; eye; ear; lung; UTI; IE	Gentamicin
Bifidobacterium	Vagina; UTI; IE; peritonitis; lung	Penicillin
Bordetella bronchiseptica	URTI; CSF (after animal contact)	Co-trimoxazole
Burkholderia cepacia, etc (formerly *Pseudomonas*)	Wounds; feet; lungs; IE; CAPD; UTI ecthyma gangrenosa; peritonitis	Ceftazidime, Clindamycin or gentamicin

Burkholderia pickettii	CSF (formerly a *pseudomonas*)	Cefalosporin
Burkholderia pseudomallei (formerly *Pseudomonas pseudomallei*)	Melioidosis: Self-reactivating septicemia + multiorgan, protean signs eg in rice-farmers, via water/soil in Papua, Thailand, Vietnam, Torres Straits	Ceftazidime (14d) + co-trimoxazole or co-amoxiclav for 3 months
Capnocytophaga ochracea and *C. sputagena*	Oral ulcer; stomatitis; arthritis Blood; cervical abscess	Penicillin or ciprofloxacin
Cardiobacterium hominis	IE (=infective endocarditis)	Penicillin + gentamicin
Chromobacterium violaceum	Nodes; eye; bone; liver; pustules	Erythromycin, chloramphenicol
Citrobacter koseri/diversus	CSF; UTI; blood; cholecystitis	Cefuroxime + gentamicin
Corynebacterium bovis/equi	IE; CSF; otitis; leg ulcer; lung	Erythromycin + rifampicin
Corynebacterium ovis	Joints; liver; muscle; granulomata	Penicillin
Corynebacterium ulcerans	Diphtheria-like ± CNS signs	Penicillin + Diphtheria antitoxin
Cyclospora cayetanensis	Diarrhea (via raspberries)	Co-trimoxazole
Edwardsiella tarda	Cellulitis; abscesses; BP↓; dysentery via penetrating fish injuries	Cefuroxime + gentamicin
Eikenella corrodens	Sinus; ears; PE post-jugular vein phlebitis (postanginal sepsis) via bites	Penicillin + gentamicin
Erysipelothrix rhusiopathiae	Erysipelas-like;	Penicillin
Eubacterium	Wounds; gynaecology sepsis; IE	Penicillin
Flavobacterium meningosepticum	Lungs; epidemic neonatal meningitis; post-op bacteremia	Penicillin
Flavobacterium multivorum	Peritonitis (spontaneous)	Cefuroxime
Gemella hemolysans	IE; meningitis after neurosurgery	Penicillin + gentamicin
Helicobacter cinaedia	Proctitis in homosexual men	Ampicillin or gentamicin
Kingella denitrificans kingae	Throat; larynx; eyelid; joint; skin	Penicillin ± gentamicin
Kurthia bibsonii/sibirica/zopfii	IE (infective endocarditis)	Penicillin
Lactobacillus	Teeth; chorioamnionitis; pyelitis	Cephalosporins, Penicillin
Megasphaera elsdenii	IE (infective endocarditis)	Metronidazole
Mobiluncus curtisii/mulieris	Vagina; uterus; septicemia in cirrhosis	Cephalosporins or ampicillin
Moraxella osloensis and *M. nonliquefaciens*	Conjunctiva; wound; vagina; UTI; CSF CNS; bone; hemorrhagic stomatitis	Penicillin
Neisseria cani	Wounds from cat bites	Amoxicillin
Neisseria cinerea/mucosa+ N. subflava; N. flavescens	IE; CNS; bone; post human bites or from peritoneal dialysis	Penicillin, cephalosporin
Pasteurella multocida	Bone; lung; CSF; UTI; pericarditis epiglottitis. Post cat/dog bite	Penicillin
Pasteurella pneumotrophica	Wounds; joints; bone; CSF	Penicillin or ciprofloxacin
Peptostreptococcus magnans	Bone; joint; wound; teeth; face	Penicillin or cephalosporins
Plesiomonas shigelloides	D&V; eye; sepsis post fishbone injury	Ciprofloxacin
Propionibacterium acnes	Face; wounds; CSF shunts; bone; IE liver granuloma (botyromycosis)	Tetracycline or penicillin
Prototheca wickerhamii/ zopfii = achlorophyllous algae	Subcutaneous granuloma; bursitis Lymphadenitis; nodules; granuloma	Amphotericin or ketoconazole
Providencia stuartii	UTI; burn or lung infections	Gentamicin
Pseudomonas maltophilia	Wounds; ear; eye; lung; UTI; IE	Co-trimoxazole
Pseudomonas putrefaciens	CSF post CNS surgery/head trauma	Cefotaxime
Rothia dentocariosa	Appendix abscess	Penicillin + gentamicin
Serratia marcescens	Wound; burns; lung; UTI; liver; CSF; bone; IE; red diaper syndrome	Imipenem, eftazidime, ciprofloxacin
Sphingomonas paucimobilis	Superficial leg ulcer; CSF; UTI	Ceftazidime
Streptococcus bovis	IE if colon cancer; do colonoscopy	Penicillin + gentamicin
Vibrio vulnificus	Wounds; muscle; uterus; fasciitis	Tetracycline, penicillin

Hematology

Alison R. Moliterno, M.D.

Contents

Relevant pages elsewhere: Transfusion (p418)

Anemia

Anemia is defined as a low hemoglobin concentration due a ↓ red cell mass. If the low Hb concentration is due to ↑ plasma volume such as in pregnancy, the anemia is then considered physiological. A low Hb is <13.5g/dL for men and <11.5g/dL for women. Anemia may be due to reduced production or ↑ loss of RBC and has many causes. The cause of the anemia will be resolved by synthesis of the history, physical examination, and inspection of the blood smear.

Symptoms Due to the underlying cause or to the anemia itself: Fatigue, dyspnea, palpitations, headache, tinnitus, anorexia, dyspepsia, bowel disturbance and angina if there is pre-existing coronary artery disease. Patients who have developed their anemia rapidly are often more symptomatic than those who have developed anemia slowly, in which case there has been time for physiologic compensations for their anemia to occur.

Signs Pallor (evident in conjunctivae) and retinal hemorrhages. In severe anemia (Hb <8g/dL), there may be signs of a hyperdynamic circulation, with tachycardia, a systolic ejection murmur and cardiac enlargement. Later, heart failure may occur and in this state, rapid blood transfusion may be fatal.

Types of anemia The first step in diagnosis is to look at the mean cell volume (MCV, *normal MCV is 80-100fL*) and the red cell distribution width (RDW, a measure of the variability of the red cell size).

Low MCV (microcytic)
• Iron-deficiency anemia (IDA, most common cause) p558.
• Anemia of inflammation.
• Thalassaemia.
• Sideroblastic anemia.

NB: Anemia of inflammation is distinguished from iron deficiency by iron studies: Serum iron, transferrin, and transferrin saturation will be reduced while ferritin will be normal or elevated. Both the anemia of inflammation and some thalassemias tend to have near normal RDWs.

Normal MCV (normocytic aaemia)
• Anemia of chronic disease
• Bone marrow failure
• Renal failure

• Hypothyroidism (or ↑MCV)
• Hemolysis (or ↑MCV)
• Pregnancy

High MCV (macrocytic anaemia)
• B_{12} or folate deficiency
• Alcohol
• Liver disease
• Reticulocytosis
• Cytotoxics, eg hydroxyurea

• Myelodysplastic syndromes
• Marrow infiltration
• Hypothyroidism
• Antifolate drugs
• Bone marrow failure states

Hemolytic anemias: Do not fall neatly into the above classification as the anemia may be normochromic, or, if the reticulocyte percentage is very high, macrocytic. Suspect a hemolytic anemia if there is a reticulocytosis (>2% of RBCs; or reticulocyte count >85 × 10⁹/L), mild macrocytosis, haptoglobin ↓ (p564), bilirubin↑, and urobilinogen↑. If the RDW is very elevated (>20), consider a microangiopathic process such as DIC or TTP.

Blood transfusion Avoid unless Hb dangerously low. The decision will depend on the severity, the cause and the underlying medical status of the patient. If risk of hemorrhage (eg active peptic ulcer), transfuse up to 8g/dL. In severe anemia with heart failure, transfusion is vital to restore Hb to safe level, eg 8–10/dL, but must be done with great care. Give packed cells *slowly* with 10–40mg furosemide IV/PO with alternate units (dose depends on previous exposure to diuretics). Check for rising JVP and basal crackles.

Iron-deficiency anemia

Iron deficiency is common (seen in up to 14% of menstruating women) and worldwide is the most frequent cause of nutritional anemias. The most common cause is blood loss, particularly menorrhagia or GI bleeding—from esophagitis, peptic ulcer, carcinoma, colitis, or diverticulitis. In the tropics hookworm (GI blood loss) is the most common cause. Poor diet may cause IDA in infants and children, those on special diets, strict vegetarians or wherever there is poverty. Iron deficiency anemia due to malabsorption (gastric surgery, gastric bypass, celiac disease, Whipple's disease, inflammatory bowel disease) is usually accompanied by other deficiency states such as folate and B_{12}.

Symptoms: Associated symptoms include ice craving (pagophagia), restless leg syndrome, and short term memory loss (adolescents).

Signs: Koilonychia (p45), atrophic glossitis, and, rarely, post-cricoid webs.

Investigations: Microcytic, hypochromic blood film showing anisocytosis and poikilocytosis (p560). Confirmed by showing serum iron↓ and ferritin↓ (more representative of total body iron) with TIBC↑. If MCV↓, and good history of menorrhagia, oral iron may be started without further tests. Otherwise investigate: Fecal occult blood, barium enema or colonoscopy, gastroscopy, microscope stool for ova. *Iron deficiency without an obvious source of bleeding mandates a careful GI workup.*

Treatment: If the MCV is low and there is a history or menorrhagia, oral iron may be started without further diagnostic workup. Oral iron eg ferrous sulfate 324mg bid or tid PO. SE: Constipation, black stools. Hb should rise by 1g/dL/wk, with a modest reticulocytosis (ie young RBC, p560). Continue until Hb is normal and for at least 3 months, to replenish stores. Parenteral iron is reserved for patients who fail oral iron trials or dialysis patients and is available as iron gluconate (well tolerated) or iron dextran (higher side effect profile).

Refractory anemia: The usual reason that iron-deficiency anemia fails to respond to iron replacement is failure of compliance, often because of GI disturbance. Altering the dose of elemental iron or the formulation of elemental iron may be helpful, or consideration of IV iron in appropriate situations. Other reasons for failure of iron supplementation include continued blood loss or malabsorption. Importantly, anemia of inflammation or thalassaemia will not respond to iron supplementation.

The anemia of chronic disease

This is associated with many diseases including infection, collagen vascular disease, rheumatoid arthritis, malignancy, and renal failure. *Investigations:* Mild normocytic anemia (eg HB >8g/dL), TIBC↓ serum iron↓, ferritin normal or ↑. *Treatment:* Treat the underlying disease. The anemia of renal failure is partly due to erythropoietin deficiency and recombinant erythropoietin is effective in raising the hemoglobin level (maintenance dose example: 50–150U/kg twice weekly; SE: Hypertension in patients with renal failure). It is also effective in raising HB and improving quality of life in those with HIV-related anemia, chemotherapy induced-anemia, chronic bone marrow failure states, and the anemia of many chronic inflammatory states.

Sideroblastic anemia

Characterized by dyserythropoiesis and iron loading (bone marrow) and sometimes hemosiderosis (endocrine, liver, and cardiac damage). It may be congenital (rare, X-linked) or acquired (usually idiopathic, part of the spectrum of the myelodysplastic disorders), but may follow alcohol or lead excess, myeloproliferative disease, malignancy, malabsorption, or anti-TB drugs. Stippled, hypochromic RBCs are seen on the blood film with sideroblasts in the marrow (erythroid precursors with iron deposited in mitochondria in a ring around the nucleus). *Treatment* is supportive; pyridoxine may occasionally be of benefit (eg 10mg/24h PO; higher doses may cause neuropathy); remove the cause if possible. In myelodysplasia, erythropoietin, with or without human granulocyte colony stimulating factor (G-CSF) may be effective, although the cost benefit of this approach is controversial.

Interpretation of iron studies

	Iron	TIBC	Ferritin
Iron deficiency	↓	↑	↓
Anemia of chronic disease	↓	↓	↑
Chronic hemolysis	↑	↓	↑
Hemochromatosis	↑	↓ (or↔)	↑
Pregnancy	↑	↑	↔
Sideroblastic anemia	↑	↔	↑

The peripheral blood film

Many primary hematological diagnoses and other systemic diagnoses can be made by careful examination of the peripheral blood film. It is also necessary for interpretation of the RBC indices.

Acanthocytes: RBCs show many spicules.

Anisocytosis: Variation in red cell size.

Basophilic stippling: Of RBCs is seen in lead poisoning, thalassaemia, and other dyserythropoietic anemias.

Blasts: Nucleated precursor cells. They are not normally seen in peripheral blood.

Burr cells: Irregularly shaped cells occurring in uremia or liver disease.

Dimorphic picture: A mixture of RBC sizes, eg partially treated iron deficiency, mixed deficiency (Fe with B_{12} or folate deficiency), post-transfusion, sidero blastic anemia.

Howell-Jolly bodies: Nuclear remnants seen in RBCs post splenectomy; rarely leukemia, megaloblastic anemia, iron-deficiency anemia, hyposplenism (eg celiac disease, neonates, thalassaemia, SLE, lymphoma, leukemia, amyloid).

Hypersegmentation: Hypersegmented neutrophils (>5 lobes to nucleus) seen in megaloblastic anemia, uremia, and liver disease.

Hypochromia: Less dense staining of RBCs seen in iron-deficiency anemia, thalassemia, and sideroblastic anemia (iron stores unusable).

Left shift: Immature white cells seen in circulating blood in any marrow out pouring, such as infection or marrow infiltration.

Leukoerythroblastic anemia: Immature cells (myelocytes, nucleated red blood cells and large platelets) seen in film. Due to extramedullary hematopoiesis associated with marrow infiltration, hypoxia, marrow fibrosis or severe anemia.

Leukemoid reaction: A marked reactive leukocytosis. Usually granulocytic and observed in severe infection, burns, acute hemolysis, metastatic cancer.

Myelocytes, promyelocytes, metamyelocytes, normoblasts: Immature cells seen in the blood in leukoerythroblastic anemia.

Normoblasts or nucleated red cells: Immature red cells, with a nucleus. Seen in leukoerythroblastic anemia, marrow infiltration, hemolysis, hypoxia.

Pappenheimer bodies: Granules of siderocytes, eg lead poisoning, carcinoma tosis, post splenectomy.

Poikilocytosis: Variation in red cell shape

Polychromasia: RBCs of different ages stain unevenly, the younger erythrocytes being bluer. An indirect assessment of reticulocytosis.

Reticulocytes: (NR: 0.8–2%; or <85×10⁹/L) Young, larger RBCs (contain RNA) signifying active erythropoiesis. ↑ in hemolysis, hemorrhage, and if B_{12}, iron or folate is given to marrow that lack these.

Rouleaux formation: Red cells stack on each other (the visual 'analogue' of a high ESR—p588).

Schistocytes: Fragmented RBCs sliced by fibrin bands observed in microan giopathic hemolytic processes (DIC, TTP, malignant hypertension).

Spherocytes: Red blood cells lacking central pallor. Observed in extravascular hemolytic processes such as autoimmune hemolysis, hereditary spherocytosis, burns.

Target cells: RBCs with central staining, a ring of pallor, and an outer rim of staining seen in liver disease, thalassemia, or sickle-cell disease-and, in small numbers, in iron-deficiency anemia.

The differential white cell count

Neutrophils 2–7.5 × 10^9/L (40–75% of the total white cell count; absolute values are more meaningful than percentages).

↑ in:
- Bacterial infections.
- Trauma; surgery; burns; hemorrhage.
- Inflammation; infarction; polymyalgia rheumatica; PAN.
- Myeloproliferative disorders.
- Steroids.
- Disseminated malignancy.

↓ in:
- Viral infections, HIV, liver disease, hepatitis C, brucellosis; typhoid; kala-azar; TB.
- Drugs, eg hydroxyurea, sulfonamides.
- Hypersplenism or neutrophil antibodies (seen in SLE and rheumatoid arthritis)- ↑ destruction.
- B$_{12}$ or folate deficiency; in bone marrow failure states, stem cell disorders- ↓ production, p584.

Lymphocytes 1.3–3.5 × 10^9/L (20–45%).

↑ in:
- Viral infections, toxoplasmosis; whooping cough; brucellosis
- Chronic lymphocytic leukemia.

Large numbers of abnormal ('atypical') lymphocytes are characteristically seen with EBV infection: These are T-cells reacting against EBV-infected B-cells. They have a large amount of clear cytoplasm with a blue rim that flows around neighboring RBCs ('dutch skirting'). Other causes of 'atypical' lymphocytes.

↓ in:
- Steroid therapy; SLE; uremia; legionnaire's disease; HIV infection; marrow infiltration; post chemotherapy or radiotherapy.

T-lymphocyte subset reference values: CD4 count: 537–1571/mm^3 (low in HIV infection). CD8 count: 235–753/mm^3; CD4/CD8 ratio: 1.2–3.8.

Eosinophils 0.04–0.44 × 10^9/L (1–6%). ↑ in: Asthma/atopy; parasitic infections (especially invasive helminths); PAN; skin disease especially pemphigus; urticaria; malignant disease (including lymphomas and eosinophilic leukemia, systemic mastocytosis); adrenal insufficiency, irradiation; Löffler's syndrome; during the convalescent phase of any infection.

The hypereosinophilic syndrome is seen when there is development of end-organ damage (restrictive cardiomyopathy; neuropathy; hepatosplenomegaly) in association with a raised eosinophil count (>1.5 × 10^9/L) for more than 6wks.

Monocytes 0.2–0.8 × 10^9/L(2–10%).

↑ in: Acute and chronic infections (eg TB; brucellosis; protozoa); malignant disease, including M4 and M5 acute myeloid leukemia (p579), and Hodgkin's disease; myelodysplasia.

Basophils 0–0.1 × 10^9/L (0–1%).

↑ in: Viral infections; urticaria; myxedema; post splenectomy; CML; UC; malignancy; systemic mastocytosis (urticaria pigmentosa); hemolysis; polycythemia rubra vera.

Macrocytic anemia

Macrocytosis (*MCV >100fL*) is a common finding; often due to alcohol (usually without any accompanying anemia).

Causes of macrocytosis (*MCV >110 fL*): Vitamin B_{12} or folate deficiency hydroxyurea.

MCV 100-110fL:
- *Drugs:* Alcohol, azathioprine, zidovudine
- Marrow infiltration
- Hemolysis
- Liver disease
- Pregnancy
- Hypothyroidism
- Myelodysplasia

Investigations

Blood film: May show hypersegmented polymorphs (B_{12}↓) or target cells (liver disease). *Other tests:* ESR (malignancy), LFT (include GGT), T4, serum B_{12}, and serum folate (or red cell folate). *Bone marrow biopsy* is indicated if the cause is not revealed by the above tests. It is likely to show 1 of these 4 states:
- Megaloblastic: B_{12} or folate deficiency (or cytotoxic drugs). (A megaloblast is a cell in which cytoplasmic and nuclear maturation are out of phase—as nuclear maturation is slow.)
- Normoblastic marrow: Liver damage, myxedema.
- ↑ erythropoiesis: Eg hemolysis.
- Abnormal erythropoiesis: Sideroblastic anemia, leukemia, aplastic anemia.

If B_{12} deficiency, consider a *Schilling test* to help to identify the cause. This determines whether a low B_{12} is due to malabsorption (B_{12} is absorbed from the terminal ileum) or to lack of intrinsic factor by comparing the proportion of an oral dose (1mcg) of radioactive B_{12} excreted in urine with and without the concurrent administration of intrinsic factor. (The blood must be saturated by giving an IM dose of 1000mcg of B_{12} first.) If intrinsic factor enhances absorption, lack of it (eg pernicious anemia, p563) is likely to be the cause.

Causes of a low B_{12} Pernicious anemia; post gastrectomy (no intrinsic factor to facilitate B_{12} absorption in the terminal ileum); dietary deficiency (vegans, children and elderly living in vegetarian households); rarely, disease of terminal ileum (where B_{12} is absorbed) eg Crohn's; resection; blind loops; diverticula; worms (*Dyphyllobothrium*). B_{12} is found in liver and all animal foods. *Body stores:* Sufficient for 3yrs.

Causes of low folate

Poor diet, heavy alcohol use, ↑ requirements (pregnancy, hemolysis, malignancy, long-term hemodialysis), malabsorption (especially celiac disease, tropical sprue), drugs (phenytoin and trimethoprim). Folate is found in green vegetables, fruit, liver. *Body stores:* Sufficient for 3 months. Maternal folate deficiency is associated with the development of fetal neural tube defects.

NB: In ill patients with megaloblastic anemia, it may be necessary to treat before the results of serum B_{12} and folate are at hand. Use large doses, eg hydroxocobalamin 1mg/24h IM, with folic acid 5mg/24h PO. Blood transfusions are very rarely needed, p418.

Folate given alone for the treatment of megaloblastic anemia when low B_{12} is the cause may precipitate, or worsen, subacute combined degeneration of the spinal cord.

Pernicious anemia

Pernicious anemia affects all cells of the body and is due to malabsorption of B_{12} resulting from atrophic gastritis and lack of gastric intrinsic factor secretion. In B_{12} deficiency, synthesis of thymidine, and hence DNA, is impaired and consequently red cell production is reduced. In addition, the CNS, peripheral nerves, gut, and tongue may be affected.

Incidence 1:1000 ↑ with advancing age

Common features
• Tiredness and weakness (90%)
• Dyspnea (70%)
• Paraesthesia (38%)
• Sore red tongue (25%)
• Diarrhea
• Mild jaundice (lemon tinge to skin)

Other features
• Retinal hemorrhages
• Prematurely grey hair
• Retrobulbar neuritis
• Mild splenomegaly
• Fever
• Neuropsychiatric (dementia)

Subacute combined degeneration of the spinal cord: This may be seen in any cause of a low B_{12}. Posterior and lateral columns are often affected, not always together. Onset is usually insidious with peripheral neuropathy. Joint-position and vibration sense are often affected first (dorsal columns) followed by distal paraesthesiae (neuropathy). If untreated, stiffness and weakness ensue. The classical triad is:
• Extensor plantars • Brisk knee jerks • Absent ankle jerks. Less common signs: Cognition↓, vision↓, absent knee jerks with brisk ankle jerks and flexor plantars, Lhermitte's sign (p338). Pain and T° sensation may be intact even when joint position sense is severely affected. CNS signs can occur without anemia.

Associations Thyroid disease (~25%), vitiligo, Addison's disease, carcinoma of stomach (so have a low threshold for endoscopy).

Tests: • Hb↓ (3–11g/dL)   • MCV >~110fL   • Hypersegmented neutrophils
• Serum B_{12} <200pg/mL • WCC & platelets↓ • Megaloblasts in the marrow

Megaloblasts are abnormal red cell precursors in which nuclear maturation is slower than cytoplasmic maturation. Antibodies to parietal cells (high sensitivity but low specificity) or to intrinsic factor (higher specificity but lower sensitivity) are present in PA. The vast majority of B_{12} deficient patients will have elevations in serum homocysteine and methylmalonic acid. However, both homocysteine and methylmalonic acid are elevated in renal disease, and hyperhomocysteinemia is present in folate deficiency. A Schilling test (p562) may be appropriate occasionally (expect it to show that <7% of an orally administered dose of labelled B_{12} is excreted-unless concurrent intrinsic factor is given).

Treatment Replenish stores with cyanocobalamin (B_{12}) 1mg IM every day for 2wks (or, if CNS signs, until improvement stops). Maintenance: 1mg IM every month for life. Initial improvement is heralded by a marked reticulocytosis (after 4–5d, but serum iron falls first). Watch for early hypokalemia and rebound thrombocytosis if severely B_{12} deficient.

Practical hints Beware of diagnosing pernicious anemia in those under 40yrs old: Look for GI malabsorption (small bowel biopsy).

1 Watch for hypokalemia in early days of therapy.
2 Pernicious anemia with high output CHF may require exchange transfusion after blood for CBC, folate, B_{12}, and marrow sampling.
3 As hematopoiesis accelerates on treatment, additional Fe and folate may be needed.
4 WBC and platelet count should normalize in 1wk. Hb rises ~1g/dL per week of treatment.
5 Dramatic rebound thrombocytosis is often observed, is transient and does not appear to be harmful.

Prognosis Complete neurological recovery is possible. Most see improvement in the first 3–6 months. Patients do best if treated as soon as possible after the onset of symptoms.

An approach to hemolytic anemia

Hemolysis is the premature breakdown of RBCs. It may occur in the circulation (intravascular) or in the reticuloendothelial system (extravascular). Normal RBCs have a lifespan of ~120d. In sickle-cell anemia, eg the lifespan may be as short as 5d. If the bone marrow does not compensate sufficiently, a hemolytic anemia will result.

Causes of hemolysis These are either genetic or acquired.

Genetic:

1 Membrane: Hereditary spherocytosis or elliptocytosis.
2 Hemoglobin: Sickling disorders (p566), thalassemia.
3 Enzyme defects: G6PD and pyruvate kinase deficiency.

Acquired:

1 Immune: Either isoimmune (hemolytic disease of newborn, blood transfusion reaction), autoimmune (warm or cold antibody mediated), or drug-induced
2 Non-immune: Trauma (cardiac hemolysis, microangiopathic anemia, p565) infection (malaria, septicemia), membrane disorders (paroxysmal nocturnal hemoglobinuria, hereditary spherocytosis, liver disease).

In searching for evidence of significant hemolysis (and, if present, its cause), try to answer these 4 questions:

• *Is there ↑ red cell breakdown?* Bilirubin↑ (unconjugated), urinary urobilinogen↑, haptoglobin↓ (binds free Hb avidly, and is then removed by the liver, so it is a good marker of hemolysis).
• *Is there ↑ red cell production?* Demonstrated by reticulocytosis, polychromasia on the blood smear, macrocytosis, marrow hyperplasia.
• *Is the hemolysis mainly extra- or intravascular?* Extravascular hemolysis may lead to splenic hypertrophy. The features of intravascular hemolysis are methemalbuminemia, free plasma hemoglobin, hemoglobinuria, low haptoglobin, and hemosiderinuria.
• *Why is there hemolysis?* See below p565.

History Ask about family history, race, jaundice, hematuria, drugs, previous anemia.

Examination Look for jaundice, hepatosplenomegaly, leg ulcers (seen in sickle-cell disease).

Investigation

• CBC, reticulocytes, bilirubin, LDH, haptoglobin, urinary urobilinogen. Films may show polychromasia, macrocytosis, spherocytes, elliptocytes, fragmented cells or sickle cells and nucleated RBCs if severe.
• Further investigations: *Direct antiglobulin test (DAT; Coombs' test)*. This will identify red cells coated with antibody or complement and a positive result usually indicates an immune cause of the hemolysis. The non-immune group are usually identifiable by associated features.
• RBC lifespan may be determined by *chromium labelling* and the major site of RBC breakdown may also be identified. *Urinary hemosiderin* (stains with Prussian Blue) indicates chronic intravascular hemolysis.
• The cause may now be obvious, but further tests may be needed. Membrane abnormalities are identified on the film, and can be confirmed by *osmotic fragility* testing. *Hb electrophoresis* will detect Hb variants. *Enzyme assays* are reserved for situations when other causes have been excluded.

Causes of hemolytic anemia

Sickle-cell disease see p566

Hereditary spherocytosis Autosomal dominant RBC membrane defect (RBCs are osmotically fragile). Hemolysis is variable. *Signs:* Splenomegaly ± ↑ risk of gallstones. RBCs show ↑fragility. *Diagnosis:* Hb 8–12g/dL. Osmotic fragility tests. Film: Many spherocytes. *Treatment:* Folate replacement; splenectomy if warranted (there are risks with ensuing hyposplenism).

Hereditary elliptocytosis Usually inherited as autosomal dominant. The degree of hemolysis is variable; splenectomy may be indicated in severe cases.

Glucose-6-phosphate dehydrogenase deficiency is the commonest RBC enzyme defect. Inheritance is sex-linked with 100 million affected in Africa, the Mediterranean, and the Middle/Far East. Neonatal jaundice occurs, but most are symptomless with normal Hb and blood film. They are susceptible to oxidative crises precipitated by drugs (primaquine, sulfonamides, ciprofloxacin), exposure to fava beans (favism) or illness. Typically there is rapid anemia and jaundice with RBC Heinz bodies (denatured Hb stained with methyl violet). *Diagnosis:* Enzyme assay. Don't do until some weeks *after* a crisis as young RBCs may have sufficient enzyme to make the results appear normal. *Treatment:* Avoid/remove precipitants; transfusion if severe.

Pyruvate kinase deficiency Usually inherited as autosomal recessive; homozygotes often have neonatal jaundice; later, chronic hemolysis with splenomegaly and jaundice. *Diagnosis:* Enzyme assay. Often well tolerated. There is no specific therapy but splenectomy may help.

Drug-induced immune hemolysis Due to formation of new RBC membrane antigens (eg penicillin in prolonged, high dose), immune complex formation (many drugs, rare), or presence of autoantibodies to the RBC: α-methyldopa, mefenamic acid, L-dopa (rare, Coombs' +ve).

Autoimmune hemolytic anemia (AIHA) *Causes:* Warm or cold antibodies. They may be primary (idiopathic) or secondary, usually to lymphoma or generalized autoimmune disease, eg SLE. *Warm AIHA:* Presents as chronic or acute anemia. *Treatment:* Steroids (± splenectomy). *Cold AIHA:* Chronic anemia made worse by cold, often with Raynaud's or acrocyanosis. *Treatment:* Keep warm. Blood transfusion is the main therapy, but chlorambucil may help. Mycoplasma and EBV may produce cold agglutinins, but hemolysis is rare.

Paroxysmal cold hemoglobinuria is caused by Donnath–Landsteiner antibody (seen in mumps, measles, chickenpox, syphilis) sticking to RBCs in cold, which causes complement-mediated lysis on rewarming.

Cardiac hemolysis Cell trauma in prosthetic aortic valves. It may indicate valve malfunction.

Microangiopathic hemolytic anemia (MAHA) Suspect if markedschistocytes and microspherocytes on the blood smear. Includes hemolytic-uremic syndrome, TTP (p260), and pre-eclampsia. Treat underlying disease; blood and fresh frozen plasma (FFP) transfusions, plasma exchange.

Paroxysmal nocturnal hemoglobinuria RBCs are unusually sensitive to complement due to loss of complement-inactivating enzymes on their surface, causing pancytopenia, abdominal pain, or thrombosis (eg Budd–Chiari syndrome) ± hemolysis. *Diagnosis:* Test for GPI[1]-linked antigen loss (CD55 and CD59). *Treatment:* Anticoagulation; blood product replacement; consider stem cell transplant.

Factors exacerbating hemolysis Infection often leads to ↑ hemolysis. Also parvoviruses cause cessation of marrow erythropoiesis. Parvovirus infection can cause acute decompensation in patients with chronic hemolytic anemias due to reticulocytopenia associated with parvovirus B_{19}.

1 GPI = glucosylphosphatidylinositol.

Sickle-cell anemia

Sickling disorders are due to the production of abnormal beta globins. An amino acid substitution in the beta globin gene (Glu → Val at position 6), results in the production of HbS rather than HbA. It is common in individuals of African descent. Approximately 10% of African Americans have sickle-cell *trait* (HbAS), which causes no disability (and may protect from *falciparum* malaria) except in hypoxia, when veno-occlusive events may occur. Symptomatic sickling occurs in heterozygotes with genes coding other analogous amino acid substitutions (eg HBSC and SD diseases). Homozygotes (CC; DD) have asymptomatic mild anemia. Individuals who are homozygous for hemoglobin S have sickle-cell anemia.

Pathogenesis HBs polymerizes when deoxygenated, causing RBCs to sickle. Sickle cells are fragile, have a shortened red cell survival, and can obstruct small vessel circulation.

Tests Hb ≈ 6–8g/dL; reticulocytes 10–20%: (hemolysis is variable); ↑bilirubin. *Hemoglobin electrophoresis:* Distinguishes SS, AS, and other HB variants. *Blood smear:* Polychromasia, nucleated red cells, sickle forms, targets. Aim for diagnosis *at birth* to aid prompt pneumococcal prophylaxis (vaccine, p158 and penicillin V).

Signs & symptoms *Early:* Anemia and jaundice, with painful swelling of hands and feet (dactylitis); also splenomegaly (rare if >10yrs, as the spleen infarcts). Youngsters with sickle cell disease may have periods of good health with acute crises (below). *Later:* Adult complications of sickle-cell anemia include recurrent vasoocclusive crisis, bone infarction and avascular necrosis, osteomyelitis, renal failure, leg ulcers, transfusional iron overload, pulmonary hypertension and stroke.

Sickle-cell crises These may be from vaso-occlusive crisis, venous thrombosis, hemolysis (rare), red cell aplasia, sequestration, or stroke.

Vaso-occlusive crisis: Common, often causing severe pain. Precipitated by cold, dehydration, infection, or physical stress. May mimic an acute abdomen or pneumonia. CNS signs: Seizures, focal signs. Transcranial Doppler can indicate risk of impending stroke (preventable by transfusion). Priapism may occur; if >24h, arrange prompt cavernosus-spongiosum shunting—prevents impotence; priapism also occurs in CML (p580).

Acute chest syndrome: Defined as fever, infiltrate on chest X-ray and chest pain. Must be monitored very closely and red cell exchange arranged if clinical status deteriorates.

Aplastic crises: These are due to parvoviruses, characterized by sudden lethargy and pallor and absent reticulocytes. Urgent transfusion is needed.

Sequestration/hepatic crises: Spleen and liver enlarge rapidly from trapped RBCs; signs: RUQ pain, INR/LFT↑, HB↓↓. Treatment includes red cell exchange tranfusion.

Management of chronic disease
- Consider hydroxyurea if frequent crises.
- Chronic blood transfusion to keep HBS level <30%, will prevent occurrence of stroke and chest syndrome but there is a high incidence of development of antibodies to red cell antigens and iron overload.
- Marrow transplant can be curative, but remains controversial.
- Splenic infarction leads to hyposplenism and appropriate prophylaxis, in terms of antibiotic and immunization should be adopted.

Prevention Genetic counseling; prenatal tests. Parental education and prompt medical attention for febrile illnesses prevents 90% of childhood deaths from infection, sequestration crises.

Management of sickle-cell crisis

Seek expert help. • Give *prompt*, generous analgesia with opiates (p412). • Crossmatch blood. CBC, reticulocytes, blood cultures, CXR. • Rehydrate with IV fluids and keep warm. • Give O_2 by mask if P_aO_2 ↓. • Empiric antibiotics for fever after culturing. • Measure HCT, reticulocytes, liver, and spleen size daily. • Give blood transfusion if HCT or reticulocytes fall sharply, or if there are CNS or lung complications—when the proportion of sickled cells should be reduced to <30%. This may require urgent exchange transfusion. *The acute chest syndrome* entails pulmonary infiltrates associated with chest pain and fever. It is a serious condition. Incidence: ~0.1 episodes/patient/yr. 13% in the landmark Vichinsky study needed ventilation, 11% had CNS symptoms, and 9% of those over 20yrs old died. Prodromal painful crisis occur ~2.5d before any abnormalities on CXR in 50% of patients. The chief causes of the infiltrates are fat embolism from bone marrow, infection with *Chlamydia*, *Mycoplasma*, or virus, and sickled RBCs. *Bronchodilators* have proved to be very effective in 20% having wheezing or obstructive pulmonary function at presentation. *Antibiotics* have an important role. *Red cell transfusion* improves oxygenation; red cell exchange should be emergently arranged if respiratory status deteriorates.

Thalassemia

Hemoglobin (Hb) is a tetramer consisting of 2 alpha and 2 beta globin molecules. Hb is heterogeneous. Adults have 95% HbA ($\alpha_2\beta_2$) and a little HbA$_2$ ($\alpha_2\delta_2$). HbF ($\alpha_2\gamma_2$) predominates in fetal life and HbA predominates after birth. HbA$_2$ and fetal hemoglobins may be relatively ↑ in beta chain disorders such as beta thalassemia and sickle cell anemia.

The thalassemias are a group of disorders resulting from reduced rate of production of one or more globin chains. This leads to an imbalance between alpha and beta chains, precipitation of excess globin chains, and anemia due to ineffective erythropoiesis and hemolysis. They are common in a band stretching from the Mediterranean to the Far East. The most important are alpha and beta thalassemia, in which there is reduced production of alpha and beta chains respectively. Since there are 2 genes for beta globin and 4 for alpha globin in each individual, there are numerous varieties of genetic defects associated with thalassemias. It is possible to correlate clinical severity with the specific genetic defect to some extent, although many other genetic and acquired factors modify the clinical phenotype.

Beta thalassemia major: This is the homozygous form in which very little beta chains are formed and results in a severe anemia presenting in the first year, often as failure to thrive. Death results in 1yr without transfusion. If adequate transfusion is given development is normal but symptoms of iron overload appear after 10yrs as endocrine failure, liver disease and cardiac toxicity. Death usually occurs at 20–30yrs due to cardiac siderosis. Long-term infusion of deferoxamine may prevent iron loading. If transfusion is inadequate there is chronic anemia with reduced growth and skeletal deformity due to bone marrow hyperplasia (bossing of skull). The smear shows very hypochromic, microcytic cells with target cells and nucleated RBCS. HbF↑, HbA$_2$ variable, HbA absent. Prevalence of carriers: Cypriot 1:7; south Italy 1:10; Greek 1:12; Turkish 1:20; English 1:100.

Betathalassemia minor: This is the heterozygous state, recognized as MCV <75fL, HbA$_2$ >3.5% and mild anemia (9–11g/dL) which is usually well tolerated but may be worsened in pregnancy.

a Thalassemia: 4 varieties are defined, depending on the number of defective alpha genes. Absence of 1 or 2 genes is common in individuals of African descent and is either undetectable or produces a mild microcytic anemia.

Hb H disease: In patients with 3 alpha gene deletions, HbH (β_4) is present at 5–30% throughout life with moderate hemolytic anemia and splenomegaly. Prognosis: Good.

Hb Barts; Infants are stillborn, or have neonatal jaundice (hydrops fetalis). They lack all alpha genes. Hb Barts is γ_4, and physiologically useless. Obstetric problems are common.

Thalassemia intermedia: This is a term used to describe individuals with thalassemia of intermediate severity who are not transfusion dependent but have severe anemia. They often have substantial splenic enlargement. Usually the explanation for the mildness of the disease is a residual ability to make beta chains.

Diagnosis Family history, CBC, MCV, smear, iron, HbA$_2$, HbF, Hb electrophoresis.

Treatment • Transfusion to keep Hb >9g/dL • Iron-chelating agent, eg deferroxamine. *Large doses of ascorbic acid also ↑ iron output but can cause cardiac failure due to sudden, rapid iron release, • Perform splenectomy if hypersplenism exists, • Give folate supplements. ↔A histocompatible marrow transplant can offer the chance of a cure in childhood.[1]

Genetic counseling should be offered. It may be particularly useful if abortion is an acceptable option.
1 D Rund 2005 *NEJM* **353** 1135.

Bleeding disorders

After trauma, 3 processes control hemorrhage: Vasoconstriction, platelet adhesion and aggregation, and fibrin deposition from activation of the coagulation cascade. Disorders of hemostasis fall into these three groups. The pattern of bleeding is important to the diagnostic approach—vascular and platelet disorders lead to prolonged bleeding from cuts, purpura, and bleeding from mucous membranes while coagulation disorders produce prolonged bleeding after injury, into joints, muscle, the GI and GU tracts.

Vascular defects. Causes may be congenital (Osler–Weber–Rendu) or acquired (senile purpura, steroids, trauma, pressure, vasculitis, diabetes, connective tissue disease, scurvy).

Platelet disorders. These may be due to quantitative or qualitative platelet defects. Causes of thrombocytopenia include:

↓ production: Marrow failure states, megaloblastosis, drugs (chemotherapy), liver disease, alcohol.

↑ destruction: Immune thrombocytopenia (ITP), infection (EBV), DIC, drugs, SLE, TTP, hypersplenism, heparin induced thrombocytopenia, pregnancy, sepsis.

Qualitative platelet defects are most frequently acquired from drugs (aspirin, Plavix®), uremia, myeloproliferative disorders, or less commonly can be due to congenital platelet disorders (Glanzmann's thrombasthenia, Bernard–Soulier).

ITP may be acute or chronic. Acute ITP is most commonly observed in children after viral infections, with rapid onset and spontaneous resolution within a year. Chronic ITP is the rule in adults, with a fluctuating course of bleeding purpura and epistaxis. Treatment is indicated when symptomatic bleeding occurs or when platelet counts are below 20,000/mcL. Treatment options include steroids, splenectomy, high-dose immune globulin, or anti-D (Winrho). Other treatments include rituxan and other immunosuppressive agents. Platelets transfusions are ineffective and should be avoided.

Coagulation disorders. Coagulation defects include congenital disorders such as hemophilia and von Willebrand's disease or acquired processes including anticoagulants, liver disease, DIC (p577), vitamin K deficiency, or acquired factor inhibitors. *Hemophilia A.* Congenital factor VIII deficiency, sex-linked recessive in one out of 10,000 male births. New mutations are common. The presentation is dependent on the severity of the deficiency and is frequently detected early in life, after surgery or trauma, or due to spontaneous bleeding into joints and muscle. Acquired hemophilia is due to factor VIII autoantibodies. These may appear in pregnancy, autoimmune diseases, or malignancy. Diagnosed by family history, bleeding history, prolongation of the aPTT, and factor VIII assay. *Management.* Seek expert advice. Avoid antiplatelet agents and IM injections. Major bleeding (hemarthrosis) requires factor VIII levels to be raised to 50% of normal. Life-threatening or CNS bleeding requires levels of 100% of normal. Both recombinant and plasma-derived factors are available. *Hemophilia B (Christmas disease)* is due to factor IX deficiency and behaves clinically like hemophilia A. *Liver disease* produces a complicated bleeding disorder, with ↓ clotting factor synthesis, dysfibrinogenemia, and ↓ clearance of circulating anti-coagulants. *Malabsorption* leads to ↓ absorption of vitamin K. Treatment: Vitamin K 10mg sq or FFP for acute hemorrhage.

The intrinsic and extrinsic pathways of blood coagulation

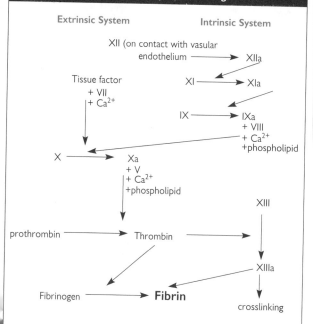

Extrinsic System   Intrinsic System

XII (on contact with vascular endothelium ⟶ XIIa

XI ⟶ XIa

Tissue factor
+ VII
+ Ca²⁺

IX ⟶ IXa
+ VIII
+ Ca²⁺
+phospholipid

X ⟶ Xa
+ V
+ Ca²⁺
+phospholipid

XIII

prothrombin ⟶ Thrombin

XIIIa

Fibrinogen ⟶ **Fibrin**

crosslinking

The fibrinolytic system The coagulation cascade simultaneously activates factors that result in fibrin dissolution by the activation of plasmin from plasminogen. The process starts by the release of tissue plasminogen activator (t-PA) from endothelial cells, a process stimulated by fibrin formation. t-PA converts inactive plasminogen to plasmin, which can then cleave fibrin, as well as several other factors.

Fibrinolytic agents

1 **Alteplase** (=rt-PA=Actilyse®; from recombinant DNA) is a fibrinolytic enzyme imitating t-PA, as above. Plasma t½ = 5min.

2 **Anistreplase** (=anisoylated plasminogen streptokinase activator complex =APSAC®) is a complex of human plasminogen and streptokinase (so anaphylaxis is possible). Plasma t½ = 90min.

3 **Streptokinase** is a streptococcal exotoxin and forms a complex in plasma with plasminogen to form an activator complex which forms plasmin from unbound plasminogen. Initially there is rapid plasmin formation which can cause uncontrolled fibrinolysis. However, plasminogen is rapidly consumed in the complex and then plasmin is only produced as more plasminogen is synthesized.

4 **Urokinase** is produced by the kidney and is found in urine. It also cleaves plasminogen.

Coagulation tests

Coagulation tests (Sodium citrate tube—beware of falsely elevated results if tube is incompletely filled or insufficiently mixed)

1 *aPTT*— activated partial thromboplastin time, measure of the intrinsic pathway. Prolonged by abnormalities in fibrinogen (I), II, VII, IX, X, XI, XII. Abnormalities can be qualitative (dysfibrinogenemia), quantitative (von Willebrand's disease, hemophilia) or acquired (heparin therapy, DIC, VIII antibodies). Also prolonged by the misnamed, lupus 'anticoagulant' as an artifact of cross-reaction with the lipid component of the test.

2 *Prothrombin time:* (PT) (expressed as a ratio compared to control: International Normalized Ratio, or INR—normal 0.9–1.2). Thromboplastin is added to test the extrinsic system. Prolonged by abnormalities in factors I, II, VII, X; warfarin, liver disease, or vitamin K deficiency.

3 *Thrombin time:* Thrombin is added to plasma to convert fibrinogen to fibrin. Prolonged in heparin treatment, DIC or dysfibrinogenemia. Reptilase time is similar to the thrombin time but is not affected by heparin, which can help distinguish heparin effect from other causes.

4 *Bleeding time:* A measure of platelet and vascular function. Prolonged in von Willebrand's disease, NSAIDs, uremia, all platelet numeric or functional defects, vascular problems (diabetes).

5 *Platelet aggregation studies:* Used to evaluate defects in platelet function. Abnormal in NSAIDs, congenital defects, myeloproliferative or myelodysplastic disorders.

6 *Mixing studies* and *Inhibitor screens:* Used for evaluating prolonged PT or aPTTs. If prolongation of the PT or aPTT is corrected by the addition of normal plasma, then a factor deficiency is established. If addition of normal plasma does not correct the clotting test, then inhibitors are suspected and further testing is required. Seek expert help for the evaluation and treatment.

Interpreting investigations into bleeding disorders

Disorder	INR	aPTT	Thrombin time	Platelet count	Bleeding time	Notes
Heparin	↔	↑↑	↑↑	↔	↔	
DIC	↑↑	↑↑	↑↑	↓	↑	FDP↑, (p576)
Liver disease	↑	↑↔	↑↔	↓↔	↔↑	↑LFTs
Platelet defect	↔	↔	↔	↔↓	↑	
Vitamin K def	↑↑	↑	↔	↔	↔	
Hemophilia	↔	↑↑	↔	↔	↔	p570
von Willebrand	↔	↑	↔	↔	↑	

Special tests may often be required. Consult a hematologist. FDP = fibrin degradation products.

Anticoagulants

Consider bleeding as a cause of any symptom in anyone on anticoagulants.

The main indications for anticoagulation
- Deep vein thrombosis/pulmonary emboli.
- To prevent embolism in atrial fibrillation or in those with mechanical heart valves.
- To prevent deep venous thrombosis/pulmonary emboli in high-risk patients (p405).

Types of anticoagulant *Standard unfractionated(~13,000 daltons)* heparin (IV or SC) is inexpensive, acts fast, and is monitored by the *activated partial thromboplastin* time (APTT). Heparin inactivates thrombin by binding to antithrombin III, leading to inactivation of coagulation enzyme Xa. Plasma infusion will not reverse the effect of heparin. *Low molecular weight heparin* preparations (5000 daltons, dalteparin, enoxaparin) $T_{1/2}$ are 2–4-fold longer than unfractionated heparin, and response is more predictable. It can be given once daily SC, no monitoring is needed, and can be used in the outpatient setting. Low molecular weight heparin inactivates factor Xa and its activity can be monitored by Xa levels. SE: Bleeding (at operative site, intracranial, retroperitoneal). CI: Uncontrolled bleeding/risk of bleeding (active peptic ulcer); endocarditis.

Warfarin. Warfarin inhibits the vitamin K dependent production of the coagulation factors II, VII, IX, and X, and the anticoagulants protein C and S. Warfarin has both a large volume of distribution and a very long $T_{1/2}$. Therapy is monitored with the INR. CI: Peptic ulcer; bleeding disorders; severe hypertension; liver failure; infective endocarditis; cerebral aneurysms; history of falls. Use with caution in the elderly and those with remote GI bleeds.

Beginning anticoagulation Heparin bolus (5000–10,000U IV over 5min) if anticoagulation is urgent, eg DVT, PE, unstable angina, MI. Giving a bolus is contraindicated (by convention) for stroke. *Infusion:* Start at 800–1400U/h. Check aPTT 4–6h after starting—aim for target of 1.5–2.5 times the upper limit of the control (target=60–80sec). Adjust as follows:[1]

PTT (sec)	Bolus (U)	Hold (min)	Rate change (U/h)	Repeat PTT
<50	5000	0	+120	4–6h
50–59	0	0	+120	4–6h
60–80	0	0	0	Next day
81–110	0	30	−50	4–6h
>110	0	60	−160	4–6h

- Start warfarin 10mg PO QD when aPTT is therapeutic on heparin. If the INR 18h after the first dose is <1.8 continue 10mg of warfarin; if INR >1.8, reduce to 5mg.
- Use the sliding scale below to keep INR in the target range. Do INR daily for 5d, then alternate days until stable, then weekly or less often.

INR	<2	2	2.5	2.9	3.3	3.6	4.1
Third dose	10mg	5mg	4mg	3mg	2mg	0.5mg	0mg
Maintenance	≥6mg	5.5mg	4.5mg	4mg	3.5mg	3mg	*

*Skip a dose; give 1–2mg the next day (if INR >4.5, skip 2 doses)
- Stop heparin when INR >2. Check platelet count if on heparin >5d.

Antidotes Consult a hematologist. Stop anticoagulation; if further steps needed, protamine sulfate can counteract heparin: 1mg IV neutralizes 100U heparin given within 15min. Maximum dose: 50mg (if exceeded, may itself have anticoagulant effect). For warfarin reversal or overdose, use phytomenadione (vitamin K): 5–10mg PO or SC for serious bleeding, 0.5–2mg for simple hematuria or epistaxis; consider 0.5mg if INR >7 without any bleeding. This takes some hours to act and may last for weeks. If serious bleeding, and INR↑, give a concentrate of activated clotting factors, activated VII or, if unavailable, infuse fresh frozen plasma.

---

1 Check with the guidelines established in your institution.

The target level represents a balance between too little anticoagulation (and risk of thrombo-embolism) and too much anticoagulation (risk of bleeding). Since the risks of thromboembolism vary with the clinical situation, optimum INR varies. Recommendations are likely to change as further trials are done: Check with a hematologist.

Choose a target INR within the range (not the range itself). This reduces the chance that the INR will stray outside the optimum range.

The incidence of fatal bleeding due to warfarin is 0.3/100 patient years. Severe bleeding is ~10-fold more common.

- Prosthetic heart valves. The degree of anticoagulation is dependent upon the location and type of prosthetic valve, the presence of atrial fibrillation or CHF, and the left atrial size. Aortic valves 2.5 (2–3) INR, mitral 3 (2.5–3.5). Caged-ball valves generally required higher INR.
- Atrial fibrillation: Important clinical parameters in determining thrombotic risk include congestive heart failure, hypertension, age >75, diabetes and previous stroke, TIA or systemic embolic event. For medium risk patients (1 or 2 risks), guidelines are an INR of 2–3, for higher risk, 2.5–3.5. An alternative for low-risk patients (0 risks) is aspirin, particularly if the risk of bleeding is high (serious co-morbidity, or difficulty with monitoring INR).
- Pulmonary embolism and above-knee DVT. Aim for INR of 2–3, and treat for 3–6 months (depends on risk of recurrence).

Leukemia and the resident

Patients with leukemia fall ill suddenly and can deteriorate rapidly. The most important acute issues are bleeding, infection and leukostasis. Unlike the differentiated cells in CLL and myeloproliferative disorders, where elevated cell counts are not usually dangerous in themselves, leukemic blasts are large and sticky, and can obstruct the small circulations in the lungs, heart, and brain. Leukemic blasts can also secrete substances that generate disseminated intravascular coagulation. Thus it is important not only to review the blood smear in patients presenting with elevated white cell counts to make the diagnosis of leukemia, it is also crucial to evaluate and treat leukemic patients who present with markedly elevated blast counts.

Neutropenic precautions and approach to febrile neutropenia: If the absolute neutrophil count is less than 500/mcL, then neutropenic precautions are as follows:
- Strict hand washing
- No rectal temperatures or unnecessary rectal examinations
- No IM injections
- Low-bacteria diet (fresh fruit and vegetables carry risk of pseudomonas)
- No fresh flowers
- Examine mouth, perineum, axillae, IV sites and indwelling catheter sites carefully
- Vital signs q 4h
- Culture urine, sputum, stool, blood (peripheral and catheter lines), CXR, CT of chest and sinuses, place PPD
- Oral candida prophylaxis

Antibiotic use in neutropenia: Treat known infections promptly. After cultures are drawn, start empiric antibiotics for fever >38.3°C or >38°C on separate occasions 1–2h apart. In the absence of fever, empiric antibiotics should also be given if the patient has hypotension, tachycardia, or a new oxygen requirement. The choice of antibiotic coverage should conform to organisms common in your community and hospital. Generally, an antipseudomonal penicillin or fourth generation cephalosporin with the addition of vancomycin (if line sepsis is suspected or if there is a high prevalence of community onset MRSA) is acceptable. Any suggestion of a fungal infection (sinusitis, thrush) mandates early antifungal therapy. If there are chest symptoms or significant hypoxia, additionally treat presumptively for pneumocytosis. Continue antibiotics until afebrile and neutrophils recover. If fever persists despite antibiotics, start antifungal therapy. If the patient has a defect in cell mediated immunity (AIDS, chronic immunsuppression for solid tumor or in the setting of bone marrow transplant) consider treatment for CMV. Recombinant human colony-stimulating factors (G-CSF, GM-CSF) usually are not useful in the treatment of neutropenic fever, although their use in individual cases may be indicated.

Hyperviscosity: If the white cell count is greater than 70–100,000/dL, WBC thrombi may form in the brain, lung, and heart. Emergent leukopheresis with concomitant high doses of cytoxan or hydroxyurea must be considered in patients with leukostasis.

Cell lysis syndrome: Hyperkalemia and hyperuricemia follows the massive destruction of cells from tumor necrosis and chemotherapy. Maintain a high urine output, alkalinize the urine, and give allopurinol before cytotoxic therapy.

Disseminated intravascular coagulation: Occurs in many leukemias and in particular, acute promyelocytic leukemia. DIC is the result of pathological thrombin formation, leading to inappropriate intravascular fibrin deposition, and platelet and clotting factor consumption. In addition to leukemia, DIC also occurs in malignancy, infection, trauma and in obstetrical disasters. DIC results in both small vessel clotting and bleeding and is associated with extensive purpura, oozing from venepuncture sites and bleeding in the brain, GI tract and lungs. The blood smear may identify schistocytes (red cell fragments). Fibrinogen and platelets are reduced, while PT, aPTT, and fibrin degradation products are elevated. Treatment of DIC includes reversal of the underlying medical condition, platelet and plasma support. Heparin may have a place in the treatment of DIC, but it is case and center dependent in its use. The use of all trans-retinoic acid (ATRA) has significantly reduced the risk of DIC in patients with acute promyelocytic anemia.

Acute lymphoblastic leukemia (ALL)

Many leukemias are associated with specific gene mutations, deletions, or translocations. ALL manifests as a neoplastic proliferation of lymphoblasts. The latest WHO classification of tumors divides ALL into precursor B lymphoblastic leukemia/lymphoblastic lymphoma and precursor T lymphoblastic leukemia/lymphoblastic lymphoma. However, the immunologic classification is still widely applied.

Immunologic classification
- *Common ALL:* 75%; defined by the presence of CD10 on the blasts. Any age may be affected, common in 2–4yr-olds.
- *T-cell ALL:* Any age but peaks in adolescent males, who present with a mediastinal mass and a high white cell count.
- *B-cell ALL:* Burkitt or Burkitt-like leukemia. Rare with a poor prognosis. Surface immunoglobulin present on the blasts.
- *Null cell ALL:* Undifferentiated, lacking the markers listed above.

Morphologic classification. The French American British (FAB) classification divides ALL into 3 types, L1, L2, L3, by microscopic appearance. It provides only limited information compared with other systems.

Signs & symptoms: Anemia, infection, bleeding, splenomegaly, lymphadenopathy, thymic enlargement, CNS involvement (cranial nerve palsies).

Common infections: Zoster, CMV, measles, candidiasis, pneumocystis pneumonia (p521), bacteremia. Consider immune globulin for patients in contact with measles or zoster when on chemotherapy.

Diagnosis: Characteristic cells in blood and bone marrow

Treatment
- *Supportive care:* Blood and platelet transfusions, IV antibiotics (p576) at first sign of infection (neutropenic regimen).
- *Chemotherapy:* As with most leukemias, patients are entered into clinical trials. A typical program is organized to achieve:
1 Remission induction: Vincristine, prednisone, L-asparaginase, and daunorubicin.
2 CNS prophylaxis: Intrathercal methotrexate; cranial irradiation
3 Consolidation: Courses of high dose chemotherapy for 2–3yrs. Relapse is common in blood, CNS and testes.

Hematological remission means no evidence of leukemia in the blood, a normal or recovering blood count, and less than 5% blasts in a normal regenerating bone marrow, and normal cytogenetics.

Bone marrow transplant (p579) is considered for patients with high risk leukemia (especially those with 9:22 translocation). Other poor prognostic indicators are adults, males, presentation with CNS signs or WBC greater than 100,000, B-cell phenotype. Cure rates in children are 70–90% while only 35% in adults and even worse in older adults. Future therapy will more specifically target leukemic cells according to their specific genetic defect.

Acute myeloid leukemia (AML)

AML arises from a normal marrow hematopoietic stem cell that has acquired genetic damage leading to aberrant proliferation and variable degrees of differentiation. It is a very rapidly progressive malignancy where survival is on the order of weeks to months if untreated.

Morphological classification is now based on the WHO criteria, which is complex and requires specialist interpretation. The WHO classification recognizes important prognostic information from cytogenetics and molecular genetics and includes five main types:
1 AML with recurrent genetic abnormalities
2 AML with multi-lineage dysplasia
3 AML and myelodysplastic syndromes, therapy related
4 AML not otherwise categorized
5 Acute leukemias of ambiguous lineage

Incidence is 1/10,000/yr and ↑ with age. AML is becoming more common as a consequence of high dose chemotherapy for both solid tumors and lymphoma.

Signs & symptoms: Anemia; infection (often Gram negative); bleeding; DIC; hepatosplenomegaly; lymphadenopathy; bone pain (sternal tenderness); leukemic infiltration of gums, testes and orbit; CNS involvement (cranial nerve palsies, cord compression).

Diagnosis: WBC is variable, and blasts are few in the peripheral blood of up to 1/3 of AML patients. Diagnosis relies therefore on bone marrow biopsy. Differentiation from ALL may be evident from microscopy, where presence of Auer rods is diagnostic for AML, but overall is secured by flow cytometric immunophenotyping and molecular methods. Molecular basis of the leukemia may dictate the specific type of treatment, and helps determine prognosis.

Complications: Infection, related both to the disease and complications of its therapy. Be alert to septicemia (p576). Oral infections are common. Both tumor lysis syndrome and leukostasis (p576) are common and must be treated.

Treatment: Supportive care: Red cell and platelet support, antibiotics, neutropenic precautions. AML itself can cause fevers, common organisms can present oddly, and candida and aspergillus are not uncommon.

Chemotherapy: Courses are intensive and include cytosine arabinoside and daunorubicin. Prognosis is better for younger patients and is also linked to specific lesions.

Bone marrow transplant: Allogeneic transplants from histocompatible siblings or from unrelated donors (accessed through national and international databases) may be indicated after remissions are obtained with chemotherapy. The idea is to destroy residual leukemic cells and the patient's own immune system with high dose cytoxan and total body irradiation, and then intravenously infuse the donor's marrow to replace the host's. BMT allows the most intensive chemotherapy regimens because marrow suppression is not an issue. Cyclosporin and methotrexate may be used to restrain the new immune system from attacking the patient's body (graft versus host disease). Complications of BMT include graft versus host disease (graft versus leukemia effect is very important to the overall success of BMT in AML); infections; venoocclusive disease; leukemia relapse. Prognosis: Allogeneic transplant survival may approach 60%. Autologous BMT in AML is intermediate between chemotherapy alone and allogeneic BMT; the role of reduced conditioning BMT is under study.

Chronic myeloid leukemia (CML)

CML is a hematopoietic stem cell disorder in which there is uncontrolled proliferation of well differentiated myeloid cells. It accounts for 15% of leukemias. As a myeloproliferative disorder (p585), it has features common to other myeloproliferative disorders including splenomegaly. However, given its unique molecular pathogenesis and natural history, it is considered separately from the other myeloproliferative disorders. It commonly presents with constitutional symptoms, but may be picked up inadvertently on routine blood work. It occurs most often in middle age with a slight male predominance.

Philadelphia chromosome (Ph[1]) A hybrid chromosome due to translocation between the long arms of chromosome 9 and 22 (t9:22). The translocation generates an oncogene, BCR/ABL, that constitutively signals within the cell, causing aberrant growth. The Philadelphia chromosome is present in granulocytes, platelet, and red cell precursors in >95% of those with CML. Those without the Philadelphia chromosome have a worse prognosis. Some patients have a masked translocation where standard cytogenetics do not reveal Ph[1], but the BCR/ABL oncogene can be detected by fluorescent in situ hybridization (FISH).

Symptoms and signs: Mostly chronic and insidiuous: Malaise, weight loss, gout, fever, night sweats, bleeding or abdominal pain. Splenomegaly, hepatomegaly, anemia, bruising.

Diagnosis: WBC is ofter markedly elevated, with an orderly left shift in the differential and an ↑ in basophils and eosinophils. Hb can be normal or low, platelets usually ↑. Leukocyte alkaline phosphatase (LAP) is reduced. Uric acid and alkaline phosphatase are ↑.

Natural history: Untreated median survival of 3–5yrs; three phases: Chronic, lasting months or years with few or any symptoms; accelerated phase, with ↑ symptoms, spleen size, and difficulty in controlling counts; blast crisis occurs uniformly and has features of acute leukemia.

Treatment

I Imatinib mesylate, a specific tyrosine kinase inhibitor, has revolutionized the management of CML. It is more effective than the previous gold standard therapy for CML, alpha-interferon, plus or minus cytarabine, in chronic phase patients. Imatinib therapy produced complete hematologic responses, major cytogenetic responses and complete cytogenetic responses in the majority of patients treated in chronic phase and improved survival over interferon when compared using historical controls. The drug is also effective in patients who have failed interferon and to some extent in both accelerated phase and blast crisis. Side effects include nausea, cramps, edema, skin rash, cytopenias and abnormal LFTs.

II The use of interferon in CML has declined dramatically with the introduction of imatinib, but it may still have a role in combination therapy.

III The role of allogeneic transplantation from a HLA matched sibling or unrelated donor must be reconsidered given the success of imatinib. This approach should be considered as first line therapy in patients in which transplant related mortality is estimated to be very low. Other patients should be offered a trial of imatinib first. The role of autologous transplantation, if any, remains to be defined in CML.

IV Treatment of transformed CML is difficult. While patients may respond to imtatinib, this is temporary. Some patients who develop a lymphoblastic transformation may respond to therapy as for ALL. Patients who develop a myeloblastic transformation rarely achieve lasting remission and allogeneic transplant offers the only hope of long term survival.

V Hydroxyurea is useful for palliative control of cell counts in patients who fail imatinib or interferon.

Chronic lymphocytic leukemia (CLL)

CLL is a monoclonal proliferation of small lymphocytes that are most frequently of B cell origin. CLL typically occurs in adults over 40yrs, with men more frequently affected than women. CLL comprises 25% of all leukemias, and is the most common hematopoeitic malignancy.

Staging correlates with survival:

0	Absolute lymphocytosis >15,000/mcL.
I	Stage 0 + enlarged lymph nodes.
II	Stage I + enlarged liver or spleen.
III	Stage II + anemia.
IV	Stage III + thrombocytopenia.

Symptoms: None in 25%, weight loss, bleeding, infection, anorexia.

Signs: Enlarged non-tender nodes, hepatosplenomegaly.

Blood smear: This is a diagnosis made by observing small, normal appearing lymph nodes, many of which fracture on the smear and are termed 'smudge cells'. May also be signs of autoimmune hemolytic anemia (spherocytes) or autoimmune thrombocytopenia (large platelets).

Complications: 1) Autoimmune hemolytic anemia 2) Infection—bacterial respiratory tract due to low immunoglobulin levels or viral due to altered cell mediated immunity 3) Bone marrow failure 4) Immune mediated thrombocytopenia.

Natural history: Some remain in Stage 0 for years without progressing. Usually, nodes slowly enlarge. Death is often via infection (pneumococcus, hemophilus, meningococcus, candida, aspergillosis) or transformation to aggressive lymphoma (Richter's syndrome).

Treatment Chemotherapy is often not required initially. Chlorambucil, effective in reducing WBC and node size ,was the mainstay of therapy, but is now being supplanted by rituxan, fludarabine and other agents in clinical trials. Steroids are useful in controlling autoimmune processes. Radiotherapy can be used for relief of lymphadenopathy or splenomegaly.

Supportive care: Transfusions, prophylactic antibiotics, immune globulin.

Prognosis is often good, depending on stage, age and molecular/immunological factors such as ZAP70 or CD38.

Hodgkin's lymphoma

Hodgkin's lymphoma (HL) is a cancer characterized by the presence of clonal malignant Reed–Sternberg cells within a reactive cellular background comprised of variable numbers of granulocytes, plasma cells, and lymphocytes. Reed–Sternberg cells are transformed B lymphocytes, many of which contain Epstein–Barr genome, suggesting an association of previous infection in the pathogenesis of HL in many patients.

Classification (in order of incidence)	Prognosis:
Nodular sclerosing	Good
Mixed cellularity*	Good
Lymphocyte predominant	Good
Lymphocyte depleted*	Poor

*Higher incidence and worse prognosis if HIV positive.

Clinical features The usual presentation is with enlarged, painless lymph nodes, usually in the neck or axillae. Rarely there may be alcohol-induced pain or features due to the mass effect of the nodes. 25% have constitutional symptoms such as fever, weight loss, night sweats (often drenching), pruritus, and loss of energy. If the fever alternates with long periods (15–28d) of normal or low temperature, it is termed a Pel–Ebstein fever (other causes of this rare fever: TB, renal cell cancer). *Signs:* Lymphadenopathy (note position, consistency, mobility, size, tenderness). Look for weight loss, anemia, hepatosplenomegaly.

Tests Lymph node biopsy for diagnosis. CBC, smear, ESR, LFTS, CXR, bone marrow biopsy, abdominal or or MRI scan. Lymphangiography is no longer used routinely. Staging laparotomy is performed if finding abdominal disease will change the therapy. It involves splenectomy with liver and lymph node biopsy.

Staging (influences treatment and prognosis.)

I   Confined to single lymph node region.
II Involvement of 2 or more regions on same side of diaphragm.
III Involvement of nodes on both sides of diaphragm.
IV Spread beyond the lymph nodes.

Each stage is subdivided into A (no systemic symptoms) or B—presence of weight loss >10% in last 6 months, unexplained fever >38°C or night sweats. These indicate more extensive disease. Pruritus is not a B symptom. Extranodal disease is indicated by a subscripted 'E' (eg IAE).

Treatment XRT for stages IA and (IA, Chemotherapy for IIA→IVB). HA patients with very large mediastinal masses also receive chemotherapy. Chemotherapy is given with an '*ABVD-type regimen (adriamycin, bleomycin, vinblastine, dacarbazine). Regimens containing nitrogen mustard such as MOPP are less common because of the frisk of sterility and secondary AML. Recently, more intensive regimens have been used, particularly for advanced disease. *Peripheral stem-cell transplantation:* Autologous or allogeneic transplantation of blood progenitor cells help restore marrow function after myeloablative therapy—as do agents which stimulate progenitor cells (eg filgrastim).

Complications of treatment Radiation-induced lung fibrosis and hypothyroidism. Chemotherapy—nausea, alopecia, infertility in men, infection due to myelosuppression, mucositis, and second malignancies, especially AML, breast cancer and non-Hodgkin's lymphoma. Autologous marrow transplant may help in relapses after chemotherapy or in previously irradiated sites.

5-yr survival Depends on stage and grade, ranging from >90% in IA lymphocyte predominant disease to <40% with IVB lymphocyte depletion.

Emergency presentations SVC obstruction—presents with JVP↑ a sensation of fullness in the head, dyspnea, blackouts, and facial edema. Arrange urgent XRT. High dose corticosteroids may also be useful.

Non-Hodgkin's lymphoma

This group includes all lymphomas without the Reed–Sternberg cell and is a very diverse group. Most are B-cell proliferations. Classification is complicated, but one helpful division is into low- and high-grade tumors. Low-grade lymphomas are more indolent but are incurable; the high-grade types are more aggressive, but long-term cure is achievable.

The low-grade group includes lymphocytic (comparable to CLL but mainly in lymphoid tissue), immunocytic, and centrocytic. The high grade lymphomas are the centroblastic, immunoblastic, and lymphoblastic.

Incidence has doubled since 1970 (to 1:10,000), perhaps from immunosuppression from sunlight exposure, HIV, HTLV-I, EBV.

The patient • Typically an adult with lymphadenopathy. • Extra-nodal spread occurs early, so presentation may be in skin, bone, gut, CNS, or lung. • Often asymptomatic. • Pancytopenia occurs (marrow dysplasia) ± hemolysis. • Infection is common. • Systemic symptoms as in Hodgkin's. Examine all over. Note nodes (if any is >10cm across, staging is advanced). Do ENT exam if GI lymphoma (GI and ENT lymphoma often coexist).

Tests, diagnosis, and staging As for Hodgkin's (staging is less important as 70% have widespread disease at presentation). Always do node biopsy, CXR, abdomen + pelvis CT, CBC, LFT, cytology of a pleural or peritoneal effusion, CSF cytology if CNS signs, or grade I or J below. **Grading** is problematic[1] NB: Survival is worse if elderly or symptomatic.

LOW	INTERMEDIATE	HIGH GRADE or SPECIAL*
A Small lymphocytic	D Follicular large	H Immunoblastic
B Follic. small cleaved	E Diffuse small cleaved	I Lymphoblastic*
C Follic. mixed cell	F Diffuse mixed	J Small noncleaved
	G Diffuse large cleaved (=Burkitt's)*	

B & G are most common; If HIV positive, the common type is J-like involving CNS, gut, marrow or liver.

Treatment Asymptomatic low-grade tumors may not need treatment and occasionally enter spontaneous remission; chlorambucil or cyclophosphamide may control symptoms. Radiation therapy can be used for local bulky disease. More aggressive disease requires combination chemotherapy, CHOP with Rituxan. Lymphoblastic lymphoma—treat as for ALL. Small noncleaved lymphomas are very aggressive and require extremely intensive therapy.

Burkitt's lymphoma This is a lymphoma occurring mainly in African children, although variants occur in the USA and Europe. It is associated with Epstein–Barr virus (EBV) infection and shows chromosomal translocations involving the immunoglobulin loci and the myc oncogene. Jaw tumors are common, usually with GI involvement. Histology shows a 'starry sky' appearance (isolated histiocytes on background of abnormal lymphoblasts). Spectacular remission may result from a single dose of a cytotoxic drug—eg cyclophosphamide.

---

1 The International Lymphoma Study Group has proposed a revised European-American classification of lymphoid neoplasla (REAL) which may be more biologically sound and more pragmatic than the above, but does away with the high-/low-grade dichotomy of the Kiel classification. The new system has the advantage of dealing with extra-nodal disease, eg of mucosa-associated lymphoid tissue—MALT (gastric MALT ls associated with *H. pylori*, and regresses when this is eradicated); it fully recognizes the heterogeneity of follicular lymphoma, and gets around the difficult distinction of diffuse large B-cell tumors into centroblastic and immunobkstic subtypes by appropriately ignoring it (it is of little clinical relevance). REAL also makes use of new genotypic analysis that can show immunoglobulin or T-cell receptor gene rearrangements, along with the association of particular lymphoma subtypes with specific chromosome breaks. Unfortunately, REAL increases the number of lymphomas it is possible to suffer from to 23. See N O'Connon 1995 *Lancet* **345** 1522 & N Harris 1994 *Blood* **84** 1361–92 & *Lancet* 1997 **349** 34&664.

Bone marrow failure

The bone marrow is responsible for hematopoiesis and, in adults, is found in the vertebrae, sternum, ribs, skull, and proximal long bones, although it may expand in anemia, eg thalassemia. All blood cells are thought to arise from an early, pluripotent stem cell which divides in an asymmetric fashion to provide a committed progenitor and other stem cells. Committed progenitors then undergo further differentiation before releasing formed elements into the blood. Bone marrow failure usually produces a pancytopenia, often with sparing of the lymphocyte count.

Causes of pancytopenia Aplastic anemia, hypersplenism, SLE, megaloblastic anemia, paroxysmal nocturnal hemoglobinuria, leukemia, myelodysplasia, drugs, liver disease.

Causes of marrow failure 1. Stem cell or erythroblast loss: Aplastic anemia—this can be toxic (eg drug, benzene), immunologic, congenital, viral (esp hepatitis B and parvoviruses) or idiopathic (most common). 2. Infiltration: From malignancy, infection (TB, MAI), 3. Fibrosis: Idiopathic myelofibrosis, HIV 4. Abnormal differentiation of a genetically damaged clone of cells, such as myelodysplastic syndromes, acute leukemia.

Aplastic anemia This presents as pancytopenia with a hypoplastic marrow (ie the marrow stops producing cells). Causes are idiopathic (50%), radiation, drugs (eg cytotoxics, chloramphenicol, anticonvulsants and gold), viruses, congenital.

Incidence: 10–20 per million per year. Presents as bleeding, anemia or infection. In approximately 50% of cases there is response to immunosuppressive therapy.

Treatment of aplastic anemia: Marrow transplantation is the best treatment for younger patients if there is a histocompatible sibling donor. In patients where transplantation in not feasible, immunosuppressive regimens are effective. Many patients respond to regimens incorporating cyclosporine, antithymocyte globulin or high dose cytoxan. Responses to androgens are rare.

Bone marrow support The symptoms of bone marrow failure are due to the pancytopenia. Red cells survive for ≈120d, platelets for an average 10d and neutrophils for 1–2d so early problems are mainly from neutropenia and thrombocytopenia.

Erythrocytes: A one unit transfusion should raise the Hb by about 1—3g/dL assuming that there are no antibodies.

Platelets: Spontaneous bleeding is unlikely if platelets >20,000/dL. Platelets require irradiation or leukocyte depletion prior to transfusion. Indications for transfusion are counts <10,000/dL and bleeding. One unit of fresh platelets should raise the count to >10,000/dL unless the patient is alloimmunized or febrile.

Neutrophils: Use 'neutropenic precautions' if the count is <500/dL. There is no role for neutrophil transfusions typically, although active fungal processes are exceptions.

Bone marrow biopsy Ideally an aspirate *and* biopsy should be taken. Biopsies may be taken from the posterior iliac crest, aspirates may be taken from anterior iliac crest or sternum. Thrombocytopenia is rarely a contraindication. Severe coagulation disorders may need to be corrected. Apply pressure afterward (lie on that side for 1–2h if platelets are low).

The myeloproliferative disorders

Polycythemia vera, essential thrombocytosis and idiopathic myelofibrosis are bone marrow disorders characterized by excess proliferation of myeloid elements—RBC, WBC, and platelets. These disorders are clonal hematopoietic stem cell disorders in which all of the circulating cells are derived from a transformed stem cell clone. The progeny of the aberrant stem cell differentiate and function normally. The 3 disorders share several features, including the fact that all may present with constitutional symptoms such as fever, weight loss, night sweats, pruritus, and malaise, and have varying degrees of extramedullary hematopoiesis, myelofibrosis and leukemic transformation. These disorders are closely related pathogenetically, many associated with a mutation in the JAK2 gene. These disorders are closely related clinically, with frequent disease evolution between different MPD subtypes over the years in a single patient.

Often these diseases are a 'panmyelosis' indicating that more than one cell line is ↑. This may generate diagnostic confusion, especially between essential thrombocytosis and polcythemia vera.

Erythrocytosis may be relative (plasma volume contraction) or absolute (↑ red cell mass). This distinction is made by red cell mass estimation using radioactive chromium. Relative erythrocytosis is often due to dehydration (alcohol or diuretics). Absolute polycythemia may be primary (polcythemia vera) or secondary from smoking, sleep apnea, chronic lung disease, tumors (fibroids, hepatoma, renal cell cancer), altitude, or rarely from high-affinity Hb.

Polycythemia rubra vera *Incidence:* 1.5/100,000/yr, peaks at 45–60yrs old. *Signs:* • elevated hemoglobin, white cells, or platelets variably affected • MCV normal or microcytic • Splenomegaly (60%). Presentation is determined by hyperviscosity (CNS signs, p576; angina; itching—typically after a hot bath) and WBC turnover (gout). It may also present with bruising, or detected incidentally after a routine CBC. *Diagnosis:* Red cell mass >125% of predicted (^{51}Cr studies). Leukocyte alkaline phosphatase (LAP) usually ↑. Erythropoietin levels are normal or low, O_2 saturation is normal. Treatment: Keep HCT <42% by phlebotomy. Iron deficiency may result from repeated phlebotomies. Hydroxyurea is used to control white cell or platelet counts if required (eg 10–20mg/kg/d PO). Prognosis: Variable—many often remain well for decades, but complications include extramedullary hematopoiesis, myelofibrosis, marrow failure, or leukemia. A particular risk is from thrombotic disorders which may derive from ↑ HCT and viscosity and/or activated white cells or platelets.

Essential thrombocytosis is defined as thrombocytosis (>600,000/mcL) in the absence of a defined stimulus, such as iron deficiency, inflammation, polycythemia vera, or idiopathic myelofibrosis. Platelet function can be abnormal and presentation may be by bleeding or thrombosis. Microvascular occlusion may lead to erythromelalgia (painful burning and erythema in fingertips and toes). *Treatment:* Hydroxyurea or anegrelide may be needed for symptoms or in high risk patients (age >60, previous thrombosis history, HTN, CAD); however, platelet count correlates poorly with the risk of thrombosis. Aspirin is useful, especially if there is any evidence of a thrombotic diathesis. Causes of a raised platelet count other myeloproliferative or inflammatory disorders, bleeding, malignancy, post-splenectomy, Kawasaki disease.

Idiopathic myelofibrosis There is intense marrow fibrosis with associated hematopoiesis in the spleen and liver (myeloid metaplasia, extramedullary hematopoiesis) causing massive splenomegaly. *Clinical features:* Variable—constitutional, splenomegaly, bone marrow failure. Smear: Leukoerythroblastic ; teardrop RBCs. Marrow tap: Dry. Treatment supportive (p584), iron and folate supplements ± splenectomy, consideration of stem cell transplantation. *Other causes of marrow fibrosis:* Any myeloproliferative disorder, lymphoma, secondary carcinoma, TB, leukemia (esp. megakaryoblastic (M7)) irradiation, SLE, HIV.

Myeloma

Myeloma is a plasma cell neoplasm which produces diffuse bone marrow infiltration and focal osteolytic lesions. An M component (M for monoclonal—not IgM) is seen on serum and/or urine electrophoresis.

Incidence 5/100,000. Peak age: 70yrs.

Classification Based on the principal neoplastic cell product:
• IgG   55%
• IgA   25%
• Light chain disease   20%.

IgD, IgE, and nonsecretory types are less common.

60% of IgG and IgA myelomas also produce free light chains which are filtered by the kidney and may be detectable as Bence Jones protein (these precipitate on heating and redissolve on boiling). They may cause renal damage or amyloidosis.

Clinical features • Bone pain/tenderness is common, often postural, eg back ribs, long bones, and shoulder. Occasionally presents as pathological fracture (but 25% have no clinical or X-ray signs of bone disease at presentation). • Fatigue (anemia, renal failure or dehydration). • Infection (poor Ig production). • Amyloid, • Neuropathy, • Viscosity: • Visual acuity-I ± hemorrhages/exudates on funduscopy. • Bleeding.

Diagnosis Abundant, clonally restricted plasma cells in marrow. Component M or urinary light chains on serum/urine electrophoresis (Bence Jones proteins) is supportive evidence. Other tests: CBC, ESR ↑, alk phos usually normal (unless healing fracture). Nonmyeloma immunoglobulins can be suppresed: Urea, creatinine, urate + Ca²⁺ ↑ in 30–50%. Bone X-rays: Punched-out lesions, osteoporosis.

Treatment Supportive: Bone pain, anemia and renal failure cause most symptoms. Give analgesia and transfusions PRN. Advise high fluid intake. Solitary lesions can be given XRT, and may heal. Bed rest tends to exacerbate hypercalcemia, so mobilization is important—this may require surgical stabilization of lytic lesions and analgesia. Pamidronate (and other newer bisphosphonates) and erythropoeitin are promising for reducing bone pain, hypercalcemia, and transfusion requirements.

Chemotherapy: None may be needed (none is curative), unless: HCT ↓ or
• Troublesome symptoms • Many osteolytic lesions • Impending fracture. • Creatinine >1.5mg/dL. • Marrow >30% plasma cells. • Serum beta-2 microglobulin >4mcg/mL. • More light chains in urine than creatinine (mcg/mL).

Optimal therapy is evolving but includes steroids, melphalan, thalidomide and other intensive chemotherapeutic regimens. The combination of vincristine doxorubicin and dexamethasone (VAD) induces remission more rapidly but does not affect survival. Autologous bone marrow transplant may offer an advantage over conventional therapy to younger patients (<65yrs). Eventually the disease becomes refractory. Monitor CBC and paraprotein.

Survival worse if BUN >28mg/dL or Hb <7.5g/dL.

Dangers
1 Hypercalcemia. Use IVNS 4–6L/d with careful fluid balance and furosemide. Consider steroids eg hydrocortisone 100mg IV q8h, Diphosphonates may be needed in refractory disease, calcitonin, mithramycin and gallium nitrate also may be useful.
2 Hyperviscosity—may need plasmapheresis.
3 Acute renal failure may be precipitated by IVP—therefore avoid IV contrast.

Paraproteinemia

Paraproteinemia refers to the presence in the circulation of immunoglobulin produced by a single clone of plasma cells or their precursors. The paraprotein is recognized as a sharp M component (M for monoclonal, not IgM) on serum electrophoresis. There are 6 major categories:

- *Multiple myeloma* (p586)
- *Waldenstrom's macroglobulinemia:* This is a lymphoplasmacytoid malignancy producing an IgM paraprotein, lymphadenopathy, and splenomegaly. CNS and ocular symptoms of hyperviscosity may occur. Chemotherapy and plasmapheresis (p588) may help.
- *Primary amyloidosis:* See below.
- *Monoclonal gammopathy* (monoclonal gammopathy of unknown significance or MGUS) is common (3% >70yr). In contrast to myeloma, in MGUS the paraprotein level is stable, immunosuppression and urine light chains are absent and there is little plasma cell marrow infiltrate.
- *Paraproteinemia in lymphoma or leukemia:* CLL.
- *Heavy chain disease:* Production of free heavy chains, causing malabsorption from infiltration of small bowel wall. It may terminate in lymphoma.

Amyloidosis

This is characterized by extracellular deposits of an abnormal protein resistant to degradation called amyloid. Various proteins, under a range of stimuli, may polymerize to form amyloid fibrils. They are shown with Congo Red staining (apple-green birefringence in polarized light).

Classification

- *Systemic:*
- Immune dyscrasia (fibrils of immunoglobulin light chain fragments, known as 'AL' amyloid).
- Reactive amyloid ('AA' amyloid—nonglycosylated protein).
- Hereditary amyloid (type I familial amyloid polyneuropathy).
- *Localized:* ↑Cutaneous. • Cerebral. • Cardiac. • Endocrine.

AL amyloid (primary amyloidosis) is associated with monoclonal proliferation of plasma cells—eg in myeloma. Clinical features include carpal tunnel syndrome, peripheral neuropathy, purpura, cardiomyopathy and macroglossia (a large tongue).

AA amyloid (secondary amyloidosis) is associated with chronic infections (eg TB, bronchiectasis), inflammation (especially rheumatoid arthritis) and neoplasia. It may affect kidneys, liver and spleen. Presents as proteinuria, nephrotic syndrome and/or hepatosplenomegaly.

The diagnosis of amyloidosis is made after Congo Red staining of affected tissue. The rectum is a common site for biopsy.

Treatment rarely helps, but AA amyloid may improve with treatment of the underlying disease.

A rare complication of amyloid is the intravascular adsorption of factor X, resulting in a prolonged PT and a serious coagulopathy.

Inflammatory markers (ESR and CRP)

The erythrocyte sedimentation rate (ESR) is a nonspecific indicator of the presence of inflammation. It measures the rate of sedimentation of RBCs in anticoagulated blood over 1h. If red cells are coated by proteins (such as IgG or fibrinogen) then the normal negative charge on the cell surface is masked and the cells will tend to stick to each other in columns (the same phenomenon as rouleaux on the blood smear, p560)—and so they will fall faster. The ESR rises with age and anemia. It is reduced in polycythemia, CHF, sickle cell anemia, trichinosis. Patients with a markedly raised ESR (>100mm/h) may have a serious malignancy, connective tissue diseases (eg giant cell arteritis), rheumatoid arthritis, renal disease, sarcoidosis, or infection.

C-reactive protein (CRP) is an acute-phase protein which is very helpful in the monitoring of inflammation. The best test is quantitative, normal <0.80mg/L. Like the ESR, it is raised in many inflammatory conditions but is much less sluggish in its response. It ↑ in h and falls within 2–3d of the inciting event. Therefore, it can be used to follow the response to therapy (eg antibiotics) or activity of disease (eg in Crohn's disease). If the CRP has fallen 3d after the onset of treatment for infection then the choice of antibiotics is probably appropriate.

CRP is raised by active rheumatic disease (rheumatoid arthritis, rheumatic fever, seronegative arthritis, vasculitis), tissue injury or necrosis (acute MI, transplanted kidney or bone marrow rejection, malignancies—esp. breast, lung, GI), burns, infection—bacterial≈viral. It is very useful for diagnosis of postoperative or intercurrent infections when the ESR may still be elevated. If the CRP has not started to fall 3d after surgery then complications must be considered (eg infection, PE). CRP is NOT raised by SLE, leukemia (fever, blast crisis, or cytotoxins), ulcerative colitis, osteoarthritis, anemia, polycythemia, or CHF. Its highest levels are seen in bacterial infections. Absence of an elevated CRP significantly reduces the pretest probability of other investigations for bacterial infection, eg bone or gallium scan, and so may be a cheaper, more comfortable alternative.

Hyperviscosity syndromes

These occur if the plasma viscosity rises to such a point that the micro-circulation is impaired. Usually relative viscosity >4 (four times the viscosity of water) is necessary to produce symptoms.

Causes; Myeloma (p586) (IgM and IgA ↑ viscosity more than the same amount of IgG because they are multimeric), Waldenstrom's macroglobulinemia, polycythemia. High leukocyte counts in leukemia may produce leukostasis, which differs from hyperviscosity per se.

Presentation: Visual disturbance, retinal hemorrhages, headaches, coma, and GU or GI bleeding.

The visual symptoms ('slow-flow retinopathy') may be described as 'looking through a watery windshield'. Other causes of slow-flow retinopathy are carotid occlusive disease and Takayasu's disease.

Treatment: Removal of as little as 1L of blood may relieve symptoms. Plasmapheresis is useful in the paraproteinemias, especially IgM, since it is mostly intravascular. Plasmapheresis for hyperviscosity due to IgG is usually less effective as it is deposited extravascularly.

The spleen and splenectomy

Splenomegaly is not uncommon and the differential diagnosis can be divided on the basis of the degree of splenic enlargement.

Massive splenomegaly: Myeloproliferative disorders (CML, PV, myelofibrosis), malaria (hyperreactive malarial splenomegaly), schistosomiasis, leishmaniasis, kala-azar, 'tropical splenomegaly' (idiopathic, in Africa and SE Asia)

Moderate splenomegaly: Infection (malaria, EBV, SBE, TB), portal hypertension, hemolytic anemia, hematologic malignancy (leukemia, lymphoma), splenic lymphoma, connective tissue disease (RA, SLE), glycogen storage diseases, common variable immunodeficiency, splenic cysts, idiopathic.

Splenomegaly can cause abdominal discomfort or more commonly pain in the left shoulder (because of the embryologic origin of the organ). It may lead to hypersplenism, defined as pancytopenia due to cells becoming trapped in the reticuloendothelial system (symptoms of anemia, infection, and bleeding). When faced with a mass in the left upper quadrant it is important to be able to recognize the spleen. The spleen moves with inspiration, enlarges toward the umbilicus, may have a notch, and 'you can't get above it' (the top margin disappears under the ribs). Ultrasound or CT may help in evaluation of the spleen. When hunting for the cause for enlargement look for lymphadenopathy and liver disease. Appropriate tests are CBC, ESR, LFTs and liver, lymph node or marrow biopsy. Aspiration or biopsy of the spleen are no longer performed.

The trend is to perform fewer splenectomies than in the past. Splenectomy may be indicated for splenic trauma or splenic cysts, or as therapy for autoimmune thrombocytopenia and autoimmune hemolytic anemia, or for the diagnosis and treatment of splenic lymphomas.

Post-splenectomy, there may be a prompt, dramatic, and transient rise in the platelet count, so patients should be mobilized early. All patients, especially children, remain at ↑ risk of infection, particularly pneumococcal septicemia. Most children are advised to take daily penicillin V until aged 20yrs. In adults, prophylaxis of 2–5yrs is recommended unless there is coexisting hematologic disease; broader spectrum agents such as amoxicillin may be more appropriate. Give adults and unvaccinated children pneumococcol (Pneumovax®) hemophilus (HiB) and meninngococcol A & C (Mengivac®) 2wks preoperatively. Warn asplenic travelers that they face an ↑ risk of tropical infections, and to adhere closely to antimalarial prophylaxis, while recognizing that is may not be effective. Counsel the patient to have standby amoxicillin to start at once if any symptoms of infection present, and to seek urgent hospital care.

Thrombophilia

Thrombophilia is a primary coagulopathy resulting in a propensity to thrombosis, and can be due to genetic predisposition or to acquired factors, or both. Thrombophilia is not rare, and needs special precautions in surgery, pregnancy, and immobilization.

Risk factors associated with venous thrombosis include stasis, inflammation, endothelial injury, and an imbalance between activated clotting factors and anticoagulants—these types of risk factors are primarily acquired and transient. While many genetic risk factors for thrombosis have been identified, they do not exert a strong effect in healthy individuals; in the setting of other acquired risks, however, they will strongly ↑ the risk of venous thrombosis.

Suspect a primary hypercoaguable state in a young patient presenting with unprovoked thrombosis. Suspicion grows if there is a personal or family history of recurrent arterial or venous thrombosis or first trimester spontaneous abortion.

Inherited thrombophilia. Acitvated protein C resistance (APC resistance) is the most common inherited risk for venous thrombosis. APC resistance is overwhelmingly due to a single nucleotide polymorphism in the factor V gene (Factor V Leiden) present in the carrier state in 5% of individuals of Northern European descent. Factor V Leiden renders factor Va resistant to cleavage by activated protein C and is associated with an mild ↑ risk of deep venous thrombosis in the heterozygous state and a marked ↑ in the homozygous state. The prothrombin 20210 polymorphism is present in approximately 2% of the Mediterranean population (carrier state) and is less strongly associated with ↑ risk of DVT than Factor V Leiden. Far less common are inherited deficiency states of antithrombin III, protein S, and protein C. *Treatment:* Those with a history of thrombosis and with inherited abnormalities should be considered for long-term anticoagulation.

Acquired thrombophilia. Common risk factors include venous stasis (after knee or hip replacement surgery), endothelial injury, congestive heart failure, bed rest, obesity, the post-operative state, indwelling catheters, cancer, heparin-induced thrombocytopenia, and certain blood disorders including myeloproliferative disorders, sickle cell anemia, PNH, and hemolytic anemias.

Cancer. There is a high risk of occult malignancy becoming evident within a year of seemingly unprovoked thrombotic events in patients less than 60yrs of age. It is not current practice, however, to investigate aggressively in a search for cancer in all patients with DVT, but rather to limit the investigation to age appropriate cancer screening. Trousseau's syndrome—migratory thrombophlebitis associated with visceral carcinoma—classically resists treatment with warfarin and requires unfractionated or low molecular weight heparin.

Antiphospholipid antibody syndrome is recurrent venous and/or arterial thrombotic events in association with an antiphospholipid antibody. There are two well-recognized aPL antibodies and three common ways of measuring them: The anticardiolipin antibody (measured with an ELISA or the dilute RVVT) and the lupus anticoagulant (a misnomer, it falsely prolongs the aPTT by interfering with the assay in vitro but is a procoagulant nonetheless) measured by the aPTT. aPL syndrome can be primary or associated with autoimmune disorders such as SLE. The annual risk of recurrent thrombosis after a confirmed thrombotic event in patients with an antiphospholipid antibody is approximately 30%. Warfarin anticoagulation with a target INR greater than 3 is effective in reducing thrombotic recurrences. Treatment during pregnancy includes both aspirin and heparin.

NB: Hypercoagulable studies performed at the time of a thrombosis can be misleading because of alterations of clotting factors due to acute illness or the thrombosis itself, and should be avoided.

Immunosuppressive drugs

Immunosuppressive drugs are used in organ and marrow transplants, rheumatoid arthritis, psoriasis, chronic hepatitis, asthma, giant cell arteritis, polymyalgia, SLE, PAN, and inflammatory bowel disease and many other autoimmune diseases.

Prednisone Steroids can be life-saving, but a number of points should be taken into consideration before initiating treatment.
- Hypertension, osteoporosis, and diabetes may be exacerbated by steroids.
- Do not stop steroids suddenly. Adrenal insufficiency may result, as endogenous production takes time to restart. p728.
- ↑ steroid dosing at times of illness/stress (eg flu or preop).
- Minimize side effects by using the lowest dose possible for the shortest amount of time. Give doses in the morning, and alternate days if possible, to minimize adrenal suppression.
- Before starting steroid treatment, extensively counsel your patient regarding the risks and benefits of steroids and the impact of steroids on their comorbidities.
- Avoid concurrent drugs bought over the counter, eg aspirin, ibuprofen; the danger is steroid-associated GI bleeds: If NSAIDs are essential ask the patient to come to you for advice. You might consider an NSAID combined with misoprostol, a prostaglandin analogue.
- Interactions: Antiepileptics (below) and rifampin.
- Strongly consider PCP prophylaxis in patients who are on other chemotherapeutic regimens, who require moderate steroid dosing for long periods of time or in patients who are otherwise immunocompromised.
- SE: TB reactivation, edema, osteoporosis, cataracts, euphoria, ↑ glucose, pneumocystis, UTI, toxoplasmosis, aspergillus, serious chicken pox/zoster, so avoid contacts (and so the need for varicella zoster immunoglobulin).
- Avoid pregnancy.

Azathioprine • SE: Peptic ulcer, marrow suppression, reduced WBC. Do CBCS.
- Interactions: Mercaptopurine and azathioprine (which metabolized to mercaptopurine) are metabolized by xanthine oxidase (XO). Azathioprine toxicity results if XO inhibitors (allopurinol) are co-administered. Genotype testing for thiopurine methyltransferase (TPMT) should be done prior to initiating azathioprine. Patients with low enzyme activity have ↑ risk of toxicity.

Cyclosporine Transplant patients usually require 6mg/kg/d; in other patients keep the dose <4mg/kg/d.
- Monitor UA and creatinine every 2wks for the 1st 3 months, then monthly if dose >2.5mg/kg/d (every 2 months if less than this). Reduce the dose if creatinine rises by >30% on 2 measurements even if the creatinine *is still in the normal* range. Stop if the abnormality persists.
- Monitor blood levels in transplant patients.
- SE: Nephrotoxicity, hepatotoxicity, edema, gum hyperplasia, tremor, paresthesia, hypertension, confusion, seizures, lymphoma, skin cancer.
- Interactions are legion. Cyclosporine is ↑ by ketoconazole, diltiazem, nicardipine, verapamil, oral contraceptives, erythromycin. Cyclosporine is ↓ by barbiturates, carbamazepine, phenytoin, rifampin. Avoid concurrent nephrotoxics: Gentamicin, amphotericin. Concurrent NSAIDS augment hepatotoxicity: Monitor LFTS.

Methotrexate Inhibits dihydrofolate reductase, which is involved in the synthesis of purines and pyrimidines. • SE: Hepatitis, lung fibrosis, CNS signs, teratogenicity.
- Methotrexate is ↑ by NSAIDs, aspirin, penicillin, probenecid.

Cyclophosphamide
- SE: Carcino- and teratogenic, hemorrhagic cystitis, marrow suppression.

Geriatric medicine

Colleen Christmas, M.D.

Contents

What is special about geriatric patients?

Many aspects regarding older adults make them a challenging and rewarding patient population to work with. Most of the care of older adults consists of chronic disease management. The course of their medical conditions will be punctuated by episodes of exacerbation of acute illness. With each successive exacerbation, prognosticating the amount of recovery becomes increasingly difficult. Another challenge in providing care to geriatric patients is that quality of life, risks of treatment, and functional disability take on greater importance in making treatment decisions.

Geriatric patients represent an incredibly heterogeneous group demographically and physiologically. From person to person the effects of lifestyle, genetic, and environmental factors produce variable results in aging of different organ systems. While one octogenarian may be active, driving, caring for grandchildren, and have well-controlled chronic conditions, the next may be severally debilitated, dependent on others for most of their care needs, and profoundly cognitively impaired. Thus the approach to geriatric patients is that it must be highly individualized.

The final principle to be considered in caring for older adults is that of intrinsic vulnerability. While exercise may ameliorate some of the adverse affects of aging on most organ systems, even the very healthy aged suffer from a reduced ability to withstand physiologic perturbation. Examples of this may include glucose metabolism that appears normal during usual situations but becomes abnormal with mild disturbance, such as a urinary tract infection. This dictates a requirement to 'stay on your toes', treat gingerly, and frequently reassess the impact of interventions in geriatric patients.

The elderly patient in the hospital

It is only in the last 200yrs that life-expectancy has risen much above 40yrs. *An aging population is a sign of successful social, health, and economic policies.*

Beware of agism. Old age is associated with disease but doesn't cause it. Any deterioration is from treatable disease *until proven otherwise.*

1 Contrary to stereotype, most old people are fit. 95% of those >65yrs and 80% of those >85yrs old do not live in institutions; about 70% of the latter can manage stairs and can bathe without help.

2 With any problem, find the cause; resist temptation to think: *This is simply aging.* Look (within reason) for treatable disease, ↓ fitness, and social factors.

3 Do not restrict treatment simply because of age. Old people vary. Age alone is a poor predictor of outcome and should not be used as a substitute for careful assessment of each patient's potential for benefit and risk.

Characteristics of disease in old age There are differences of emphasis in the approach to old people compared with young people.

1 *Multiple pathology:* Several disease processes may coincide: Find out which impinge on each complaint (eg senile cataract + arthritis = falls).

2 *Multiple causes:* One problem may have several causes. Treating each alone may do little good; treating all may be of much benefit.

3 *Non-specific presentations:* Some presentations are common in old people—incontinence; immobility; instability (falls); and delerium/confusion. Any disease may present with these. Also, typical signs and symptoms may be absent (MI without chest pain; pneumonia, but no cough, fever, or sputum).

4 *Rapid worsening if treatment is delayed:* Complications are common.

5 *More time is required for recovery:* Impairment in homeostatic mechanisms leads to loss of 'physiological reserve'.

6 *Impaired metabolism and excretion of drugs:* Doses may need lowering, not least because there is often less tolerance to side effects.

7 *Social factors:* These are central in aiding recovery and return to home.

Special points in caring for the elderly

In the history: Assess all disabilities, then:
- *Home details* (eg stairs; access to toilet?).
- *Medication* What? When? Assess understanding and concordance. How many different tablets can they cope with? Which are the most important drugs? You may have to ignore other desirable remedies, or enlist the help of a friend, a spouse, or a pharmacist (who can batch morning, noon, and night doses in compartmentalized containers so complex regimens may be reduced to 'take the morning compartment when you get up, the noon compartment before lunch, etc.').
- *Social network* (regular visitors; family and friends).
- *Care details* What services are available?—Meals delivered; home care nurse; community psychiatric agency; physical therapist—who else is involved in the care? Speak to others (relatives; loved ones, neighbors; caregivers; personal physician).

On examination:
- Do BP lying and standing (postural hypotension may lead to falls).
- Rectal exam: Impaction may lead to overflow incontinence.
- Detailed CNS examination is often needed, eg if presentation is non-specific.

Make a care plan:
- Include nutrition. Is the patient able to eat the food that is delivered?
- Involve a multi-disciplinary team. The physician cannot be expected to cover all of the bases, so should rely on other health care professionals and their expertise.

Beyond the hospital: Planning successful discharges (how to live and be frail in the community)

Start planning discharge from day 1. A very common question on rounds is: 'Will this patient do OK at home?—we've got them as good as we can, but is discharge safe?' In answering this take into account:

- Most patients want to go home promptly. If not, find out why.
- Is the home suitable for a frail person? Stairs? Toilet on same floor?
- If toilet access is difficult, can they transfer from chair to commode?
- Can they open a can, use the phone, turn on a microwave, cook soup?
- Does the patient live alone?
- Does the caregiver have family support? Is he/she already exhausted by other duties (eg young children at home)?
- Is the family supportive—in theory or in practice?
- Are the neighbors friendly? 'But I would not trouble them.'
- Are social services and community geriatric services well integrated? Proper *case management programs* with defined responsibilities, entailing integration of social and geriatric services really can help.

Frailty, falls, and postural hypotension

Frailty is a syndrome that best incorporates the notion of ↑ vulnerability to insults and subsequent exaggerated effects of insults. A phenotype has been described[1] where 3 or more of 5 recognized characteristics describe this syndrome:
- Unintended weight loss of 10 or more pounds over the previous 12 months.
- Poor grip strength.
- Self-reported poor endurance and exhaustion.
- Slow walking time.
- Low physical activities level .

Studies demonstrate that frailty is ↑ with aging and is associated with higher rates of health care utilization, disability, and mortality[1].

The biologic mechanisms contributing to the development of frailty are just beginning to be unraveled, with the hopes that discovery of such mechanisms will lead to interventions that favorably alter the clinical course.

Falls are common (30% of those >65yr fall in a year) and this may be the start of a fatal course of events. There are many causes. 10% are related to loss of consciousness or dizziness. For most, there is no clear single cause, and many factors compete.

History: Exact circumstances of fall. Find out about any CNS, cardiac, or musculoskeletal abnormalities. Drugs, eg causing: Postural hypotension; sedation; arrhythmia, eg tricyclics; parkinsonism, eg neuroleptics, including metoclopramide and prochlorperazine. Alcohol.

Examination: For causes: Postural hypotension; arrhythmias; detailed neurological examination, including cerebellar signs, parkinsonism, proximal myopathy, gait, watch patient get up from chair, test for Romberg's sign; mechanical instability in knees.

Consequences: Cuts; bruises; fractured ribs (± pneumonia) or limbs, especially neck of femur; head injury (± subdural hematoma).

Management: The patient's confidence may be shattered even if there is no serious injury. Look for causes and treat. Consider physical therapy—include learning techniques on how to get up from floor. Occupational therapists may advise on reducing household hazards, and adding aids. Exercise and balance training can prevent falls.

Postural hypotension is important because it is common and a cause of falls and poor mobility. Typical times are after meals, on exercise, and on getting up at night. May be transient with illness (eg flu).

Causes: Leg vein insufficiency; autonomic neuropathy; drugs (diuretics, nitrates, antihypertensives, antidepressants, sedatives). Red cell mass may be low. *Management:* Reduce or stop drugs if possible. Counsel patient to stand up slowly in stages. Try compression stockings. Reserve fluid-retaining drugs fludrocortisone 0.1mg PO daily, ↑ as needed) in those severely affected when other measures fail.

1. Fried LP, Tangen CM, Walston JB, *et al.* 2001. Frailty in older adults: evidence for a phenotype. *J Gerontol* **56** M146.

Impairment, disability, and stroke rehabilitation

Doctors are experts at diagnosing disease and identifying impairment. But we are slow to see the patient's perspective. Considering the concepts of impairment and disability may help.

Impairment refers to systems or parts of the body that do not work. 'Any loss or abnormality of psychological, physiological or anatomical structure or function.'[1] For example, following stroke, paralysis of the right arm or aphasia would be impairment.

Disability refers to things people cannot do. 'Any restriction or lack (resulting from an impairment) of ability to perform an activity in the manner, or within the range, considered normal for a human being.'[1] For example, following stroke, difficulties in 'activities of daily living' (eg with dressing, walking).

Making use of these distinctions Two people with the same impairment (eg right hemiparesis) may have different disabilities (eg one able to dress, the other unable). The disabilities are likely to determine the quality of the person's future. Treatment may usefully be directed at reducing disabilities. For example, Velcro® fasteners in place of buttons may enable a person to dress.

Three stages of management

Assessment of disability: Traditional 'medical' assessment focuses on disease and impairment. Full assessment requires a thorough understanding of disability. Discuss detailed assessments with expert therapists, the patient, and relatives to help define their problems.

Who can help? Hospital doctors are part of a large team. Involve other members of the team early, including nurses, occupational and physical therapists, social workers, and the primary care physician. Also, there are self-help organizations for most chronic diseases aimed both for patients and their care-givers.

Generate solutions to problems: A list of disabilities is the key. Rehabilitation should look at each disability (eg unable to undress). Uncover the origin of the disability (in terms of disease and impairment). Mutual goals should be agreed upon with the patient and relatives in accordance with their wishes. At every visit, review, renew, and adapt goals.

Rehabilitation after stroke

▶Good care consists of attention to detail. The principles of rehabilitation are those of any chronic disease and are best carried out in specialist inpatient stroke units (they reduce morbidity and institutionalization).

Special points in early management: Watch the patient drink a glass of water: If they cough or gag, they should be kept NPO for several days.

▶*Maintenance IV fluids should (almost) always be ordered at the same time as making someone NPO.* The optimal use of nasogastric (NG) and percutaneous endoscopic gastrostomy (PEG) tubes is controversial though a randomized clinical trial demonstrated no benefit compared to NPO in the 1st week after a dysphagic stroke. Consider consulting with the speech and swallowing service.

Avoid injuring the extremities of patient through careless lifting.

Ensure good bladder and bowel care through frequent toileting. Avoid early catherization, which may prevent return to continence.

Position the patient to minimize spasticity.

1 WHO 1989 Tech Report No 779, *Health of the Elderly*

Urinary incontinence

Incontinence is never normal though it occurs in up to 30% of the elderly at home and 50% in long-term care. It is transient in 30%–40% of patients and the causes are multiple and frequently coexist.

Intrinsic urinary tract malfunction can result in: *Detrusor overactivity*, involuntary contractions of the bladder, *detrusor underactivity*, failure of adequate bladder contraction, *stress incontinence*, abnormally low urethral resistance, or *obstruction*, abnormally high urethral resistance.

Causes of transient incontinence are often (but not always) outside the urinary tract. Remember *'DIAPPERS'*: **D**elirium; **I**nfection of the urine (not asymptomatic bacteriuria); **A**trophic urethritis and vaginitis (responds to estrogen); **P**harmaceuticals (sedatives, anticholinergics, antipsychotics, antidepressants, narcotics, α-adrenergics, diuretics, ACE inhibitors), **P**sychological (severe depression); **E**xcess urine (↑ input; ↑ production—diuretics, EtOH, ↑ glucose, ↑ calcium; mobilized peripheral edema), **R**estricted mobility (arthritis, pain, gait disorders), **S**tool impaction.

Points in the history Urgency (the abrupt need to void or a spontaneous emptying of the bladder without warning) suggests detrusor overactivity. Leakage during stress maneuvers (eg coughing, laughing, sneezing) suggests ↓ urethral resistance. Prostatism suggests obstruction. Ask about other medical illnesses—cancer, DM, UTIs, h/o pelvic XRT. A 2-7-d voiding diary is useful. The patient should record the time, volume, situation and associated symptoms whenever urine is passed.

Physical examination A comprehensive physical examination is vital. Look for abnormal affect, functional impairment (eg ↓ mobility, vision, etc), CHF, orthostasis, peripheral edema, atrophic vaginitis. Test perianal sensation and reflexes (anal wink, S4–5; bulbocavernosus, S2–4). Do a rectal exam for resting and voluntary anal tone, fecal impaction and prostate enlargement. The cough stress test is useful (especially in women). Check the post-void residual (PVR) by in/out, 'straight' catheter or ultrasound estimation, after a voluntary void (normal: <50–100mL).

Investigations Chemistry panel, CA^{2+}, urinalysis and culture. In selected patients, consider renal U/S, urine cytology, urodynamic studies.

Treatment is aimed at the cause. Specific measures may include: Altered timing of medications, compression stockings during the day to ↓ nocturnal mobilization of edema, and behavioral techniques such as frequent voiding (eg Q2–3h—refer to the voiding diary for guidance) to avoid bladder overdistention and involuntary contraction. Pelvic floor, or 'Kegel' exercises (voluntary contraction of the external urethral sphincter for 10 seconds x ~50/d) can help stress incontinence in women. Drugs with anticholinergic or α-adrenergic antagonist activity may be useful (see table opposite). Surgery, prostheses (eg penile clamps), intravaginal pessaries, external collecting devices (indwelling or condom catheters) and absorbent pads are reserved for refractory incontinence.

Complications Perineal rash, decubitus ulcers, indwelling catheters and UTIs, social stigmatization, anxiety/depression, ↓ sexual activity, institutionalization.

Drugs for urinary incontinence Start with the lowest dose, then titrate up until symptoms improve or intolerable side effects develop. The expected benefits are small.

Detrusor overactivity	
Propantheline	7.5–30mg PO 3–4 times a day
Oxybutynin	2.5–5mg PO 3–4 times a day
Imipramine	25–50mg PO 1–3 times a day
Stress incontinence	
Phenylpropanolamine	25–50mg PO 2–3 times a day
Outlet obstruction	
Prazosin	1–2mg PO 2–4 times a day
Phenoxybenzamine	5–10mg PO daily (for short-term use only)

Polypharmacy

Geriatric patients disproportionately consume prescription and non-prescription medications. Additionally, geriatric patients have poorer tolerance for adverse drug effects and more commonly suffer from the harms of medications than their younger counter parts. Thus trying to minimize the total number of drugs consumed is both a laudable and a formidable goal.

Drugs that should be avoided because safer alternatives exist include COX-2 inhibitors and non-COX specific NSAIDs and meperidine. Benzodiazepines and non-benzodiazepine sleeping agents should be avoided for insomnia. Drugs to treat Alzheimer's disease have demonstrated little, if any, meaningful clinical benefit; their use should be considered carefully as a trial in an individual. Atypical antipsychotics do not offer benefit over older, less expensive agents for behavioral problems in dementia. Finally, any new drug must also be very carefully considered. In seeking FDA approval for release, must drugs have not been tested on the average geriatric patient with multiple comorbidities and medications. Most certainly they have not been tested on the most frail elderly. Only after a drug has been on the market and used in large numbers of 'average' people do many of the serious toxicities become apparent. Many elderly are seriously injured as the result of new medications. Adhere to the adage, 'start low, go slow' with any new medicine.

Costs, ability to take, and potential toxicity are important determinants in selecting drugs. Opportunities to get 'double duty' from medications should be explored. For example, a person with neuropathic pain and depression may derive good benefit from nortriptyline at bedtime for both of these problems rather than gabapentin 3 times a day and an SSRI once a day.

Finally, the selection of medications must consider the overall treatment goals for each individual and whether or not data exists that the considered medication will reasonably further those goals.

Examination of mental state

The examination of cognitive functions is important in every patient. Much can be accomplished by careful observation during the course of the history and physical examination. For more detailed assessment of specific cognitive functions, you should have a set of questions (and tasks) with which to test the patient. Use these whenever an altered mental state is contributing to the clinical problem. A description of each of the tests performed, and the patient's response, is more useful for the clinical record than a 'score' on a question set. Before starting, tell the patient that you are going to test their thinking. Reassure them that it is a standard part of the examination.

Components of the mental state examination

Level of arousal Eg, alert, drowsy, asleep but responds to voice/touch/gentle shake/pain. Rouses for x seconds, then falls back to sleep.

Orientation Ask the patient's name, the place where you are located, and the time (day of the week, date, month, year, season).

Attention Recite months of the year forward and backward. If unable try days of the week, the word 'world'.

Memory distant Names of children, where they grew up, jobs. *Recent* Describe news events, details of recent illness, dinner last night. *Learning* Give 3 objects to remember (eg 'glass, a duck, and a shoe'). Make sure they can repeat them without prompting after a 30s delay without distractions. Ask them again in 3–5min (don't forget!).

Speech Fluency, naming, repetition, comprehension.

Calculation Serial 7s. How many quarters in $1.50? Nickels in $1.10? Simple addition, multiplication, etc.

Reading Read aloud (eg lunch menu), then describe what they read.

Writing Write a sentence, eg about the weather.

Construction Draw the numbers inside a circle as if it were a clock. Copy intersecting pentagons. Copy a cube.

Left/right discrimination

Praxis Salute. Pretend to comb, roll dice, deal a pack of cards.

'Frontal' functions Copy a sequence of 3 hand movements; *Go/No-go task*: 'Every time I tap my hand twice, you tap once. When I tap once, you do nothing.' *Word lists*: 'In one minute, tell me all of the words that you can think of that begin with the letter F.'

Cortical sensation Graphesthesia Ask the patient to identify numbers, drawn in each palm. *Stereognosis* identify objects (eg comb, quarter, nickel, pen) placed in each hand without looking. Note: These terms refer to normal functions. 'Agraphesthesia' and 'astereognosis' are abnormal.

Sometimes a complex multidimensional question can be used as a screening test for cognitive dysfunction. For example:

600

'Pretend that you are looking at a clock. The little hand is on the 7 and the big hand is on the 3. What time will it be in 15min?'

A correct response on this task ('7:30') requires many faculties, including attention, language comprehension, calculation, visual memory, and construction. In selected patients, in whom mental state is not the issue, this may be sufficient to satisfy yourself that there are no gross cognitive abnormalities. ►Never document that the mental status is normal unless you have tested it.

Approach to dementia

▶An altered mental state is due to a treatable illness until proved otherwise.

Dementia is not a part of normal aging. It is a syndrome, with many causes, of progressive impairment of cognition with the preservation of clear consciousness.

Clinical features The key to diagnosis is a good history (usually requiring an informant) of progressive impairment of memory and other cognitive functioning, together with objective evidence of such impairment. The history should go back at least several months, and usually years. Typically the patient has become increasingly forgetful, and has performed normal tasks (eg cooking, shopping, finances, work) with ↓ competence. Sometimes the patient appears to have changed personality eg uncharacteristically rude or aggressive.

Points in the history

• Baseline personality, education, profession • Duration of illness • Onset (abrupt or insidious) • Comorbid disease • PMH: Poor nutrition, head trauma, depression or other psychiatric illness • Medications (incl. PRNs) • Toxins (occupational, EtOH) • Risk factors for infections (HIV, syphilis) • Family history of depression, dementia or other degenerative disease

Epidemiology Incidence ↑ with age. Very rare <55yr. 5–10% prevalence >65yr; up to 50% >85yr. In the USA there are ~4 million people with Alzheimer's disease at a cost of ~$90 billion/yr year.

Causes Definitive diagnosis requires a pathological specimen (biopsy or autopsy). Premorbid diagnoses are often mistaken. *Alzheimer's disease (AD)* is the most common cause of dementia (55–70% of all cases). *Vascular dementia:* 5–25% of all cases. Essentially multiple small strokes. Usually evidence of vasculopathy (high BP, previous strokes); sometimes of focal neurological damage; onset sometimes sudden and deterioration may be 'stepwise.' Optimize vascular risk factors. *Lewy body disease* is characterized by Lewy bodies in the brainstem and cortex. There are fluctuating but persisting cognitive deficits, parkinsonism, and hallucinations.

Less common causes HIV (*not uncommon* in those known to have HIV); progressive multifocal leukoencephalopathy; Pick's disease; progressive supranuclear palsy; Parkinson's disease; Jakob-Creutzfeldt disease; Huntington's disease; Wernicke–Korsakoff disease.

Initial assessment *For all patients with progressive dementia*: Careful history (as above); CNS exam (including mental state); CBC, ESR, chemistry, TSH, B₁₂, syphilis serology, drug levels; CT or MRI of the brain. *For selected patients*: Neuropsychology testing; psychiatric examination; EEG; HIV testing; LP; toxic screen.

Management Treat any treatable cause. Treat concurrent illnesses (these may contribute significantly to confusion). In most people the dementia remains and will progress. Involve relatives and social services.

Potentially treatable dementias

The frequency of reversible dementias that present to memory specialists is somewhere between 0% and 30%. The reason to investigate dementia is to find one of the causes that can be fixed.

Drug toxicity Check *all* medications.

Chronic metabolic disturbance Organ failure (heart, kidney, liver, lungs); Wilson's disease; obstructive sleep apnea; dialysis encephalopathy (?aluminum toxicity); heavy metals (eg lead).

Normal pressure hydrocephalus is thought to be due to impaired CSF absorption, causing dementia, gait apraxia, and urinary incontinence. Disproportionately large ventricles on CT/MRI. Diagnosis is difficult to confirm, though some patients benefit from CSF shunts (eg ventriculoperitoneal). Good prognosticators for response to shunting include: Short duration of symptoms; more prominent gait disorder than dementia; known etiology (eg history of subarachnoid hemorrhage, head trauma); altered CSF dynamics (with invasive monitoring).

Intracranial mass Tumors (especially meningiomas); subdural hematoma.

Infection Syphilis; Lyme; chronic meningitis (TB, fungal, parasitic).

Connective tissue disease SLE; sarcoidosis; primary angiitis of the CNS and other vasculitides.

Endocrine Hypo-/hyperthyroidism; parathyroid; adrenal and pituitary disease; insulinoma.

Nutritional Deficiencies of B_{12}, nicotinamide (pellagra), thiamine.

Psychiatric Pseudodementia of depression.

Alzheimer dementia (AD)

This is the worst neuropsychiatric disorder of our times. Suspect Alzheimer's disease in adults with any persistent, acquired deficit of memory and cognition—eg as revealed in the mental test score and other neuropsychometric tests. Onset may be from 40 years (or earlier, eg in Down's syndrome)—so the notions of 'senile' and 'pre-senile' dementia are irrelevant.

Diagnosis is often haphazard. Specialist assessment with neuroimaging for all would be ideal (this would help rule out frontal lobe and Lewy body dementias, and Pick's disease).

Histology (rarely used)
- Deposition of β–amyloid protein in cortex (a few patients have mutations in the amyloid precursor protein).
- Neurofibrillary tangles and an ↑ number of senile plaques.

Presentation Early (stage I) in AD there is failing memory and spatial disorientation. In stage II (follows after several years) personality changes (eg ↑ aggression and focal parietal signs—dysphasia, apraxia, agnosia, and acalculia). Parkinsonism may occur. In stage III the patient becomes apathetic, wasted, bedridden and incontinent. Seizures and spasticity are common. **Mean survival** 7 years from onset.

Management *Theoretical issues:* Potential strategies:
- Preventing the breakdown of acetylcholine, eg donepezil, below.
- Augmenting nerve growth factor (NGF), which is taken up at nerve endings, and promotes nerve cell repair.
- Stimulating nicotinic receptors which may protect nerve cells.
- Inhibition of the enzymes that snip-out β–amyloid peptide from amyloid precursor protein (APP), so preventing fibrils and plaques.
- Anti-inflammatories to prevent activation of microglial cells to secrete neurotoxins (eg glutamate, cytokines) which stimulate formation of APP.
- Regulation of calcium entry (mediates the damage of neurotoxins).
- Preventing oxidative damage by free radicals.

603

Practical issues: Treat concurrent illnesses (they contribute significantly to confusion). In most people the dementia remains and will progress. Involve relatives and community services.

Consult with an expert; if the dementia is mild or moderate, consider ↑ acetylcholine availability by inhibiting acetylcholinesterase (eg donepril 5mg PO every night at bedtime, ↑ to 10mg after 1 month). Effects may be minimal, but subtle cognitive changes can cause significant behavioral improvement even without 'objective' ↑ in bedside tests of cognition. The need for institutional care may be delayed.

Prevention There are no clear ways to avoid this disease. HRT and controlling vascular risk factors may offer some protection.

Preventive geriatrics

Although even the most fit elderly will have continued declines in most organ systems with aging, evidence clearly supports that exercise can ameliorate many of these losses substantially. It may help improve range of movement and function and ↓ pain associated with knee osteoarthritis. It has been shown to both treat osteoporosis and in retrospective studies prevent osteoporosis. Exercise, particularly exercises that incorporate some aspect of balance training, have been shown to reduce falls, even in high- risk individuals. As with their younger counterparts, exercise may lower BP and favorably alter lipid profiles. Clearly the most fit individuals tend to have the longest life expectancy and longest period of functional independence. Epidemiologic studies demonstrate that improving fitness state is associated with beneficial effects on mortality, even when this change is enacted in older age.

Though the best exercise regimen has not been firmly established, most elderly are remarkably sedentary and will gain substantially simply from reducing their inactivity by altering lifestyle. Examples of this include watching less television, taking the stairs rather than the elevator, parking further away from the entrance of stores, and walking up and down every aisle in the grocery store. Walking is an inexpensive exercise that has functional relevance. The physician may assist in improving fitness by endorsing exercise and identifying barriers and facilitators to exercise with patients.

Most authorities endorse screening examinations for older individuals similar to those of younger individuals when the projected life expectancy is greater than 5yrs and when such screening (and subsequent decisions based on the results) is consistent with the overall goals of care of the individual. Though accurate prognosis is extremely difficult in patients with severe chronic conditions that exacerbate and remit, some evidence suggests that most physicians tend to underestimate life expectancy in the elderly when considering these decisions. Be particularly cautious of the risk of ageism. For example, the life expectancy of an 85-year-old woman who is in the top quartile of functional status is nearly 10-yrs. Screening decisions about patients with cognitive impairment are particularly vexing and must take into careful consideration the ability of the patient to participate in the testing, the risks of such testing, the ability of the patient to undergo treatments if a disease is found, and most of all the overarching goals of care.

Prevention of injury in the elderly would include assessment for falls, discussions about firearms, particularly if a demented individual is in the home, use of seat belts in cars, evaluation for continued ability to drive, and home safety assessment.

Smoking cessation reduces the risk of lung cancer at any age. Though not proven for 1° prevention of CAD, it continues to have an important role in prevention of MI in patients with established CAD. Thus, cessation of smoking is important to endorse and encourage even in the elderly.

Finally, several periodic immunizations are advised in the elderly, though their benefits for all subgroups is often debated. Pneumococcal vaccination is recommended at least once over the age of 65yrs, with consideration of revaccination in certain subgroups. Influenza vaccination is advised annually for all elderly, though likely the most effect approach to preventing influenza in nursing homes is to aggressively immunize staff. Periodic (every 10yrs) revaccination for tetanus is also advised.

Biochemistry

Stephen D. Sisson, M.D.

Contents

On being normal in the society of numbers

Laboratory medicine reduces our patients to a few easy-to-handle numbers: this is the discipline's great attraction—and its greatest danger. The normal range (reference interval) is usually that which includes 95% of patients. If variation is randomly distributed, 2.5% of our results will be 'too high', and 2.5% 'too low' on an average day, when dealing with apparently normal people. This statistical definition of normality is the simplest. Other definitions may be *normative*—ie stating what an upper or lower limit *should* be. For example, the upper end of the reference interval for LDL cholesterol may be given as 130mg/dL because this is what preventative cardiologists state to be the *desired* maximum, while the risk of CHD ↑ above 100mg/dL (and even 70mg/dL). The WHO definition of anemia in pregnancy is an Hbg of <11g/dL, which makes 20% of mothers anemic. This 'lax' criterion has the presumed benefit of triggering actions which result in fewer deaths by hemorrhage. So do not just ask 'What is the normal range?'—also question about who set the range, for what population, and for what reason.

The essence of laboratory medicine

Only do a test if the result will influence management. Make sure you look at the result! Explain to the patient where this test fits in to his or her overall plan of management. Do not interpret laboratory results except in the light of clinical assessment.

If there is disparity: trust clinical judgement and repeat the test.

Reference intervals (normal ranges) are usually defined as the interval, symmetrical about the mean, containing 95% of results on the population studied. The more tests you run, the greater the probability of an 'abnormal' result of no clinical significance.

Artifacts Delayed analysis for plasma potassium.

Anion gap (AG) Reflects unmeasured anions.

Biochemistry results: major disease patterns ($\uparrow$ = raised, $\downarrow$ = lowered)

Dehydration: Urea$\uparrow$, albumin$\uparrow$ (useful to plot change in a patient's condition). Hematocrit (PCV)$\uparrow$, creatinine$\uparrow$; also urine volume$\downarrow$; skin turgor$\downarrow$.

Renal failure: Creatinine$\uparrow$, urea$\uparrow$, AG$\uparrow$, K$^+\uparrow$, PO$_4^{3-}\uparrow$, HCO$_3^-\downarrow$.

Thiazide and loop diuretics: Sodium$\downarrow$, potassium$\downarrow$, bicarbonate$\uparrow$, urea$\uparrow$.

Bone disease:	Ca^{2+}	PO_4^{3-}	Alk phos
Osteoporosis	Normal	Normal	Normal
Osteomalacia	$\downarrow$	$\downarrow$	$\uparrow$
Paget's	Normal	Normal	$\uparrow\uparrow$
Myeloma	$\uparrow$	$\uparrow$, normal	Normal
Bone metastases	$\uparrow$	$\uparrow$, normal	$\uparrow$
1° Hyperparathyroidism	$\uparrow$	$\downarrow$, normal	Normal, $\uparrow$
Hypoparathyroidism	$\downarrow$	$\uparrow$	Normal
Renal failure (low GFR)	$\downarrow$	$\uparrow$	Normal, $\uparrow$

Hepatocellular disease: Bilirubin$\uparrow$, AST$\uparrow$ (alk phos slightly$\uparrow$, albumin$\downarrow$).

Cholestasis: Bilirubin$\uparrow$, γGT$\uparrow\uparrow$ alk phos$\uparrow\uparrow$, AST$\uparrow$.

Myocardial infarct: AST$\uparrow$, LDH$\uparrow$, CK$\uparrow$, troponin T/I $\uparrow$.

Diabetes mellitus: Glucose$\uparrow$, (bicarbonate$\downarrow$ if acidotic).

Addison's disease: Potassium$\uparrow$, sodium$\downarrow$.

Cushing's syndrome: May show potassium$\downarrow$, bicarbonate$\uparrow$, sodium$\uparrow$.

Conn's syndrome: May present with potassium$\downarrow$, bicarbonate$\uparrow$ (and high BP). Sodium normal or $\uparrow$.

Diabetes insipidus: Sodium$\uparrow$, plasma osmolality$\uparrow$, urine osmolality $\downarrow$ (both hypercalcemia and hypokalemia may cause nephrogenic diabetes insipidus).

Inappropriate ADH secretion: Na$^+\downarrow$ with normal or low urea and creatinine, plasma osmolality $\downarrow$. Urine osmolality $\uparrow$ (and > than plasma osmolality), urine Na $\uparrow$ (>20mmol/L).

Excess alcohol intake: Evidence of hepatocellular disease. Early evidence in γGT $\uparrow$, MCV$\uparrow$, ethanol in blood before lunch.

Some immunodeficiency states: Normal serum albumin but *low* total protein (low as immunoglobulins are missing—also making crossmatching difficult because expected hemagglutinins are absent;).

Life-threatening biochemical derangements (See p609)

The laboratory and ward tests

Laboratory staff like to have contact with you.

10 tips to better laboratory results

1 Interest someone from the laboratory in your patient's problem.
2 Fill in the request form fully.
3 Give clinical details, not your preferred diagnosis.
4 Ensure that the lab knows who to contact.
5 Label specimens as well as the request form.
6 Follow the hospital labeling routine for crossmatching.
7 Find out when analyzers run, especially batched assays.
8 Talk with the lab before requesting an unusual test.
9 Be thoughtful: don't 'shoot the messenger'.
10 Plot results graphically: abnormalities show sooner.

Artifacts and pitfalls in laboratory tests

- Do not take blood sample from an arm which has IV fluid running into it.
- Repeat any unexpected result before acting on it.
- For clotting time do not sample from a heparinized IV catheter.
- Serum K^+ is overestimated if sample is old or hemolyzed (this occurs if venipuncture is difficult).
- If using Vacutainers, fill *plain* tubes first—otherwise, anticoagulant contamination from previous tubes can cause errors.
- Total calcium results are affected by albumin concentration.
- INR may be overestimated if citrate bottle is under filled.
- Drugs may cause *analytic* errors (eg prednisolone cross-reacts with cortisol). Be suspicious if results are unexpected.
- Food may affect result, eg bananas raise urinary HIAA.

Using dipsticks Store dipsticks in a closed container in a cool, dry place, not refrigerated. If improperly stored, or past expiration date, do not use. For urine tests, dip the dipstick briefly in urine, run edge of strip along container and hold strip horizontally. Read at the specified time—check instructions for the type of stick.

Urine specific gravity (SG) can be measured by dipstick. It is not a good measure of osmolality. Causes of low SG (<1.003) are: diabetes insipidus, renal failure. Causes of high SG (>1.025) are: diabetes mellitus, adrenal insufficiency, liver disease, heart failure, acute water loss. Hydrometers underestimate SG by 0.001 per 3°C above 16°C.

Sources of error in interpreting dipstick results

Bilirubin: False positive: phenothiazines. False negative: urine not fresh, rifampicin.

Urobilinogen: False negative: urine not fresh. (Normally present in urine due to metabolism of bilirubin in the gut by bacteria and subsequent absorption.)

Ketones: L-dopa affects color (can give false positive). 3-hydroxybutyrate gives a false negative.

Blood: False positive: myoglobin, profuse bacterial growth. False negative: ascorbic acid.

Urine glucose: Depends on test. Pads with glucose oxidase are not affected by other reducing sugars (unlike Clinitest®) but can give false positive to peroxide, chlorine; and false negative with ascorbic acid, salicylate, L-dopa.

Protein: Highly alkaline urine can give false positive.

Blood glucose: Sticks use enzymatic method and are glucose specific. A major source of error is applying too little blood (a large drop to cover the pad is necessary), and poor timing. Reflectance meters ↑ precision but introduce new sources of error.

Laboratory results: When to take action NOW

- On receiving a dangerous result, first check the name and date.
- Go to the bedside. If the patient is conscious, turn off any IVF (until fluid is checked: a mistake may have been made) and ask the patient how he or she is. *Any seizures, faints, collapses, or unexpected symptoms?*
- Be skeptical of an unexpectedly wildly abnormal result with a well patient. Could the specimens have got mixed up? Is there an artifact? Was the sample taken from the 'drip' arm? A low calcium, eg may be due to a low albumin. Perhaps the lab is using a new analyzer with a faulty wash cycle? *When in doubt, repeat the test.*

The values chosen below are somewhat arbitrary and must be taken as a guide only. Many results less extreme than those below will be just as dangerous if the patient is old, immunosuppressed, or has some other pathology such as pneumonia.

Plasma biochemistry (beware electrocardiological ± CNS events, eg seizures)

Calcium (corrected for albumin) >14mg/dL If shortening Q–T interval on ECG, then dangerous hypercalcemia.

Calcium (corrected for albumin) <8mg/dL + symptoms such as tetany or long Q–T = *Dangerous hypocalcemia.*

Glucose <60mg/dL = *Hypoglycemia. Glucose 50mL 50% IV if coma.*

Glucose >400mg/dL = *Severe hyperglycemia. Is parenteral insulin needed?*

Potassium <2.5mEq/L = *Dangerous hypokalemia, esp. if on digoxin.*

Potassium >6.5mEq/L = *Dangerous hyperkalemia.*

Sodium <120mEq/L = *Dangerous hyponatremia.*

Sodium >155mEq/L = *Dangerous hypernatremia.*

Blood gases

P_aO_2 <60mmHg = Severe hypoxia. Give O_2.

pH <7.1 = Dangerous acidosis.

Hematology results

Hbg <7g/dL with low mean cell volume (<75fL) or history of bleeding. *This patient may need urgent transfusion (no spare capacity).*

Platelets <40 × 10⁹/L *May need a platelet transfusion; consult a hematologist.*

Plasmodium falciparum seen Start antimalarials now.

CSF results

>1 neutrophil/mm³ *Consider meningitis.*

Positive Gram stain *Talk to a microbiologist; urgent broad spectrum therapy.*

Conflicting, equivocal, or inexplicable results Get prompt help; repeat test.

Intravenous fluid therapy

If fluids cannot be given orally, they are normally given intravenously. Alternatives are via a central venous line or subcutaneously.

Three principles of fluid therapy

1 Maintain normal daily requirements. About 2500mL fluid containing roughly 100mEq sodium and 70mEq potassium per 24h is required. A good regimen is 5% dextrose in ½ normal saline with 20–30mEq of potassium per liter of fluid administered at 84cc/H. Post-operative patients may need more fluid and more saline depending on operative losses. If the serum sodium is rising, then more dextrose and less saline is required.

2 Replace additional losses. The amount and type of fluid lost is a guide (check fluid charts, drainage bottles, etc.). Remember that febrile patients have ↑ insensible losses too. In practice, the problem is usually whether to give saline or dextrose. Most body fluids (eg vomitus) contain salt, but less than plasma, and thus replacement will require a mixture of saline and dextrose. Hypotensive patients require resuscitation with saline, or a colloidal plasma expander, eg Dextran® or Haemaccel®, but not dextrose (caution in liver failure, see below). Note that Dextran® interferes with platelet function and may prolong bleeding. Patients with acute blood loss require transfusion with packed cells or whole blood. As a holding measure, colloid or saline may be used while blood is being cross matched. If more than 1L is required then O-negative or group-specific blood should be used.

3 Special cases. Patients with *heart failure* are at greater risk of pulmonary edema if given too much fluid. They also tolerate saline less well since Na⁺ retention accompanies heart failure. If IV fluids must be given, use with care. Patients with *liver failure*, despite being edematous and often hyponatremic, have ↑ total body sodium, and saline should not be used in resuscitation; salt-poor albumin solution or blood should be given.

A note on fluids. *0.9% saline ('normal saline')* has about the same sodium content as plasma (150mEq/L) and is isotonic with plasma. *5% dextrose* is isotonic, but only contains 50g/L (dextrose is glucose), and is a way of giving water, since the liver rapidly metabolizes all the glucose, leaving only water. It provides little energy.

More concentrated glucose solutions exist, and may be used in the treatment of hypoglycemia. They are hypertonic and irritant to veins. Therefore, care in their use is needed, and infusion sites should be inspected regularly, and flushed with saline after use.

Examine patients regularly to assess fluid balance, and look for signs of heart failure, which can result if excess fluid is given. Excessive dextrose infusion may lead to water overload.

Daily weighing helps to monitor overall fluid balance, as will fluid balance charts.

Acid–base balance

Arterial blood pH is closely regulated in health to 7.40 ± 0.05 by various mechanisms including bicarbonate, other plasma buffers, and the kidney. Acid–base disorders needlessly confuse many people, but if a few simple rules are applied, then interpretation and diagnosis are easy.

• pH <7.35 is an acidosis; pH >7.45 is an alkalosis.
• CO_2 is an acidic gas (normal concentration 35–45mmHg).
• HCO_3^- is alkaline (normal concentration 22–28Eq/L).
• 1° changes in HCO_3^- are termed *metabolic*, and of CO_2 *respiratory*.

1 Look at the pH: If the pH is lower than normal, an acidosis is present. If the pH is higher than normal, an alkalosis is present. Note that a normal pH does not exclude an acid–base disorder; both an acidosis and alkalosis may be present.
2 Is the CO_2 abnormal? If so, is the change in keeping with the pH (ie if there is an acidosis, is CO_2 raised)? If so it is a *respiratory* problem. If there is no change, or an *opposite* one, then the change is likely to be compensatory.
3 Is the HCO_3^- abnormal, and if so, is the change in keeping with the pH? If so the problem is a *metabolic* one.

An example

pH 7.05, CO_2 15mmHg, HCO_3^- 8.0mEq/L.

There is an *acidosis*, and the CO_2 is low (which would raise pH). Thus the CO_2 is likely compensatory. However, the HCO_3^- is low, and is thus the cause; ie a *metabolic acidosis* is present.

Metabolic acidosis *pH ↓, HCO_3^- ↓*

To help diagnosis, determine the anion gap (AG)—this estimates unmeasured anions (including phosphates, sulfates, and negatively charged proteins—they are hard to measure directly). The anion gap is calculated as the difference between plasma cations (Na^+ is the dominant plasma cation; some include the potassium as well) and anions (Cl^- and HCO_3^-): Normal range: 12 ± 2mEq/L (if potassium included, add 4mEq/L).

When presented with a primary metabolic acidosis, the body will attempt to compensate by hyperventilating, which will lower the pCO_2 and combat the fall in serum pH. However, some patients will have coexisting respiratory disorders, and may present with an inappropriate compensatory response. In a patient who presents with a 1° metabolic acidosis, we can use the serum HCO_3 to predict what the pCO_2 should be in the normal host with the following equation:

$$1.5(HCO_3) + 8 ± 2 = pCO_2$$

If the measured pCO_2 is not close to what we predict, a second disorder coexists (if the pCO_2 is less than predicted, we have a respiratory alkalosis; if the pCO_2 is higher than predicted, we have a respiratory acidosis). The limit of respiratory compensation for a metabolic acidosis is pCO_2 of approx. 20. *Do not use this equation when the primary disorder is not a metabolic acidosis*

Causes of metabolic acidosis and increased anion gap:
Due to ↑ production of fixed/organic acids. HCO_3^- falls and unmeasured anions associated with the acids accumulate. Mnemonic for differential diagnosis is 'MUDPILES':
• M: Methanol
• U: Uremia
• D: Diabetic ketoacidosis (also include alcoholic ketoacidosis and starvation ketosis). 'D' also stands for drugs (eg biguanides such as metformin; nucleoside reverse transcriptase inhibitors such as d4T)
• P: Paraldehyde
• I: Ischemia (via production of Lactate) 'I' also stands for iron and isoniazid, two uncommon causes of anion gap metabolic acidosis

- L: Lactate
- E: Ethylene glycol/ethanol
- S: Salicylates.

Causes of metabolic acidosis and normal anion gap:

Due to loss of bicarbonate or ingestion of H^+ ions (Cl^- is retained, thus the anion gap does not change). Mnemonic for differential diagnosis is 'DURHAM'
- D: Diarrhea
- U: Ureteral diversion
- R: Renal tubular acidosis
- H: Hyperalimentation
- A: Addison's disease. 'A' also stands for acetazolamide or amphotericin
- M: Miscellaneous (pancreatic fistulae, ammonium chloride ingestion).

Causes of metabolic acidosis and low anion gap

Mnemonic for differential diagnosis is 'BAM'
- B: Bromism
- A: Albumin (low serum albumin)
- M: Multiple myeloma.

Metabolic alkalosis $pH\uparrow$, $HCO_3^-\uparrow$
- Vomiting
- Nasogastric suction
- K^+ depletion (diuretics)
- Burns
- Conn's syndrome
- Cushing's syndrome
- Renal artery stenosis
- Licorice ingestion
- Bartter's syndrome
- Ingestion of base (citrate, acetate).

Respiratory acidosis $pH\downarrow$ $CO_2\uparrow$

Any lung (eg chronic obstructive pulmonary disease), neuromuscular (eg amyotrophic lateral sclerosis), or physical cause (eg pneumothorax) of respiratory failure. Obstructive sleep apnea is a common cause of respiratory acidosis. Narcotics, which suppress the central respiratory drive, can cause a respiratory acidosis.

Look at the P_aO_2. It will probably be low. Is oxygen therapy required?

Use O_2 with care if chronic obstructive pulmonary disease (COPD) is the underlying cause, as too much oxygen may make matters worse.

Respiratory alkalosis $pH\uparrow$, $CO_2\downarrow$

A result of hyperventilation.

CNS causes: Stroke, subarachnoid hemorrhage, meningitis.

Other causes: Anxiety, high altitude, fever, pregnancy, drugs, eg salicylates. Pulmonary embolus often causes a respiratory alkalosis with hypoxemia. Sepsis and salicylates cause both a respiratory alkalosis and metabolic acidosis.

Terminology: To aid understanding, we have used the terms acidosis and alkalosis, where a purist would sometimes have used acid-, alkal-emia.

Kidney function

The kidney controls the elimination of many substances. It also makes erythropoietin, renin, and 1,25-dihydroxycholecalciferol (ie vitamin D). Filtered sodium is exchanged with potassium and hydrogen ions by exchanges and channels in the distal tubule. Glucose spills over into urine when plasma concentration is above renal threshold for reabsorption ($\approx$200mg/dL, but varies from person to person, and is lower in pregnancy).

Creatinine clearance is a measure of glomerular filtration rate (GFR)—the volume of fluid filtered by glomeruli per minute. About 99% of this fluid is reabsorbed. Creatinine, once filtered, is only slightly reabsorbed. Thus:

[Creatinine]^{plasma} × creatinine clearance = [creatinine]^{urine} × urine flow rate

To measure creatinine clearance (normal value is $\approx$125mL/min). Collect urine over 24h. At the start, void and discard urine; from then on, and at end of 24h, void into the bottle. Take sample for plasma creatinine once during 24h. Use formula above. Major sources of error are calculation (eg units) and failure to collect all urine. If urine collection is unreliable, use formula:

$$\text{Creatinine Clearance (mL/min)} = \frac{(140 - \text{age in years}) \times (\text{wt in kg})}{72 \times \text{serum creatinine in mg/dL}}$$

For women, multiply above by 0.85. Unreliable if: unstable renal function; very obese; edematous. (The protein: creatinine ratio in a spot morning urine is an alternative way to monitor chronic renal decline.)

Abnormal kidney function

There are 3 major biochemical pictures.

- **Low GFR** (classic acute renal failure)
  Plasma biochemistry: The following are raised: urea, creatinine, potassium, hydrogen ions, urate, phosphate, anion gap.
  The following are lowered: calcium, bicarbonate.
  Other findings: Oliguria.
  Diagnosis: Low GFR (creatinine clearance).
  Causes: Early acute oliguric renal failure, long-standing chronic renal failure.
- **Tubular dysfunction** (damage to tubules)
  Plasma biochemistry: The following are lowered: potassium, phosphate, urate, bicarbonate. There is acidosis. Urea and creatinine are normal.
  Other findings (highly variable): Polyuria with glucose, amino acids, proteins (lysozyme, β_2-microglobulin), and phosphate in urine.
  Diagnosis: Test renal concentrating ability.
  Cause: Recovery from acute renal failure. Also: Hypercalcemia, hyperuricemia, myeloma, pyelonephritis, hypokalemia, Wilson's disease, galactosemia, heavy metal poisoning.
- **Chronic renal failure:** As GFR reduces, creatinine, urea, phosphate and urate all ↑. Bicarbonate (and Hb) ↓. Eventually potassium increases and pH ↓. There may also be osteomalacia.

Assessment of renal failure may need to be combined with other investigations to reach diagnosis, eg urine microscopy, radiology, or renal biopsy (in glomerulonephritis), or ultrasound.

Urate and the kidney

Causes of hyperuricemia High levels of urate in the blood (hyperuricemia) may result from ↑ turnover or ↓ excretion of urate. Either may be drug-induced.

- *Drugs:* Cytotoxics; thiazides; pyrazinamide.
- *Increased cell turnover:* Lymphoma; leukemia; psoriasis; hemolysis; muscle death (rhabdomyolysis). *Tumor lysis syndrome.*
- *Reduced excretion:* Primary gout; chronic renal failure; lead nephropathy; hyperparathyroidism; pre-eclampsia.
- *In addition:* Hyperuricemia may be associated with hypertension and hyper-lipidemia. Urate may be raised in disorders of purine synthesis such as the Lesch–Nyhan syndrome.

Hyperuricemia and renal failure Severe renal failure from any cause may be associated with hyperuricemia, and very rarely this may give rise to gout. Sometimes the relationship of cause and effect is reversed so that it is the hyperuricemia that causes the renal failure. This can occur following cyto-toxic treatment (*tumor lysis syndrome*), eg in leukemia; and in muscle necrosis.

How urate causes renal failure In some instances, ureteric obstruction from urate crystals occurs. This responds to retrograde ureteral catheteriza-tion and lavage. More commonly, urate precipitates in the renal tubules. This may occur at plasma levels ≥ 20mg/dL.

Prevention of renal failure Before starting chemotherapy, ensure good hydration; consider alkalinization of the urine and initiate allopurinol (a xanthine oxidase inhibitor), which prevents a sharp rise in urate following chemotherapy. There is a remote risk of inducing xanthine nephropathy.

Treatment of hyperuricemic acute renal failure Prompt rehydration and alkalinization of the urine after excluding bilateral ureteral obstruction. Once oliguria is established, hemodialysis is required and should be used in preference to peritoneal dialysis.

Gout (See p370)

Electrolyte physiology

Most sodium is extracellular and is pumped out of the cell by the sodium pump, in exchange for K^+, which requires energy from ATP. Sodium is the major extracellular cation; potassium is the major intracellular cation.

Osmolarity is the number of osmoles per *liter* of solution.

Osmolality is the number of osmoles per kilogram of solvent (*normal:* 280–300).

A *mole* is the molecular weight expressed in grams.

To estimate plasma osmolality: $2(Na^+)$ + urea/2.8 + glucose/18. If the measured osmolality is greater than this (ie measured osmolality is more than 10mmol/L higher than the estimated osmolality, an osmolar gap is said to exist). If an osmolar gap is present, consider: diabetes mellitus, high blood ethanol, methanol, or ethylene glycol.

Fluid compartments For 70kg man: *total fluid* = 42L (60% body weight). *Intracellular fluid* = 28L (67% body fluid), *extracellular fluid* = 14L (33% body fluid). *Intravascular component* = 5L of blood (3L plasma).

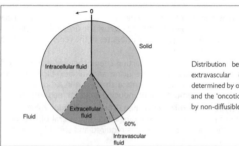

Distribution between intra- and extravascular compartments is determined by osmotic equilibrium, and the 'oncotic pressure' exerted by non-diffusible proteins.

Fluid balance over 24h is roughly:

Input (mL water)	Output (mL water)
Drink: 1500	Urine: 1500
In food: 800	Insensible loss: 800
Metabolism of food: 200	Stool: 200
Total: **2500**	Total: **2500**

Control of sodium *Renin* is produced by the juxtaglomerular apparatus in response to ↓ renal blood flow, and catalyses the conversion *angiotensinogen* (a peptide made by the liver) to *angiotensin I*. This is then converted by angiotensin-converting enzyme (ACE), which is located in the lung and blood vessels) to *angiotensin II*. The latter has several important actions including efferent renal arteriolar constriction (so ↑ perfusion pressure); peripheral vasoconstriction; and stimulation of the adrenal cortex to produce *aldosterone*, which activates the sodium pump in the distal renal tubule leading to reabsorption of sodium and water from the urine, in exchange for potassium and hydrogen ions.

High GFR results in high sodium loss.

High renal tubular blood flow and hemodilution ↓ sodium reabsorption in the proximal tubule.

Control of water Controlled mainly by sodium concentration. ↑Plasma osmolality stimulates thirst, and the release of antidiuretic hormone (ADH) from the posterior pituitary, which ↑ the passive water reabsorption from the renal collecting duct by opening water channels to allow water to flow from the hypotonic luminal fluid into the hypertonic renal interstitium.

Natriuretic peptide

Secretory granules have long been known to exist in the atria, and if homogenized atrial tissue is injected into rats, their urine volume (and Na^+ excretion) rises. This is evidence of endocrine action via the effects of atrial natriuretic peptide (ANP). BNP is a similar hormone originally identified from pig brain (hence the B). Most of the BNP is secreted from ventricular myocardium. Plasma BNP is closely related to left ventricular pressure. In myocardial infarction and left ventricular dysfunction, these hormones can be released in large quantities. Secretion is also ↑ by tachycardia, glucocorticoids, and thyroid hormones. Vasoactive peptides (endothelin-1, angiotensin II) also influence secretion. ANP and BNP both ↑ GFR and ↓ renal Na^+ resorption; they also ↓ preload by relaxing smooth muscle. ANP partly blocks secretion of renin and aldosterone.

BNP as a biomarker of heart failure[1] As plasma BNP reflects myocyte stretch, BNP is used to diagnose heart failure. ↑BNP distinguishes heart failure from other causes of dyspnea more accurately than left ventricular ejection fraction, ANP, and N-terminal ANP (sensitivity: >90%; specificity: 80–90%). BNP is highest in decompensated heart failure, intermediate in left ventricular dysfunction but no acute heart failure exacerbation, and lowest in those without heart failure or left ventricular dysfunction.

What BNP threshold for diagnosing heart failure? If BNP >100ng/L, this 'diagnoses' heart failure better than other clinical variables or clinical judgment in on-call settings (history, examination, and CXR). BNP can be used to 'rule out' heart failure if <50ng/L (negative predictive value (PV) 96%, ie the chance of BNP being <50ng/L given that heart failure is absent in 96%). In those with heart failure, BNP is higher in systolic dysfunction than in isolated diastolic dysfunction (eg hypertrophic or dilated cardiomyopathy), and is highest in those with systolic *and* diastolic dysfunction.

Threshold (ng/L)	Sensitivity (%)	Specificity (%)	Positive PV	Negative PV	Accuracy (%)
≥50	97	62	71	96	79
≥80	93	74	77	92	83
≥100	90	76	79	89	83
≥125	87	79	80	87	83
≥150	85	83	83	85	84[2]

BNP ↑ in proportion to right ventricular dysfunction, eg in 1° pulmonary hypertension, cor pulmonale, PE, and congenital heart disease, but rises are less than in left ventricular disorders.

Prognosis in heart failure: The higher the BNP, the higher the cardiovascular and all-cause mortality (independent of age, NYHA class, previous MI and LV ejection fraction). ↑BNP in heart failure is also associated with sudden death. Serial testing may be important: persistently high BNP levels despite vigorous anti-failure treatment predict adverse outcomes. In one study, those with heart failure randomized to get N-terminal BNP-guided (rather than symptom-guided) therapy had fewer adverse events.

Prognosis in angina and MI: BNP has some prognostic value here (adverse left ventricular remodelling; LV dysfunction; death post-MI).

Prognosis in COR pulmonale/primary pulmonary hypertension: BNP is useful.

Cautions with BNP A BNP >50ng/L does not exclude other coexisting diseases such as pneumonia. Also, assays vary, so consult with your lab.

1 Lemos J 2003 *Lancet* **362** 316.   2 Maisel A *N Engl J Med* 2002 **347** 161.

Sodium: hyponatremia

Signs & symptoms depend on severity and rate of change in serum sodium, and include: confusion, seizures, hypertension, cardiac failure, edema, anorexia, nausea, muscle weakness.

Diagnosis See tree in diagram OPPOSITE. The key question is: Is the patient dehydrated? History and urinalysis are your guides.

Causes of hyponatremia (For a full list, see the diagram OPPOSITE.)
• *Diuretics*, especially thiazides.
• *Water excess*, either orally, or as excess 5% dextrose IV.
• *Pseudohyponatremia*: (1) If serum volume↑ from high lipids or protein, Na^+ falls, but plasma osmolalitity is ↔. (2) If plasma glucose ≥200mg/dL, make a correction. Add 1.8 to Na^+ for every 100 that glucose is above 100mg/dL to correct. (3) Na^+ will be ↓ if blood is from an arm with a dextrose IV.

Management Don't base treatment on plasma Na^+ concentration alone. The presence of symptoms, duration, and state of hydration influence treatment. If possible, correct the underlying cause. If chronic: fluid restriction, or cautious rehydration with saline if dehydrated, is often sufficient if asymptomatic, although demeclocycline may be required. If symptomatic, saline may be given, but do not correct chronic changes rapidly (max 15mEq/dL/day rise in serum sodium). Acute hyponatremia may be treated with saline infusion and furosemide. *Hypervolemic hyponatremia* (cirrhosis, CHF) treat the underlying disorder. *In emergency* (seizures, coma), consider IVF of 0.9% saline or hypertonic saline (eg 1.8% saline) at 70mEq Na^+/h. Aim for a gradual ↑ in plasma sodium to ≈125mmol/L. Can combine with furosemide. Watch for heart failure, and central pontine myelinolysis. Seek expert help.

Syndrome of inappropriate ADH secretion (SIADH) An important, but over-diagnosed, cause of hyponatremia. The diagnosis requires concentrated urine (sodium >20mEq/dL & osmolality >500mosmol/kg) in the presence of hyponatremia (<125mEq/dL) or low plasma osmolality (<260mmol/kg), and the absence of hypovolemia, edema, or diuretics.

Causes: Malignancy, eg lung small-cell; pancreas; prostate; lymphoma.
CNS disorders: Meningoencephalitis; abscess; stroke; subarachnoid hemorrhage, subdural hemorrhage; head injury; Guillain–Barré; vasculitis, eg SLE.
Chest disease: TB; pneumonia; abscess; aspergillosis.
Metabolic disease: Porphyria; trauma.
Drugs: Opiates; chlorpropamide; psychotropics; SSRIs; cytotoxics.
Treatment: Treat the cause, fluid restrict, occasionally demeclocycline.

Hypernatremia

Signs & symptoms Look for thirst, confusion, coma, and fits—with signs of dehydration: dry skin, ↓skin turgor, postural hypotension, and oliguria if water deficient. Laboratory features: ↑PCV, ↑albumin, ↑urea.

Causes Usually due to water loss in excess of sodium loss; typically implies impaired access to water:
- Fluid loss without water replacement (eg diarrhea, vomiting, burns).
- Incorrect IV fluid replacement (excessive saline).
- Diabetes insipidus. Suspect if large urine volume. This may follow head injury, or CNS surgery, especially pituitary.
- Osmotic diuresis.
- Primary aldosteronism: suspect if BP↑, K^+↓, alkalosis (HCO₃↑).

Management: Give water orally if possible; if not, dextrose 5% IV slowly (~4L/24h) guided by urine output and plasma Na^+. Some authorities recommend 0.9% saline (esp. if hypovolemic) as this causes less marked fluid shifts and is hypotonic in a hypernatremic patient. Avoid hypotonic solutions.

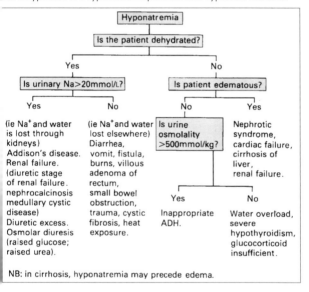

NB: in cirrhosis, hyponatremia may precede edema.

Potassium

General points Most potassium is intracellular, and thus serum potassium levels are a poor reflection of total body potassium. The concentrations of K^+ and H^+ ions in extracellular fluid tend to vary together. This is because these ions compete with each other in the exchange with sodium which occurs across most cell membranes (sodium is pumped out of the cell) and in the distal tubule of the kidney (sodium is reabsorbed from the urine). Thus, if H^+ ion concentration is high, fewer K^+ ions will be excreted into the urine. Similarly K^+ will compete with H^+ for exchange across cell membranes and extracellular K^+ will accumulate. Insulin and catecholamines both stimulate K^+ uptake into cells by stimulating the Na^+/K^+ pump.

Hyperkalemia

A plasma potassium >6.5mEq/dL needs urgent treatment but first ensure that this is not an artifact (eg due to hemolysis inside the collection tube).

Signs & symptoms Cardiac arrhythmias. Sudden death. *ECG:* Tall peaked T waves; small P wave; wide QRS complex becoming sinusoidal, VF. (see OPPOSITE.)

Causes
- Oliguric renal failure
- K^+-sparing diuretics
- Rhabdomyolysis, burns, tumor lysis
- Metabolic acidosis (DM)
- Excess K^+ therapy
- Addison's disease
- Massive blood transfusion
- Drugs, eg ACEI, potassium-sparing diuretics

- Artifact. Hemolysis of sample; delay in analysis—K^+ leaks out of RBCs; thrombocythemia—platelets leak K^+ as sample clots in tube.

Treatment Treat underlying cause.

Hypokalemia

If K^+ <2.5mEq/dL, urgent treatment is required. Note that hypokalemia exacerbates digoxin toxicity.

Signs & symptoms Muscle weakness, hypotonia, cardiac arrhythmias, cramps, and tetany. *ECG:* Small or inverted T waves; prominent U wave (after T wave); prolonged P–R interval; depressed ST segment.

Causes
- Diuretics
- Vomiting and diarrhea
- Pyloric stenosis
- Villous adenoma rectum
- Intestinal fistulae
- Cushing's syndrome/steroids/ACTH
- Conn's syndrome
- Alkalosis
- Purgative and licorice abuse
- Renal tubular failure.

If on diuretics, then ↑bicarbonate is the best indication that hypokalemia is likely to have been long-standing. Magnesium may be low, and hypokalemia is often difficult to correct until magnesium levels are normalized. In hypokalemic periodic paralysis, intermittent weakness lasting up to 72h appears to be caused by K^+ shifting from extra- to intracellular fluid. Suspect Conn's syndrome if hypertensive, hypokalemic alkalosis in someone not taking diuretics.

Treatment *If mild:* (>2.5mEq/dL, no symptoms) give oral K^+ supplement. If taking a thiazide diuretic, hypokalemia >3.0mEq/dL rarely needs treating. *If severe:* (<2.5mEq/dL, dangerous symptoms) give IV potassium cautiously, not more than 20mEq/h, and not more concentrated than 40mEq/L. Do not give potassium if oliguric.

Never give potassium as a fast 'stat' bolus dose.

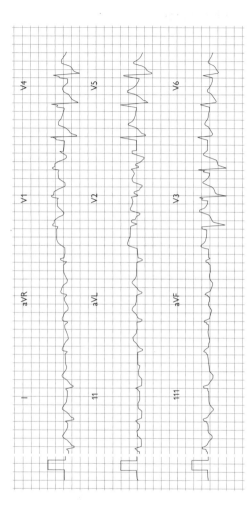

ECG 13—hyperkalemia—note the flattening of the P-waves, prominent T-waves, and widening of the QRS complex.

Calcium: physiology

General points About 40% of plasma calcium is bound to albumin. Usually it is total plasma calcium that is measured although it is the unbound, ionized portion that is important. Therefore, *adjust total calcium level for albumin as follows:* add 0.8 to the measured calcium for every 1 unit that albumin is below 4.0 (perform the reverse if albumin is elevated). However, many factors affect binding (eg other proteins in myeloma, cirrhosis, individual variation) so be cautious in your interpretation. If in doubt over an abnormal calcium, check the ionized calcium.

The control of calcium metabolism

• *Parathyroid hormone (PTH):* A rise in PTH causes a rise in plasma Ca^{2+} and a ↓ in plasma PO_4^{3-}. This is due to $\uparrow Ca^{2+}$ and $\uparrow PO_4^{3-}$ reabsorption from bone; and $\uparrow Ca^{2+}$ but ↓ PO_4^{3-} reabsorption from the kidney. PTH secretion enhances active vitamin D formation. PTH secretion is itself controlled by ionized plasma calcium levels.

• *Vitamin D:* Calciferol (Vitamin D_3), and ergocalciferol (Vitamin D_2) are biologically identical in their actions. Serum vitamin D is converted in the liver to 25-hydroxy vitamin D (25(OH) vitamin D). In the kidney, a second hydroxyl group is added to form the biologically active 1,25-dihydroxy vitamin D (1,25(OH)$_2$ vitamin D), also called calcitriol, or the much less active 24,25(OH)$_2$ vitamin D. Calcitriol production is stimulated by ↓Ca^{2+}, ↓ PO_4^{3-}, and PTH. Its actions include $\uparrow Ca^{2+}$ and $\uparrow PO_4$ absorption from the gut; $\uparrow Ca^{2+}$ and $\uparrow PO_4^{3-}$ reabsorption in the kidney; enhanced bone turnover; and inhibition of PTH release. Disordered regulation of 1,25(OH)$_2$ vitamin D underlies familial normocalcemic hypercalciuria which is a major cause of calcium oxalate renal stone formation.

• *Calcitonin:* Made in C-cells of the thyroid, this causes a ↓ in plasma calcium and phosphate, but its physiological role is unclear. It is a marker to detect recurrence or metastasis in medullary carcinoma of the thyroid.

• *Thyroxine:* May $\uparrow$plasma calcium although this is rare.

• *Magnesium:* ↓Mg^{2+} prevents PTH release, and may cause hypocalcemia.

Hypocalcemia

Apparent hypocalcemia may be an artifact of hypoalbuminemia (above).

Signs & symptoms Tetany, depression, perioral paresthesias, carpopedal spasm (wrist flexion and fingers drawn together) especially if brachial artery occluded with BP cuff (*Trousseau's sign*), neuromuscular excitability, eg tapping over parotid (facial nerve) causes facial muscles to twitch (*Chvostek's sign*). Cataract if chronic Ca^{2+}↓. ECG: Q–T interval↑.

Causes It may be a consequence of thyroid or parathyroid surgery. *If phosphate raised,* then either chronic renal failure, hypoparathyroidism, pseudohypoparathyroidism, or acute rhabdomyolysis. If phosphate ↔ or ↓ then either osteomalacia (high alkaline phosphatase), over-hydration or pancreatitis. In respiratory alkalosis, the total Ca^{2+} may be normal, but ionized Ca^{2+}↓ and the patient may have symptoms because of this.

Treatment If *symptoms are mild,* give calcium 5mmol/6h PO. Do daily plasma calcium levels. If necessary add calcitriol (ie vitamin D). If *symptoms are severe,* give 10mL of 10% calcium gluconate (2.25mmol) IVF over 30min (bolus injections are only needed very rarely). Repeat as necessary. If due to respiratory alkalosis, correct the alkalosis.

Hypercalcemia

Signs & symptoms 'Bones, stones, groans, and psychic moans'. Abdominal pain; vomiting; constipation; polyuria; polydipsia; depression; anorexia; weight loss; tiredness; weakness; BP↑; confusion; fever; renal stones; renal failure; corneal calcification; cardiac arrest. ECG: Q–T interval↓.

Causes & diagnosis Most commonly malignancy (myeloma, bone metastases, PTHrP↑) and 1° hyperparathyroidism. Others include sarcoidosis, vitamin D intoxication, and familial benign hypocalciuric hypercalcemia (rare; defect in calcium-sensing receptor). Pointers to malignancy are: ↓albumin, ↓Cl⁻, ↓K⁺, alkalosis, ↓ PO_4^{3-}, ↑alkaline phosphatase. Other investigations (eg isotope bone scan, CXR, ESR) may also be of diagnostic value.

Treat the underlying cause. If Ca^{2+} >14mg/dL, and severe abdominal pain, vomiting, fever, or confusion, aim to reduce calcium as follows:

• Blood tests: Measure urine and electrolytes, Mg^{2+}, creatinine, Ca^{2+}, PO_4^{3-}, alkaline phosphatase.
• Fluids: Rehydrate with IVF 0.9% saline, eg 4–6L in 24h as needed. Correct hypokalemia/hypomagnesemia (mild metabolic acidosis needs no treatment). This will reduce symptoms, and ↑renal Ca^{2+} loss. Monitor urine and electrolytes.
• Diuretics: Furosemide 40mg/12h PO/IV, once rehydrated. Avoid thiazides.
• Bisphosphonates: A single dose of pamidronate will lower Ca^{2+} over 2–3d. Maximum effect is at 1wk. They inhibit osteoclast activity, and so bone resorption.
• Steroids: Occasionally used, eg prednisolone 40–60mg/d for sarcoidosis.
• Salmon calcitonin: Now rarely used. More side effects than bisphosphonates, but quicker onset. Again inhibits osteoclasts.
• Other: Chemotherapy may ↓Ca^{2+} in malignant disease, eg myeloma.

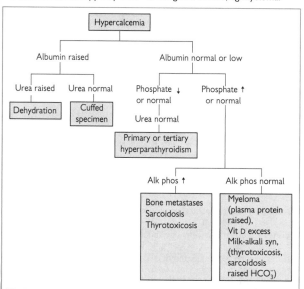

NB: The best discriminating features between bone metastases and hyperparathyroidism (the 2 commonest causes of hypercalcemia) are low albumin, low chloride, alkalosis (all suggesting metastases). Raised plasma PTH strongly supports hyperparathyroidism.

Magnesium

Magnesium is distributed 65% in bone and 35% in cells; plasma concentration tends to follow that of Ca^{2+} and K^+. Magnesium excess is usually caused by renal failure, but rarely requires treatment in its own right.

Magnesium deficiency causes paresthesias, seizures, tetany, and arrhythmias. Digitalis toxicity may be exacerbated. *Causes:* Severe diarrhea; ketoacidosis; alcohol; total parenteral nutrition (monitor weekly); accompanying hypocalcemia; accompanying hypokalemia (especially with diuretics) and hypophosphatemia. *Treatment:* If needed, give magnesium salts, PO or IV.

Hypermagnesemia is usually iatrogenic, or excessive antacids. *Features:* Neuromuscular depression, ↓BP, CNS depression, coma.

Zinc

Zinc deficiency This may occur in parenteral nutrition or, rarely, from a poor diet (too few cereals and dairy products; anorexia nervosa; alcoholism). Rarely it is due to a genetic defect. *Signs & symptoms:* Look for red, crusted skin lesions especially around nostrils and corners of mouth. *Diagnosis:* Therapeutic trial of zinc (plasma levels are unreliable as they may be low, eg in infection or trauma, without deficiency).

Selenium

An essential element present in cereals, nuts, and meat. Low soil levels in some parts of Europe and China cause deficiency states. Required for the antioxidant glutathione peroxidase, which ↓harmful free radicals. It is also antithrombogenic, and is required for sperm motility proteins. Deficiency may ↑ the frequency of neoplasia and atheroma, and may lead to a cardiomyopathy or arthritis. Serum levels are a poor guide. Toxic symptoms may also be found with overenergetic replacement.

Plasma proteins

Electrophoresis distinguishes a number of bands (see figure OPPOSITE).

Albumin is synthesized in the liver; $t_{1/2} \approx 20d$. It binds *bilirubin*, *free fatty acids*, *calcium*, and some *drugs*. *Low albumin* results in edema. *Causes:* Liver disease, nephrotic syndrome, burns, protein-losing enteropathy, malabsorption, malnutrition, late pregnancy, artifact (eg from arm with IVF), posture (5g/L higher if upright), genetic variations, malignancy. *High albumin—Causes:* Dehydration; artifact (eg stasis).

α1 zone: α_1-antitrypsin, thyroxine-binding globulin, and high-density lipoprotein (HDL). α_1-antitrypsin deficiency (autosomal recessive) leads to cirrhosis and emphysema: unopposed phagocyte proteases. Accelerated age-related decline in FEV$_1$ from a normal of ~35mL/yr to 80mL/yr, exacerbated by smoking. Signs: dyspnea; weight↓; cor pulmonale; PCV↑; LFT↑ (hepatocytes cannot secrete the protein).

α2 zone: α_2-macroglobulin, ceruloplasmin, very low density lipoprotein (VLDL), and haptoglobin.

β zone: Transferrin, low-density lipoprotein (LDL), fibrinogen, C3 and C4 complement. Reduced in active nephritis, glomerulonephritis, and SLE.

γ zone: Immunoglobulins, factor VIII, C-reactive protein (CRP), and α-fetoprotein. *Diffusely raised* in: chronic infections, liver cirrhosis, sarcoidosis, SLE, RA, Crohn's disease, TB, bronchiectasis, PBC, hepatitis, and parasitemia. It is *low* in: nephrotic syndrome, malabsorption, malnutrition, immune deficiency (severe illness, diabetes mellitus, renal failure, malignancy, or congenital).

Paraproteinemia. (See p587)

Acute phase response The body responds to a variety of insults with, among other things, the synthesis, by the liver, of a number of proteins normally present in serum in small quantities)—eg α_1-antitrypsin, fibrinogen, complement, haptoglobin, and CRP. An ↑ density of the α_1- and α_2-fractions, often with a reduced albumin level, is characteristic of conditions such as infection, malignancy (especially α_2-fraction), trauma, surgery, and inflammatory disease.

CRP Levels help monitor inflammation/infection. Normal <0.5mg/dL. Like the ESR, it is raised in many inflammatory conditions, but changes more rapidly; increases in hours and falling within 2–3d of recovery. Therefore, it can be used to follow the response to therapy (eg antibiotics) or disease activity (eg Crohn's disease). CRP values in mild inflammation 10–50mg/L; active bacterial infection 50–200mg/L; severe infection or trauma >200mg/L; see BELOW. CRP levels also predict outcome in patients with cardiovascular disease if measured using a highly sensitive assay. Low risk <1mg/dL; moderate risk 1–3; and high risk >3mg/L.

Urinary proteins
If urinary protein loss >0.15g/24h, then pathological.

Albuminuria Usually caused by renal disease. Microalbuminuria (albumin excretion between 3–300mg/d may be seen with diabetes or hypertension).

Bence Jones protein consists of light chains excreted in excess by some patients with myeloma. They are not detected by dipsticks and may occur with normal serum electrophoresis.

CRP	
Marked elevation	*Normal-to-slight elevation*
Bacterial infection	Viral infection
Abscess	Steroids/estrogens
Crohn's disease	Ulcerative colitis
Connective tissue diseases	SLE
(except SLE)	Atherosclerosis
Neoplasia	
Trauma	
Necrosis (eg MI)	

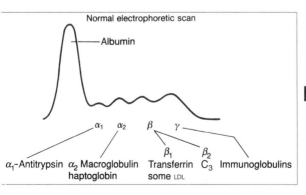

Normal electrophoretic scan

— Albumin

α_1 α_2 β γ

β_1 β_2

α_1-Antitrypsin α_2 Macroglobulin   Transferrin C_3 Immunoglobulins
haptoglobin   some LDL

625

Plasma enzymes

Reference intervals vary between laboratories.

Raised levels of specific enzymes can be a useful indicator of a disease. However, remember that most can be raised for other reasons too. The major causes of *raised enzymes* are given below.

Alkaline phosphatase
- Liver disease (suggests cholestasis).
- Bone disease (isoenzyme distinguishable, reflects osteoblast activity) especially Paget's, growing children, healing fractures, osteomalacia, metastases, 1° hyperparathyroidism, and renal failure.
- Pregnancy (placenta makes its own isoenzyme).

Alanine-amino transferase (ALT; SGPT)
- Liver disease (suggests hepatocyte damage). Also raised in shock.

α-amylase
- Acute pancreatitis (not chronic pancreatitis as little tissue remaining).
- Severe uremia, diabetic ketoacidosis.

Aspartate-amino transferase (AST; SGOT)
- Liver disease (suggesting hepatocyte damage).
- Myocardial infarction.
- Skeletal muscle damage and hemolysis.

Creatine kinase (CK)
- Myocardial infarction (isoenzyme 'CK-MB'. MI diagnosed if CK-MB>6% total CK, or CK-MB mass >99 percentile of normal).
- Muscle damage (rhabdomyolysis; prolonged running; hematoma; seizures; IM injection; defibrillation; bowel ischemia; myxedema; dermatomyositis)—and *drugs* (eg statins). A raised CK does not necessarily mean an MI.

Gamma-glutamyl transferase (GGT, γGT)
- Liver disease (particularly alcohol-induced damage, cholestasis, drugs).

Lactate dehydrogenase (LDH)
- Myocardial infarction.
- Liver disease (suggests hepatocyte damage).
- Hemolysis, pulmonary embolism, and tumor necrosis.

Tumor markers

Tumor markers are rarely sufficiently specific to be of diagnostic value. Their main value is in monitoring the course of an illness and the effectiveness of treatment. Reference ranges vary between laboratories.

Alpha-fetoprotein ↑In hepatocellular CA, germ cell tumors (not pure seminoma) hepatitis; cirrhosis; pregnancy; open neural tube defects.

CA 125 Raised in carcinoma of the ovary, uterus, breast, and hepatocellular carcinoma. Also raised in pregnancy, cirrhosis, and peritonitis.

CA 15-3 Raised in carcinoma of the breast and benign breast disease.

CA 19-9 Raised in colorectal and pancreatic carcinoma, and cholestasis.

Carcino-embryonic antigen (CEA) ↑In gastrointestinal neoplasms, especially colorectal CA. Also cirrhosis, pancreatitis, and smoking.

Human chorionic gonadotrophin Raised in pregnancy and germ cell tumors.

Neurone specific enolase (NSE) Raised in small-cell carcinoma of lung and neuroblastoma.

Placental alkaline phosphatase (PLAP) Raised in pregnancy, carcinoma of ovary, seminoma, and smoking.

Prostate specific antigen (PSA) See BOX.

Prostate specific antigen (PSA)

As well as being a marker of prostate cancer, PSA is (unfortunately) raised in benign prostatic hypertrophy. 25% of large benign prostates give PSA up to 10mcg/L; levels may be higher if recent ejaculation; therefore, avoid ejaculation for 24h prior to measurement. Other factors causing raised PSA: recent rectal examination, prostatitis, and UTI (PSA levels may not return to base-line for some months after the latter).[1] Plasma reference interval is age specific, an example of the top end of the reference interval for total PSA is:

Healthy males of age (yrs)	PSA mcg/L
40–50	2.5
50–59	3.5
60–69	5.0
70–79	6.5
80–89	7.5

The above is a rough guide only; different labs have different reference ranges, and populations vary. More specific assays, such as free PSA/total PSA index, and PSA density, are also becoming available, which may partly solve these problems. It is shown to illustrate the common problem of interpreting a PSA of ~8—and as a warning against casual requests for PSAs in the (vain) hope of simple answers. The following indicates the proportion of patients with a raised PSA and benign hypertrophy or carcinoma.

	PSA mcg/L	
Benign prostatic hypertrophy	<4 in 91%	
	4–10 in 8%	PSA will be ~50% lower
	>10 in 1%	after 6 months on 5α
Prostate carcinoma	<4 in 15%	reductase inhibitors
	4–10 in 20%	
	>10 in 65%	

1 Up to six months in one study. G Aus 2003 *Urology* **62** 278

The porphyrias

The acute porphyrias are rare genetic diseases caused by errors in the pathway of heme biosynthesis resulting in the toxic accumulation of porphobilinogen and δ-aminolaevulinic acid (porphyrin precursors). Characterized by acute neurovisceral crises, due to the ↑ production of porphyrin precursors, and their appearance in the urine. Some forms have cutaneous manifestations. Prevalence: 1–2/100,000.

Acute intermittent porphyria A low-penetrant autosomal dominant condition (porphobilinogen deaminase gene); 28% have no family history (*de novo mutations*). ~10% of those with the defective gene have neurovisceral symptoms. Attacks are intermittent, more common in women, and may be precipitated by many drugs (see below). Urine porphobilinogens are raised during attacks and often (50%) between them (the urine may go deep red on standing). Fecal porphyrin levels are normal. There are no skin manifestations.

Variegate porphyria and hereditary coproporphyria Autosomal dominant, characterized by photosensitive blistering skin lesions and/or acute attacks. The former is prevalent in Afrikaners in South Africa. Porphobilinogen is high only in an attack, and other metabolites may be detected in feces.

Features of an acute attack Colic ± vomiting ± fever ± WCC↑—so mimicking an acute abdomen (anesthesia can be disastrous here)—also:

- Hypotension
- Hyponatremia
- Hypokalemia
- Hypotonia
- Proteinuria
- Psychosis/odd behavior
- Peripheral neuritis
- Paralysis
- Seizures
- Sensory impairment
- Sight may be affected
- Shock (± collapse).

Drugs to avoid in acute intermittent porphyria are legion (they may precipitate above symptoms ± quadriplegia), they include: *alcohol*; *several anesthetic agents* (barbiturates, halothane); *antibiotics* (chloramphenicol, sulfonamides, tetracyclines); *painkillers* (pentazocine); *oral hypoglycemics*; *contraceptive pill*.

Treatment of an acute attack
- Remove precipitants, then:
- IV fluids to correct electrolyte imbalance.
- High carbohydrate intake (eg Hycal®) by NG tube if necessary.
- IV haematin is probably the treatment of choice in most centers now.
- Nausea controlled with prochlorperazine 12.5mg IM.
- Sedation if necessary with chlorpromazine 50–100mg PO/IM.
- Pain control with: aspirin, dihydrocodeine, or morphine.
- Seizures can be controlled with diazepam.
- Treat tachycardia and hypertension with propranolol.

Non-acute porphyrias

Porphyria cutanea tarda, erythropoietic protoporphyria, and *congenital erythropoietic porphyria* are characterized by cutaneous photosensitivity alone, as there is no overproduction of porphyrin precursors, only porphyrins.

Alcohol, lead, and iron deficiency cause abnormal porphyrin metabolism.

Offer genetic counseling to all patients and their families.

Radiology

Clifford R. Weiss, M.D., Ari M. Blitz, M.D., Katarzyna J. Macura, M.D., PhD

Contents

General considerations: Help the radiologist help you!

Radiology is a powerful part of the diagnostic and therapeutic tool set and has become central to the diagnosis of many medical and surgical conditions. For many diagnostic questions there are any number of imaging tests which may be of use. In general the rule is to perform less expensive and more readily available examinations (such as plain film and ultrasound) before progressing on to more expensive ones (such as CT and MRI). However, a hospital bed is an expensive resource, and if a more expensive test can make or exclude a diagnosis quickly, performing it early may save time and money and may prevent patient complications.

Deciding what test (or tests) to order and in what sequence can be quite difficult given the range of imaging tests currently available. Furthermore, most imaging tests can be tailored to maximize sensitivity and specificity depending on the patient's underlying disease process and suspected diagnosis. These considerations fall within the scope of radiology and involving a radiologist early in the decision-making process can greatly speed up the diagnostic process, saving clinician and patient time and money.

When communicating with a radiologist, it is important to realize that many imaging findings are nonspecific and can be interpreted differently depending on the clinical setting. Hence, it is of utmost importance to provide relevant clinical information when ordering the imaging study, to allow the radiologist to answer the question the clinical team has in mind.

So for any radiologic study ask yourself: How can I help the radiologist help me?

Provide the radiologist with relevant clinical history

Clinical information allows the radiologist to perform the appropriate test, to modify the imaging procedure to ↑ specificity in the characterization of pathology, to advise an alternative test that may be more appropriate, and to interpret the imaging findings in the context of the clinical information at hand. The clinical history that should be provided is essentially what is normally put in the first line of a good internal medicine presentation. It is important to include the patient's age, sex, significant underlying diseases, past surgical history, if relevant, current symptoms prompting the examination (with as much spatial/anatomic localization as possible), and the suspected diagnosis or differential diagnosis. For example: '65-year-old woman with a past medical history of pancreatic cancer, now with acute onset shortness of breath and tachycardia, suspect pulmonary embolus'.

Ask the radiologist for advice

Radiologists are imaging specialists, and should be used for consultations. Radiologists are aware of the availability of advanced technologies at the particular institution, of the appropriate preparation for a study, of equipment limitations, and of contraindications for a given study. It is essential to consult radiologists when determining which diagnostic test would be most appropriate. The radiologist may suggest a technique that the clinician may not be aware of. What is considered to be the 'best diagnostic study' for a given disease process can vary somewhat from institution to institution, depending on equipment, availability, and local expertise. The radiologist will know details.

Determine the urgency of the study

This question is essential to nighttime/off-hours radiology, in order to help the radiologist triage studies. Nonessential studies performed when the radiology department is understaffed can make it very difficult to provide essential care to critically ill patients. The levels of urgency can be divided into the following:

- *Emergent:* The patient is unstable/critically ill or rapidly deteriorating. The diagnosis is uncertain and management will rapidly change depending on the imaging findings.
- *Urgent:* The patient is stable but the management of the patient could significantly and rapidly change depending on the imaging findings.
- *Standard:* The patient is stable but there is a diagnostic dilemma which may or may not change long term management.

Prepare a patient before the procedure

The following questions should be considered:

- Is the patient aware that they are to have the study, and are they willing to have the study? Is the patient able to undergo the procedure? One standard question is: Is the patient too heavy to fit on the imaging table? Can the patient be moved?
- Is the study contraindicated for any reason? Contraindications will vary from imaging modality to modality and from organ system to organ system.
- Is the patient properly prepped for the procedure? Do they need to be NPO? Do they need to have a full bladder or a Foley catheter in place? Do they need to receive oral contrast before coming down for their procedure (and if so, how much and how long beforehand)? Are they going to receive IV contrast, and if so do they have appropriate IV access? Does the patient need consent? If so, is the patient consentable? Does the patient need to be well hydrated for the procedure? Do any medications need to be given before the procedure either as premedication or as part of procedure, or do any medications need to be stopped?

Radiography (x-rays, plain films)

Image obtained by transmitting x-rays (ionizing radiation) through the body to a detector (film or a photo-sensitive plate in digital image systems). The image obtained represents a shadowgram as the body absorbs different amounts of radiation depending on the density of the tissue. Denser tissues, such as bone absorb more radiation and appear white as only limited to no x-rays reach the film, and less dense tissues such as lung absorb less radiation and appear dark as more x-rays reach the film and expose the photo-sensitive cells.

Although this modality does use ionizing radiation, doses are fairly low, and other than early pregnancy there is essentially no contraindication to obtaining a radiograph. Because radiographs can be obtained almost anywhere there is also no weight limitation, although heavier patients require more radiation and create noisier films.

Considerations

- **'One view is no view.'** Because these are two-dimensional representations of three-dimensional structures, two orthogonal views should be obtained, if possible.
- **Not all radiographs are equal.** Radiographs done on stationary equipment within a radiology department are generally of higher-quality than are radiographs done portably. This is due to the presence of a better grid system and the ability to better position the patient on the stationary system. Thus, if the patient can be easily moved to radiology department they should be.
- **Order coned (organ-specific) radiographs.** Radiographs are most diagnostic in the center of the x-ray beam where the photons are parallel. Thus if the area of interest is the wrist, order wrist series not a forearm series, so that the wrist will be adequately included in the center of the filed of view.
- **Do not skip the radiograph.** Radiographs are excellent screening tools, are often diagnostic, and usually should be obtained before other more expensive and time consuming imaging modalities. (One glaring exception to this rule is skull radiographs which are obsolete and have been replaced by CT.)

There are 4 basic steps in interpreting any radiograph

1 **Check the technical accuracy of the film.** Is the film named, dated, right/left orientated, and marked as to whether AP (anteroposterior), PA (posteroanterior), erect, or supine. X-ray beam penetration is important: ideally vertebral bodies are visible through heart on a CXR. If the film is under penetrated diffuse 'whitening' effect and poor anatomical detail is present. Check for rotation (eg asymmetry of clavicles on a CXR) as this may affect the appearances of normal structures (eg the hila).

2 **Describe the abnormalities seen.** This may be a change in the appearance of normally visualized structures, or an area of ↑ opacity or translucency. Plain films identify the interfaces between different densities. These interfaces occur, and are visible on the film, only when two different tissue densities are immediately adjacent to each other. These densities are:

- Gas/air
- Fat (normal adipose tissue, lipomas, oily deposits, etc.)
- Soft tissue (like muscle, tendon, ligament, water, visceral organs, blood vessels, nerves, etc.)
- Calcified structures (bone, calcified granulomas, tumoral calcinosis, etc.)
- Metallic structures (surgical clips, radiodense markers in central lines bullet fragments)

A border is seen at an interface of two densities, eg heart (water) and lung (air); this 'silhouette' is lost if air in the lung is replaced by consolidation (water). This is the *silhouette sign* and can be used to localize pathology (eg right middle lobe pneumonia or collapse causing loss of distinction of the right heart border).

3 Translate the abnormalities into gross pathology (eg pleural fluid, consolidation, collapse).

4 Suggest a differential diagnosis

Develop a structured approach so as not to miss any major abnormality.

Treat the patient, not the film.

The chest film

(FIGS. 18.1–18.7)

Things to keep in mind before you start

- *Order the best possible exam:* Upright PA and lateral views are always preferable whenever possible (shallow inspiration in supine/sitting patients → crowded lung markings may simulate disease)
- *Double-check the name on the film.*
- *Look thoroughly and systematically.* Examine all the structures, including abdomen, bones, mediastinum, lungs together (to judge symmetry), and lungs separately.
- *Compare to old examinations when possible.* Age and progression of findings can be crucial to diagnosis and treatment.
- *Localize the findings:* Always look at both PA and lateral views. You need two views to localize any chest findings.

Lines and hardware: If you look at these up front, you won't forget them. All lines and hardware need to be identified and examined for correct location and potential complications. Examples include: prosthetic valves, ICDs/pacers, vagus nerve stimulators, Swan–Ganz catheters, central lines (check for tip location and for pneumothorax), endotracheal tubes (check for tip location and possible endobronchial intubation), chest tubes, NG tubes, feeding ('Dobhoff') tubes (check tip location), sternal wires (are these intact?).

The diaphragm: Check lung expansion (normally 6 ± 1 anterior ribs or 9 ± 1 posterior ribs). Overinflation may be reflected in flattened diaphragms, suggesting COPD or asthma. Right hemidiaphragm is higher than the left by up to 3 cm in 95% of cases. The lateral costophrenic angles should be sharp and acute and may be ill-defined in hyperinflation or with effusion. On a lateral view, the right hemidiaphragm is the one that passes through the heart shadow to the anterior chest wall while the left ends at the posterior heart border.

The root of the neck and trachea: The trachea is central, but slight deviation to the right may be seen inferiorly. A paratracheal line is commonly <5mm, its thickening and nodularity suggests paratracheal lymphadenopathy/mass.

Mediastinum and heart: Look for the landmarks. The cardio-thoracic ratio is the ratio of the heart width to the chest width. It should be <50% (essential to have a PA film as the heart is magnified on AP or supine films). Observe patterns of cardiac enlargement. Mediastinal widening may be due to aortic aneurysm or dissection, mediastinal fluid, enlarged lymph nodes, thymus, thyroid or tumor.

The hila: Composed of pulmonary arteries and veins with nodes and airways. Left is higher than right (~1 cm) 95% of the time but is of equal density. Look for change in density and rounded configuration. This could be due to tumor, enlarged lymph nodes, hypoinflation or just rotated film.

The lung fields:

↑ *translucency may be due to:*
- Pneumothorax—absent vascular markings and visceral pleura/lung edge visible.
- Bullous change—ie emphysema.
- Chronic pulmonary embolus—localized oligemia (regional lack of visualization of pulmonary blood vessels) .
- Hyperinflation in COPD.
- Absent anterior chest wall structures—ie mastectomy or Poland's syndrome.

Abnormal opacities may be classified as:
- Consolidation: Lobar or segmental opacity plus air bronchogram but little volume change (unlike collapse).

- Collapse/atelectasis: Volume loss causes shift of the normal landmarks (hila, fissures, diaphragm, etc.).
- Pulmonary nodules ('coin' lesions): Calcified pulmonary nodules are almost never tumors but usually represent granulomata (exceptions are metastatic osteosarcomas and chondrosarcomas).
- 'Ring' shadows: Either airways with peribronchial 'cuffing' (pulmonary edema, bronchiectasis), or cavitating lesions, eg abscess (bacterial, fungal) or tumor.
- Linear opacities: Septal lines (Kerley's B lines —interlobular lymphatics seen in low-pressure pulmonary edema, lymphangitic spread of tumor, or interstitial lung disease — eg pulmonary fibrosis). Discoid atelectasis—linear band of atelectasis.

Acute conditions not to miss

- Pneumothorax, especially tension pneumothorax (see a thin white line of visceral pleura with no lung markings peripheral to it; if tension pneumothorax, lung may be severely collapsed with mediastinal shift to the opposite side, scooping of the ipsilateral hemidiaphragm, and may also see subcutaneous air/subcutaneous emphysema)
- Widened mediastinum in a patient with chest pain and/or history of trauma— may represent aortic aneurysm or dissection, traumatic transection, and mediastinal hematoma.
- Free air in the abdomen seen under the right hemidiaphragm.

Don't:

- Succumb to 'satisfaction of search'. After identifying one example of pathology on the image, don't give up your search until you have thoroughly examined the whole film, including all the corners; there may be two or more important findings!
- Fail to give an adequate history to the radiologist and to check the radiologist's final interpretation. Basic imaging interpretation is easy, but subtle abnormalities require the trained eye of a radiologist.
- Forget to recheck danger areas. Apices, AP (aorto-pulmonary) angle, retrocardiac region, and paratracheal area.

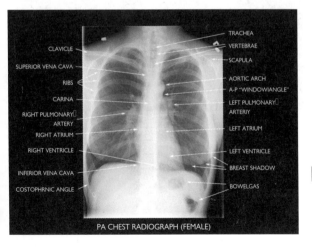

PA CHEST RADIOGRAPH (FEMALE)

TRACHEA
VERTEBRAE
SCAPULA
CLAVICLE
SUPERIOR VENA CAVA
AORTIC ARCH
RIBS
A-P "WINDOW/ANGLE"
CARINA
LEFT PULMONARY ARTERIY
RIGHT PULMONARY ARTERY
LEFT ATRIUM
RIGHT ATRIUM
RIGHT VENTRICLE
LEFT VENTRICLE
INFERIOR VENA CAVA
BREAST SHADOW
COSTOPHRNIC ANGLE
BOWELGAS

Fig. 18.1

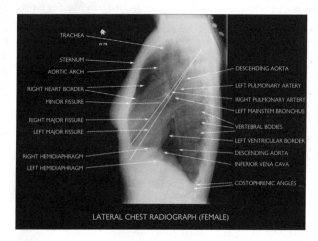

Fig. 18.2

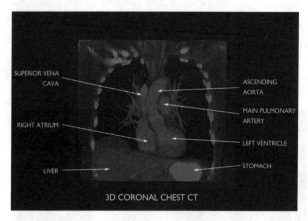

Fig. 18.3

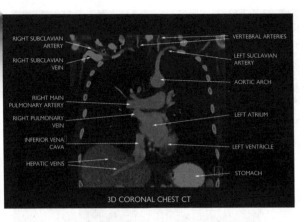

Fig. 18.4

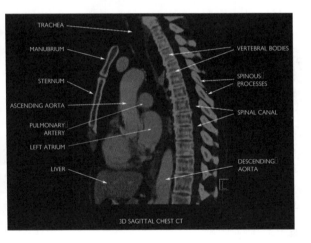

Fig. 18.5

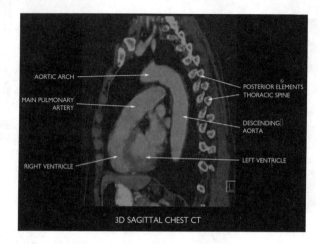

Fig. 18.6

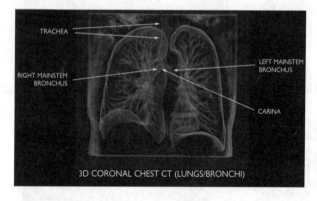

Fig. 18.7

The abdominal film (FIGS 18.8–18.12)

Things to keep in mind before you start

- *Order the best possible exam:* A true abdominal series of radiographs includes 3 films:
  1 UPRIGHT PA Chest (to look for free air under the diaphragms)
  2 UPRIGHT Abdomen AFTER at least 5min of upright positioning to allow air to percolate superiorly and appear
  3 SUPINE Abdomen.
- *Double-check the name, date and time on the film:* Make sure the patient's name matches and that you are looking at the appropriate time point.
- *Plain films only identify the interfaces between tissues of different densities.* Interfaces made by adjacent tissues which are the same density cannot be seen. For example you cannot see the interface between two adjacent loops of fluid filled small bowel. What you can identify are abnormal contours and mass effects created by the underlying pathology (ie loops of small bowel displaced by a large pelvic mass).
- *Look thoroughly and systematically:* Develop a repeatable method by which you look at all abdominal films; review by organ system.
- *Compare new vs. old findings:* Compare to prior films whenever possible, as age and progression of findings can be crucial to diagnosis and treatment.
- *Don't forget the patient:* While abdominal radiographs can offer valuable clues to diagnosis, it is possible for a very sick patient to have a normal appearing abdominal series of radiographs.

Observe the gas pattern and position. Small bowel is recognized by its central position and valvulae conniventes, thin folds that reach from one wall to the other. Larger bowel is more peripheral and the haustrae, colonic folds, extend only partially across. Abnormal position may point to pathology eg centrally displaced loops in ascites; bowel displaced to the left lower quadrant by splenomegaly. Look for dilated bowel loops, defined as >3cm diameter for the small bowel, and as >6cm diameter for the large bowel. Also look for air-fluid levels in the bowel on upright film.

- If the dilated loops are the small bowel only, it is a probable small bowel obstruction
- If the dilated loops are the large bowel only, it may be a large bowel obstruction or a cecal or sigmoid volvulus when x-ray shows a large 'bean' shaped loop of large bowel arising from pelvis.
- If the dilated loops are seen in the small and large bowel, it may be an adynamic ileus, a large bowel obstruction with an incompetent ileocecal valve, gastroenteritis, or excessive aerophagia.
- Localized peritoneal inflammation can cause a localized dilatation of bowel in response to inflammatory irritation (focal ileus). This may be seen on the plain film as a 'sentinel loop' of intraluminal gas and can provide a clue to the site of pathology.

Look for extraluminal/extraintestinal gas. Look everywhere. Look in the portal vein territory (peripheral liver) or biliary system (central liver and gallbladder) where air may be seen after passing a stone, after ERCP, or with gas-forming biliary infection or with bowel necrosis). Look at the GU system (entero-vesical fistula, pyelonephritis), in the peritoneum (double wall sign-visualization of the outer wall of bowel loops caused by gas outside the bowel loop and normal intraluminal gas), triangle sign (represents a triangular pocket of air between two loops of bowel and the abdominal wall), football sign (a large collection of air, which seems to outline the entire abdominal cavity, air surrounding the falciform ligament, may have the appearance of the laces of the football), the colonic wall (pneumatosis coli, infective colitis) or in a subphrenic abscess. Free air can be detected on the left lateral decubitus radiograph, as free air collects around the inferior edge of the liver, which forms the least dependent part of the abdomen in that position.

Look for calcification in the abdomen or pelvis. Calcification in arteries (atherosclerosis, the eggshell calcification in an aneurysm), lymph nodes, phleboliths (smooth, round), renal calcification or ureteric stones (usually jagged; look along the line of the ureter), adrenal (TB), pancreatic (chronic pancreatitis), liver or spleen granulomas, gallstones (only 10% radio-opaque), bladder (stone, tumor, TB, schistosomiasis), uterus fibroids, dermoid cyst of the ovary which may contain teeth.

Bones of spine and pelvis. Look for metastases (osteolytic or osteoblastic), Paget's disease—'picture frame vertebral body', osteomalacia, collapse, osteoarthritis, hyperparathyroidism—'rugger-jersey' spine, ankylosing spondylitis—'bamboo spine'.

Soft tissues. The psoas lines are obliterated in retroperitoneal inflammation, hemorrhage or peritonitis. Note kidney size and shape (normally 2–3 vertebral bodies length and parallel to the psoas line).

Acute conditions not to miss:
• Pneumoperitoneum—this usually means perforation unless recent instrumentation.
• Portal venous air (peripheral liver) and/or pneumatosis (air in the wall of bowel, usually colon)—this often means necrotic bowel.

Don't:
• Forget to look for lower lung pathology on the upright abdominal film.

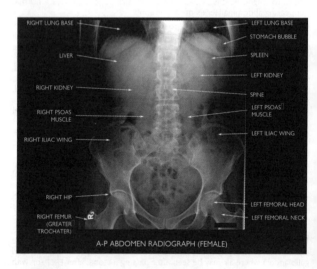

A-P ABDOMEN RADIOGRAPH (FEMALE)

Fig. 18.8

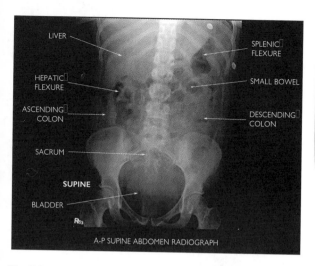

Fig. 18.9

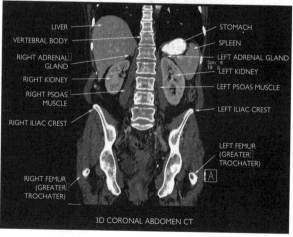

Fig. 18.10

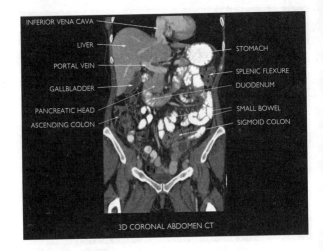

Fig. 18.11

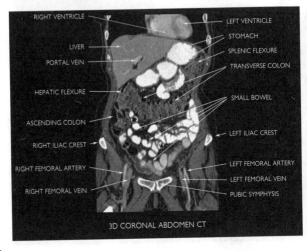

642   Fig. 18.12

Chest and abdominal radiography

Although in many cases CT and MRI have replaced many of the traditional plain film imaging series, chest and abdominal radiography should be the first step in chest and abdominal imaging. They are fast, inexpensive and are excellent screening tools and in most cases these will suffice.

Skull /sinus radiography: Except when looking for radio-opaque foreign bodies in the head (orbits, face etc.) skull radiographs should not be ordered. CT is far more sensitive and specific and is standard of care for head imaging.

Skeletal radiography: Plain film evaluation is often the first method of examination of the extremities and demonstrates fractures, joint effusions, radiodense foreign matter, and lytic or sclerotic bone lesions. Even if MR and CT are requested for further evaluation, comparison to plain films is often essential for accurate diagnosis of skeletal abnormalities, and will be needed by the radiologist.

Spine radiography: Although often obtained in acute trauma to assess for acute fracture, multidetector CT has largely replaced spine radiography in this area as it is far more sensitive and specific than radiography, and multiplanar reconstructions can be performed. If traumatic spinal injury is strongly suspected CT should be the first imaging test obtained, followed by MRI as needed.

Fluoroscopy

Fluoroscopy is a real-time, moving radiograph. This modality does use ionizing radiation the dose of which ↑ with ↑ patient weight, and with ↑ study length. It should also be noted there is in fact a weight limit on the fluoroscopy table, and this should be confirmed with fluoroscopy team prior to sending the patient to radiology.

GI studies with contrast. In all of these studies radiopaque contrast (either barium or water soluble contrast depending on perforation and aspiration risks) is introduced by mouth, feeding tube, or enema in order to evaluate the GI tract.

Upper GI series is performed for evaluation of the esophagus, stomach, and duodenum. *The upper GI series with small bowel follow through* continues to follow the contrast though the entire small bowel. Indications for these studies include: • The diagnosis of perforation of the esophagus or stomach (post-traumatic or iatrogenic). • The evaluation of gastric outlet obstruction. • The evaluation of bowel obstruction. • The evaluation of GI bleeding or of Crohn's disease when endoscopy is normal. • The evaluation of malabsorption syndromes. • The evaluation of small bowel motility. • The evaluation of surgical anastomosis in a post-op patient.

Cine-esophagram is a method for investigating dysphagia when motility and pharyngeal coordination need to be observed. This is a very specialized study in which a patient is asked to swallow barium containing solids and liquids of various consistencies under direct fluoroscopic visualization. These studies are filmed for detailed review and are often performed in conjunction with clinical speech and swallowing specialists.

Enteroclysis is a rarely performed procedure used for more detailed evaluation of the small bowel. The indications are the same as for a small bowel series. Enteroclysis is more sensitive in the evaluation of tiny small bowel tumors and mucosal lesions. However, this study involves the placement of a naso-duodenal tube to deliver special contrast mix with cellulose for a 'see-through' effect, and a higher dose of radiation.

Barium enema is commonly performed with the 'double contrast' (barium and air) technique which provides a more detailed examination of surface mucosal pattern. Cleansing the colon is the single most important determinant of quality of barium enemas. Indications include:
• Demonstration of structural lesions (eg tumor, diverticula, polyps, ulcers, fistulae, perforation). • Evaluation of colonic obstruction. • Failed colonoscopy.

Intravenous pyelography (IVP). In the past, this examination was used to evaluate for renal masses, collecting system and obstruction. However IVP has essentially been replaced by CT urography and MRI.

Percutaneous transhepatic cholangiography is used to confirm dilated biliary ducts in obstructive jaundice in combination with external drainage or internal drainage (using an endoprosthesis across the stricture).

Angiography. Angiography involves the use of intravenous contrast dye to visualize arterial and venous disease (atheromatous stenosis and thrombosis, embolism, aneurysms, AV fistulae and angiomatous malformations), and may be combined with interventions eg balloon dilatation, stenting, embolization, thrombolysis etc.

Pulmonary angiography is used for visualization of emboli and vascular abnormalities and assessment of right heart pressures. It is the historic 'gold standard' procedure for diagnosis of PE but has been largely replaced by CT pulmonary angiography.

Cerebral angiography is used for the evaluation of intra- and extracranial vascular disease such as atherosclerosis, aneurysms, and arteriovenous malformations.

Visceral angiography is used to evaluate the patency of the visceral arterial supply in cases of suspected ischemic bowel. It is also used to locate the source of GI bleeding (acute or chronic) and to treat these areas by selectively infusing drugs or embolic material into the bleeding territory.

Renal angiography is used for the investigation of renal hypertension (2° to atheroma or fibromuscular hyperplasia) and can guide vascular interventions, eg balloon angioplasty, stenting.

Peripheral angiography is used for the evaluation of peripheral vascular disease.

It is important to realize that CT and MR angiography have replaced many of the diagnostic angiographic studies listed above and that much of the angiographic work that is performed today is therapeutic rather than purely diagnostic.

Contrast reactions: There are many types of contrast agents that can be administered intravenously, including high osmolar, low osmolar, ionic, and nonionic contrast media. All of the contrast media for the x-ray based studies (angiography, CT, IVP) are iodine based. Any contrast agent administered intravenously can cause adverse reactions. Reactions include hives, bronchospasm, cardio-pulmonary compromise from anaphylaxis. Adverse reactions occur in ~1/1000 patients and death by anaphylaxis in 1/40,000. Risk factors for contrast reaction should always be reviewed prior to imaging. With a history of mild to moderate prior reaction to IV contrast, the patient may require pre-medication with steroids. A common regimen includes prednisone 40mg PO, 24h, 12h, and 1h before the procedure and a single dose of diphenhydramine 50mg PO 1h before the procedure. When the patient has a history of severe anaphylactic reaction to IV contrast, iodine based contrast is absolutely contraindicated. It is important to note that there is no proven link between seafood and contrast allergies.

Contrast mediated nephrotoxicity: Risk factors include congestive heart failure, diabetes, pre-existing renal insufficiency, age greater than 70, concurrent nephrotoxic medications, high dose hyperosmolar IV contrast, diuretic medications, or dehydration. IV 0.9% saline 1mL/kg/hr 4–6h before contrast administration and 12–24h after exposure, significantly reduces the risk of contrast nephrotoxicity in patients with mild renal insufficiency. Acetylcysteine dosed 600mg PO BID for 24h before contrast administration and continued for 48h after contrast, along with hydration, is superior to hydration alone in preventing nephrotoxicity[1]. When possible, it is beneficial to discontinue nephrotoxic medications and diuretics for at least 24h after contrast administration. Low osmolar contrast media are less nephrotoxic than high osmolar contrasts in patients with renal insufficiency. Alternative imaging modalities such as magnetic resonance, ultrasound, and nuclear scintigraphy should be considered in patients at high risk of developing contrast nephropathy.

1 Brick, R. et al. Acetylcysteine for prevention of contrast nephropathy: meta analysis. *Lancet* 2003; **303**: 598–603.

Ultrasound (sonography)

Ultrasound uses the reflections of high-frequency sound waves to construct an image of a body organ. This modality is extremely powerful tool, which can be tailored to any number of diagnostic and interventional uses. It does not use ionizing radiation to produce images; hence it is safe even in early stages of pregnancy. Furthermore ultrasound is completely portable. There are essentially no contraindications to ultrasound, although very obese people may have a limited examination.

Ultrasound is the imaging modality of choice in obstetrics and is often the first line of investigation of abdominal organs and pelvic lesions. Ultrasound is often used to guide needle aspiration, or biopsy of masses and collections. However, it is very operator-dependent and reliability of results may vary. The use of color Doppler allows the assessment of vascular patency and direction of flow through vessels. Pulsed Doppler ultrasound can be used in quantitative analysis of flow.

Abdominal scan (including renal and right upper quadrant) may be used to assess: 1) The liver—size and texture (eg fatty liver, shrunken cirrhotic liver), masses within it (cysts vs. tumor). 2) The biliary system (dilation in obstructive jaundice, although the cause, ie stone vs. tumor, is less reliably seen). 3) Doppler of the portal and splanchnic veins is used to rule out thrombosis and assess direction of flow in the portal veins in cirrhosis. 4) The gallbladder (inflammatory thickening and gallstones). 5) The pancreas (pseudocysts, abscesses and sometimes tumor, note that the pancreas is often poorly seen, being obscured by bowel gas). 6) The aorta and major vessels for aneurysm. 7) The kidneys (size, texture, hydronephrosis, cystic disease, stones, tumor, perinephric fluid collections, renal vascular patency). 8) The appendix for suspected appendicitis in pediatric patients, pregnant women and thin adults. Note that right upper quadrant and abdominal ultrasounds require that the patient remain NPO between 4–8h prior to the examination in order to allow the gallbladder to expand, and in order to minimize abdominal gas. Also, a quantitative serum β-HCG should be obtained before all pelvic ultrasounds performed in young women in order to evaluate for ectopic pregnancy as the interpretation of this examination varies widely depending on the levels of β-HCG.

Pelvic scan may be used to assess: 1) Obstetric pathology—ultrasound is the standard imaging technique for monitoring of normal and abnormal pregnancy, fetal growth and organ development, localization of the placenta, and ectopic pregnancy. 2) Ovaries (masses—tumors, cysts, torsion). 3) Uterus (masses—fibroids, cysts, endometrial polyps, hyperplasia). **Pelvic ultrasounds in female patients require transabdominal scan (TA) and transvaginal scan (TV). For a TA scan a full bladder either due to oral intake of water or due to filling of the bladder via a Foley catheter is needed. For a TV scan, patient needs to consent.

Testicular scan. Useful for the evaluation of testicular masses, infections (epididymitis, orchitis), torsion.

Vascular scan. Duplex/Doppler evaluation can be used to assess arterial and venous patency throughout the body. 1) Arterial (carotid and peripheral arterial stenosis, fistulae, aneurysm). 2) Venous (lower extremity venous ultrasound with compression is the standard of care for the assessment of deep venous thrombosis).

Thyroid scan. Used to distinguish cyst from solid nodule/tumor. May not be able to characterize nodule as benign or malignant. Used for guidance for percutaneous biopsy.

Ultrasound-guided biopsy/drainage (including paracentesis and thoracentesis) can be performed throughout the body. Ultrasound provides guidance and safe access to avoid injury to adjacent organs, and its use is the standard of care for most percutaneous procedures.

Computed tomography (CT, CAT) scan

To produce a computed tomography (CT) image a rotating x-ray tube and detectors are used to scan a patient as she/he is passed through the scanner gantry. The scans from each 360° rotation are then processed to produce cross-sectional images which can subsequently be post-processed to provide 2D and 3D reconstructions of body organs in different projections. This modality is X-ray based and uses ionizing radiation.

CT scanners produced after the early 1990s use spiral acquisition algorithms. In fact, most scanners currently are designed as multi-detector or 'multislice' scanners. Multidetector imaging allows for faster scanning, thinner slices, higher imaging resolution, and better 3D reconstruction from the entire volume of scanned body part.

CT can be performed with or without IV or oral contrast. Oral contrast should always be given prior to abdominal or pelvic scanning in order to help delineate the bowel (the exception are protocols for renal stone studies and CT angiography). In order to fill as much of the bowel as possible the general rule is to give oral contrast early and often. IV contrast is used to differentiate enhancing vascular structures and lesions from non-enhancing nonvascular structures. The contrast used for CT is similar to that used in angiographic procedures, therefore standard precautions and consent are utilized.

Tissue density measurements (expressed as Hounsfield units) can be used to differentiate between tissue types (air, fat, muscle, blood, fluid, bone). In Hounsfield units, bone has attenuation of +1000, water is 0, air is –1000, fat is <0 and the remaining tissues fall between depending on tissue composition.

Head CT. CT is the first line diagnostic procedure for intracranial processes. CT can diagnose hydrocephalus, intracranial hemorrhage (subdural, epidural, subarachnoid, intraparenchymal), masses/intracerebral edema, and cerebral atrophy. CT is indicated in the setting of moderate to severe head trauma to assess intracranial structures as well as the cranial bones, and provides an excellent assessment of the extent and location of intracranial hemorrhage. If injury to the region of the face is suspected a separate facial CT should be ordered evaluate for facial fractures and intraorbital pathology. Although unenhanced head CT is often normal within the 1st 6h after ischemic infarction it should still be ordered on all patients suspected of presenting with ischemic stroke to assess for the presence of hemorrhage (a contraindication to the administration of thrombolytic agents), of alternative diagnoses (such as intracranial mass) and mass effect and edema which may alter the treatment plan. Contrast enhanced multidetector CT perfusion and cerebral/cervical angiography is an exquisitely sensitive modality for assessment of acute infarction, as well as assessing for cerebrovascular embolic sources. The combination of unenhanced and contrast enhanced CT may soon become the modality of choice for the assessment of ischemic infarction, due to its widespread availability and speed.

Neck CT. Contrast enhanced CT of the neck is useful to assess for traumatic damage, abscess, neoplasm and for vascular disease (CT angiography).

Chest CT. CT is the modality of choice for the evaluation of thoracic abnormalities. Non-contrast chest CT is able to demonstrate small lesions such as pneumonias, pleural deposits, and pulmonary nodules which are not visible on plain radiography. High resolution chest CT is used to assess and diagnose lung parenchymal disease (eg emphysema, interstitial lung disease). Contrast enhanced chest CT is used to evaluate lung and pleural masses as well as mediastinal masses and thoracic adenopathy. CT angiography is the modality of choice for the assessment of pulmonary embolism, aortic aneurysm and aortic dissection, as well as post trauma when aortic injury is suspected. ECG–gated, multidetector CT is also being used to perform coronary angiography and to assess cardiac function.

Abdominal CT: CT is also the modality of choice for the evaluation of nearly all abdominal pathology in both solid and luminal organs. With few exceptions (such as renal stone protocols) abdominal CT should be performed with both oral and intravenous contrast. This provides the most contrast between abdominal structures, allows for evaluation of post-trauma injuries (eg active hemorrhage, parenchymal organ and hollow organ injuries), infection/abscess, masses, adenopathy, and vascular disease throughout the abdomen. Unenhanced CT is the modality of choice when evaluating a patient for renal stones. CT can be used to assess for bowel disease such as obstruction, cancer, perforation/pneumoperitoneum, and inflammatory/infectious disease. CT is usually not the modality of choice for the evaluation of purely pelvic pathology especially in female patients (ie GU-origin). Both ultrasound and MRI are more sensitive and specific, have higher resolution within the pelvis, and do not irradiate the gonads. CT is useful in assessing pelvic adenopathy, GI tract and skeletal abnormalities.

Musculoskeletal CT. CT examination is generally reserved for operative planning for complex fractures or to further evaluate or characterize osseous lesions. As in other areas of the body, contrast enhanced CT is excellent for evaluating possible soft tissue abscess in these regions.

Spine CT. If equivocal plain film findings or severe pain are present CT scan to assess the osseous structure of the spinal column should be considered. In most major trauma centers cervical spine CT has nearly completely replaced plain radiography when cervical spine trauma is strongly suspected.

CT Angiography. High-resolution, contrast enhanced, multidetector CT is able to produce 3D reconstructed images of nearly every arterial territory. CT has already begun to replace cerebral, carotid, thoracic, pulmonary arterial, abdominal, renal and peripheral diagnostic angiography in both emergent and non-emergent settings.

Magnetic resonance imaging (MRI)

MRI uses a combination of powerful magnetic fields and radiofrequency waves to image protons within the soft tissues of the body and is able to provide high contrast between different types of soft tissues. Tissues are excited in the magnetic field and can be identified via specific signal characteristics that are registered by a computer and transformed into images. MR is a very diverse technique which uses pulse sequences to produce various tissue weightings (eg T1, T2, proton density) to allow for superior soft tissue characterization. No ionizing radiation is used in this procedure. There are no known biological hazards to humans from being exposed to magnetic fields of the strength used in medical imaging today. Most facilities prefer not to image pregnant women. This is due to the fact that there has not been much research done in the area of biological effects on a developing fetus. The first trimester in a pregnancy is the most critical and the decision of whether or not to scan a pregnant patient is made on a case-by-case basis with consultation between the MRI radiologist and the patient's obstetrician. The benefit of performing the scan must outweigh the risk, however small, to the fetus and mother. Informed consent is usually obtained before the procedure.

Although MRI is an extremely powerful technique which is advancing rapidly, it is limited by a lack of portability, its relatively slow speed of imaging, requirement to lay still (patient's motion distorts imaging), highly variable and specific imaging protocols tailored to the clinical questions, limitation in the field of view that can be imaged at high resolution (scan focused on the organ of interest can generate more detail) and by many absolute and relative contraindications.

MRI machines are noisy, and some patients become disoriented, suffering claustrophobia and sometimes panic. Thorough discussion of the procedure and sedation may be needed to comfort the patient.

Contraindications to MRI: The specific contraindications to MRI will vary from institution to institution.
- *Absolute contraindications:*
  - Non-MRI compliant aneurysm clips or other surgical clips placed in the last 6wks
  - Neurostimulator device
  - Pacemaker or defibrillator (this may vary)
  - Cochlear implant
  - Metallic ocular foreign body (suspect this in patients with a welding history—evaluate with orbit x-ray)
  - Other metallic implanted devices such as insulin pumps
  - Metallic shrapnel
  - Obesity >the maximum table allowance (will vary, usually <350lb).
- *Relative contraindications:*
  - Claustrophobia
  - Unstable patients (only MR compatible life support equipment can be used in the scanning area)
  - Dependance on infusion pumps.

Gadolinium contrast: Gadolinium is a very safe contrast agent in patients with normal renal function. It is completely unrelated to CT/angiographic iodinated contrast, and gadolinium allergies are extremely rare. Gadolinium is avoided in pregnant patients and in patients with renal failure (see BOX).

> Nephrogenic Systemic Fibrosis/Nephrogenic Fibrosing Dermopathy (NSF/NFD) is a newly described complication of gadolinium in patients with renal failure.
>
> NSF/NFD is seen in patients that have noticeably advanced renal failure. The disease causes fibrosis of the skin and connective tissues throughout the body. Patients develop skin thickening that may prevent bending and extending joints, resulting in decreased mobility of joints. In addition, patients may experience fibrosis that has spread to other parts of the body such as the diaphragm, muscles in the thigh and lower abdomen, and the interior areas of lung vessels. The clinical course of NSF/NFD is progressive and may be fatal.
>
> Before gadolinium is administered to patients with renal failure, your institution's policy regarding NSF/NFD should be consulted.

Head/neck MRI. MRI is the modality of choice for the evaluation of tumors and infections of the head (both intra and extra cranially), face and neck. MRI is also indicated in the evaluation of demyelinating disease (eg multiple sclerosis). MRI with diffusion weighted and perfusion imaging is an exquisitely sensitive modality for assessment of acute infarction and can demonstrate a region of infarction and its ↓ or delayed perfusion within minutes of onset of symptoms. MR angiography (MRA) can be performed to evaluate the carotid and vertebral arteries as well as the circle of Willis for atherosclerotic disease, stenosis and aneurysm. MR venography is used for the assessment of venous sinus thrombosis.

Spine MRI. If neurologic findings relating to the spine are present or if demyelination, infection or neoplasm involving the spinal canal are suspected, MRI is the modality of choice for the evaluation of the spinal cord and the surrounding CSF spaces. If MRI is unavailable or contraindicated, CT myelography can be considered.

Chest MRI. MRI is less sensitive in the evaluation of lung parenchyma when compared to CT. However, MRI can be used to assess mediastinal masses, chest wall tumors, and breast masses. MRI and MRA (MR angiography) is frequently used in the evaluation of the thoracic aorta for aneurysm and/or dissection. ECG gated cardiac MRI is also indicated for the evaluation of myocardial function, of structural/congenital anomalies of the heart (eg repaired tetralogy of Fallot), and of cardiac tumors (eg myxoma). Furthermore, MRI's abilities to distinguish healthy myocardium from diseased or scarred myocardium allows for the evaluation of right ventricular dysplasia, hypertrophic cardiomyopathy, and for the detection of infarcted, stunned, and normal myocardium.

Abdominal MRI. MRI of the abdomen can be used for the evaluation of mass or infection within any of the solid abdominal organs and, to a lesser degree, hollow organs. MRI is most often used for the evaluation of lesions that are poorly seen on CT (eg metastatic disease), for the characterization of lesions that are indeterminate with other modalities (eg 'complex' renal cysts or 'indeterminate' liver or adrenal lesions), and for patients who are unable to be evaluated with CT (eg allergy to iodinated contrast). MRI is often used to assess the biliary tree (MRCP) to evaluate pancreatic ductal anomalies (eg divisum) or for diagnosis of biliary obstruction. MRA of the abdomen is used for the evaluation of the renal arteries, celiac trunk, superior and inferior mesenteric arteries, for stenosis and atherosclerotic disease. MRA is also used to assess aortic dissection or aneurysm.

Pelvic MRI. MRI is a sensitive and specific modality for the evaluation of both the male and female pelvis. In both men and women MRI can be used to evaluate for abscess, lymphadenopathy, carcinomas of the colon and rectum, carcinomas of the bladder, and pelvic soft tissue masses. In the post-operative setting, MRI can be used to distinguish between post-operative changes and tumor recurrence, and monitor response to therapy. In the female pelvis MRI is the modality of choice for the evaluation of uterine anomalies (eg Müllerian duct anomalies, adenomyosis), for the assessment of adnexal masses, and the radiologic staging of cervical and endometrial cancer. It can also be used to evaluate pelvic organ prolapse. In the male pelvis, endorectal MRI is used for staging of prostate cancer

Musculoskeletal MRI. MRI is the modality of choice when examination of ligaments and tendons is necessary and is also the best means of examination of the bone marrow and soft tissue masses. MRI, therefore, is commonly used for the evaluation of joints for ligamentous injury, cartilaginous injury, meniscal tears, or arthritic changes. MRI is most often ordered for the evaluation of the knees to evaluate meniscal tears, ACL and PCL tears, cartilaginous injury and for degenerative changes. MRI is also the modality of choice for the evaluation of the shoulder joints, and is typically ordered for the evaluation of rotator cuff tears or for other traumatic or degenerative changes in the shoulder. MR arthrography of the shoulder is most useful for the evaluation of labral tears. MRI is used for the evaluation of suspected radiographically occult fractures, palpable soft tissue masses, and in the staging of primary neoplasms of the bone and soft tissue. MR angiography of the extremities can be performed with or without the use of IV gadolinium for the evaluation of peripheral vascular disease.

Radioisotope scanning (nuclear medicine)

Radioisotope scanning involves the administration of a small amount of radioactive tracer and plotting its distribution throughout the body in general and in the organ that is to be studied in particular.

The radioactive tracer consists of a ligand (nonradioactive) which is complexed to a radionuclide. Technetium-99m (^{99}Tcm) is the most common tracer used in nuclear medicine imaging centers; others include Indium-111 (^{111}In), Iodine-123 (^{123}I), Gallium-67 (^{67}Ga) (all gamma ray emitters). The gamma rays emitted by the radioisotope are transformed into analogue and/or digital information by a gamma camera. Imaging performed by a rotating gamma camera is termed Single Photon Emission Computed Tomography or SPECT.

Anatomic modalities such as CT or MRI provide anatomical details but rarely allow assessment of the functional significance of the anatomical abnormalities. Radioisotope studies provide physiological/functional information. Correlative imaging provides complimentary information of greater clinical relevance than either type of test individually. Many SPECT cameras have been combined with CT scanners in order to provide fusion images which display both function and anatomy simultaneously.

Bone scan. ^{99}Tcm-MDP (methylene diphosphonate) is the commonly used radiotracer; it is retained in areas with ↑ osteoblastic activity. Common indications: Assessment of metastatic disease from a known primary, Assessment of extent of Paget's disease, Diagnosis of occult or stress fractures, Identification of osteoid osteoma, Characterization of metabolic bone disease. Note that bone scanning it typically negative in cases of multiple myeloma.

Cardiac scan. *Myocardial perfusion imaging* is used mainly to evaluate atypical chest pain, to assess the extent of ischemic heart disease, and to assess viable myocardium prior to revascularization. Dipyridamole, adenosine or dobutamine are used as stressors if arthritis, abnormal ECG (left bundle branch block, or on digoxin with changes to the ECG) preclude exercise, or those in whom the exercise test is inconclusive. SPECT imaging is performed after injection of ^{201}Tl (Thallium-201), or ^{99}Tcm-MIBI (methoxy isobutyl isonitrile). *Radionudide ventriculography (MUGA):* ECG—gated imaging is performed after radiolabeled red blood cells and provides objective and reproducible data on ventricular ejection fractions, regional wall motion abnormalities and information on ventricular aneurysms.

Lung scan (V/Q). ^{99}Tcm -MAA (macroaggregates of albumin) is commonly used to assess perfusion (Q) and ^{133}Xe is used to assess ventilation (V). V/Q scanning relies on the physiological principle of reduction in segmental perfusion with maintained normal ventilation in pulmonary embolism. Matched reduction in perfusion and ventilation can be seen in parenchymal lung disorders. Scans are always interpreted with a current CXR and reports are in the form of probabilities: High probability (>80% likelihood of PE), low probability (<20% likelihood of PE), intermediate probability (~20–80% likelihood of PE) or 'very low probability' (<5% likelihood of PE). Note that CT pulmonary angiography is both sensitive and specific technique for the assessment of acute pulmonary embolism.

Liver scan. ^{99}Tcm-tin or sulfur colloid are taken up by macrophages (Kupffer cells in liver) and may be used to assess diffuse liver disease.

Hepatobiliary scan (HIDA). ^{99}Tcm—mebrofenin is taken up by the hepatocytes, and secreted into the bile, then disperses with the bile into the bile ducts, the gallbladder, and the intestine. This test is used mainly to diagnose acute cholecystitis, for diagnosing biliary leaks post surgery and for quantitative information on gallbladder kinetics (ie assessment of chronic cholecystitis) when used in conjunction with an IV infusion of cholecystokinin (CCK).

Thyroid scan. ^{99}Tcm-pertechnetate or ^{123}I-Iodide may be used for assessment of solitary thyroid nodules, for assessment of congenital hypothyroidism and localization of ectopic thyroid tissue, diagnosis of autonomous functioning thyroid adenomas and for the differentiation of Graves' from multinodular goiter. ^{131}I scans are useful in the assessment and follow-up of patients with thyroid cancer.

Parathyroid scan. ^{99}Tcm -MIBI is used to localize a parathyroid adenoma once a biochemical diagnosis of primary hyperparathyroidism is made.

Adrenal scan. Pheochromocytomas and other tumors of neuroectodermal origin can be localized using ^{123}I-MIBG (metaiodobenzylguanidine).

Renal scan. Radioisotope scanning and computer-assisted analysis of the images of the kidneys (renography) provides vital functional information. Standard renography with ^{99}Tcm-DTPA or ^{99}Tcm-MAG3 (Mertiatide) provides data on split renal function, and uptake and excretory patterns of each kidney. Diuretic renography performed by injecting furosemide at the end of a standard renogram helps to distinguish physiological dilatation of the renal pelvis from obstructive nephropathy. Captopril renography performed by repeating the standard renogram after administration of PO captopril (25–50mg) helps to confirm renovascular disorder (unilateral better than bilateral). ^{99}Tcm -DMSA (dimethyl succinic acid), a renal cortical imaging agent, is useful in chronic pyelonephritis; renal scarring, cortical cysts, and tumors.

Inflammation/infection scan. ^{111}In-oxine labeled leukocytes are typically used to evaluate osteomyelitis (in conjunction with either a phase bone scan using ^{99}Tcm-MDP or a marrow scan using ^{99}Tcm-sulfur colloid). However, leukocytes radiolabeled with ^{111}In-oxine or ^{99}Tcm-HMPAO can also be used for the evaluation of fever of unknown origin; localization of abscesses (5–10d old) evaluation of chronic inflammation, assessment of mediastinal lymphomas, prosthetic infection (especially hip) and assessment of patients with inflammatory bowel disease.

Lymphangiography is useful to differentiate venous edema from lymphatic edema and to diagnose lymphatic obstruction.

Esophageal transit and gastric emptying studies help to assess upper GI motility.

Radiolabeled red blood cell scans are useful in the localization of active upper GI bleeding.

Meckel's scans help to localize abnormal functioning ectopic gastric mucosa (as in Meckel's diverticulum).

Positron emission tomography (PET)

Molecules labeled with positron-emitting radionuclides are injected, and post-annihilation event photon paths are analyzed by crystal detectors to produce 3D images of glucose metabolism ^{18}F- FDG (fluorodeoxyglucose).

Currently PET is used primarily for the evaluation of recurrent/metastatic tumors, for assessing tumor response to chemo/radiation therapy, and for assessing an unknown lesion's metabolic activity/neoplastic potential—eg a newly appearing lung nodule. Studies are frequently performed in a hybrid PET/CT scanner for accurate physiologic/anatomic correlation.

PET can also be used to determine the site of epileptogenic foci, where there is no anatomic lesion which could be demonstrated by MRI. PET can also be used to diagnose dementia (even before symptoms start), and distinguish Alzheimer's from other dementias (symmetrical hypometabolism in parietal and temporal lobes not the frontal lobes, which are affected in Pick's dementia, for example).

PET development is currently one of the most active areas of research within radiology and its indications and uses continue to expand.

Practical procedures

Rosalyn W. Stewart, M.D., M.S., C. Mathew Stewart, M.D., PhD

Contents

There is no substitute for learning by experience. It is better to wait for someone to come and assist you with a non-urgent procedure when you are not fully confident in your skills, than to try on your own.

General considerations

- Always obtain informed consent; explain the procedure, the indications, risks, and alternatives.
- Getting consent for life-saving emergency procedures is not necessary.
- Universal precautions should be practiced and proper sterile technique is essential.
- Sedation and analgesia, when required, should be planned in advance
- Assess for presence of coagulapathy or need to modify medications (eg heparin drip)

Suturing

- Assess for foreign-body (consider X-ray), deep tissue damage, injury to nerve, blood vessels or tendons.
- Anesthetize wound with topical anesthetic, local, or regional anesthetic.
- Clean wound with copious sterile normal saline irrigation.
- Select suture type, or use liquid stitches (if using glue, no need to anesthetize wound).
- Size indicated by a '0', the more '0's the smaller (4–0 is <3–0).
- Apply topical antibiotic and sterile dressing, if near joint, immobilize with a splint.
- Consider need for tetanus prophylaxis.

Body region	Size of suture	Removal (days)
Scalp	Staple, or 4, 5–0	5–7
Face	6–0	3–5
Trunk	4, 5–0	5–7
Extremities	4, 5–0	7
Joints	4–0	10–14
Hand	5–0	7
Foot	3, 4–0	7–10

Nasogastric tube insertion

Indication

Aspirate stomach contents for diagnosis (eg assess for GI bleeding) or treatment (eg treatment of ileus, obstruction), or for feeding/medication.

Contraindications

• Facial or basilar skull fractures, esophageal stricture, history of caustic ingestion, penetrating cervical spine wounds, choanal atresia, recent surgery to upper GI tract, Zenker's diverticulum.

Complications

• Pain, tracheal intubation, esophagitis, retro- or nasopharyngeal necrosis, perforation of the stomach.

Equipment

• Towel for covering patient's clothes, emesis basis, nasogastric tube, cup of water and straw, lubricating gel, vasoconstrictor spray, catheter-tip syringe, stethoscope.

Technique

• Put patient in sitting position, have towels over chest and an emesis basin in lap.
• For unconscious patient, put them in left lateral decubitis position with head turned downward to help prevent aspiration.
• Apply topical anesthetic to nares and pharynx.
• Select tube: 16 = large, 12 = medium, 10 = small.
• Estimate length: Put tip at nose, loop tube over ear lobe and then down to xiphoid as well as umbilicus. Mark the latter spot with tape before insertion.
• Spray topical vasoconstrictor.
• Give patient water with a straw to drink and support the patient's head to prevent them pulling away.
• Insert lubricated tube along floor of nose with the natural curve pointing down, at 60–90 degree angle to plane of face, and advance toward occiput.
• Have patient swallow some water and flex head slightly, when patient swallows, advance tube into esophagus and then into stomach.
• The patients should be able to speak, if unable, you may have just intubated the trachea inadvertently. Coughing and gagging may also indicate there may be trachael intubation.
• Advance to the pre-determined distance.
• Connect a 60cc catheter-tip syringe to lumen and while auscultating over left upper quadrant, push air into tube. A bubble of air should be heard immediately.
• Secure tube.

Placing an IV catheter

1 Ask for help until you are experienced.

2 Set up a tray Swab to clean skin. Find: IV catheters; gauze to stop bleeding from unsuccessful attempts; tape and sterile barrier to secure the catheter; flush.

3 Set up the first bag of fluid.

4 Explain procedure to patient. Place the tourniquet around the arm.

5 Search hard for the best vein (palpable, not just visible). Don't be in a hurry. Rest the arm below the level of the heart to aid filling. Ask the patient to clench and unclench their fist.

6 Sit comfortably—with the patient lying (helps prevent syncope).

7 Tap the vein to make it prominent. Avoid sites spanning joints.

8 Clean the skin You may use local anesthetic (or Emla® cream). Use a fine needle to raise a bleb of lidocaine. Wait 15s.

After it is in: (1) Connect fluid tube; check flow. (2) Fix catheter firmly with tape. (3) Bandage a loop of the tube to the arm. (4) Check the flow rate. (5) Explain that no needle is left in the arm, but that care needs to be taken.

If you fail after three attempts or are having trouble putting in an IV—**get help.**

Hypotensive patients need fluid quickly.

• If the patient may need blood quickly, use a large size catheter.

▶'**The IV is no longer working**' Ask yourself:

• Is there fluid in bag and tubing?

• Inspect the IV: Take bandage off.

• Is the 'IV' still needed?

• Is the infusion pump working?

• Are there kinks in the tube?

Inflamed IV sites need prompt attention. The catheter should be removed and another placed at a different site.

Catheterizing bladders

Catheters *Size* (in French gauge): 12 = small; 16 = large. Usually a 12 or 14 is right. Use the smallest you can. *Shape: Foley* is typical; *coudé (elbow)* catheters have an angled tip to ease around enlarged prostates but are more risky. *Condom catheters*♂ have no in-dwelling parts, and are preferred by nurses and patients (less pain, less restriction of movement), even though they may leak and fall off.

Catheter problems: • Infection (don't use antibiotics unless systemically ill). Consider bladder irrigation, eg 0.9% saline or chlorhexidine 0.02% (may irritate). • *Bladder spasm* may be painful. Try reducing the water in the balloon.

Methods of catheterizing bladders

Per urethrae This route is used to relieve urinary retention, to monitor urine output in critically ill patients, or to collect urine for diagnosis uncontaminated by urethral flora. It is contraindicated in urethral injury (eg pelvic fracture) and acute prostatitis. Catheterization introduces bacteria into the bladder, so aseptic technique is essential.

• Lie the patient supine in a well-lit area: Women with knees flexed and hips abducted with heels together. Use a gloved hand to prep urethral meatus in a pubis-to-anus direction, holding the labia apart with the other hand. With uncircumcised men, retract the foreskin; use a gloved hand to hold the penis still and off the scrotum. The hand used to hold the penis or labia should not touch the catheter (use forceps if needed).

• Put sterile lidocaine 2% gel on the catheter tip and ≤10mL into the urethra (≤5mL if ♀). In men, stretch the penis perpendicular to the body to eliminate any urethral folds that may lead to false passage.

• Use steady *gentle* pressure to advance the catheter. Significant obstructions encountered should prompt withdrawal and reinsertion. With prostatic hypertrophy, a *coudé* tip catheter may get past the prostate.

• Insert fully; wait until urine emerges before inflating the balloon. Remember to check the balloon's capacity before inflation. Pull the catheter back so that the balloon comes to rest at the bladder neck.

• Remember to reposition the foreskin in uncircumcised men to prevent edema of the glans after the catheter is inserted.

Central venous catheter cannulation

Indications
- Emergency access
- Central venous pressure monitoring
- Large volume parenteral fluid administration
- Delivery of parenteral fluids (nutrition, hyperosmolar)
- Delivery of medications (chemotherapy)
- Alternative for repetitive venous cannulations
- Procedures (hemodialysis, plasmapharesis)
- Cardiac catherization, temporary transvenous pacemaker.

Contraindications
- Abnormal or distorted anatomy
- Bleeding diathesis
- Burns
- Cellulitis
- Pneumothorax/hemothorax on contralateral side
- Uncooperative patient.

Complications
- Infection, bleeding, arterial perforation, pneumothorax, hemothorax, thrombosis, catheter fracture, air embolism.

Equipment
- Central line kit
- Sterile gloves, sterile gown, hair cover, mask, eye protection
- Sterile drape
- Sterile gauze pads
- Needle driver
- Suture scissors
- Suture on a cutting needle
- Occlusive dressing
- Completed X-ray request form.

Access locations
- Internal jugular
- Subclavian
- Femoral.

Technique (Seldinger technique)
- Position patient, clean and prep site, drape in sterile fashion.
- Flush central venous catheter with sterile saline, flush all ports.
- Insert finder needle while applying negative pressure and locate vessel.
- Once blood return insert guide wire through needle into the vein.
- Remove needle while holding onto the guide wire.
- Enlarge entry site with dilator.
- Pass catheter over guide wire and into vessel.
- Remove guide wire.
- Secure catheter with suture.
- Apply sterile dressing.
- Obtain a post procedure central line placement X-ray.

Approaches
Internal jugular:

- Position patient in 15–20 degree Trendelenburg position.
- Turn head to contralateral side and hyperextend the neck to tense the sternocleidomastoid muscle. The internal jugular vein is anterior and lateral to the carotid. It travels under the apex of the triangle formed by the sternal and clavicular heads of sternocleidomastoid muscle and the clavicle.
- Anesthetize with needle directed toward the ipsilateral nipple and the junction of the medial third and middle third of the clavicle.

- Puncture skin at this site and direct needle caudally toward the ipsilateral nipple.
- When blood flow is obtained, continue with the Seldinger technique.
- The right side is preferred because there is no thoracic duct, there is a straight course to the right atrium, and the dome of the lung's pleura is usually lower.

Subclavian:
- Position patient in Trendelenburg position with a towel roll under the thoracic spine, between the scapulae to hyperextend the back.
- Anesthetize at the distal third of the clavicle.
- Aim needle under the clavical toward the sternal notch.
- When blood flow is obtained, continue with the Seldinger technique.

Femoral:
- Palpate the femoral artery pulse at the midpoint between the anterior superior iliac spine and the symphysis pubis. The vein is parallel and immediately medial to the artery.
- Anesthetize the skin and subcutaneous tissue.
- Puncture needle at this site.
- When blood flow is obtained, continue with the Seldinger technique.

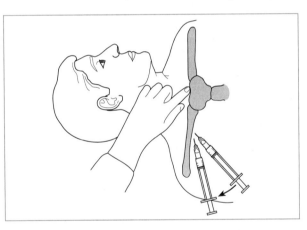

Fig 19.1 Right subclavian vein puncture – infraclavicular approach.

Paracentesis

Indications
- Diagnosis (cytology for neoplasia, culture for spontaneous bacterial peritonitis)
- Therapeutic relief from ascites, including relief of pain, or respiratory compromise.

Contraindications
- Coagulopathy
- Pregnancy
- Evidence of abdominal wall skin infection or bowel obstruction.

Complications
- Bleeding. Rare complication caused by injury to large vessels of abdominal wall, the inferior epigastric vessels, or to mesenteric vessels. Avoid injury to epigastric vessels by staying midline or lateral to the rectus abdominus. Hemodynamic instability after paracentesis requires emergency investigation and may require an exploratory laparotomy.
- Infection. Ascites leak may ↑ chances of peritonitis.
- Injury to nearby structures. Bowel and bladder injuries most likely. Bowel injuries are minimized by careful technique and patient positioning. Bowel injuries lead to delayed peritonitis and sepsis. Risk of bowel injury during procedures is ↑ near abdominal scars due to possible adhesion of bowel to previous abdominal incision. Bladder injuries minimized by voiding or placing a Foley catheter prior to procedure.
- Hypotension from rapid changes in pressure and fluid of abdominal cavity, rarely by intravascular shift to abdominal compartment.

Equipment
- Paracentesis kit.

Technique
- Place patient in supine position. Tap out the ascites, marking a point where fluid has been identified, avoiding scars or vessels.
- Clean the skin.
- Anesthetize skin at the insertion site. The ideal site is midline, 1–2cm below the umbilicus. Do not use a midline site if a previous midline incision is present (due to risk of bowel adhesion to abdominal wall). The lateral site is between the anterior-superior iliac crest and the lateral border of the rectus abdominus, at the level of the umbilicus.
- Insert a 21G needle on a 20mL syringe into the skin and advance while aspirating until fluid is withdrawn.
- Remove the needle and apply a sterile dressing.
- Send fluid for microscopy, culture, and cytology.

Thoracentesis

Indications
- Diagnosis (malignancy, infection, inflammation)
- Therapeutic.

Contraindications
- Local skin infection,
- Uncooperative patient.

Complications
- Bleeding, infection, pneumothorax, hemothorax, pulmonary contusion or laceration, diaphragm, spleen, or liver puncture, bronchopleural fistula, re-expansion pulmonary edema.

Equipment
- Thoracentesis kit
- Sterile gauze pad
- Iodine
- Fenestrated drape
- Oxygen by nasal cannula
- Specimen collection tubes and/or vacuum bottles.

Technique
- Position patient sitting on edge of bed resting head and extended arms on a bedside table. If the patient is unable to sit, place the patient in the lateral decubitis position.
- Confirm location of fluid by percussion, auscultation, and chest X-ray.
- Locate needle insertion site, 1–2 interspaces below the fluid level, but not below 8th rib.
- Mark site with a marker.
- Prep and drape area with proper sterile technique.
- Anesthetize skin and then insert needle until it touches the superior border of a rib while aspirating and advancing. Move needle over the superior margin of the rib and anesthetize the intercostals muscle layers.
- Insert the thoracentesis needle in the same tract as the anesthesia needle.
- Draw off 10–30mL of pleural fluid.
- Send fluid to the lab for *chemistry* (protein, glucose, pH, LDH, amylase); *bacteriology* (microscopy and culture, AFB stain, TB culture); *cytology*.
- If large volume removal is needed, use the Seldinger technique and insert catheter through the needle and into the chest.
- Get a post-procedure chest X-ray.

Inserting a chest tube

NB: This is a sterile procedure.

Indications
• Hemothorax, trauma
• Chylothorax
• Empyema
• Effusion
• Pneumothorax.

Contraindications
• Previous thoracic surgery
• Pulmonary blebs
• Osscilator ventilation
• Prior pleural adhesions.

Complications
• Scar formation
• Injury to lung or surrounding organs

• Bleeding
• Pain
• Pheumothorax.

Equipment
• Chest tube kit
• Sterile gloves, sterile gown, hair cover mask, eye protection
• Sterile drape
• Sterile gauze pads
• Needle driver
• Suture scissors
• Iodine
• 1% lidocaine

• Scalpel
• Suture
• Chest tube: 10–14F usually; 28–30F if trauma or hemothorax
• Pleurivac container with water seal
• Connection tubes
• Petroleum gauze
• Occlusive dressing
• Completed X-ray request form.

Technique
• Obtain pre-procedure X-ray to confirm location for chest tube insertion.
• Choose insertion site: 4th–6th intercostals space, anterior to mid-axillary line
  • In the 'safe triangle', see figure OPPOSITE
  • A more posterior approach, eg the 7th space posterior, may be required to drain a loculated effusion
  • The 2nd intercostals space in the mid-clavicular line may be used for apical pheumothoraces
  • The posterior and anterior approaches are more uncomfortable.
• Infiltrated down to the pleura with 10–20cc of 1% lidocaine.
  • Verify that either air or fluid can be aspirated from the proposed insertion site.
• If not do not proceed.
  • Wait 3min for the anesthetic to have an effect.
• Make 2cm incision above anesthetized rib to avoid neurovascular bundle under rib.
  • Blunt dissect with forceps down to the pleura.
  • Puncture pleura with scissors or forceps.
  • If inserting large bore tube (>24F), then sweep a finger inside chest to clear adherent lung and exclude obstructing structures (eg in blunt abdominal trauma, stomach in the chest).
• Before inserting the chest tube, remove the metal trochar completely and introduce the tube atraumatically using forceps to advance it.
• Advance the tip upwards to the apex of lung (or base of lung if draining an effusion). Stop when you meet resistance.

• Attach the chest tube to the drainage container with water seal.
  • Ensure that the chest tube is bubbling with respiration.
• With large/medium bore tubes, the incision should be closed with a mattress suture or suture across the incision.
  • Purse string sutures are not recommended as they may lead to scarring and ↑ wound pain.
• Fix the chest tube with a second suture tied around the chest tube.
• Cover with petroleum gauze and occlusive dressing.

- Secure the tube with tape to prevent slippage.
- Obtain post-placement X-ray to observe the position of the tube.
- Give PO/IV/IM analgesia.

Tension pneumothorax

- In a tension pneumothorax air is drawn into the intra-pleural space, with each breath, but cannot escape due to a valve-like effect of the tiny flap in the parietal pleura. The ↑ pressure progressively compresses the heart and the other lung.
- Give the patient 100% oxygen.
- Insert a large bore IV cannula through an intercostals space anywhere on the affected side.
  - Usually 2nd intercostals space in the midclavicular lilne.
  - Remove the stylet, which will allow the trapped air to escape, usually with audible hiss.
- Secure IV cannula with tape.
- Insert chest tube as above.
  - Chest tube is to continue to release air from the pleural space.

The 'safe triangle' for insertion of a chest tube

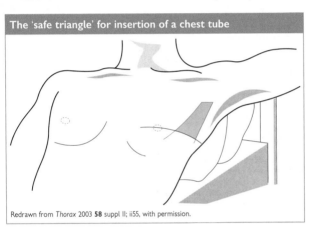

Redrawn from *Thorax* 2003 **58** suppl II; ii55, with permission.

Lumbar puncture (LP)

Indication
- Suspected CNS infection
- Suspected subarachnoid hemorrhage
- Disease diagnosis: Pseudotumor cerebri, Guillian-barre syndrome, multiple sclerosis, systemic lupus erythematosis, meningeal carcinomatosis
- Infusion: Antibiotics, chemotherapy, contrast (myelography/cisternography).

Contraindication
- Local skin infection
- ↑ intracranial pressure (except pseudotumor cerebri)
- Supratentorial mass lesions (CT first)
- Platelet count <50,000/severe bleeding diathesis
- Unstable patient.

Complications: Pain shooting pains in the lower extremities, infection, bleeding, spinal fluid leak, hematoma, spinal headache (10–20%), brain herniation from supratentorial mass or extreme pressure.
- Spinal headache usually occurs 24–48h after LP with resolution over hours to 2wks.
- Constant dull bilateral ache more frontal than occipital that is positional – worse with upright.
- Blood patch (injection of 20cc of autologous venous blood into the epidural space) causes immediate relief in 95%.

Equipment
- Spinal tray
- Sterile gloves
- Fenestrated drape
- Anesthetic cream.

Technique
- Apply local anesthetic cream if sufficient time is available.
- Position patient near edge of bed/table in the lateral decubitis or sitting position. Flex spine anteriorly (flex hips, knees, and neck).
- Locate L3–L4 interspace at the level of the iliac crests.
- Open spinal tray in a sterile manner, prepare skin at the selected interspace with antiseptic solution and cover with a fenestrated drape.
- Anesthetize skin with 1% lidocaine.
- Using the spinal needle, puncture the skin in the midline just caudal to the palpated spinous process, angle needle about 15° cephalad toward the umbilicus.
- Advance needle about 3–4cm then withdraw stylet to check for CSF flow. If no fluid replace stylus and advance a fraction then repeat.
- Usually there a slight 'pop' felt as the needles penetrates the dura; advance 1–2mm further.
- If resistance is felt (bone) withdraw needle slightly and change its angle.
- Once fluid is obtained place end of stopcock with the attached manometer onto the needle hub to measure the opening pressure.
- Normal opening pressure 50–200mmH$_2$O; elevated >250mmH$_2$O
- Note color of fluid as well as opening pressure.
- Opening pressure can only reliably be measured while patient is lying quietly on their side in an unflexed position (have patient straighten legs and relax; this will help prevent an artificially elevated pressure).
- Turn stopcock to allow the CSF to flow into the test tubes; label tubes in the order collected.
- Collect 2–3cc of CSF in each of 3–4 tubes.
- Send tubes for appropriate studies.

Tube 1	**Tube 2**	**Tube 3**	**Tube 4**
Bacteriology Culture and Gram stain	Biochemistry Glucose Protein	Hematology Cell count and differential	Optional Viral studies PCR Metabolic studies VDRL Fungus TB Electrophoresis Cytology

- Replace stylus and withdraw the needle
- Cover with sterile dressing and have patient lay supine for next 2h.

NB: CSF normal values

Lymphocytes $<5/\text{mm}^3$
Glucose 60–70% blood glucose
Protein 15–45mg%

Bloody tap: This is an artifact due to piercing a blood vessel, which is indicated by fewer red cells in successive tubes and no yellowing of CSF (xanthochromia).

If the patient's blood count is normal, the rule of thumb is to subtract from the total CSF WCC (per mcL) one white cell for every 1000RBCs. To estimate the true protein level, subtract 10mg/L for every 1000RBCs/mm^3 (be sure to do the count and protein estimation on the same tube). Note: High protein levels in CSF make it appear yellow.

Subarachnoid hemorrhage: Xanthochromia (yellow supernatant on spun CSF). Red cells in equal numbers in all tubes. RBCs can provoke an inflammatory response most marked after 48h.

Raised protein: Meningitis; MS; Guillain–Barré syndrome.

Very raised CSF protein: Spinal block; TB; or severe bacterial meningitis.

Method of defining the interspace between the 3rd and 4th lumbar vertebrae

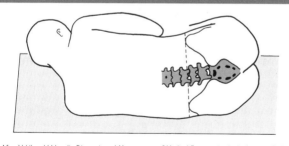

After Vakil and Udwadia *Diagnosis and Management of Medical Emergencies* 2nd edn, OUP, Delhi.

Cricothyroidotomy

This is an emergency procedure to overcome upper airway obstruction above the level of the larynx.

Indications Upper airway obstruction when endotracheal intubation not possible, eg irretrievable foreign body; facial edema (burns, angioedema); maxillofacial trauma; infection (epiglottitis).

Procedure Lie the patient supine with neck extended (eg pillow under shoulders). Run your index finger down the neck anteriorly in the midline to find the notch in the upper border of the thyroid cartilage: Just below this, between the thyroid and cricoid cartilages, is a depression—the cricothyroid membrane.

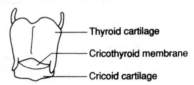

— **Thyroid cartilage**

— **Cricothyroid membrane**

— **Cricoid cartilage**

Needle cricothyroidotomy: Pierce the membrane with large-bore cannula (14G) attached to syringe: Withdrawal of air confirms position lidocaine may or may not be required). Slide cannula over needle at 45° to skin in sagittal plane. Use a Y-connector or improvise connection to O_2 supply and give 15L/min: Use thumb on Y-connector to allow O_2 in over 1s and CO_2 out over 4s ('transtracheal jet insufflation').

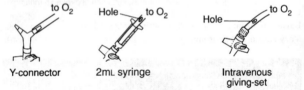

| Y-connector | 2mL syringe | Intravenous giving-set |

Surgical cricothyrotomy: Smallest tube for prolonged ventilation is 6mm. Introduce high-volume low-pressure cuff tracheostomy tube through horizontal incision in membrane.

Complications Local hemorrhage; posterior perforation of trachea ± esophagus; laryngeal stenosis; tube blockage; subcutaneous tunnelling.

Emergency needle pericardiocentesis

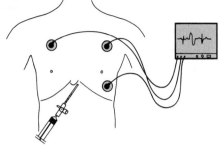

- *Equipment*: 20mL syringe, long 18G cannula, 3-way tap, ECG monitor, skin cleanser.
- If time allows, use aseptic technique, and, if conscious, local anesthesia technique and sedation, eg with midazolam: Titrate up to 0.07mg/kg IV—start with 2mg over 1min, 1mg in elderly.
- Ensure you have IV access and full resuscitation equipment at hand.
- Introduce needle at 45° to skin just below and to left of xiphisternum, aiming for tip of left scapula. Aspirate continuously and watch ECG. Frequent ventricular ectopics or an injury pattern (ST segment↓) on ECG imply myocardial penetration—withdraw slightly.
- Evacuate pericardial contents through the syringe and 3-way tap. Removal of only a small amount of fluid (eg 20mL) can produce marked clinical improvement. If you are not sure whether the fluid you are aspirating is pure blood (eg on entering a ventricle), see if it clots (heavily blood-stained pericardial fluid does not clot).
- You can leave the cannula *in situ* temporarily, for repeated aspiration. If there is reaccumulation, pericardiectomy may be needed.
- Send fluid for microscopy and culture, as needed, including tests for TB.

Complications: Laceration of ventricle or coronary artery (± subsequent hemopericardium); aspiration of ventricular blood; arrhythmias (ventricular fibrillation); pneumothorax; puncture of aorta, esophagus (± mediastinitis), or pericarditis.

Cardioversion/defibrillation

Indications Ventricular fibrillation or tachycardia, fast AF (p120), supraventricular tachycardias if other treatments (p118) have failed or there is hemodynamic compromise.

The aim is to completely depolarize the heart using a direct current.

• Unless critically ill, conscious patients require sedating medication.

Procedure (for monophasic defibrillators)

Do not wait for a crisis before familiarizing yourself with the defibrillator.

• Set the energy level (eg 200J for ventricular fibrillation or ventricular tachycardia; 100J for atrial fibrillation; 50J for atrial flutter).

• Place pads on chest, 1 over apex and 1 below right clavicle (less chance of skin arc than jelly).

• **Make sure no one else is touching the patient or the bed**.

• Disconnect oxygen circuit tubing during shock delivery.

• Press the button(s) on the electrode(s) to give the shock.

• Watch ECG. Repeat the shock at a higher energy if necessary.

NB: For AF and SVT, it is necessary to synchronize the shock on the R-wave of the ECG (by pressing the 'SYNC' button on the machine). This ensures that the shock does not initiate a ventricular arrhythmia. *If the SYNC mode is engaged in VF, the defibrillator will not discharge!*

• It is only necessary to anesthetize the patient if conscious.

• After giving the shock, monitor ECG rhythm. Consider anticoagulation, as the risk of emboli is ↑. Get an up-to-date 12-lead ECG.

Inserting a temporary cardiac pacemaker

Possible indications in the setting of acute myocardial infarction

• *Complete AV block:* With inferior MI (right coronary artery occlusion) pacing may only be needed if symptomatic; spontaneous recovery may occur.

• with anterior MI (representing massive septal infarction).

• *Second degree block:* Wenckebach (p117) implies decremental AV node conduction; may respond to atropine in inferior MI; pace if anterior MI. Type 2 block is usually associated with distal fascicular disease and carries high risk of complete heart block, so pace in both types of MI.

• *First degree block:* Observe carefully: 40% develop higher degrees of block.

• *Bundle branch block:* Pace prophylactically if evidence of trifascicular disease (p124) or non-adjacent bifascicular disease.

• *Sino-atrial disease + serious symptoms:* Pace unless responds to atropine.

Other indications where temporary pacing may be needed

• Drug poisoning, eg with β-blockers, digoxin, or verapamil.

• Symptomatic bradycardia, unresponsive to atropine.

• Suppression of drug-resistant VT and SVT (overdrive pacing; do on ICU).

• Asystolic cardiac arrest with P-wave activity (ventricular standstill).

• During or after cardiac surgery—eg around the AV node or bundle of His.

Method and technique for temporary pacing Learn from an expert.

• *Preparation:* Monitor ECG; have a defibrillator to hand. Create a sterile field and ensure that the pacing wire fits down the cannula easily. Insert a peripheral cannula.

• *Insertion:* Place the cannula into the subclavian or internal jugular vein (p658). Pass the pacing wire through the cannula into the right atrium. It will either pass easily through the tricuspid valve or loop within the atrium. If the latter occurs, it is usually possible to flip the wire across the valve with a combined twisting and withdrawing movement. Advance the wire slightly. At this stage the wire may try to exit the ventricle through the pulmonary outflow tract. A further withdrawing and rotation of the wire will aim the tip at the apex of the right ventricle. Advance slightly again to place the wire in contact with the endocardium. Remove any slack to ↓risk of subsequent displacement.

- Checking the threshold: Connect the wire to the pacing box and set the 'demand' rate slightly higher than the patient's own heart rate and the output to 3V. A paced rhythm should be seen. Find the pacing threshold by slowly reducing the voltage until the pacemaker fails to stimulate the tissue (pacing spikes are no longer followed by paced beats). The threshold should be less than 1V, but a slightly higher value may be acceptable if it is stable—eg after a large infarction.
- Setting the pacemaker: Set the output to 3V or over 3 times the threshold value (whichever is higher) in 'demand' mode. Set the rate as required. Suture the wire to the skin, and fix with a sterile dressing.
- Check the position of the wire (and exclude pneumothorax) with a CXR.

Recurrent checks of the pacing threshold are required over the next few days. The formation of endocardial edema can be expected to raise the threshold by a factor of 2–3.

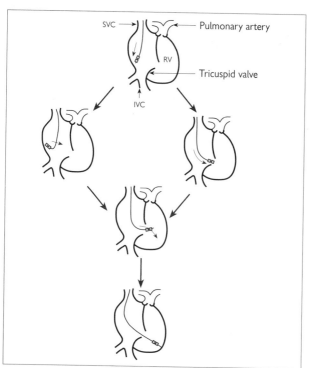

Emergency medicine

Arjun S. Chanmugam, M.D. and Neel Vibhaker, M.D.

▶ To manage an emergency condition, you must be prepared to treat and diagnose at virtually the same time.

Patients that present with an emergency condition generally fall into two categories. They will either have a life-threatening condition or an organ-threatening condition. Knowledge of some basic disease processes and an understanding of how to approach patients who may be critically ill is of importance in managing their care. Recognizing that an emergent condition is present is the key first step, and the second step is to activate the appropriate resources as quickly as possible. Remember, if you suspect an emergent condition, ask for help as soon as possible, even if you are not sure whether there is an emergency.

Contents

Introduction to emergencies

Patients who have an emergent condition require immediate intervention. As stated above, recognition is the critical first step. Any patient who has a problem with their airway, who has any trouble breathing or who has difficulty maintaining their blood pressure (A, B, Cs) should be considered as having a potential medical emergency. The next step is to activate the appropriate resources to support the patient, which means asking for help and applying 'Oh MI'—Oxygen, cardiac Monitoring and an Intravenous catheter. While providing the patient with as much support as possible, consider the potential threats to life and the potential threats to any organ system. This list must be considered as soon as possible in order to provide the patient with the correct medical interventions. By continuing to consider the potential life threats and the organ threats, the well prepared provider will be in a better position to craft the all important management plan; the plan of action.

When developing your management plan, two data sources must be used. The subjective data, which includes all the historical elements including the patient's version of the events leading to presentation, the medical record, and comments from other people. The second data set is the objective data, the physical findings as well as any laboratory, radiological, or other studies. Very often the heart of the diagnosis lies in the subjective data while the objective data confirms the diagnostic suspicion.

The key to good management is to identify any abnormality, any source of concern, or to put it another way, any red flag. Every red flag must be appropriately addressed. Whenever new data is acquired, regardless of the source, the treatment plan must be modified to incorporate the new data and the evolving condition of your patient.

Continuous re-evaluation is critically important, because by definition an emergent condition is a state that can change dramatically and quickly. To that end, remember to dynamically review the temperature, pulse rate and quality, respiratory rate and pattern, BP, oxygen saturation as well as the most important vital sign of all, the mental status. All this should be done in the context of the preliminary assessment which is listed on the facing page.

Preliminary assessment (primary survey)

Airway   Assessment: Any signs of airway obstruction? Ascertain patency.

Management: Establish a patent airway

Key: Protect cervical spine if injury possible, especially in the presence of a change in mental status

Breathing   Assessment: Determine respiratory rate, check bilateral chest movement, percuss, and auscultate.

Management: If no respiratory effort, treat as arrest (p674), intubate, and ventilate. If breathing is compromised, give high concentration O_2, manage according to findings, eg relieve tension pneumothorax.

Circulation   Assessment: Check pulse and BP; check capillary refill; look for evidence of hypoperfusion

Management: Peripheral or central IV catheters, fluids (crystalloids or blood products), measure urine output consider central venous pressure measurement, consider pressors

if no cardiac output, treat as arrest

Disability   Assess 'level of consciousness' with AVPU score (alert? Responds to voice? To pain? Unresponsive?); check pupils: Size, equality, reactions. *Glasgow Coma scale*, if time allows.

Exposure   Undress patient, but cover to avoid hypothermia.

Quick history from relatives or significant others may assist with diagnosis: *Events* surrounding onset of illness, contributing issues, evidence of overdose/suicide attempt, any suggestion of trauma? *Past medical history:* Especially diabetes, asthma, COPD, alcohol, opiate or street drug abuse, epilepsy or recent head injury; recent travel. *Medication:* Current drugs. *Allergies.*

Once appropriate ventilation and circulation support are adequate, a more complete history, examination, along with more thorough investigations, should be undertaken as part of the appropriate management.

Cardiorespiratory arrest

Confirm absence of pulse, BP, and/or respirations.

Causes MI; PE; trauma; tension pneumothorax, electrocution; shock (septic, cardiogenic, neurogenic, hypovolemic and anaphylactic); hypoxia; hypercapnia; hypothermia; electrolyte/acid/base imbalance; drugs, eg digoxin.

Basic life support Request help immediately. Check for responsiveness. Ask someone to call the arrest team and bring the automatic external defibrillator. Note the time. Place patient in a supine position. Consider a precordial thump (in witnessed arrests; recheck carotid pulse). Begin CPR as follows (ABC):

Airway: Open airway. If no contraindications use head tilt ± chin lift. Clear the mouth.

Breathing: Assess breathing, if inadequate give 2 breaths, each inflation ~1s long. Use specialized bag and mask system (eg Ambu® system) if available and 2 resuscitators present. Otherwise, mouth-to-mouth breathing.

Chest compressions: Give 30 compressions to 2 breaths (30:2), pediatrics (15:2). CPR should not be interrupted except to give shocks or to intubate. Use the heel of hand with straight elbows. Center over the lower half of the sternum. Aim for 4 to 5cm compression at 100/min. Allow the chest to return to normal position. Push hard and push fast.

Advanced life support For algorithm & details, see OPPOSITE. Notes:
- Place defibrillator paddles on chest as soon as possible and set monitor to read through the paddles if delay in attaching leads. Assess rhythm: Is this VF/pulseless VT? The following assumes monophasic defibrillator.
- In VF/VT, defibrillation must occur without delay: 200;300;360J (biphasic 120,150, 200).
- Asystole and electromechanical dissociation (synonymous with pulseless electrical activity) are rhythms with a worse prognosis compared to VF/VT, but potentially remediable (see box OPPOSITE). Treatment may be life-saving.
- Obtain IV access and intubation if possible.
- Look for reversible causes of cardiac arrest, and treat accordingly.
- Check for pulse if ECG rhythm compatible with a cardiac output.
- Reassess ECG rhythm. All shocks now 360J (biphasic 200). Repeat defibrillation if still VF/VT. However, if 3 shocks have already been administered consider vasopressin or epinephrine prior to another defibrillation attempt.
- Send someone to find the patient's chart and the patient's usual doctor. These may give clues as to the cause of the arrest.
- If IV access fails, naloxone, atropine, diazepam(valium) epinephrine, and lidocaine (NAVEL) may be given down the tracheal tube but absorption is unpredictable. Give 2–3 times the IV dose diluted in ≥10mL 0.9% saline followed by 5 ventilations to assist absorption. Intracardiac injection is not recommended.

When to stop resuscitation: This is one of the most difficult decisions to make and there are no definitive recommendations. Consider stopping resuscitation after 20min if there is refractory asystole or electromechanical dissociation. In general, in those patients without myocardial disease, resuscitations are often continued until core temperatures are >33°C and pH and potassium are normal.

After successful resuscitation:
- 12-lead ECG; CXR, comprehensive metabolic panel, glucose, blood gases, CBC, CK/troponin.
- Transfer to appropriate unit such as a CCU/ICU.
- Monitor vital signs.
- Whatever the outcome, explain to relatives what has happened.

When 'do not resuscitate' may be a valid decision
- If a patient's condition is such that resuscitation is unlikely to succeed.

- If a mentally competent patient has consistently stated or recorded the fact that he or she does not want to be resuscitated.
- If the patient has signed an advanced directive forbidding resuscitation.
- *Ideally, involve patients & relatives in the decision **before** the emergency.* When in doubt, resuscitate.

Cardiac arrest: 2005 guidelines for advanced life support

Management of Cardiac Arrest[1]

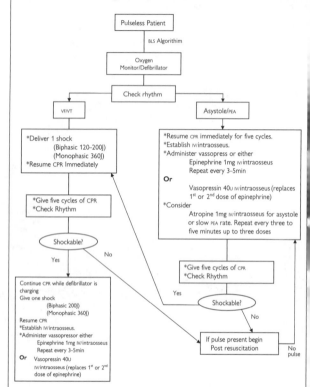

Do not interrupt CPR for >10s, except to defibrillate.

Resistant VT/VF consider:

- Amiodarone 300mg IV (peripherally if no central access). A further 150mg may be given, followed by an infusion of 1mg/min for 6h, then 0.5mg/min for 6h. Magnesium sulphate infusion can be considered as a 2g bolus.
- Alternatives to amiodarone are:
  - Lidocaine 100mg IV; can repeat once; then give 2–4mg/min IVI.
  - Procainamide 30mg/min IV to a total dose of 17mg/kg.
- Seek expert advice from a cardiologist.

Asystole with P waves: Start external pacing (percutaneous transthoracic pacing through special paddles). If unavailable, use atropine 0.6mg/5min IV while awaiting further help.

Treat acidosis with good ventilation. Sodium bicarbonate may worsen intracellular acidosis and precipitate arrhythmias, so use only in severe acidosis after prolonged resuscitation (eg 50mL of 8.4% solution by IVI).

676

1 Ref: 2005 American Heart Association Guidelines for CPR and ECC, *Circulation*, Vol 12, Issue 24 suppl, December 13, 2005. American Heart Association, 2005.

Headache

Life threatening considerations
- Meningitis
- Encephalopathy
- Intracranial bleed.

Organ threatening causes
- Narrow angle glaucoma
- Temporal arteritis (ESR↑)
- Severe anemia

Other potential causes
- Tension headache
- Migraine
- Cluster headache
- Post-traumatic
- Drugs (nitrates, calcium channel antagonists)
- Carbon monoxide poisoning or anoxia

Signs of meningismus?
- Meningitis (may not have fever or rash)
- Subarachnoid hemorrhage.

Decreased conscious level or localizing signs?
- Encephalitis/meningitis
- Stroke
- Cerebral abscess
- Subarachnoid hemorrhage
- Tumor
- Subdural hematoma.

Papilledema?
- Tumor
- Severe hypertension
- Benign intracranial hypertension
- Any CNS infection, if prolonged (eg >2wks)—eg TB meningitis.

Others
- Paget's disease (alk phosp ↑↑↑)
- Sinusitis
- Altitude sickness
- Cervical spondylosis.

Worrying features or 'red flags'
- First or worst headache—*consider subarachnoid hemorrhage*
- Thunderclap headache—*consider subarachnoid hemorrhage*
- Unilateral headache and eye pain—*cluster headache*
- Unilateral headache and ipsilateral symptoms—*migraine, tumor, vascular*
- Cough-initiated headache—*raised ICP/venous thrombosis*
- Persisting headache ± scalp tenderness in over 50s—*temporal arteritis*
- Headache with fever or neck stiffness—*meningitis*
- Change in the pattern of 'usual headaches'
- Decreased level of consciousness.

Two other vital questions:
- Where have you been? (Malaria)
- Might you be pregnant? (Eclampsia; especially if proteinuria and BP↑).

Shortness of breath: Emergency presentations

Wheezing?
- Asthma
- COPD
- Heart failure
- Anaphylaxis.

Stridor? (Upper airway obstruction)
- Foreign body or tumor
- Acute epiglottitis
- Anaphylaxis
- Trauma, eg laryngeal fracture
- Angioedema.

Crepitations?
- Heart failure
- Pneumonia
- Bronchiectasis
- Fibrosis.

Chest clear?
- Pulmonary embolism
- Hyperventilation
- Metabolic acidosis, eg diabetic ketoacidosis (DKA)
- Anemia
- Drugs, eg salicylates
- Shock (may cause air hunger)
- Central causes.

Others
- Pneumothorax—pain, ↑ resonance
- Pleural effusion.

Chest pain: Differential diagnosis

First exclude any potentially life-threatening causes, by virtue of history, brief examination, and limited investigations. Then consider other potential causes.

Immediate life-threatening
- Acute myocardial infarction
- Angina/acute coronary syndrome
- Aortic dissection
- Tension pneumothorax
- Pulmonary embolism
- Esophageal rupture

Others
- Pneumonia
- Empyema
- Chest wall pain
  - Muscular
  - Rib fractures
  - Bony metastases
  - Costochondritis
- Pleurisy
- Gastro-oesophageal reflux
- Pericarditis
- Esophageal spasm
- Herpes zoster
- Cervical spondylosis
- Intra-abdominal
  - Cholecystitis
  - Peptic ulceration
  - Pancreatitis
- Sickle-cell crisis
- Although cardiac pain is usually described as a dull pressure or a substernal pressure that radiates to jaw, neck or arm, and is usually associated with exertion, not all cardiac chest pain presents classically. It is worthwhile to consider obtaining CXR, ECG, CBC, CMP, and 'cardiac' enzymes, including troponin on all patients who are at risk. Cardiac chest pain can, and does at times, present atypically, so please consider options such as short stay units or observation units for low risk patients. Cardiac monitoring in appropriate inpatient units is indicated for higher risk patients.

Discuss options with a colleague, and the patient.

Remember, just because the patient's chest wall is tender to palpation, doesn't mean the cause of the chest pain is musculoskeletal. Make sure you have excluded all potential life-threatening causes.

Coma

Definition *Unarousable unresponsiveness.*

Causes

Metabolic: Drugs, poisoning, eg carbon monoxide, alcohol, tricyclics
Hypoglycemia, hypergylcemia (ketoacidotic, or HONK)
Hypoxia, CO_2 narcosis (COPD)
Sepsis
Hypothermia
Myxedema, Addisonian crisis
Hepatic/uremic encephalopathy

Neurological: Trauma
Infection meningitis (p336); encephalitis, eg Herpes simplex
give IV acyclovir if the slightest suspicion (p337), tropical:
Malaria (do thick films), typhoid, rabies, trypanosomiasis
Tumor: Cerebral/meningeal tumor
Vascular, subdural/subarachnoid hemorrhage, stroke,
hypertensive encephalopathy
Epilepsy: Non-convulsive status (p344) or post-ictal state

Immediate management see OPPOSITE (and coma CNS exam, p684)
- Assess airway, breathing, and circulation. Consider intubation if GCS <8. Support the circulation if required (ie IV fluids). Give O_2 and treat any seizures. Protect the cervical spine.
- Check blood glucose in all patients. Give 50mL 50% dextrose IV immediately if presumed hypoglycemia.
- IV thiamine if any suggestion of Wernicke's encephalopathy (consider giving glucose first).
- IV naloxone for opiate intoxication (may also be given IM or via ET tube); IV flumazenil for benzodiazepine intoxication *if* airway compromised, and patient not known to be chronically dependent on benzodiazepines. Caution must be exercised when administering flumazenil to a patient who has benzodiazepine dependency as it may precipitate seizures.

Examination
- Vital signs are vital—obtain full set, including temperature.
- Signs of trauma—hematoma, laceration, bruising, CSF/blood in nose or ears, fracture 'step' deformity of skull, subcutaneous emphysema, 'raccoon eyes'.
- Stigmata of other illnesses: Liver disease, alcoholism, diabetes, myxedema.
- Skin for needle marks, cyanosis, pallor, rashes, poor turgor.
- Smell the breath (alcohol, hepatic fetor, ketosis, uremia).
- Meningismus but do *not* move neck unless cervical spine is cleared.
- Heart/lung exam for murmurs, rubs, wheeze, consolidation, collapse.
- Abdomen/rectal for organomegaly, ascites, bruising, peritoneal signs, melena.
- Are there any foci of infection (abscesses, bites, middle ear infection?)
- Any features of meningitis: Neck stiffness, rash, focal neurology?
- Note the *absence* of signs, eg *no* pin-point pupils in a known heroin addict, or a diabetic patient whose breath does *not* smell of acetone.

Quick history from family, ambulance staff, bystanders: Abrupt or gradual onset? Suicide note present? Was there any seizure activity? Be highly suspicious of cervical spinal injury and consider spinal immobilization if there is uncertainty. Recent complaints—headache, fever, vertigo, depression? Recent medical history—sinusitis, otitis, neurosurgery, ENT procedure? Past medical history—diabetes, asthma, ↑BP, cancer, epilepsy, psychiatric illness? Drug or toxin exposure (especially alcohol or other recreational drugs)? Any recent travel?

Critical considerations: In all undiagnosed coma patients or in those with focal neurological signs, a CT scan is very helpful. A lumbar puncture may be needed for meningitis or subarachnoid hemorrhage.

Management of coma[1]

ABC of life support

↓

O_2, IV access

↓

Stabilize cervical spine

↓

Blood glucose

↓

Control seizures

↓

Consider IV glucose, thiamine, naloxone, or flumazenil

↓

Brief examination, obtain history

↓

Investigations

ABG, CBC, CMP, LFT, ESR, CRP, TOTAL CK

Ethanol, toxic screen, drug levels

Blood cultures, urine culture

CXR

↓

Reassess the situation and plan further investigations

1 *Check pupils every few minutes during the early stages,* particularly if trauma is the likely cause. Doing so is the quickest way to find a localizing sign (so helpful in diagnosis, but remember that false localizing signs *do* occur)—and observing *changes* in pupil behavior (eg becoming fixed and dilated) is the quickest way of finding out just how bad things are.

The Glasgow coma scale (GCS)

The GCS was first developed to assess consciousness in trauma patients. This scale is now often used in a variety of situations to quantify in a reliable, objective way the conscious state of a person. It can be used by medical and nursing staff for initial and continuing assessment. Three areas are examined when obtaining a GCS score and includes the motor response, verbal response and eye response.

Best motor response This has 6 grades:

6 Follows command. The patient obeys a command to complete a simple task upon your request.

5 Localizing response to pain: The patient responds to pain by reaching towards the painful stimuli.

4 Withdraws to pain: The patient retreats from the painful stimuli in some fashion, without attempting to localize the response

3 Flexor response to pain: The patient responds to painful stimuli by abnormally flexing the upper limbs.

2 Extensor posturing to pain: The painful stimulus causes limb extension (adduction, internal rotation of shoulder, pronation of forearm)—decerebrate posture.

1 No response to pain.

Note that it is the best response of any limb which should be recorded.

Best verbal response This has 5 grades:

5 Oriented: The patient knows who they are, where they are, and why they are where they are, the year, season, and month.

4 Confused conversation: The patient responds to questions in a conversational manner but there is some disorientation and confusion.

3 Inappropriate speech: Random or exclamatory articulated speech, but no conversational exchange.

2 Incomprehensible speech: Moaning but no words.

1 None.

Record level of best speech.

Eye opening This has 4 grades:

4 Spontaneous eye opening.

3 Eye opening in response to speech: Any speech, or shout, not necessarily request to open eyes.

2 Eye opening in response to pain: Painful stimuli results in eye opening.

1 No eye opening.

An overall score is made by adding the individual scores from the 3 areas assessed. For example: A person who is dead has no response to pain + no verbalization + no eye opening would have a GCS= 3. A severely ill patient would have a GCS 8 or lower; a moderate injury, GCS 9–12; minor injury, GCS 13– In general, 'less than equal to 8, intubate'.

NB: An abbreviated coma scale, AVPU, is sometimes used in the initial assessment ('primary survey') of the critically ill:

• A = alert
• V = responds to vocal stimuli
• P = responds to pain
• U = unresponsive.

The neurological examination in coma

A patient that appears to have an altered level of consciousness has a problem in one of two areas Altered level of consciousness implies either (1) a diffuse, bilateral, cortical dysfunction (usually producing loss of awareness with normal arousal) or (2) damage to the ascending reticular activating system (ARAS) located throughout the brainstem from the medulla to the thalami (usually producing loss of arousal with unassessable awareness). The brainstem can be affected directly (eg pontine hemorrhage) or indirectly (eg compression from trans-tentorial or cerebellar herniation secondary to a mass or edema).The following are areas to be examined in patients with altered level of consciousness.

• Level of consciousness; describe using *objective* words Such as 'unarousable', responds to questions, responds to pain.
• Respiratory pattern—Cheyne–Stokes (p71), hyperventilation (acidosis, hypoxia, or rarely, neurogenic), ataxic or apneustic (breath-holding) breathing (brainstem damage with grave prognosis).
• Eyes—almost all patients with ARAS pathology will have eye findings.

Visual fields—in light coma, test fields with visual threat. No blink in 1 field suggests hemianopsia and contralateral hemisphere lesion.

Pupils *Normal direct & consensual* = intact midbrain. *Midposition (3–5mm) non-reactive ± irregular* = midbrain lesion. *Unilateral dilated & unreactive ('fixed')* = 3rd nerve compression. *Small, reactive* = pontine lesion ('pinpoint pontine pupils') or drugs. *Horner's syndrome* = ipsilateral lateral medulla or hypothalamus lesion, may precede uncal herniation. Beware patients with false eyes or who use eye drops for glaucoma.

Extraocular movements (EOMs)—observe resting position and spontaneous movement; then test the vestibulo-ocular reflex (VOR) with either the *Doll's-head maneuver* (normal if the eyes keep looking at the same point in space when the head is quickly moved laterally or vertically) or *ice water calorics* (normal if eyes deviate towards the cold ear with nystagmus to the other side). If present, the VOR exonerates *most* of the brainstem from the VII nerve nucleus (medulla) to the III (midbrain). *Don't move the head unless the cervical spine is cleared.*

Fundi—papilledema, subhyaloid hemorrhage, hypertensive retinopathy, signs of other disease (eg diabetic retinopathy).

• Examine for CNS asymmetry (tone, spontaneous movements, reflexes).

Shock

Definition: Circulatory insufficiency resulting in inadequate tissue perfusion. Shock can be classified into four categories (1) hypovolemic (caused by inadequate circulating volume); (2) cardiogenic (caused by inadequate cardiac pump function); (3) distributive (caused by peripheral vasodilatation and maldistribution of blood flow ie sepsis); and (4) obstructive (caused by extra cardiac obstruction to blood flow). *Shock is often manifested by BP <90mmHg. a weak pulse, evidence of end organ dysfunction, such as cool or mottled skin, oliguria , hepatic insufficiency or altered mental status. However the signs of shock can be subtle depending on the cause of shock.*

- **Hypovolemia:** *Bleeding:* Trauma, ruptured aortic aneurysm, ruptured ectopic pregnancy. *Fluid loss:* Vomiting (eg GI obstruction), diarrhea (eg cholera), burns, pools of sequestered (unavailable) fluids ('third spacing', eg in pancreatitis). *Heat exhaustion* may cause hypovolemic shock (also hyperpyrexia, oliguria, rhabdomyolysis, unconsciousness↓, hyperventilation, hallucination, incontinence, collapse, coma, pin-point pupils, LFTs↑, and DIC, p576).

- **Cardiogenic:** *Heart dysfunction* that includes dysrhythmias, tachyarrhythmias, or bradyarrhythmias. Overt pump failure is another cause of cardiogenic shock and can result from acute coronary syndromes, myocarditis, or cardiomyopathie as well as acute valvular dysfunction (especially regurgitant lesions) or rupture of ventricular septum or ventricular wall.

- **Obstructive shock:** Pathology that prevents blood flowing from the heart includes pericardial disease (tamponade), tension pneumothorax, pulmonary emboli, pulmonary hypertension or other cardiac tumor as well as obstructive valvular disease (aortic or mitral stenosis).

- **Distributive shock:** Blood is maldistributed throughout the body in this type of shock and includes septic shock, anaphylactic shock, neurogenic shock as well as vasodilator drugs and acute adrenal insufficiency.

- **Sepsis:** Gram –ve (or +ve) septicemic shock from endotoxin-induced vasodilatation may be sudden and severe, with shock and coma but no signs of infection (fever, WBC↑). • **Neurogenic:** Eg post-spinal surgery. • **Endocrine failure:** Addison's disease or hypothyroidism. • **Iatrogenic:** Drugs, eg anesthetics, antihypertensives.

Assessment ABC.

- **ECG:** Rate, rhythm, ischemia? • *General:* Cold and clammy—cardiogenic shock or fluid loss. Look for signs of anemia or dehydration—skin turgor, postural hypotension? Warm and well perfused, with bounding pulse—septic shock. Any features suggestive of anaphylaxis—history, urticaria, angioedema, wheeze? • *CVS:* Usually tachycardic (unless on beta-blocker, or in spinal shock) and hypotension. But in the young and fit or pregnant women, the systolic BP may remain normal, although the *pulse pressure* will narrow, with up to 30% blood volume depletion. Difference between arms—aortic dissection? • *JVP or central venous pressure:* If raised, cardiogenic shock likely. • *Check abdomen:* Any signs of trauma, or aneurysm? Any evidence of GI bleed?—check for melena.

Management If BP unrecordable, call the cardiac arrest team.

See OPPOSITE for general management. Specific measures:

- **Anaphylaxis** (p688) • **Cardiogenic shock** (p696) • **Septic shock:** (if no clue to source): IV cefuroxime 1.5g/8h (after blood culture) or gentamicin p498 (do levels; reduce in renal failure) + antipseudomonal penicillin, eg ticarcillin (as Timentin®, max dose 3.1g/4h IVI). Give colloid, or crystalloid, by IVI. Refer to ICU if possible for monitoring ± inotropes (eg dopamine in 'renal' dose of 2–5mcg/kg/min IVI). Goal directed therapy now includes measurement of lactic acid, CVP, urine output, and hematocrit. • **Hypovolemic shock:** Fluid replacement: Saline or colloid initially; if bleeding use blood; risks and benefits. Titrate against BP, CVP, urine output. Treat the underlying cause. If severe hemorrhage, exsanguinating, or more than 1L of fluid required to maintain BP, consider using group-specific blood, or O Rh–ve blood. Correct electrolyte abnormalities. Acidosis often responds to fluid replacement.

• **Heat exposure (heat exhaustion):** Sponge bath + fanning; avoid ice and immersion. Resuscitate with high-sodium IVI, such as 0.9% saline ± hydrocortisone 100mg IV. Dantrolene seems ineffective. Chlorpromazine 25mg IM may be used to stop shivering. Stop cooling when core temperature <39°C.

Management of shock

If BP unrecordable, call the cardiac arrest team
↓
ABC (including high-flow O₂)
↓
Raise foot of the bed
↓
IV access × 2 (wide bore; get help if this takes >2min)
↓
Identify and treat underlying cause
↓
Infuse crystalloid *fast* to raise BP
(unless cardiogenic shock)
↓
Seek expert help early
↓
Investigations

• CBC, CMP, ABG, glucose, CRP • Cross-match and check clotting • Blood cultures, urine culture, ECG, CXR • Others: Lactate, echo, abdominal CT, US
↓
Consider arterial line, central venous line, and
bladder catheter (aim for a urine flow >30mL/h)
↓
Further management: • Treat underlying cause if possible • Fluid replacement as dictated by BP, CVP, urine output • Don't overload with fluids if cardiogenic shock • If persistently hypotensive, consider inotropes

NB: *Remember that higher flow rates can be achieved through peripheral lines than through 'standard' gauge central lines.*

If cause unclear: R as hypovolemia—most common cause, and reversible.

Ruptured abdominal aortic aneurysm: Aim for a systolic BP of ~90mmHg.

SIRS, sepsis, and related syndromes

The pathogenesis of sepsis and septic shock is becoming increasingly understood. The 'systemic inflammatory response syndrome' (SIRS) is the early phase of septic shock and is thought to involve the cytokine cascades, free radical production, and the release of vasoactive mediators. SIRS is defined as the presence of 2 or more of the following features:

• Temperature >38°C or <36°C   • Tachycardia >90 bpm
• Respiratory rate >20 breaths/min
• WBC >12 x 10⁹/L or <4 x 10⁹/L, or >10% immature (band) forms

Related syndromes include:

Sepsis: SIRS occurring in the presence of infection. If SIRS continues then severe sepsis can result.

Severe sepsis: Sepsis with evidence of organ hypoperfusion eg hypoxemia, oliguria, lactic acidosis, or altered cerebral function.

Septic shock: Severe sepsis with hypotension (systolic BP <90mmHg) despite adequate fluid resuscitation, or the requirement for vasopressors/inotropes to maintain BP. If sepsis progresses the patient may end up with multiorgan dysfunction syndrome (MODS)

Septicemia was used to denote the presence of multiplying bacteria in the circulation, but has been replaced with the definitions above.

Anaphylactic shock

Type I IgE-mediated hypersensitivity reaction. Release of histamine and other agents causes: Capillary leak; wheeze; cyanosis; edema (larynx, lids, tongue, lips); urticaria. More common in atopic individuals. An *anaphylactoid reaction* results from direct release of mediators from inflammatory cells, without involving antibodies, usually in response to a drug, eg N-acetylcysteine.

Common precipitants
- Drugs, eg penicillin, and contrast media in radiology
- Latex
- Stings, eggs, fish, peanuts, strawberries.

Signs and symptoms
- Itching, erythema, urticaria, edema
- Wheeze, laryngeal obstruction, cyanosis
- Tachycardia, hypotension.

Management of anaphylaxis

Secure the airway—give 100% O_2
Intubate if respiratory obstruction imminent
↓

Remove the cause; raising the feet may help restore the circulation
↓

Give epinephrine SQ
0.3mg (ie 0.3mL of 1:1000)
Repeat every 5min, if needed as guided by BP, pulse, and respiratory function, until better
↓

Secure IV access
↓

Diphenhydramine 25–50mg IV and solumedrol 125mg IV
↓

IVI (0.9% saline, eg 500mL over ¼h; up to 2L may be needed)
Titrate against blood pressure
↓

If wheeze, treat for asthma (p702)
May require ventilatory support
↓

If still hypotensive, admission to ITU and an IVI of adrenaline may be needed ± aminophylline and nebulized albuterol: Get expert help.

Further management
- Admit to ward. Monitor ECG.
- Continue benadryl[1] 25–50mg/4–6h PO/IV if itching.
- Suggest a 'Medic-alert' bracelet naming the culprit allergen.
- Teach about self-injected epinephrine (eg 0.3mg, Epipen®) to prevent a fatal attack.
- Skin-prick tests showing specific IgE help identify which allergens to avoid.

Note

Epinephrine (adrenaline) is given SQ and NOT IV unless the patient is severely ill, or has no pulse. The IV dose is **different:** 100mcg per min—titrating with the response. This is 1mL of *1:10,000 solution* per min. Stop as soon as a response has been obtained.

Acute myocardial infarction

A common medical emergency, and prompt appropriate treatment saves lives and myocardium. If in doubt, seek immediate help.

Pre-hospital management

Arrange an emergency ambulance. Aspirin 325mg PO (unless clear contraindication). Analgesia, eg morphine 5–10mg IV (avoid IM injections, as risk of bleeding with thrombolysis). Sublingual NTG unless hypotensive.

Management See OPPOSITE for acute measures.

Thrombolysis effective in reducing mortality if given early. Greatest benefit is seen if given <12h of the onset of chest pain, but some benefit up to 24h. The door to needle time for thrombolysis should be <90min (<60min if possible).

Indications for thrombolysis: Presentation within *12h* of chest pain with:
• ST elevation >2mm in 2 or more chest leads or
• ST elevation >1mm in 2 or more limb leads or
• Posterior infarction (dominant R waves and ST depression in V_1–V_3)
• New onset left bundle branch block.
Presentation within *12–24h* if continuing chest pain and/or ST elevation.

Thrombolysis contraindications: (consider urgent angioplasty instead)
• Internal bleeding
• Prolonged or traumatic CPR
• Heavy vaginal bleeding
• Acute pancreatitis
• Active lung disease with cavitation
• Recent trauma or surgery (<2wks)
• Cerebral neoplasm
• Severe hypertension (>200/120mmHg)
• Suspected aortic dissection
• Previous allergic reaction
• Pregnancy or <18wks postnatal
• Severe liver disease
• Esophageal varices
• Recent head trauma
• Recent hemorrhagic stroke.

Relative CI: History of severe hypertension; peptic ulcer; history of CVA; bleeding diathesis; anticoagulants.

Streptokinase (SK) is the usual thrombolytic agent. Dose: 1.5 million units in 100mL 0.9% saline IVI over 1h. SE: Nausea; vomiting; hemorrhage; stroke (1%); dysrhythmias. Any hypotension usually responds to slowing down or stopping the infusion. Also watch for allergic reactions and anaphylaxis (rare). Do not repeat unless it is within 4d of the first administration.

Alteplase (rt-PA) may be indicated if the patient has previously received SK (>4d) or reacted to SK. Dose: 15mg IV bolus, then 0.75mg/kg (max 50mg) over 30min, then 0.5mg/kg (max 35mg) over 60 min. Accelerated rt-PA has benefit if given within 6h, especially in younger patients with anterior MI. Standard rt-PA is given to patients presenting at 6–12h. *Tenecteplase* is given by bolus injection (over 10s), which in some cases may be an advantage. Dose: 30mg IV (max 50mg) if wt<60kg, 35mg IV (max 50mg) if wt 60–69kg, 40mg IV (max 50mg) if wt 70–79kg, 45mg IV (max 50mg) if wt 80–89kg, 50mg IV (max 50mg) if wt>90kg.

Complications
• Recurrent ischemia or failure to reperfuse (usually detected as persisting pain and ST-segment elevation in the immediate aftermath of thrombolysis): Additional analgesia, GTN, β-blocker, consider re-thrombolysis or do angioplasty if ↑ or new ST segment elevation.
• Stroke.
• Pericarditis: Analgesics, try to avoid NSAIDs.
• Cardiogenic shock p696 and heart failure p692.

Right ventricular infarction
• Confirm by demonstrating ST elevation in RV3/4, and/or echo. NB: RV4 means that V_4 is placed in the right 5th intercostal space in the midclavicular line.
• Treat hypotension and oliguria with fluids.
• Avoid nitrates and diuretics.
• Intensive monitoring and inotropes may be useful in some patients.

Management of an acute MI

Attach ECG monitor and record a 12-lead ECG

↓

High-flow O_2 by face mask (caution, if COPD)

↓

IV access

Bloods for CBC, CMP, glucose, lipids, cardiac enzymes

↓

Brief assessment

History of cardiovascular disease; risk factors for IHD

Contraindications to thrombolysis?

Examination: Pulse, BP, JVP, cardiac murmurs, signs of heart failure, peripheral pulses, scars from previous cardiac surgery

↓

Aspirin 325mg if not given previously that day and no contraindications

↓

Next consider morphine unless hypotensive

↓

NTG 0.4mg sublingually unless hypotensive

↓

β-blocker, eg metoprolol 5mg IV (unless asthma or left ventricular failure)

↓

Thrombolysis see OPPOSITE

↓

CXR

Do not delay thrombolysis while waiting unless aneurysm suspected

↓

Consider DVT prophylaxis

↓

Continue medication except calcium channel antagonists (unless specific indication)

If pain is uncontrolled, especially if continuing ST elevation, consider re-thrombolysis with rt-PA (no bolus), tenecteplase, or rescue angioplasty.

Acute coronary syndrome (ACS) (without ST-elevation)

ACS includes unstable angina, evolving myocardial infarction (MI), and non-Q wave or subendocardial MI. Although the underlying pathology is similar, management differs and, therefore, ACS is usually divided into 2 classes:
• ACS with ST segment elevation or new LBBB (acute MI p690).
• ACS without ST segment elevation (unstable angina or non-Q wave MI).

ACS is associated with a greatly ↑ risk of MI (up to 30% in the 1st month). Patients should be managed medically until symptoms settle. They are then investigated by angiography with a view to possible angioplasty or surgery (CABG).

Assessment

Brief history: Previous angina, relief with rest/nitrates, history of cardiovascular disease, risk factors for IHD.

Examination: Pulse, BP, JVP, cardiac murmurs, signs of heart failure, peripheral pulses, scars from previous cardiac surgery.

Investigations ECG: ST depression; flat or inverted T waves; or normal. CBC, CMP, glucose, lipids, cardiac enzymes. CXR.

Measurement of cardiac troponins helps predict which patients are at risk of a cardiac event, and who can be safely discharged early. Note that 2 different forms of troponin are measured: Troponin T and troponin I: They have different reference intervals (consult your lab).

Management

See OPPOSITE for acute management

The aim of drug therapy is twofold:
1 Anti-ischemic, eg β-blocker, nitrate, calcium channel antagonist.
2 Antithrombotic, eg aspirin, low molecular weight heparin, abciximab, which interfere with platelet activation, and so reduce thrombus formation.

Further measures:
• Wean off NTG infusion when stabilized on oral drugs.
• Stop heparin when pain-free for 24h, but give at least 3–5d therapy.
• Check serial ECGs and cardiac enzymes for 12–72h.
• Address modifiable risk factors: Smoking, hypertension, hyperlipidemia, diabetes.
• Gentle mobilization.

If symptoms recur, refer to a cardiologist for urgent angiography and angioplasty or CABG.

Prognosis Overall risk of death ~1–2%, but ~15% for refractory angina despite medical therapy. Risk stratification can help predict those most at risk and allow intervention to be targeted at those individuals. The following are associated with an ↑ risk:
• Hemodynamic instability: Hypotension, pulmonary edema
• T-wave inversion or ST segment depression on resting ECG
• Previous MI
• Prolonged rest pain
• Older age
• Diabetes mellitus.

Indications for consideration of invasive intervention:
• Poor prognosis, eg pulmonary edema
• Refractory symptoms
• Positive exercise tolerance tests (ETT) at low workload
• Non-Q wave MI.

Acute management of ACS without ST-segment elevation

Admit to CCU and monitor closely

↓

High-flow O$_2$ by face mask

↓

Analgesia:
eg morphine 5–10mg IV + metoclopramide 10mg IV

↓

Nitrates: NTG spray or sublingual tablets as required

↓

Aspirin: 160–325mg if not given previously that day and no contraindications *reduces risk of MI and death*

↓

β-blocker: Eg metoprolol 50–100mg/8h or atenolol 50–100mg/24h
If β-blocker contraindicated (asthma, COPD, LVF, bradycardia, coronary artery spasm), give rate-limiting calcium antagonist (eg verapamil [1] *80-120mg/8h PO, or diltiazem 60-120mg/8h PO)*

↓

Low molecular weight heparin
(eg enoxaparin 1mg/kg/12h or dalteparin 120u/kg/12h SC)
Alternatively: Unfractionated heparin 5000U IV bolus then IVI
Check APTT 6-hourly. Alter IVI rate to maintain APTT at 1.5-2.5 times control

↓

IV nitrate if pain continues
(eg NTG 50mg in 50mL 0.9% saline at 2–10mL/h)
titrate to pain, and maintain systolic BP >100mmHg

↓

Record ECG while in pain

↓

High-risk patients

(persistent or recurrent ischemia, ST-depression, diabetes, ↑troponin)
Infusion of a GPIIb/IIIa antagonist (eg tirofiban) and, ideally, urgent angiography. Addition of clopidogrel may also be useful

↓

Optimize drugs: β-blocker; Ca^{2+} channel antagonist; ACE-i nitrate.
Intensive statin regimens, *starting at top dosages,* may ↓ long- and short-term mortality/adverse events, eg by stabilizing plaques.

↓

If symptoms fail to improve, refer to a cardiologist for urgent angiography ± angioplasty or CABG

Low-risk patients

(no further pain, flat or inverted T-waves, or normal ECG, **and** *negative troponin)*
May be discharged if a repeat troponin is negative.
Treat medically and arrange further investigation eg stress test, angiogram.

---

1 Do not use verapamil and a β-blocker together (can cause asystole).

Severe pulmonary edema (X-RAY PLATE 2)

Causes
- Cardiovascular—usually left ventricular failure—post-MI, or ischemic heart disease. Also mitral stenosis, arrhythmias, and malignant hypertension.
- ARDS (p174, any cause, eg trauma, malaria, drugs), look for predisposing factors, eg trauma, post-op, sepsis. *Is aspirin overdose or glue-sniffing/drug abuse likely?* Ask friends/relatives.
- Fluid overload.
- Neurogenic, eg head injury.

Differential diagnosis Asthma/COPD, pneumonia, and pulmonary edema are often hard to distinguish, especially in the elderly, where that may co-exist. Do not hesitate to treat all 3 simultaneously (eg with albuterol nebulizer, furosemide IV, morphine, fluoroquinolone).

Symptoms Dyspnea, orthopnea (eg paroxysmal), pink frothy sputum. NB: Drugs; other illnesses (recent MI/COPD or pneumonia).

Signs Distressed, pale, sweaty, pulse↑, tachypnea, pink frothy sputum, pulsus alternans, JVP↑, fine lung crackles, triple/gallop rhythm (p50), wheeze (cardiac asthma). Usually sitting up and leaning forward. Quickly examine for possible causes.

Investigations
- CXR (X-RAY PLATE 2)—cardiomegaly, signs of pulmonary edema: Look for shadowing (usually bilateral), small effusions at costophrenic angles, fluid in the lung fissures, and Kerley B lines (linear opacities).
- ECG—signs of MI.
- CMP; 'cardiac' enzymes, ABG.
- Consider echo.

Management

Begin treatment before investigations. See OPPOSITE.

Monitoring progress: BP; heart rate; cyanosis; respiratory rate; JVP; urine output, ABG.

Once stable and improving:
- Daily weights; BP and pulse/6h. Repeat CXR.
- Change to oral furosemide or bumetanide.
- If on large doses of loop diuretic, consider the addition of a thiazide or metolazone 2.5–5mg daily PO).
- ACE-i if left ventricular failure—also consider echo. If ACE-i contraindicated, consider hydralazine and nitrate.
- Also consider β-blocker and spironolactone.
- Is the patient suitable for cardiac transplantation?
- Consider digoxin ± warfarin, especially if AF.

Management of heart failure

Sit the patient upright

↓

Oxygen
100% if no pre-existing lung disease

↓

IV access and monitor ECG
Treat any arrhythmias, eg AF (p120)

↓

Investigations while continuing treatment
see OPPOSITE

↓

Morphine 2.5–5mg IV slowly
Caution in liver failure and COPD

↓

Furosemide 40–80mg IV slowly
Larger doses required in renal failure

↓

NTG spray 2 puffs SL or 2 × 0.3mg tablets SL
Don't give if systolic BP <90mmHg

↓

Necessary investigations, examination, and history

↓

If systolic BP ≥100mmHg, start a nitrate infusion
eg isosorbide dinitrate 2-10mg/h IVI; keep systolic BP ≥90mmHg

↓

If the patient is worsening: Further dose of furosemide 40–80mg
*Consider ventilation (invasive or non-invasive eg CPAP; get help)
or ↑ nitrate infusion*

↓

If systolic BP <100mmHg, treat as cardiogenic shock (p696),
ie consider a Swan-Ganz catheter and inotropic support

↓

If systolic BP is >180mmHg, consider treating for hypertensive LVF (p132)

Cardiogenic shock

This has a high mortality. Ask a senior physician's help both in formulating an *exact* diagnosis and in guiding treatment.

Cardiogenic shock is shock caused primarily by the failure of the heart to maintain the circulation. It may occur suddenly, or after progressively worsening heart failure.

Causes
- Arrhythmias
- Cardiac tamponade
- Tension pneumothorax
- MI
- Myocarditis; myocardial depression (drugs, hypoxia, acidosis, sepsis)
- Valve destruction (endocarditis)
- Pulmonary embolus
- Aortic dissection

Management

If the cause is MI prompt revascularization (thrombolysis or acute angioplasty) is vital; see p690[1] for indications and contraindications.
- Manage in coronary care unit, if possible.
- Investigation and treatment may need to be done concurrently.
- See OPPOSITE for details of management.
- *Investigations* ECG, CMP, CBC, CK, CK-MB, troponin, ABG, CXR, echo. If indicated, CT thorax (aortic dissection) and $\dot{V}/\dot{Q}$ scan or pulmonary angiogram for PE.
- *Monitor* CVP, BP, ABG, ECG; urine output. Do a 12-lead ECG every hour until the diagnosis is made. Consider a Swan–Ganz catheter to assess pulmonary wedge pressure and cardiac output, and an arterial line to monitor pressure. Catheterize for accurate urine output.

Cardiac tamponade

Essence: Pericardial fluid collects → intrapericardial pressure rises → heart cannot fill → pumping stops.

Causes: Trauma, lung/breast cancer, pericarditis, myocardial infarct, bacteria, eg TB. *Rarely:* Urea↑, radiation, myxedema, dissecting aorta, SLE.

Signs: Falling BP, a rising JVP, and muffled heart sounds = Beck's triad; JVP↑ on inspiration (Kussmaul's sign); pulsus paradoxus (pulse fades on inspiration). Echocardiography may be diagnostic. CXR: Globular heart; left heart border convex or straight; right cardiophrenic angle <90°. ECG: Electrical alternans.

Management: This can be very difficult. Everything is against you: Time, physiology, and your own confidence, as the patient may be too ill to give a history, and signs may be equivocal—but bitter experience has taught us not to equivocate for long.

Request the presence of your senior at the bedside (do not make do with telephone advice). With luck, prompt pericardiocentesis (p667) brings swift relief. While awaiting this, give O_2, monitor ECG, and set up IVI. Take blood for group and save.

1 SHOCK trial 2003 V Menon *Congest Heart Fail* **9** 35. NNT for acute angioplasty = 5.

Management of cardiogenic shock

Oxygen
Titrate to maintain adequate arterial saturations
↓
Morphine 2.5–5mg IV for pain and anxiety
↓
Investigations and close monitoring
(see OPPOSITE)
↓
Correct arrhythmias (p116–122), CMP abnormality
or acid–base imbalance
↓
Optimize filling pressure
if available measure pulmonary capillary wedge pressure (PCWP)

If PCWP <15mmHg fluid load   *If PCWP >15mmHg*
↓   ↓
Give a plasma expander   Inotropic support
100mL every 15min IV   *eg dobutamine 2.5-10mcg/kg/min IV*
Aim for PCWP of 15-20mmHg   *Aim for a systolic BP >80mmHg*
↓   ↓

Consider 'renal dose' dopamine
2-5mcg/kg/min IV (via central line only)
↓
Consider intra-aortic balloon pump if you expect the underlying
condition to improve, or you need time awaiting surgery
↓
Look for and treat any reversible cause
MI or PE—consider thrombolysis;
surgery for: Acute VSD, mitral, or aortic regurgitation

Wide complex tachycardia

ECG shows rate of >100bpm and QRS complexes >120ms.

Principles of management

If in doubt, treat as ventricular tachycardia (the most common cause).

Identify the underlying rhythm and treat accordingly.

Differential

- Ventricular tachycardia (VT) including torsade de pointes.
- SVT with aberrant conduction, eg AF, atrial flutter.
- Pre-excited tachycardias, eg AF, atrial flutter, or AV re-entry tachycardia with underlying WPW (p118).

(NB: Ventricular ectopics should not cause confusion when occurring singly but if >3 together at a rate of >120, this constitutes VT.)

Identification of the underlying rhythm may be difficult, seek expert help. Diagnosis is based on the history: If IHD/MI the likelihood of a ventricular arrhythmia is >95%, a 12-lead ECG, and the lack of response to IV adenosine (p118).

ECG findings in favour of VT:

- Fusion beats or capture beats (ECG p123).
- Positive QRS concordance in chest leads.
- Marked left axis deviation or rightwards axis.
- AV dissociation (occurs in 25%) or 2 : 1 or 3 : 1 AV block.
- QRS complex >160ms.
- Any atypical bundle-branch-block pattern.

Management Give high-flow O_2 by mask and monitor O_2 saturations.

- Connect patient to a cardiac monitor and have a defibrillator to hand.
- Assess CVS: Consciousness↓, BP <90, oliguria, angina, pulmonary edema.
- Obtain 12-lead ECG (request CXR) and obtain IV access.

If hemodynamically unstable

- Synchronized DC shock.
- Correct any hypokalemia and hypomagnesemia: 20–40mEq/h IV with cardiac monitoring, 1–2gm IV magnesium sulfate over 30min.
- Follow with amiodarone 150mg IV over 10min.
- For refractory cases procainamide or sotalol may be considered.

If hemodynamically stable

- Correct hypokalemia and hypomagnesemia: As above.
- Amiodarone 150mg IV over 10 min. Alternatively lidocaine 50mg (2.5mL or 2% solution) IV over 2min, repeated every 5min up to 200mg.
- If this fails, use synchronized DC shock.

After correction of VT

- Establish the cause (via the history and tests above).
- Maintenance anti-arrhythmic therapy may be required. If VT occurs after MI, give IV amiodarone or lidocaine infusion for 12–24h; if 24h after MI, also start oral anti-arrhythmic: Sotalol (if good LV function) or amiodarone (if poor LV function).
- Prevention of recurrent VT: Surgical isolation of the arrhythmogenic area or implantation of tiny automatic defibrillators may help.

Ventricular fibrillation (ECG p123). Use non-synchronized DC shock (there is no R wave to trigger defibrillation, p668).

Ventricular extrasystoles (ectopics) are the most common post-MI arrhythmia but they are also seen in healthy people (often >10/h). Patients with frequent ectopics post-MI have a worse prognosis, but there is no evidence that anti-dysrhythmic drugs improve outcome, indeed they may ↑ mortality.

Torsade de pointes: A form of VT, with a constantly varying axis, often in the setting of long-QT syndromes (ECG p123). This can be congenital or acquired, eg from drugs (eg some anti-dysrhythmics, tricyclics, antimalarials, newer antipsychotics and terfenadine). Torsade in the setting of congenital long-QT syndromes can be treated with high doses of β-blockers.

In acquired long-QT syndromes, stop all predisposing drugs, correct hypokalemia, and give $MgSO_4^{2+}$ (1–4g IV). Alternatives include: Overdrive pacing.

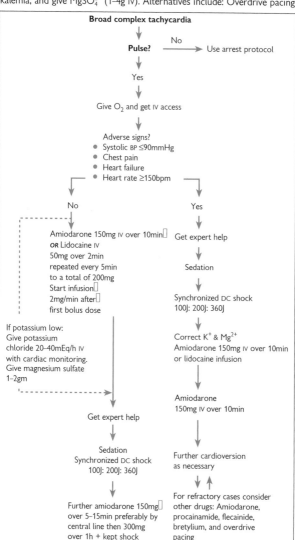

Broad complex tachycardia

Pulse? → No → Use arrest protocol

↓ Yes

Give O₂ and get IV access

Adverse signs?
- Systolic BP ≤90mmHg
- Chest pain
- Heart failure
- Heart rate ≥150bpm

No / Yes

No branch:
Amiodarone 150mg IV over 10min
OR Lidocaine IV
50mg over 2min
repeated every 5min
to a total of 200mg
Start infusion
2mg/min after
first bolus dose

If potassium low:
Give potassium
chloride 20–40mEq/h IV
with cardiac monitoring.
Give magnesium sulfate
1–2gm

Get expert help

Sedation
Synchronized DC shock
100J: 200J: 360J

Further amiodarone 150mg
over 5–15min preferably by
central line then 300mg
over 1h + kept shock

Yes branch:
Get expert help

Sedation

Synchronized DC shock
100J: 200J: 360J

Correct K⁺ & Mg²⁺
Amiodarone 150mg IV over 10min
or lidocaine infusion

Amiodarone
150mg IV over 10min

Further cardioversion
as necessary

For refractory cases consider
other drugs: Amiodarone,
procainamide, flecainide,
bretylium, and overdrive
pacing

Narrow complex tachycardia

ECG shows rate of >100bpm and QRS complex duration of <120ms.

Differential diagnosis
- Sinus tachycardia: Normal P-wave followed by normal QRS.
- *Atrial tachyarrhythmias:* Rhythm arises in atria, AV node is a bystander.
  - Atrial fibrillation (AF): Absent P-wave, irregular QRS complexes.
  - Atrial flutter: Atrial rate ~260–340bpm. Saw-tooth baseline, due to continuous atrial electrical activity. Ventricular rate often 150bpm (2:1 block).
  - Atrial tachycardia: Abnormally shaped P-waves, may outnumber QRS.
  - Multifocal atrial tachycardia: 3 or more P-wave morphologies, irregular QRS complexes.
- *Junctional tachycardia:* AV-node is part of the pathway. P-wave either buried in QRS complex or occurring after QRS complex.
  - AV nodal re-entry tachycardia.
  - AV re-entry tachycardia, includes an accessory pathway, eg WPW (p118).

Principles of management See algorithm OPPOSITE.
- If the patient is compromised, use DC cardioversion.
- Otherwise, identify the underlying rhythm and treat accordingly.
- Vagal maneuvers (carotid sinus massage, Valsalva maneuver) transiently ↑ AV block, and may unmask an underlying atrial rhythm.
- If unsuccessful, give adenosine which causes transient AV block. It has a short half-life (10–15s) and works in 2 ways:
  - by transiently slowing ventricles to show the underlying atrial rhythm;
  - by cardioverting a junctional tachycardia to sinus rhythm.

Give 6mg IV bolus into a large vein, followed by saline flush, while recording a rhythm strip. If unsuccessful, give 12mg, then 12mg at 2min intervals. Warn about SE: Transient chest tightness, dyspnea, headache, flushing. *CI:* Asthma, $2^{nd}/3^{rd}$-degree AV block or sinoatrial disease (unless pacemaker). *Interactions:* Potentiated by dipyridamole, antagonized by theophylline.

Specifics *Sinus tachycardia:* Identify and treat underlying cause.

Supraventricular tachycardia: If adenosine fails, use diltiazem 20mg IV over 2min. NB: NOT if on a β-blocker. If no response, a further 5mg IV over 3min (if age <60yrs). Alternatives: Metoprolol 5mg IV or sotalol 20–120mg IV (over 10min); or amiodarone. If unsuccessful, use DC cardioversion.

Atrial fibrillation/flutter: Manage along standard lines (p120).

Atrial tachycardia: Rare; may be due to digoxin toxicity. Withdraw digoxin, consider digoxin-specific antibody fragments. Maintain K^+ at 4–5mmol/L.

Multifocal atrial tachycardia: Most commonly occurs in COPD. Correct hypoxia and hypercapnia. Consider verapamil if rate remains >110bpm.

Junctional tachycardia: Where antegrade conduction through the AV node occurs, vagal maneuvers are worth trying. Adenosine will usually cardiovert a junctional rhythm to sinus rhythm. If it fails or recurs, β-blockers (or verapamil—**not** with β-blockers, digoxin, or class I agents such as quinidine). If this does not control symptoms, consider radiofrequency ablation.

Wolff–Parkinson–White (WPW) syndrome (ECG p121) Caused by congenital accessory conduction pathway between atria and ventricles. Resting ECG shows short P–R interval and widened QRS complex due to slurred upstroke or 'delta wave'. 2 types: WPW type A (+ve δ wave in V_1), WPW type B (–ve δ wave in V_1). Patients present with SVT which may be due to an AVRT, (p118) pre-excited AF, or pre-excited atrial flutter. Risk of degeneration to VF and sudden death. ℞ flecainide, propafenone, sotalol, or amiodarone. Refer to cardiologist for electrophysiology and ablation of the accessory pathway.

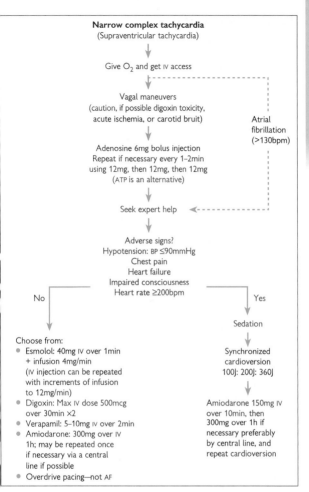

Narrow complex tachycardia
(Supraventricular tachycardia)

↓

Give O$_2$ and get IV access

↓

Vagal maneuvers
(caution, if possible digoxin toxicity,
acute ischemia, or carotid bruit)

Atrial
fibrillation
(>130bpm)

↓

Adenosine 6mg bolus injection
Repeat if necessary every 1–2min
using 12mg, then 12mg, then 12mg
(ATP is an alternative)

↓

Seek expert help ◄- - - - - -

↓

Adverse signs?
Hypotension: BP ≤90mmHg
Chest pain
Heart failure
Impaired consciousness
Heart rate ≥200bpm

No ────────────────┘ └──────────── Yes

Sedation

↓

Choose from:
- Esmolol: 40mg IV over 1min
  + infusion 4mg/min
  (IV injection can be repeated
  with increments of infusion
  to 12mg/min)
- Digoxin: Max IV dose 500mcg
  over 30min ×2
- Verapamil: 5–10mg IV over 2min
- Amiodarone: 300mg over IV
  1h; may be repeated once
  if necessary via a central
  line if possible
- Overdrive pacing—not AF

Synchronized
cardioversion
100J: 200J: 360J

↓

Amiodarone 150mg IV
over 10min, then
300mg over 1h if
necessary preferably
by central line, and
repeat cardioversion

Acute severe asthma

The severity of an attack is easily underestimated.

An atmosphere of calm helps.

Presentation Acute breathlessness and wheeze.

History Ask about usual and recent treatment; previous acute episodes and their severity and best peak expiratory flow rate (PEFR). Have they been admitted to ICU?

Differential diagnosis Acute infective exacerbation of COPD, pulmonary edema, upper respiratory tract obstruction, pulmonary embolism, anaphylaxis.

Investigations PEF—but may be too ill; arterial blood gases; CXR (to exclude pneumothorax, infection); CBC; CMP.

Assessing the severity of an acute asthmatic attack

Severe attack:
- Unable to complete sentences
- Respiratory rate >25/min
- Pulse rate >110 beats/min
- Peak expiratory flow <50% of predicted or best.

Life-threatening attack:
- Peak expiratory flow <33% of predicted or best
- Silent chest, cyanosis, feeble respiratory effort
- Bradycardia or hypotension
- Exhaustion, confusion, or coma
- Arterial blood gases: Normal/high P_aCO_2 >36mmHg
  P_aO_2 <60mmHg
  low pH, eg <7.35.

Treatment Life-threatening or severe asthma, see OPPOSITE.
- Albuterol 5mg nebulized, ipratropium bromide 500mcg nebulized, with oxygen.
- If PEF remains <75%, repeat albuterol and give prednsione 60mg PO.
- Monitor oxygen saturation, heart rate, and respiratory rate.

Discharge

Patients, before discharge, must have:
- Been on discharge medication for 24h.
- Had inhaler technique checked.
- Peak flow rate >75% predicted or best with diurnal variability <25%.
- Steroid and bronchodilator therapy.
- Own a PEF meter and have management plan.
- Follow-up appointment within 1wk.
- Respiratory clinic appointment within 4wks.

Drugs used in acute asthma

Albuterol (β_2-agonist) *SE:* Tachycardia, arrhythmias, tremor, $K^+\downarrow$.

Aminophylline (Inhibits phosphodiesterase; $\uparrow$[cAMP]). *SE:* Pulse$\uparrow$; arrhythmias, nausea, seizures. The amount of IV aminophylline may need altering according to the individual patient: Always check the BNF. Monitor ECG.
- *Factors which may necessitate reduction of dose:* Cardiac or liver failure, drugs which $\uparrow$ the half-life of aminophylline, eg cimetidine, ciprofloxacin, erythromycin, contraceptive steroids.
- *Factors which may require $\uparrow$dose:* Smoking, drugs which shorten the half-life, eg phenytoin, carbamazepine, barbiturates, rifampin.
- Serious toxicity (BP$\downarrow$, arrhythmias, cardiac arrest) can occur. Measure plasma K^+: Theophyllines may cause $K^+\downarrow$. Don't load patients already on oral preparations.

Immediate management of acute severe asthma

Assess severity of attack (see above). Warn ICU if attack severe.

Start treatment immediately (prior to investigations).
• Sit patient up and give high-dose O_2 in: 100% via non-rebreathing bag.
• Albuterol 5mg (or terbutaline 10mg) plus ipratropium bromide 0.5mg nebulized with O_2.
• Hydrocortisone 100mg IV or prednisone 60mg PO.
• CXR to exclude pneumothorax.

If life-threatening features (above) present:
• Inform ICU.
• Add magnesium sulphate ($MgSO_4$) 1.2–2g IV over 20min.
• Give albuterol nebulizers every 15min, or 10mg continuously per hour.

Further management

If improving • 40–60% O_2.
  • Consider oral prednisone 10–60mg with taper.
  • Nebulized albuterol every 4h.
  • Monitor peak flow and oxygen saturations.

If patient not improving after 15–30min
  • Continue 100% O_2 and steroids.
  • Hydrocortisone 100mg IV or prednisone 60mg PO if not already given.
  • Give albuterol nebulizers every 15min, or 10mg continuously per hour.
  • Continue ipratropium 0.5mg every 4–6h.

If patient still not improving
  • Discuss with ICU staff.
  • Repeat albuterol nebulizer every 15min.
  • $MgSO_4$ 1.2–2g IV over 20min, unless already given.
  • Consider aminophylline; if not already on a theophylline, load with eg 6mg/kg IV over 20min, then 500mcg/kg/h, eg in a small adult: 750mg/24h; large adult 1200mg/24h. Adjust dose according to plasma theophylline, if available. Do levels if infusion lasts >24h. Alternatively, give salbutamol IV, eg 3–20mcg/min. IPPV may be required.
• If no improvement, or life-threatening features are present, consider transfer to ICU, accompanied by a doctor prepared to intubate.

Monitoring the effects of treatment
• Repeat PEF 15–30min after initiating treatment.
• Pulse oximeter monitoring: Maintain S_aO_2 >92%.
• Check blood gases within 2h if: Initial P_aCO_2 was normal/raised or initial P_aO_2 <60mmHg or patient deteriorating.
• Record PEF pre- and post-β-agonist in hospital at least 4 times.

Once patient is improving
• Wean down and stop aminophylline over 12–24h.
• Reduce nebulized albuterol and switch to inhaled β-agonist.
• Initiate inhaled steroids and stop oral steroids if possible.
• Continue to monitor PEF. Look for deterioration on reduced treatment and beware early morning dips in PEF.
• Look for the cause of the acute exacerbation and admission.

Acute exacerbations of COPD

Common medical emergency especially in winter. May be triggered by viral or bacterial infections.

Presentation ↑ cough, breathlessness, or wheeze. ↓ exercise capacity.

History Ask about usual/recent treatments (especially home oxygen), smoking status, and exercise capacity (may influence a decision to ventilate the patient).

Differential diagnosis Asthma, pulmonary edema, upper respiratory tract obstruction, pulmonary embolus, anaphylaxis.

Investigations
- Peak expiratory flow (PEF)—but may be too ill.
- Arterial blood gases.
- CXR to exclude pneumothorax and infection.
- CBC; CMP.
- ECG.
- Blood cultures (if febrile).
- Send sputum for culture.

Management
- Look for a cause, eg infection, pneumothorax.
- See OPPOSITE for acute management.
- Prior to discharge, coordinate steroid reduction, home oxygen, smoking, pneumococcal & flu vaccinations (p158).

Treatment of stable COPD p172

Non-pharmacological:	Stop smoking, encourage exercise, treat poor nutrition or obesity, influenza, vaccination.
Pharmacological:	
• Mild	Short-acting β$_2$-agonist or ipratropium PRN.
• Moderate	Regular short-acting β$_2$-agonist and/or ipratropium. Consider corticosteroid trial.
• Severe	Combination therapy with regular short-acting β$_2$-agonist and ipratropium. Consider corticosteroid trial. Assess for home nebulizers.

More advanced disease:
- Consider pulmonary rehabilitation in moderate/severe disease.
- Consider long-term oxygen therapy if P_aO_2 <55mmHg (p172).
- Indications for surgery: Recurrent pneumothoraces; isolated bullous disease; lung volume reduction surgery (selected patients).
- Assess social circumstances and support required. Identify and treat depression.

Management of acute COPD

Controlled oxygen therapy
Start at 24–28%; vary according to ABG.
Aim for a P_aO_2 >60mmHg with a rise in P_aCO_2 <12mmHg
↓

Nebulized bronchodilators:
Albuterol 5mg/4h and ipratropium 500mcg/6h
↓

Steroids
IV hydrocortisone 200mg or oral prednisone 60mg
↓

Antibiotics:
Use if evidence of infection, eg amoxicillin 500mg/8h PO
↓

Physiotherapy to aid sputum expectoration
↓

If no response:
Repeat nebulizers and consider IV aminophylline[1]
↓

If no response:
1. Consider nasal intermittent positive pressure ventilation
(NIPPV) if respiratory rate >30 or pH <7.35.
It is delivered by nasal mask and a flow generator
↓

2. Consider intubation[2] & ventilation if pH <7.26 and P_aCO_2 is rising
↓

3. Consider a respiratory stimulant drug, eg doxapram
1.5–4mg/min IV *SE: Agitation, confusion, tachycardia, nausea*
Only for patients who are not suitable for mechanical ventilation
A short-term measure only

Oxygen therapy

• The greatest danger is hypoxia, which probably accounts for more deaths than hypercapnia. *Don't leave patients severely hypoxic.*
• However, in some patients, who rely on their hypoxic drive to breathe, too much oxygen may lead to a reduced respiratory rate, and hypercapnia, with a consequent fall in conscious level.
• Therefore, care is required with O_2, especially if there is evidence of CO_2 retention. Start with 24–28% O_2 in such patients. Reassess after 30min.
• Monitor the patient carefully. Aim to raise the P_aO_2 above 60mmHg with a rise in P_aCO_2 <12mmHg.
• In patients without evidence of retention at baseline use 28–40% O_2, but still monitor and repeat ABG.

705

1 Aminophylline: Do not give a loading dose to patients on maintenance methylxanthines theophyllines/aminophylline). Load with 250mg over 20min, then infuse at a rate of ~500mcg/kg/h. Check plasma levels if given for >24h. ECG monitoring is required.
2 A decision to ventilate will depend on the patient's premorbid state—exercise capacity, home oxygen, and comorbidity. Ask about this information before you need to make this decision.

Pneumothorax (X-RAY PLATE 6)

Tension pneumothorax requires immediate relief (see below). Do not delay management by obtaining a *CXR*.

Causes Often spontaneous (especially in young thin men) due to rupture of a subpleural bulla. Other causes: Asthma; COPD; TB; pneumonia; lung abscess; carcinoma; cystic fibrosis; lung fibrosis; sarcoidosis; connective tissue disorders (Marfan's syndrome, Ehlers–Danlos syndrome); trauma; iatrogenic (subclavian CVP line insertion, pleural aspiration or biopsy, percutaneous liver biopsy, positive pressure ventilation).

Clinical features *Symptoms:* There may be no symptoms (especially in fit young people with small pneumothoraces) or there may be sudden onset of dyspnea and/or pleuritic chest pain. Patients with asthma or COPD may present with a sudden deterioration. Mechanically ventilated patients may present with hypoxia or an ↑ in ventilation pressures. *Signs:* Reduced expansion, hyper-resonance to percussion and diminished breath sounds on the affected side. *With a tension pneumothorax, the trachea will be deviated away from the affected side and the patient will be very unwell.*

Investigations *A CXR should not be performed if a tension pneumothorax is suspected, as it will delay immediate necessary treatment.* Otherwise, request an expiratory film, and look for an area devoid of lung markings, peripheral to the edge of the collapsed lung (X-RAY PLATE 6). *Ensure the suspected pneumothorax is not a large emphysematous bulla.* Check ABG in dyspneic patients and those with chronic lung disease.

Management Depends on whether it is a primary or secondary (underlying lung disease) pneumothorax, size and symptoms—see OPPOSITE.
- Pneumothorax due to trauma or mechanical ventilation requires a chest tube.
- Aspiration of a pneumothorax, BELOW.
- Insertion and management of a chest tube, p662.

Surgical advice: Arrange if: Bilateral pneumothoraces; lung fails to expand after intercostal drain insertion; 2 or more previous pneumothoraces on the same side; or history of pneumothorax on the opposite side.

Tension pneumothorax (X-RAY PLATE 6)

This is a medical emergency.

Essence: Air drawn into the pleural space with each inspiration has no route of escape during expiration. The mediastinum is pushed over into the contralateral hemithorax, kinking and compressing the great veins. Unless the air is rapidly removed, cardiorespiratory arrest will occur.

Signs: Respiratory distress, tachycardia, hypotension, distended neck veins, trachea deviated away from side of pneumothorax. ↑ percussion note, reduced air entry/breath sounds on the affected side.

Treatment:

To remove the air, insert a large-bore (14–16G) needle into the 2nd intercostal interspace in the midclavicular line on the side of the suspected pneumothorax.

Do this *before* requesting a CXR.

Then insert a chest tube, p662.

Chest tube drainage
- Use a small tube (10–14F) unless blood/pus is also present.
- Never clamp a bubbling tube.
- Tubes may be removed 24h after the lung has re-expanded and air leak has stopped (ie the tube stops bubbling). This is done during expiration or a valsalva maneuver.
- If the lung fails to re-expand within 48h, or if there is a persistent air leak, specialist advice should be obtained, as suction or surgical intervention may be required.
- If suction is required, high volume, low pressure (–10 to –20cm H_2O) systems are required.

Pneumonia
(X-RAY PLATE 5 & 8)

An infection of the lung parenchyma. Incidence of community-acquired pneumonia is 12 per 1000 adults. Of these, 1 will require hospitalization, and mortality in these patients is still 10%.

Common organisms
- *Streptococcus pneumoniae* is the most common cause (60–75%).
- *Mycoplasma pneumoniae* (5–18%).
- *Staphylococcus aureus*.
- *Hemophilus influenzae*.
- *Legionella* species and *Chlamydia psittaci*.
- Gram-negative bacilli, often hospital-acquired or immunocompromised eg *Pseudomonas* especially in those with COPD.
- Viruses including influenza account for up to 15%.

Symptoms
- Fever, rigors, malaise, anorexia, dyspnea, cough, purulent sputum (classically 'rusty' with pneumococcus), hemoptysis, and pleuritic chest pain.

Signs
- Fever, cyanosis, herpes labialis (pneumococcus), confusion, tachypnea, tachycardia, hypotension, signs of consolidation (diminished expansion, dull percussion note, ↑ tactile vocal fremitus/vocal resonance, bronchial breathing), and a pleural rub.

Investigations
- CXR (X-RAY PLATE 5 & 8).
- Oxygen saturation arterial blood gases if S_aO_2 <92% or severe pneumonia.
- CBC, CMP, LFT, CRP, atypical serology.
- Blood and sputum cultures.
- Pleural fluid may be aspirated for culture.
- Bronchoscopy and bronchoalveolar lavage if the patient is immunocompromised or on ICU.

Severity
Core adverse features 'CURB' score:
- Confusion;
- BUN >20mg/dL;
- Respiratory rate ≥30/min;
- BP <90/60mmHg).

A score >2 indicates severe pneumonia. Other features ↑ the risk of death are: Age ≥50yrs; co-existing disease; bilateral/multilobar involvement; P_aO_2 <60mmHg or S_aO_2 <92%.

Management See OPPOSITE.

Complications

Pleural effusion, empyema, lung abscess, respiratory failure, septicemia, pericarditis, myocarditis, cholestatic jaundice, renal failure.

Management of pneumonia

Oxygen to maintain P_aO_2 >60mmHg
Caution if history of COPD

↓

Treat hypotension and shock p686

↓

Investigations
see OPPOSITE

↓

Antibiotics
see BELOW

↓

Intravenous fluids may be required
(anorexia, dehydration, shock)

↓

Analgesia for pleuritic chest pain, eg acetaminophen 1g/6h or NSAID

↓

Some patients may need intubation and a period of ventilatory support

Antibiotics p159

Community-acquired

Mild	*Streptococcus pneumoniae* *Haemophilus influenzae* *Mycoplasma pneumoniae*	Amoxicillin 500mg–1.0g/8h PO + erythromycin 500mg/6h PO or fluoroquinolone if IV required: Ampicillin 500mg/6h + erythromycin 12.5mg/kg/6h IVI
Severe	As above	Augmentin IV or cephalosporin IV (eg Cefuroxime 1.5g/8h IV) AND erythromycin as above
Atypical	*Legionella pneumophilia*	Clarithromycin 500mg/12h PO/IVI ± rifampin
	Chlamydia species	Tetracycline
	Pneumocystis jiroveci	High-dose co-trimoxazole

Hospital acquired

	Gram −ve bacilli Pseudomonas Anaerobes	Aminoglycoside IV + anti- pseudomonal penicillin IV or 3rd gen cephalosporin IV

Aspiration

	Strep. pneumoniae Anaerobes	Cefuroxime 1.5g/8h IV + metronidazole 500mg/8h IVI

Neutropenic patients

	Gram +ve cocci Gram −ve bacilli	Aminoglycoside IV + antipseudomonal penicillin IV or 3rd gen cephalosporin IV
	Fungi	Consider antifungals after 48h

3rd gen = 3rd generation, eg cefotaxime

Massive pulmonary embolism (PE)

Always suspect pulmonary embolism (PE) in sudden collapse 1–2wks after surgery. Mortality ranges from 0.7 to 6.0 per 100,000 persons.

Mechanism Venous thrombi, usually from DVT, pass into the pulmonary circulation and block blood flow to lungs. The source is often occult.

Risk factors
- Malignancy
- Surgery—especially pelvic
- Immobility
- Birth control pills (there is also a slight risk attached to HRT)
- Previous thromboembolism and inherited thrombophilia, p590.

Prevention Early post-op mobilization is the simplest method; consider:
- Antithromboembolic stockings.
- Low molecular weight heparin prophylaxis SC.
- Avoid contraceptive pill if at risk, eg major or orthopedic surgery.
- Recurrent PEs may be prevented by anticoagulation, vena caval filters are of limited use, and should be combined with anticoagulation.

Signs and symptoms
- Acute dyspnea, pleuritic chest pain, hemoptysis, and syncope.
- Hypotension, tachycardia, gallop rhythm, JVP↑, loud P_2, right ventricular heave, pleural rub, tachypnea, and cyanosis. AF.

Classically, PE presents 10d post-op, with collapse and sudden breathlessness while straining at stool—but PE may occur after any period of immobility, or with no predisposing factors. Breathlessness may be the only sign. Multiple small emboli may present less dramatically with pleuritic pain, hemoptysis, and gradually ↑ breathlessness.

▶Look for a source of emboli—especially DVT (is a leg swollen?).

Investigations
- CMP, CBC, baseline clotting.
- ECG (commonly normal or sinus tachycardia); right ventricular strain pattern V1–3 (p93), right axis deviation, RBBB, AF, may be deep S-waves in I, Q-waves in III, inverted T-waves in III ('S_I Q_{III} T_{III}').
- CXR—often normal; ↓ vascular markings, small pleural effusion. Wedge-shaped area of infarction.
- ABG: Hyperventilation + gas exchange↓: P_aO_2↓, P_aCO_2↓, pH often↑.
- CT pulmonary angiography is sensitive and specific in determining if emboli are in pulmonary arteries. If helical CT is unavailable, a *ventilation-perfusion ($\dot{V}/\dot{Q}$) scan* can aid diagnosis. If $\dot{V}/\dot{Q}$ scan is equivocal, pulmonary angiography or bilateral venograms may help.
- D-dimer blood test, ↑ if thrombosis present. May help in excluding a PE.

Management See OPPOSITE for immediate management.
- Try to prevent further thrombosis with compression stockings.
- Heparin should be given for ≥5d, and until INR >2. Then stop.
- If obvious remedial cause, 6wks' treatment with warfarin may be sufficient. Otherwise, continue for at least 3–6 months (long-term if recurrent emboli, or underlying malignancy).
- Is there an underlying cause, eg thrombophilic tendency (p590), malignancy (especially prostate, breast, or pelvic cancer), SLE, or polycythemia?

If good story and signs, make the diagnosis. Start treatment (OPPOSITE) before definitive investigations.

Management of massive pulmonary embolism

Oxygen, 100%

↓

Morphine 10mg IV with antiemetic
if the patient is in pain or very distressed

↓

►If critically ill, consider immediate surgery

↓

IV access and start heparin
either unfractionated heparin 80 units/kg bolus
then 18 units/kg/h IV as guided by APTT (p574)
or low molecular weight heparin, eg enoxaparin 1mg/kg SC q12h

↓

| What is the systolic BP? |

<90mmHg
Start rapid fluid resuscitation

↓

If BP still↓ after 500mL colloid,
dobutamine 2.5–10mcg/kg/min IV;
aim for systolic BP >90mmHg

If BP still↓, consider norepinephrine

If the systolic BP <90mmHg after
30–60min of standard treatment,
clinically definite PE and no CI
(p690), consider thrombolysis.

>90mmHg
Start warfarin
10mg/24h PO (p574)

↓

Confirm diagnosis

Acute upper gastrointestinal bleeding

Causes

Common: • Gastric/duodenal ulcer • Gastritis • Mallory–Weiss tear (esophageal tear due to vomiting) • Esophageal varices • Portal hypertensive gastropathy • Drugs: NSAIDs, aspirin, thrombolytics, anticoagulants.

Rarer: • Hemobilia • Nose bleeds (swallowed blood); esophageal/gastric malignancy • Esophagitis • Angiodysplasia • Hemangiomas • Ehlers–Danlos or Peutz–Jeghers' syndrome • Bleeding disorders • Aorto-enteric fistula (in those with an aortic graft).

Signs & symptoms Hematemesis, or melena, dizziness (especially postural), fainting, abdominal pain, dysphagia? Postural hypotension, hypotension, tachycardia (not if on β-blocker), ↓JVP, ↓urine output, cool and clammy, signs of chronic liver disease; telangiectasia or purpura; jaundice (biliary colic + jaundice + melena suggests hemobilia). NB: Ask about previous GI problems, drug use, and alcohol intake.

Management *Assess whether patient is in shock:*
• Cool & clammy to touch (especially nose, toes, fingers) ↓capillary refill.
• Pulse >100bpm
• JVP <1cm H_2O
• Systolic BP <100mmHg
• Postural drop
• Urine output <30mL/h.

If not in shock: Insert 2 big cannulae; start slow saline IV to keep lines patent; check bloods and monitor vital signs + urine output. Aim to keep Hb >8g/dL. NB: Hb may not fall until circulating volume is restored.

If in shock: See OPPOSITE for management

Variceal bleeding: Resuscitate then proceed to urgent endoscopy for banding or sclerotherapy. Give octreotide 50mcg/h IVI for 2–5d. If massive bleed or bleeding continues, pass a Sengstaken–Blakemore tube. A bleed is the equivalent of a large protein meal so start treatment to avoid hepatic encephalopathy. Esomeprazole 40mg PO may also be helpful in preventing stress ulceration.

Endoscopy Within 4h if you suspect variceal bleeding; within 12–24h if shocked on admission or significant comorbidity. Endoscopy can identify the site of bleeding, estimate the risk of rebleeding (rebleeding doubles mortality) and can be used to administer treatment. *Risk of rebleeding:* Active arterial bleeding seen (90% risk); visible vessel (70% risk); adherent clot/black dots (30% risk). *No site of bleeding identified:* Bleeding site missed on endoscopy; bleeding site has healed (Mallory–Weiss tear)nose bleed (swallowed blood); site distal to 3rd part of the duodenum (Meckel's diverticulum, colonic site).

Rebleeds Serious event: 40% of patients who rebleed will die. If 'at risk' maintain a high index of suspicion. If a rebleed occurs, check vital signs every 15min and call senior cover. To prevent rebleeding in endoscopically-proven high risk cases, IVI omeprazole has been tried, eg 80mg followed by an infusion of 8mg/h for 72h, then 20mg/24h PO for 8wks.

Signs of a rebleed:
• Rising pulse rate.
• Falling JVP ± ↓ hourly urine output.
• Hematemesis or melena.
• Fall in BP (a late and sinister finding) and ↓ conscious level.

Acute drug therapy Following successful endoscopic therapy in patients with **major** ulcer bleeding, IV omeprazole (80mg stat followed by 8mg/h for 72h) is recommended. There is no firm evidence to support the use of somatostatin or antifibrinolytic therapy in the majority of patients.

Immediate management if hypotensive with GI bleed

Protect airway and keep NPO
↓
Insert two large-bore cannulae *14-16G*
↓
Draw bloods
CBC, CMP, LFT, glucose, clotting screen
Cross-match 6 units
↓
Give high-flow O$_2$
↓
Rapid IV colloid infusion
Up to 1L
↓
If remains hypotensive, give blood
Group specific or O Rh-ve until cross-match done
↓
Otherwise slow saline infusion[1]
To keep lines open
↓
Transfuse as dictated by hemodynamics
↓
Correct clotting abnormalities
Vitamin K, FFP, platelet concentrate
↓
Set up CVP line to guide fluid replacement
Aim for >5cm H$_2$O CVP may mislead if there is ascites or CCF
A Swan-Ganz catheter may help
↓
Catheterize and monitor urine output
Aim for >30mL/h
↓
Monitor vital signs every 15min until stable, then hourly
↓
Notify surgeons of all severe bleeds
↓
Urgent endoscopy for diagnosis ± control of bleeding

Poor prognostic signs:

- Age >60
- Systolic BP <100mmHg
- Bradycardia or rate >100bpm
- Bleeding diathesis

- Chronic liver disease
- Consciousness level↓
- Significant co-morbidity

1 Avoid saline in patients with decompensated liver disease (ascites, peripheral edema) as it worsens ascites, and despite a low serum sodium, patients have a high body sodium. Use whole blood, or salt-poor albumin for resuscitation, and 5% dextrose for maintenance.

Acute liver failure

Fulminant liver failure is assumed to be potentially reversible. Therefore, treatment is supportive and designed to buy time for the patient's liver to regenerate.

Management

- Seek expert help. Is transfer to a liver unit appropriate? p210
- Nurse with a 20° head-up tilt in ICU.
- Treat the cause if known (eg acetaminophen overdose, p738).
- Caution with secretions and blood if hepatitis suspected.
- Check blood glucose 1–4 hourly and give 50mL 50% dextrose IV if <3.5mmol/L. Give 10% dextrose IV, 1L/12h to avoid hypoglycemia.
- NGT to avoid aspiration and remove any blood (bleeding varices) from stomach. Protect the airway with an endotracheal tube.
- Monitor temperature; pulse; RR; BP; pupils; urine output.
- Daily lab blood glucose; INR; CMP; LFT; ammonia; blood cultures, and EEG. The INR (or PT) is the best measure of liver synthetic function.
- Avoid FFP unless bleeding or undergoing a surgical procedure. Some centers give vitamin K daily. Platelet transfusions may be required if thrombocytopenic and bleeding.
- Daily weights (ascites).
- Minimize absorption of nitrogenous substances and worsening of coma by restricting protein and emptying the bowel with lactulose and magnesium sulfate enemas. Aim for 2 soft stools/d.
- Consider neomycin 1g/6h PO to reduce numbers of bowel organisms.
- Consider N-acetylcysteine. Even in non-acetaminophen liver failure, this can improve oxygenation and clotting profiles.
- Watch renal function carefully. Consider hemodialysis if water overload or acute renal failure develops.
- Reduce acid secretion and risk of gastric stress ulcers, eg with cimetidine IV or a proton pump inhibitor. Cimetidine dose by slow IV injection: 300mg over >5min; may be repeated every 8h (or use IVI in 0.9% saline).
- Avoid sedatives (but diazepam is used for seizures), or other drugs with hepatic metabolism.
- Treat sepsis aggressively, and don't forget the risk of spontaneous bacterial peritonitis.

NB: Attempts to correct acid–base balance are often harmful.

MeningitisND

Do not delay treatment, it may save a life.

Make sure the referring physician gives a dose of antibiotic before sending the patient to you if possible.

Presentation
- Headache
- Meningismus: Neck stiffness, photophobia, Kernig's sign, Brudzinski's sign, headache
- Conscious level ↓, coma
- Petechial (non-blanching) rash—may only be 1 or 2 spots
- Seizures (~20%)
- Focal neurological signs (~20%).

Common organisms
- Meningococcus
- Pneumococcus
- *Hemophilus influenzae* (especially children)
- *Listeria monocytogenes*.

Management
- Careful examination: Pay attention to the neurological exam; look for rashes; assess GCS.
- If shocked, resuscitate with fluids and oxygen.
- If ICP raised, summon help immediately and inform neurosurgeons.
- Start antibiotics (below) immediately.

Investigations
- CMP, CBC, LFT, glucose, coagulation screen.
- Blood culture, throat swabs (one for bacteria, one for virology), stool culture for viruses.
- Lumbar puncture (p664) if safe. Don't forget to measure the opening pressure! **Contraindications** are: Suspected intracranial mass lesion, focal signs, papilledema, trauma, or middle ear pathology. Major coagulopathy. Send samples for cell count and differential, C&S, Gram stain, protein estimation, glucose, and to virology.
- CT head before LP if mass lesion or raised ICP suspected.
- CXR.

Antibiotics

Local policies vary. If in doubt ask. The following are suggestions only, where the organism is unknown:
- <50yrs: Vancomycin 1g IV/12h + ceftriaxone 2g IV over >2min as 1 daily dose.
- >50yrs: Vancomycin 1g IV/12h + ceftriaxone 2g IV over >2min daily + ampicillin 2g IV/4h (for *Listeria*).
- Acyclovir if herpes encephalitis suspected.
- Once organism isolated, seek urgent microbiological advice.

Further measures
- There is some evidence that high dose steroids may reduce neurological complications. Therefore, some centers recommend the administration of dexamethasone 10mg IV before or with the 1st dose of antibiotics (but do not delay giving antibiotics), then every 6h for 4d. Avoid in patients with shock.
- General supportive measures.
- Remember meningitis is a notifiable disease.
- Inform local public health officer for contact tracing.
- Antibiotic prophylaxis for family and close contacts (depends on the organism—ask a microbiologist). p336.

Typical CSF in meningitis

	Pyogenic	Tuberculous	Viral ('aseptic')
Appearance	Often turbid	Often fibrin web	Usually clear
Predominant cell	Polymorphs	Mononuclear	Mononuclear
Cell count/mm³	eg 90–1000+	10–1000/mm³	50–1000/mm³
Glucose	<½ plasma	<½ plasma	>½ plasma
Protein (g/L)	>1.5	1–5	<1
Organisms	In smear and culture	Often absent in smear	Not in smear or culture

(There are no hard-and-fast rules)

Cerebral abscess

Suspect this in any patient with ICP↑, especially if there is fever or ↑WBC. It may follow ear, sinus, dental, or periodontal infection; skull fracture; congenital heart disease; endocarditis; bronchiectasis.

Signs: Seizures, fever, localizing signs, or signs of ↑ICP. Coma. Signs of sepsis elsewhere (eg teeth, ears, lungs, endocarditis).

Investigations: CT/MRI (eg 'ring-enhancing' lesion); ↑WBC, ↑ESR; biopsy.

Treatment: Urgent neurosurgical referral; treat ↑ICP (p722). If frontal sinuses or teeth are the source, the likely organism will be *Strep. milleri* (microaerophilic), or oropharyngeal anaerobes. In ear abscesses, *B. fragilis* or other anaerobes are most common. Bacterial abscesses are often peripheral; toxoplasma lesions (p520) are deeper (eg basal ganglia). Remember the possibility of underlying immunosuppression.

Status epilepticus

This means seizures lasting for >30min, or repeated seizures without intervening consciousness. Mortality and the risk of permanent brain damage ↑ with the length of attack. Aim to terminate seizures lasting more than a few min as soon as possible (<20min).

Status usually occurs in known epileptics. If it is the 1st presentation of epilepsy, the chance of a structural brain lesion is high (>50%). Diagnosis of tonic–clonic status is usually clear. Non-convulsive status (eg absence status or continuous partial seizures with preservation of consciousness) may be more difficult: Look for subtle eye or lid movement. An EEG can be very helpful. *Could the patient be pregnant* (any pelvic mass)? If so, eclampsia is the likely diagnosis, check the urine and BP: Call a senior obstetrician—immediate delivery may be needed.

Investigations
- Bedside glucose, the following tests can be done once ℞ has started.
- Glucose, blood gases, CMP, Ca^{2+}, CBC, ECG.
- Consider anticonvulsant levels, toxicology screen, LP, culture blood and urine, EEG, CT, carbon monoxide level.
- Pulse oximetry, cardiac monitor

Treatment See OPPOSITE. Basic life support—and these agents:

1 Lorazepam ~2mg as a slow bolus (≤2min) into a large vein. Beware respiratory arrest during the last part of the injection. Have full resuscitation facilities to hand for all IV benzodiazepine use. (Alternative: Diazepam but it is less long-lasting—give 10mg IV over 2min; if needed, repeat at 5mg/min, until seizures stop or 20mg given—or significant respiratory depression occurs.) The rectal route is an alternative for diazepam if IV access is difficult.

While waiting for this to work, prepare other drugs. If seizures continue …

2 Phenytoin infusion: 15mg/kg IVI, at a rate of ≤50mg/min. (Don't put diazepam in same line: They don't mix.) Beware BP↓ and do not use if bradycardic or heart block. Requires BP and ECG monitoring. 100mg/6–8h is a maintenance dose (check levels). If seizures continue …

3 Dexamethasone 10mg IV if vasculitis/cerebral edema (tumor) possible.

4 General anesthesia expert guidance on ICU.

As soon as seizures are controlled, start oral drugs (p346). Ask what the cause was, eg hypoglycemia, pregnancy, alcohol, drugs, CNS lesion or infection, hypertensive encephalopathy, inadequate anticonvulsant dose (p344).

Management of status epilepticus

Open and maintain the airway, lay in recovery position
Remove false teeth if poorly fitting, insert oral/nasal airway, intubate if necessary

↓

Oxygen, 100% + suction (as required)

↓

IV access and take blood
CMP, LFT, CBC, glucose, calcium,
Toxicology screen if indicated, anticonvulsant levels

↓

Thiamine 100mg IV over 10min if alcoholism or malnourishment suspected. Unless glucose known to be normal IV glucose 50mL 50%

↓

Correct hypotension with fluids

↓

Slow IV bolus phase—to stop seizures: Eg lorazepam 2–4mg

↓

IV infusion phase: If seizures continue, start phenytoin,15mg/kg IVI, at a rate of ≤50mg/min. Monitor ECG and BP. 100mg/6–8h is a maintenance dose (check levels). Alternative: Diazepam infusion: 100mg in 500mL of 5% dextrose; infuse at ~40mL/h as opposite

↓

General anesthesia phase: Continuing seizures require expert help with paralysis and ventilation with continuous EEG monitoring in ICU

Never spend longer than 20min on someone with status epilepticus without having help at the bedside from a neurologist.

Head injury

If the pupils are unequal, diagnose rising intracranial pressure (ICP), eg from extradural hemorrhage, and summon urgent neurosurgical help (p335). Retinal vein pulsation at fundoscopy helps exclude ICP↑.

Initial management (See OPPOSITE.) Write full notes. Record times.
- Involve neurosurgeons at an early stage, especially with comatosed patients, or if raised ICP suspected.
- Examine the CNS. Chart pulse, BP, T°, respirations + pupils every 15min.
- Maintain C-spine immobilization until an adequate exam can be done.
- Assess antegrade amnesia (loss from the time of injury, ie post-traumatic) and retrograde amnesia—its extent correlates with the severity of the injury, and it never occurs without antegrade amnesia.
- Meticulous care to bladder & airway.

Who needs a CT head?

If any of the following are present, a CT is required immediately:
- GCS <13 at any time, or GCS 13 or 14 at 2h following injury
- Focal neurological deficit
- Suspected open or depressed skull fracture, or signs of basal skull fracture
- Post-traumatic seizure
- Vomiting >once
- Loss of consciousness OR any of the following:
  - Age ≥65
  - Coagulopathy
  - 'Dangerous mechanism of injury' eg RTA, fall from great height
  - Confusion of >30min.

When to ventilate immediately:
- Coma ≤8 on Glasgow coma scale (GCS; p684)
- P_aO_2 <70 mmHg in air (<100 mmHg with O_2) or P_aCO_2 >45mmHg
- Spontaneous hyperventilation (P_aCO_2 <26mmHg)
- Respiratory irregularity.

Ventilate before neurosurgical transfer if:
- Deteriorating level of consciousness
- Bilateral fractured mandible
- Bleeding into mouth, eg skull base fracture
- Seizures.

Risk of intracranial hematoma in adults
- Fully conscious, no skull fracture = <1 : 1000
- Confused, no skull fracture = 1 : 100
- Fully conscious, skull fracture = 1 : 30
- Confused, skull fracture = 1 : 4.

Criteria for admission
- Difficult to assess (child; postictal; alcohol intoxication).
- CNS signs; severe headache or vomiting; fracture.
- Loss of consciousness does **not** require admission if well, and a responsible adult is in attendance.

Drowsy trauma patients (GCS <15 to >8) smelling of alcohol: Alcohol is an unlikely cause of coma if plasma alcohol <50mg/dL. If unavailable, estimate blood alcohol level from the osmolar gap, p616. **Never assume signs are just alcohol**.

Complications Early: Extradural/subdural hemorrhage, seizures.
Late: Subdural, p335; seizures; diabetes insipidus; parkinsonism; dementia.

Indicators of a bad prognosis ↑ age, decerebrate rigidity, extensor spasms, prolonged coma, hypertension, hypoxemia, T° >39°C. 60% of those with loss of consciousness of >1 month will survive 3–25yrs, but may need daily nursing care.

Immediate management plan

ABC
↓

Oxygen, 100%
Intubate and hyperventilate if necessary
NB: *Beware of a cervical spine injury*
↓

Stop blood loss and support circulation
Treat for shock if required (p686)
↓

Treat seizures with diazepam
↓

Assess level of consciousness (GCS)
Antegrade and retrograde amnesia
↓

Rapid examination survey
↓

Investigations
CMP, *glucose*, CBC, *blood alcohol, toxicology screen*, ABG & *clotting*
↓

Neurological examination
↓

Brief history
When? Where? How? Had a fit? Lucid interval? Alcohol?
↓

Evaluate lacerations of face or scalp
*Palpate deep wounds with sterile glove to check for
step deformity. Note obvious skull/facial fractures*[1]
↓

Check for CSF leak, from nose (rhinorrhea) or ear
Any blood behind the ear drum?
*If either is present, suspect basilar skull fracture: Do CT
Give tetanus toxoid, and refer at once to neurosurgeons*
↓

Palpate the neck posteriorly for tenderness and deformity
*If detected, or if the patient has obvious head injury,
or injury above the clavicle with loss of consciousness,
immobilize the neck and get cervical spine radiographs*
↓

Radiology
As indicated: Cervical spine, CXR; CT of head

Raised intracranial pressure (ICP↑)

There are 3 types of cerebral edema:
- Vasogenic: ↑ capillary permeability—tumor, trauma, ischemia, infection.
- Cytotoxic—cell death, from hypoxia.
- Interstitial (eg obstructive hydrocephalus).

Because the cranium defines a fixed volume, brain swelling quickly results in ↑ICP which may produce a sudden clinical deterioration. Normal ICP is 0–10mmHg. The edema from severe brain injury is probably both cytotoxic and vasogenic.

Causes
- Primary or metastatic tumors.
- Head injury.
- Hemorrhage (subdural, extradural, subarachnoid; intracerebral, intraventricular).
- Meningoencephalitis; brain abscess.
- Hydrocephalus; cerebral edema; status epilepticus.

Signs & symptoms
- Headache; drowsiness; vomiting; seizures. History of trauma.
- Listlessness; irritability; drowsiness; falling pulse and rising BP (Cushing's response); coma; Cheyne–Stokes respiration; pupil changes (constriction at first, later dilatation—do not mask these signs by using agents, such as tropicamide, to dilate the pupil to aid fundoscopy).
- Papilledema is an unreliable sign, but venous pulsation at the disc may be absent (absent in ~50% of normal people, but loss of it is a useful sign).

Investigations
- CMP, CBC, LFT, glucose, serum osmolality, clotting, blood culture, CXR
- CT head
- Then consider lumbar puncture if safe. Measure the opening pressure!

Treatment
The goal is to ↓ICP and avert secondary injury. Urgent neurosurgery is required for the definitive treatment of ↑ICP from focal causes (eg hematomas). This is achieved via a craniotomy or burr hole. Also, an ICP monitor (or bolt) may be placed to monitor pressure. Surgery is generally not helpful following ischemic or anoxic injury.

Holding measures are listed OPPOSITE.

Herniation syndromes *Uncal herniation* is caused by a lateral supratentorial mass which pushes the ipsilateral inferomedial temporal lobe (uncus) through the temporal incisura and against the midbrain. The 3rd nerve, travelling in this space, gets compressed causing a dilated ipsilateral pupil, then ophthalmoplegia (a fixed pupil localizes a lesion poorly but is 'ipsilateralizing'). This may be followed (quickly) by contralateral hemiparesis (pressure on the cerebral peduncle) and coma from pressure on the ascending reticular activating system (ARAS) in the midbrain.

Cerebellar tonsil herniation is caused by ↑pressure in the posterior fossa forcing the cerebellar tonsils through the foramen magnum. Ataxia, VI nerve palsies, and +ve Babinski (upgoing plantars) occur first, then loss of consciousness, irregular breathing, and apnea. This syndrome may proceed very rapidly given the small size of, and poor compliance in, the posterior fossa.

Subfalcian (cingulate) herniation is caused by a frontal mass. The cingulate gyrus (medial frontal lobe) is forced under the rigid falx cerebri. It may be silent unless the anterior cerebral artery is compressed and causes a stroke—eg contralateral leg weakness ± abulia (lack of decision-making).

Immediate management plan

ABC

↓

Correct hypotension and treat seizures

↓

Brief examination, history if available
Any clues, eg meningococcal rash, previous carcinoma

↓

Elevate the head of the bed to 30–40°

↓

If intubated, hyperventilate to ↓P_aCO_2 (eg to 26mmHg)
This causes cerebral vasoconstriction and reduces ICP almost immediately

↓

Osmotic agents (eg mannitol) can be useful *pro tem* but
may lead to rebound ↑ICP after prolonged use (~12–24h)
*Give 20% solution 1-2g/kg IV over 10-20min (eg 5mL/kg). Clinical effect is
seen after ~20min and lasts for 2-6h. Follow serum osmolality—aim for
about 300mosmol/kg but don't exceed 310*

↓

Corticosteroids are *not* effective in reducing ICP
except for edema surrounding tumors
eg dexamethasone 10mg IV and follow with 4mg/6h IV/PO

↓

Fluid restrict to <1.5L/d

↓

Monitor the patient closely, consider monitoring ICP

↓

Aim to make a diagnosis

↓

Treat cause or exacerbating factors
eg hyperglycemia, hyponatremia

↓

Definitive treatment if possible

Diabetic ketoacidosis (DKA)

Hyperglycemic ketoacidotic coma occurs mainly in type I diabetes: It may be the initial presentation for a newly diagnosed diabetic patients. Precipitants include: Infection, surgery, MI, non-compliance, or wrong insulin dose. The diagnosis requires the presence of ketosis and metabolic acidosis

Signs & symptoms
- Polyuria, polydipsia, lethargy, anorexia, hyperventilation, ketotic breath, dehydration, vomiting, abdominal pain, coma.

Investigations
- Lab glucose, CMP, HCO_3^-, amylase, osmolality, ABG, CBC, urine and blood cultures, serum ketones.
- Urine tests: Ketones, CXR.
- To estimate plasma osmolarity: $2[Na^+] + [(urea) mg/dL]/2.8 + [(glucose) mg/dL]/18$.

Keypoints in the treatment of diabetic ketoacidosis

Treat dehydration aggressively with IVF.
- *Plasma glucose* is usually high, but not always, especially when insulin therapy is instituted.
- *High WBC* may be seen in the absence of infection.
- *Infection:* Often there is no fever. Do urine & blood cultures, and CXR. Start broad-spectrum antibiotics early if infection is suspected.
- *Hyponatremia: Pseudohyponatremia is* common, due to osmolar compensation for the hyperglycemia. corrected plasma $[Na^+]$ = measured Na + 1.6 (Glucose-100).
- *Ketoacidosis:* Blood glucose may return to normal long before ketones are cleared from the bloodstream. A rapid reduction in the amount of insulin administered in response to a ↓ in serum glucose may lead to lack of clearance and return to DKA. This may be avoided by maintaining a constant rate of insulin, eg 0.1U/kg/h IVI, and co-infusing D5W to when plasma glucose falls below 250–300mg/dL during the extended insulin regimen.
- *Acidosis* can be present without gross elevation of glucose; when this occurs consider other causes as well (eg salycilates, lactic acidosis).
- *Serum amylase* is often raised and non-specific abdominal pain is common, even in the absence of pancreatitis.

Management See OPPOSITE. Dehydration is more life-threatening than hyperglycemia — so its correction takes precedence.
- Monitor electrolytes carefully, especially potassium levels (which may fall during therapy), glucose, creatinine, HCO_3^-, hourly initially. Aim for a fall in glucose of 90mg/dL per hour, and correction of the acidosis. The use of venous HCO_3^- can be used as a guide to progress, and may prevent the need for repeated arterial blood gas sampling. K^+ disturbance may cause dysrhythmias.
- Flow chart of vital signs, fluids inputs and output (urine output) and ketones; insert foley catheter if no urine passed for >4h. Monitoring CVP may sometimes be helpful in guiding fluid replacement.
- Find and treat infection (lung, skin, perineum, urine after cultures).

NB: If acidosis is severe (pH <7), some give IV bicarbonate. This remains controversial because of effects on the Hb-dissociation curve and cerebral circulation—discuss with your senior resident.

Complications Cerebral edema, aspiration pneumonia, hypokalemia, hypomagnesemia, hypophosphatemia, thromboembolism.

Talk with the patient: Ensure there are no further preventable episodes or other complicating issues.

Other emergencies: Hyperosmolar non-ketotic coma & hypoglycemia p726.

Management plan

IV access and start fluid (0.9% saline IVF) replacement immediately

↓

Check plasma glucose: Usually >200mg/dL
if so give 4–8U (0.1U/KG) regular insulin IV

↓

Investigation precipitating cause

↓

*Labs electroltyes, glucose, CMP, osmolality, blood gases, CBC,
serum ketones,blood culture, mg, phos, Ca, CXR, EKG
Urine tests: Ketones, urine C&S;*

↓

Insulin sliding scale (below)

↓

Continue fluid replacement, K⁺ replacement

↓

Check glucose and CMP, regularly (hourly initially)

↓

Continue the investigation of causes

Fluid replacement

- Give 1 liter (L) of 0.9% saline immediately. Then, typically, 1L over the next hour, 1L over 2h, 1L over 4h, then 1L over 6h.
- Use dextrose saline or 5% dextrose when blood glucose is <259–300mg/dL.
- Those >65yrs or with CHF need less saline and more cautious fluid delivery.

Potassium replacement

- Total body potassium is invariably low, and plasma K⁺ falls as K⁺ enters cells with treatment.
- Don't add K⁺ to the first bag. Less will be required in renal failure or oliguria. Determine Urine output prior to K replacement. Check CMP hourly initially, and replace as K+ as needed.

Other diabetic emergencies

Hypoglycemic coma Usually *rapid* onset; may be preceded by odd behavior (eg aggression), sweating, pulse↑, seizures.

Management: Give 20–30g dextrose IV eg 200–300mL of 10% dextrose. This is preferable to 50–100mL 50% dextrose which harms veins. Expect prompt recovery. Glucagon 1mg IV/IM is nearly as rapid as dextrose but will not work in intoxicated patients. Dextrose IVI may be needed for severe prolonged hypoglycemia. Once conscious, give sugary drinks and a meal.

Hyperglycemic hyperosmolar non-ketotic coma Those with type-2 diabetes are at risk of this. The history is longer (eg 1wk), with marked dehydration and glucose >800mg/dL. Acidosis is absent as there has been no switch to ketone metabolism—the patient is often old, and presenting for the first time. The osmolality is >340mosmol/kg. Focal CNS signs may occur. The risk of DVT is high, so give *full* heparin anticoagulation (p574).

Rehydrate over 48h with 0.9% saline IVI, eg at ½ the rate used in ketoacidosis. Wait an hour before giving any insulin (it may not be needed, and you want to avoid rapid changes). If it is needed, 1U/h might be a typical initial dose. Look for the cause, eg MI, or bowel infarct.

Hyperlactatemia is a rare but serious complication of DM (eg after septicemia or biguanide use). Blood lactate: >5mmol/L. Seek expert help. Give O_2. Treat any sepsis vigorously.

Thyroid emergencies

Myxedema coma *Signs & symptoms:* Looks hypothyroid; >65yrs; hypothermia; hyporeflexia; glucose↓; bradycardia; coma; seizures.

History: Prior surgery or radioiodine for hyperthyroidism.

Precipitants: Infection; MI; stroke; trauma.

Examination: Goiter; cyanosis; heart failure; precipitants.

Treatment: Preferably in intensive care.
- Take venous blood for: T3, T4, TSH, CBC, CMP, cultures, cortisol.
- Take arterial blood for P_aO_2.
- Give high-flow O_2 if cyanosed. Correct any hypoglycemia.
- Give T3 (triiodothyronine) 5–20mcg IV slowly. Be cautious: This may precipitate manifestations of undiagnosed ischemic heart disease.
- Give hydrocortisone 100mg/8h IV—vital if pituitary hypothyroidism is suspected (ie no goiter, no previous radioiodine, no thyroid surgery).
- IVI 0.9% saline. Be sure to avoid precipitating LVF.
- If infection suspected, give antibiotic, eg cefuroxime 1.5g/8h IVI.
- Treat *heart failure* as appropriate (p128).
- Treat *hypothermia* with warm blankets in warm room. Beware complications (hypoglycemia, pancreatitis, arrhythmias). p742.

Further therapy: T3 5–20mcg/4–12h IV until sustained improvement (eg ~2–3d) then thyroxine (T4=levothyroxine) 50mcg/24h PO. Continue hydrocortisone. Give IV fluids as appropriate (hyponatremia is dilutional).

Hyperthyroid crisis (thyrotoxic storm) *Sign & symptoms:* Severe hyperthyroidism: Fever, agitation, confusion, coma, tachycardia, AF, vomitting and diarrhea, goiter, thyroid bruit, 'acute abdomen' picture.

Precipitants: Recent thyroid surgery or radioiodine; infection; MI; trauma.

Diagnosis: Confirm with technetium uptake if possible, but do not wait for this if urgent treatment is needed.

Treatment: Enlist expert help from an endocrinologist. See OPPOSITE.

Management plan for thyrotoxic storm

IVI 0.9% saline, 500mL/4h. NG tube if vomiting.

↓

Take blood for: T3, T4, cultures (if infection suspected).

↓

Sedate if necessary (eg chlorpromazine 50mg PO/IM).

↓

If no contraindication, give propranolol 40mg/8h PO (maximum IV dose: 1mg over 1min, repeated up to 9 times at ≥2min intervals).

↓

High-dose digoxin may be needed to slow the heart, eg 1mg over 2h IVI.

↓

Antithyroid drugs: Propylthiouracil (PTU 50–200mg q 4h).

↓

Hydrocortisone 100mg/6h IV or dexamethasone 4mg/6h PO.

↓

Treat suspected infection with eg cefuroxime 1.5g/8h IV.

↓

Adjust IV fluids as necessary; cool with sponging ± acetaminophen.

Addisonian crisis

Signs & symptoms: May present in shock (tachycardia; peripheral vasoconstriction; postural hypotension; oliguria; weak; confused; comatose)—typically (but not always!) in a patient with known Addison's disease, or someone on long-term steroids who has forgotten to take tablets. An alternative presentation is with hypoglycemia.

Precipitating factors: Infection, trauma, surgery.

Management: If suspected, treat before biochemical results.
- Take blood for cortisol (10mL heparin or clotted) and ACTH if possible (10mL heparin, to go straight to laboratory).
- Hydrocortisone sodium succinate 100mg IV stat.
- IVI: Use a plasma expander first, for resuscitation, then 0.9% saline.
- Monitor blood glucose: The danger is hypoglycemia.
- Blood, urine, sputum for culture.
- Give antibiotics (eg cefuroxime 1.5g/8h IVI).

Continuing treatment
- Glucose IV may be needed if hypoglycemic.
- Continue IV fluids, more slowly. Be guided by clinical state.
- Continue hydrocortisone sodium succinate 100mg IV/IM every 6h.
- Change to oral steroids after 72h if patient's condition good. The ACTH stimulation test (cosyntropin) is impossible while on hydrocortisone.
- Fludrocortisone is needed only if hydrocortisone dose <50mg/d and the condition is due to adrenal disease.
- Search for the cause, once the crisis is over.

Hypopituitary coma

Usually develops gradually in a person with known hypopituitarism. Rarely, the onset is rapid due to infarction of a pituitary tumor (pituitary apoplexy)—as symptoms include headache and meningismus, subarachnoid hemorrhage is often misdiagnosed.

Presentation: Headache; ophthalmoplegia; consciousness↓; hypotension; hypothermia; hypoglycemia; signs of hypopituitarism (p300).

Tests: T4; cortisol; TSH; ACTH; glucose. Pituitary fossa CT/MRI.

Treatment:
- Hydrocortisone sodium succinate 100mg IV/6h.
- Only after hydrocortisone begun: T3 10mcg/12h PO.
- Prompt surgery is needed if the cause is pituitary apoplexy.

Pheochromocytoma emergencies

Stress, abdominal palpation, parturition, general anesthetic, or contrast media used in radiography may produce dangerous *hypertensive crises* (pallor, pulsating headache, hypertension, feels 'about to die').

Treatment Get help.
- Phentolamine 2–5mg IV. Repeat to maintain safe BP.
- Labetalol is an alternative agent (p130).
- When BP controlled, give phenoxybenzamine 10mg/24h PO (↑ by 10mg/d as needed, up to 0.5–1mg/kg/12h PO); SE: Postural hypotension; dizziness; tachycardia; nasal congestion; miosis; idiosyncratic marked BP drop soon after exposure. The idea is to ↑ the dose until the blood pressure is controlled and there is no significant postural hypotension. A β_1-blocker may also be given at this stage.
- Surgery is usually done electively after a period of 4–6wks to allow full alpha blockade and volume expansion. When admitted for surgery the phenoxybenzamine dose is ↑ until significant postural hypotension.

Acute renal failure (ARF)—management

Seek expert help promptly: BP, urinary sediment, serum K⁺, creatinine, and ultrasound **must** be rapidly known. Have them at hand. p250.

Definition Acute (over hours or days) deterioration in renal function, characterized by a rise in serum creatinine and urea, often with oliguria or anuria.

Causes
• Hypovolemia
• Low cardiac output
• Sepsis
• Drugs
• Obstruction
• Other eg hepatorenal syndrome, vasculitis.

Investigations
• CMP, Ca^{2+}, PO_4^{3-}, CBC, ESR, CRP, INR, LFT, CK, LDH, protein electrophoresis, hepatitis serology, autoantibodies, blood cultures.
• Urgent urine microscopy and cultures. White cell casts suggest infection, but are seen in interstitial nephritis, and red cell casts an inflammatory glomerular condition.
• USS of the renal tract.
• ECG, CXR.

Management See OPPOSITE for acute measures. Underlying principles are:

3 **Treat precipitating cause** Treat acute blood loss with blood transfusion, and sepsis with antibiotics (p374). ARF is often associated with other diseases that need more urgent treatment. For example, someone in respiratory failure *and* renal failure may need to be managed in the ICU, not a renal unit, to ensure optimal management of the respiratory failure.

4 **Treat life-threatening hyperkalemia** See OPPOSITE.

5 **Treat pulmonary edema, pericarditis, and tamponade** (p696) Urgent dialysis may be needed. If in pulmonary edema, and no diuresis, consider removing a unit of blood, before dialysis commences.

6 **Treat volume depletion** if necessary. Resuscitate quickly; then match input to output. Use a large-bore line in a large vein (central vein access can be risky in obvious volume depletion).

7 **Treat sepsis**

8 **Further care**
  • Has obstruction been excluded? Examine for masses PR and *per vaginam*; arrange urgent ultrasound; is the bladder palpable? Bilateral nephrostomies relieve obstruction, provide urine for culture, and allow pyelography to
  • determine the site of obstruction.
  • If worsening renal function but dialysis independent, consider renal biopsy.
  • Diet: High in calories (2000–4000kcal/d) with adequate high-quality protein. Consider nasogastric feeding or parenteral route if too ill.

Prognosis Depends on cause (ATN mortality: Surgery or trauma—60%, medical illness—30%, pregnancy—10%). Oliguric ARF is worse than non-oliguric—more GI bleeds, sepsis, acidosis, and higher mortality.

Urgent dialysis if :
• K⁺ persistently high (>6.0meq/L).
• Acidosis (pH <7.2).
• Pulmonary edema and no substantial diuresis.
• Pericarditis. (In tamponade, only dialyse *after* pressure on the heart is relieved.)
• High catabolic state with rapidly progressive renal failure.

Management

Catheterize to assess hourly urine output, and establish fluid charts
↓
Assess intravascular volume BP, JVP, skin turgor, fluid
balance sheet, weight, CVP, attach to cardiac monitor
consider inserting a central venous cannula
↓
Investigations *(see OPPOSITE)*
↓
Identify and treat hyperkalemia—see below
Use a cardiac monitor
↓
If dehydrated
Fluid challenge: 250–500mL of colloid or saline over 30min
↓
Reassess
Repeat if still fluid depleted. Aim for a CVP of 5–10cm H_2O
↓
Once fluid replete, continue fluids at 20mL + previous hour's
urine output per hour
↓
If volume overloaded. Consider urgent dialysis
A nitrate infusion, furosemide or 'renal dose' dopamine may help in the
short term, especially to make space for blood transfusion etc.
but does not alter outcome
↓
Correct acidosis with sodium bicarbonate IV
↓
If clinical suspicion of sepsis, take cultures, then treat vigorously
Do not leave possible sources of sepsis (eg IV lines) in situ if not needed
↓
Avoid nephrotoxic drugs, eg NSAIDs, ACE-inhibitors, gentamicin.
Check Medication Sheet for all drugs given.

Hyperkalemia

The danger is ventricular fibrillation. A K^+ >6.5meq/L will usually require
urgent treatment, as will those with ECG changes:
• Tall 'tented' T-waves ± flat P-waves ± ↑ P–R interval (p620).
• Widening of the QRS complex—leading eventually, and dangerously, to a
sinusoidal pattern and VF/VT.

Treatment:
• 10mL calcium gluconate (10%) IV over 2min, repeated as necessary if
severe ECG changes. This provides cardio-protection. It does not change
serum potassium levels.
• Insulin + glucose, eg: 10 units regular insulin + 50mL of glucose 50% IV.
Insulin moves K^+ into cells.
• Nebulized albuterol (2.5mg) also makes K^+ enter cells.
• Polystyrene sulfonate resin (eg Kayexalate, 15g/8h in water) orally or, if
vomiting makes the PO route problematic, as a 30g enema (followed by
colonic irrigation, after 9h, to remove K^+ from the colon).
• Dialysis.

Acute poisoning—general measures

Diagnosis comes mainly from history. The patient may be reluctant or unwilling to tell the truth about what has been taken. Pill identification is occasionally helpful and texts such as the PDR may be useful. Multiple ingestions are common. While awaiting the results of the serum and urine toxicological screen, certain physical findings may help to narrow the potential drugs ingested. *Fast or irregular pulse:* Albuterol, antimuscarinics, tricyclics, quinine, or phenothiazine poisoning.

- *Respiratory depression:* Opiate or benzodiazepine toxicity.
- *Hypothermia:* Phenothiazines, barbiturates.
- *Hyperthermia:* Amphetamines, MAOIs, cocaine, or ecstacy (p736).
- *Coma:* Benzodiazepines, alcohol, opiates, tricyclics, or barbiturates.
- *Seizures:* Recreational drugs, hypoglycemic agents, tricyclics, phenothiazines, or theophyllines.
- *Constricted pupils:* Opiates or insecticides (organophosphates, p736).
- *Dilated pupils:* Amphetamines, cocaine, quinine, or tricyclics.
- *Hyperglycemia:* Organophosphates, theophyllines, or MAOIs.
- *Hypoglycemia:* Insulin, oral hypoglycemics, alcohol, or salicylates.
- *Renal failure:* Salicylate, acetaminophen, or ethylene glycol.
- *Metabolic acidosis:* Alcohol, ethylene glycol, methanol, acetaminophen, or carbon monoxide poisoning—p736.
- *↑Osmolality:* Alcohols (ethyl or methyl); ethylene glycol p612.

Management See OPPOSITE for a general guide to management
- *Take blood* as appropriate (p734). Always check acetaminophen and salicylate levels.
- *Empty stomach* if appropriate (p734).
- *Consider specific antidote* (p736) or oral activated charcoal (p734).
- *If you are not familiar with the poison* get more information. Call your local Poison Control Center.

Continuing care Measure temperature, pulse, BP, and blood glucose regularly. Use a continuous ECG monitor. If unconscious, nurse semi-prone, turn regularly, keep eyelids closed. A urinary catheter will be needed if the bladder is distended, or renal failure is suspected, or forced diuresis undertaken. Take to ICU, eg if respiration↓.

Psychiatric assessment Be sympathetic despite the hour! Interview relatives and friends if possible. Aim to establish:
- *Intentions at time:* Was the act planned? What precautions against being found? Did the patient seek help afterwards? Does the patient think the method was dangerous? Was there a final act (eg suicide note)?
- *Present intentions.*
- *What problems* led to the act: Do they still exist?
- *Was the act* aimed at someone?
- Is there a *psychiatric disorder* (depression, alcoholism, personality disorder, schizophrenia, dementia)?
- What are his *resources* (friends, family, work, personality)?

The assessment of suicide risk: The following ↑ the chance of future suicide: Original intention was to die; present intention is to die; presence of psychiatric disorder; poor resources; previous suicide attempts; socially isolated; unemployed; male; >50yrs old.

Referral to psychiatrist: This depends partly on local resources. Ask advice if presence of psychiatric disorder or high suicide risk.

Emergency care

ABC, clear airway

↓

Consider ventilation (if the respiratory rate is <8/min, or P_aO_2 <60mmHg, when breathing 60% O_2, or the airway is at risk, eg GCS <8)

↓

Treat shock (p686)

Further management

↓

Assess the patient

↓

History from patient, friends, or family is vital

↓

Features from the examination may help (see OPPOSITE)

↓

Investigations

Glucose, CMP, CBC, LFT, INR, ABG, ECG, acetaminophen, and salicylate levels
Urine/serum toxicology, specific assays as appropriate

↓

Monitor

$T°$, pulse & respiratory rate, BP, O_2 saturations, urine output ± ECG

↓

Treatment

Supportive measures: May need catheterization
↓Absorption: Consider gastric lavage ± activated charcoal, p734

Consider naloxone if unconscious level and pin-point pupils

733

Acute poisoning—specific points

Plasma toxicology For all unconscious patients, acetaminophen and aspirin levels and blood glucose are required. The necessity of other assays depends on the drug taken and the index of suspicion. Be guided by the poison information service. More common assays include: Digoxin; methanol; lithium; iron; theophylline. Toxicological screening of urine, especially for recreational drugs, may be of use in some cases.

Gastric lavage In general only of use if presentation within 40min of ingestion and if a potentially toxic dose of a drug has been taken. Lavage beyond this time frame may make matters worse. *Do not empty stomach* if petroleum products or corrosives such as acids, alkalis, bleach, have been ingested (*exception:* Paraquat), or if the patient is unconscious or unable to protect their airway (unless intubated). Never induce vomiting.

Gastric emptying and lavage Gastric emptying and lavage is contraindicated in patients who have a change in mental status, who are comatose, or have an absent gag reflex. These patients may require endotracheal intubation prior to insertion of a nasogastric tube. If conscious, get verbal consent.
- Monitor O_2 by pulse oximetry.
- Have suction apparatus to hand and working.
- Position the patient in left lateral position.
- Raise the foot of the bed by 20cm.
- Pass a lubricated tube (14mm external diameter) via the nares, asking the patient to swallow.
- Confirm position in stomach—blow air down, and auscultate over the stomach.
- Siphon the gastric contents. Check pH with litmus paper.
- Perform gastric lavage using 300–600mL tepid water at a time.
- Repeat until no tablets in siphoned fluid.
- Leave activated charcoal (50g in 200mL water) in the stomach unless alcohol, iron, Li^+, or ethylene glycol ingested.
- When pulling out tube, occlude its end (prevents aspiration of fluid remaining in the tube).

Activated charcoal reduces the absorption of many drugs from the gut when given as a single dose of 50g with water, eg salicylates, acetaminophen. It is given in repeated doses (50g 4 hourly) to ↑ elimination of some drugs from the blood, eg carbamazepine, dapsone, theophyllines, quinine, digoxin, phenytoin, phenobarbitone (phenobarbital), & paraquat. Lower doses are used in children.

Some specific poisons and their antidotes

Benzodiazepines Flumazenil (for respiratory arrest) 200mcg over 15s; then 100mcg at 60s intervals if needed. Usual dose range: 300–600mcg IV over 3–6min (up to 1mg; 2mg if on ITU). May provoke seizures.

β-blockers Severe bradycardia or hypotension. Try atropine up to 3mg IV. Give glucagon 2–10mg IV bolus + 5% dextrose if atropine fails (± an atropine infusion of 50mcg/kg/h). If unresponsive, consider pacing or an aortic balloon pump.

Cyanide This fast-killing poison has affinity for Fe^{3+}, and inhibits the cytochrome system, ↓aerobic respiration. *3 phases:* • Anxiety ± confusion • Pulse↑ or ↓ • Seizures ± shock ± coma. *Treatment:* 100% O_2, GI decontamination; if consciousness↓ give ampule of amyl nitrate for inhalation (if no IV established), 10cc of 3% solution sodium nitrate IV and 50cc of 25% solution of sodium thiosulfate. *Get expert help.* p741.

Carbon monoxide Despite hypoxemia skin is pink (or pale), not blue as carboxyhemoglobin (COHb) displaces O_2 from Hb binding sites. *Symptoms:* Headache, vomiting, pulse↑, tachypnea, and, if COHb >50%, fits, coma, & cardiac arrest. Remove the source. Give 100% O_2. Metabolic acidosis usually responds to correction of hypoxia. If severe, anticipate cerebral edema. Give mannitol IV (p722). Confirm diagnosis with a heparinized blood sample (COHb >10%) quickly as levels may soon return to normal. Monitor ECG. *Hyperbaric O_2 may help: Discuss with the poisons service if is or has been unconscious, pregnant, COHb >20%, or failing to respond.*

Digoxin *Symptoms:* Cognition↓, yellow-green visual halos, arrhythmias, nausea, & anorexia. If serious arrhythmias are present, correct hypokalemia, and inactivate with digoxin-specific antibody fragments (Digibind®). If load or level is unknown, give 20 vials (800mg)—adult or child >20kg. Consult Poison Control. Dilute in water for injections (4mL/38mg vial) and 0.9% saline (to make a convenient volume); give IVI over ½h, via a 0.22mcm-pore filter. If the amount of digoxin ingested is known, Poison Control will tell you how many vials of Digibind® to give, eg if 25 tabs of 0.25mg ingested, give 10 vials; if 50 tabs, give 20 vials; if 100 tabs, give 40 vials.

Heavy metals Enlist expert help.

Iron Deferoxamine 15mg/kg/h IVI; max 80mg/kg/d. NB: Gastric lavage if iron ingestion in last hour; consider whole bowel irrigation.

Oral anticoagulants If major bleed, treat with vitamin K, 5mg slow IV; give prothrombin complex concentrate 50U/kg IV (or if unavailable, fresh frozen plasma 15mL/kg IVI). If it is vital that anticoagulation continues, enlist expert help. Warfarin can normally be restarted within 2–3d.

NB: Coagulation defects may be delayed for 2–3d following ingestion.

Opiates (Many analgesics contain opiates.) Give naloxone eg 0.8–2mg IV; repeat every 2min until breathing adequate (it has a short $t_{1/2}$, so it may need to be given often or IM; max 10mg). Naloxone may precipitate features of opiate withdrawal—diarrhea and cramps which will normally respond to diphenoxylate and atropine (Lomotil®—eg 2 tablets/6h PO). Sedate as needed. High-dose opiate misusers may need methadone (eg 10–30mg/12h PO) to combat withdrawal.

Phenothiazine poisoning (eg chlorpromazine) No specific antidote. *Dystonia (torticollis, retrocollis, glossopharyngeal dystonia, opisthotonus):* Try benztropine 1–2mg IV/IM. Treat *shock* by raising the legs (± plasma expander IVI, or dopamine IVI if desperate). Restore body temperature. *Monitor ECG.* Avoid lidocaine in dysrhythmias. Use diazepam IV for prolonged seizures (p718). *Neuroleptic malignant syndrome* consists of: Hyperthermia, rigidity, extrapyramidal signs, autonomic dysfunction (labile BP, pulse↑, sweating, urinary incontinence), mutism, confusion, coma, WBC↑, CPK↑; it may be treated with cooling. Dantrolene has been tried.

Carbon tetrachloride poisoning this solvent, used in many industrial processes, causes vomiting, abdominal pain, diarrhea, seizures, coma, renal failure, and tender hepatomegaly with jaundice and liver failure. IV acetylcysteine may improve prognosis. Seek expert help.

Organophosphate insecticides inactivate cholinesterase—the resulting ↑ in acetylcholine causes the SLUD response: **S**alivation, **l**acrimation, **u**rination, and **d**iarrhea. Also look for sweating, small pupils, muscle fasciculation, coma, respiratory distress, and bradycardia. *Treatment:* Wear gloves; remove soiled clothes. Wash skin. Take blood (CBC & serum cholinesterase activity). Give atropine IV 2mg every 10min till full atropinization (skin dry, pulse >70, pupils dilated). Up to 3d' treatment may be needed. Also give pralidoxime 30mg/kg slowly. Repeat as needed every 30min; max 12g in 24h. Even if fits are not occurring, diazepam 5–10mg IV seems to help.

Paraquat poisoning (Found in weed-killers.) This causes D&V, painful oral ulcers, alveolitis, and renal failure. Diagnose by urine test. Give activated charcoal *at once* (100g followed by a laxative, then 50g/3–4h, ± antiemetic). *Get expert help.* Avoid O_2 early on (promotes lung damage).

Ecstasy poisoning Ecstasy is a semi-synthetic, hallucinogenic substance (MDMA, 3,4-methylenedioxymethamphetamine). Its effects range from nausea, muscle pain, blurred vision, amnesia, fever, confusion, and ataxia to tachyarrhythmias, hyperthermia, hyper/hypotension, water intoxication, DIC, K^+↑, acute renal failure, hepatocellular and muscle necrosis, cardiovascular collapse, and ARDS. There is no antidote and treatment is supportive. Management depends on clinical and lab findings, but may include:
- Administration of activated charcoal and monitoring of BP, ECG, and temperature for at least 12h (rapid cooling may be needed).
- Monitor urine output and CMP (renal failure p252), LFT, creatinine kinase, platelets, and coagulation (DIC p576). Metabolic acidosis may benefit from treatment with sodium bicarbonate.
- Anxiety: Diazepam 0.1–0.3mg/kg PO. Max IV does over 2min.
- Narrow complex tachycardias in adults: Consider metoprolol 5–10mg IV.
- Hypertension can be treated with nifedipine 5–10mg PO or phentolamine 2–5mg IV. Treat hypotension conventionally (p686).
- Hyperthermia: Attempt to cool, if rectal T° >39°C. Consider dantrolene 1mg/kg IV (may need repeating: Discuss with your senior and a poison unit, p732). Hyperthermia with ecstasy is akin to serotonin syndrome, and propranolol, muscle relaxation and ventilation may be needed.

Snakes *Snake envenomation:* There are two types of poisonous snakes in the US, the pit viper (rattlesnake) and the elapid(coral snake) For suspected envenomations, consider giving 1–2 vials of specific antivenom as soon as possible. To locate antisera for exotic snakes, call a regional poison control center (800-222-1222). CroFab is now available for pit viper bites and 4–6 vials should be given if there is evidence of local or systemic reaction *Management:* Avoid active movement of affected limb (so use splints/slings). *Avoid incisions and tourniquets.* Get help.

Salicylate poisoning

Aspirin is a weak acid with poor water solubility. It is present in many over-the-counter preparations. Anaerobic metabolism and the production of lactate and heat are stimulated by the uncoupling of oxidative phosphorylation. Effects are dose-related, and potentially fatal:
• 150mg/kg: Mild toxicity • 250mg/kg: Moderate • >500mg/kg: Severe toxicity.

Signs & symptoms Unlike acetaminophen, many early features. Vomiting, dehydration, hyperventilation, tinnitus, vertigo, sweating. Rarely; lethargy or coma, seizures, vomiting, ↓BP and heart block, pulmonary edema, hyperthermia. Patients present initially with respiratory alkalosis due to a direct stimulation of the central respiratory centers and then develop a metabolic acidosis. Hyper- or hypoglycemia may occur.

Management Correct dehydration. Gastric lavage if within 1h, activated charcoal (may be repeated, but is of unproven value).
• Acetaminophen and salicylate level, glucose, CMP, LFT, INR, ABG, HCO_3^-, CBC. Salicylate level may need to be repeated after 2h, due to continuing absorption if a potentially toxic dose has been taken.
• Levels over 700mg/L are potentially fatal.
• Monitor urine output, and blood glucose. If severe poisoning: Salicylate levels, blood pH, and CMP. Consider urinary catheter and monitoring urine pH. Beware hypoglycemia.
• If plasma level >500mg/L (3.6mmol/L), consider alkalinization of the urine, with IV sodium bicarbonate. Aim to make the **urine** pH 7.5–8.5. NB: Monitor serum K^+ as hypokalemia may occur.
• Consider dialysis if plasma level >700mg/L, and if renal or heart failure, seizures, severe acidosis, or persistently ↑plasma salicylate. ECG monitor.
• Discuss any serious cases with the local toxicological service or national poisons information service.

Acetaminophen poisoning

140mg/kg, or 12g in adults may be fatal. However, prompt treatment can prevent liver failure and death.

Signs & symptoms None initially, or vomiting ± RUQ pain. Later: Jaundice and encephalopathy from liver damage (the main danger) ± renal failure.

Management *General measures* p732, lavage if >12g (or >140mg/kg) taken within 1h. Give activated charcoal if <8h since ingestion. Specific measures:
• Glucose, CMP, LFT, INR, ABG, HCO_3^-, FBC. Blood level at 4h post-ingestion.
• If <8h since overdose and plasma acetaminophen is above the line on the graph OPPOSITE, start N-acetylcysteine.
• If >8h and suspicion of large overdose (>7.5g) err on the side of caution and start acetylcysteine, stopping it if acetaminophen level below the treatment line and INR and ALT are normal.
• Acetylcysteine is given by IVI: 140mg/kg in 200mL of 5% dextrose over 15min. Then 50mg/kg in 500mL of 5% dextrose over 4h. Then 100mg per kg/16h in 1L of 5% dextrose. Rash is a common SE: Treat with chlorpheniramine (=chlorphenamine), and observe; do not stop unless anaphylaxis, ie shock, vomiting, wheeze occurs (≤10%).
• If ingestion time is unknown, or it is staggered, or presentation is >15h from ingestion, treatment *may* help. Get advice.
• The graph may mislead if HIV+ve (hepatic glutathione↓), or if long-acting acetaminophen has been taken, or if pre-existing liver disease or induction of liver enzymes has occurred. Beware glucose↓; ward-test hourly; INR/12h.
• Next day do INR, CMP, LFT. If INR rising, continue acetylcysteine until <1.4.
• If continued deterioration, discuss with the liver team.

Do not hesitate to get expert advice. *Criteria for transfer to ICU:*
- *Encephalopathy* or *ICP↑*. Signs of CNS edema: BP >160/90 (sustained) or brief rises (systolic >200mmHg), bradycardia, decerebrate posture, extensor spasms, poor pupil responses. ICP monitoring can help, p722.
- *INR* >2.0 at <48h—or >3.5 at <72h (so measure INR every 12h). Peak elevation: 72–96h. LFTs are *not* good markers of hepatocyte death. If INR is *normal* at 48h, the patient may go home.
- *Renal impairment* (creatinine >2.2mg/dL). Monitor urine flow. Daily CMP and serum creatinine (use hemodialysis if >2.4mg/dL).
- *Blood pH* <7.3 (lactic acidosis → tissue hypoxia). • *Systolic BP* <80mmHg.

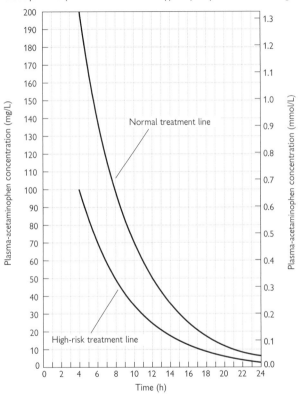

Patients whose plasma-acetaminophen concentrations are above the **normal treatment line** should be treated with acetylcysteine by intravenous infusion (or, provided the overdose has been taken **within 10–12hrs**, with methionine by mouth). Patients on enyzme-including drugs (eg carbamazepine, phenobarbital, phenytoin, rifampicin, and alcohol) or who are malnourished (eg in anorexia, in alcoholism, or those who are HIV-positive) should be treated if their plasma-acetaminophen concentrations are above the **high-risk treatment line**. (We thank Dr Alun Hutchings for permission to reproduce this graph.)

Burns

Resuscitate and arrange transfer for all major burns. (>25% partial thickness in adult and >20% in children). Assess site, size, and depth of the burn. Referral is still warranted in cases of full thickness burns >5%, partial thickness burns >10% in adults or >5% in children or the elderly, burns of special sites, chemical and electrical burns and burns with inhalational injury.

Assessment *Burn size* is important to assess (see table) as it influences the magnitude of the inflammatory response (vasodilatation, ↑ vascular permeability) and thus the fluid shift from the intravascular volume. The size must be estimated to calculate fluid requirements. Ignore erythema.

Burn depth determines healing time/scarring; assessing this may be hard, even when experienced. The big distinction is whether the burn is partial thickness (painful, red, and blistered) or full thickness (insensate/painless and white/grey). **NB:** Burns can evolve, particularly over the 1st 48h.

Resuscitation *Airway:* Beware of upper airway obstruction developing if hot gases inhaled. Suspect if history of fire in enclosed space, soot in oral/nasal cavity, singed nasal hairs of hoarse voice. A flexible laryngo/bronchoscopy is useful. Involve anesthesiologist early and consider early intubation.

Breathing: Exclude life-threatening chest injuries (eg tension pneumothorax) and constricting burns. Give 100% O_2 if carbon monoxide poisoning is suspected (mostly from history, may have cherry-red skin, measure carboxyhemoglobin (COHb) and compare to nomograms). With 100% O_2 $t_{1/2}$ of COHb falls from 250min to 40min (consider hyperbaric oxygen if pregnant; CNS signs; >20% COHb). SpO_2 measured by pulse oximeter is unreliable. Do escharotomy if thoracic burns impair chest excursion.

Circulation: Partial thickness burns >10% burns in a child and >15% in adults require IV fluid resuscitation. Put up 2 large-bore (14G or 16G) IV lines. Do not worry if you have to put these through burned skin, intraosseous access is valuable in infants. Secure them well: They are literally lifelines.

Use a *burns calculator* flow chart or a formula, eg: *Parkland formula* (popular): 4 × weight (kg) × % burn=mL Lactated Ringers in 24h, half given in 1st 8h.

Muir and Barclay formula: [weight (kg) × %burn]/2=mL colloid (eg Haemaccel®) per unit time. Time periods are 4h, 4h, 4h, 6h, 6h, and 12h.

Either formula is acceptable but must use appropriate fluid ie crystalloid for Parkland not colloid. **NB:** A meta-analysis (somewhat flawed) suggests the use of colloid (albumin) can cause ↑ mortality (slightly); it is also expensive. Replace fluid from the time of burn, not from the time first seen in hospital.

Formulae are only guides: Adjust IVI according to clinical response and urine output; aim for >0.5mL/kg/h (>1mL/kg/h in children), ~50% more in electrical burns & inhalation injury. Monitor T° (core & surface); catheterize the bladder.

Treatment Do *not* apply cold water to extensive burns: This may intensify shock. If transferring to a burns unit, do not burst blisters or apply any special creams as this can hinder assessment. Simple saline gauze or Vaseline® gauze is suitable; cling film is useful as a temporary measure and relieves pain. Use morphine in IV aliquots and titrate for good analgesia. Ensure tetanus immunity. Antibiotic prophylaxis is not routine.

Definitive dressings There are many dressings for partial thickness burns, including biological (pigskin, cadaveric skin), synthetic (Mepitel®, Duoderm®) and silver sufadiazine cream (Flamazine®). Major full thickness burns benefit from early tangential excision and split-skin grafting as the burns wound is a major source of inflammatory cytokines causing SIRS (systemic inflammatory response syndrome) and from an ideal medium for bacterial growth.

Smoke inhalation

Initially there is laryngospasm that leads to hypoxia and straining (leading to petechiae), then hypoxic cord relaxation leads to true inhalation injury. Free radicals, cyanide compounds, and carbon monoxide accompany thermal injury. Cyanide compounds (generated from burning plastic in particular) bind reversibly with ferric ions in enzymes, so stopping oxidative phosphorylation, causing dizziness, headaches, and seizures. Tachycardia and dyspnea soon give way to bradycardia and apnea. Carbon monoxide is generated later in the fire as oxygen is depleted; the COHb level does not correlate well with the severity of poisoning.

▸▸ 100% O_2 is given to elute both cyanide and CO.
▸▸ Involve ICU/anesthesiologist early: Early ventilation may be useful, consider repeated bronchoscopic lavage.
▸▸ Enroll expert help in cyanide poisoning, there is no single regimen suitable for all situations. Clinically mild poisoning may be treated by rest, O_2, and amyl nitrite 0.2–0.4mL via an Ambu® bag. IV antidotes may be used for moderate poisoning: Sodium thiosulphate is a common first choice. More severe poisoning may require eg hydroxocobalamin, sodium nitrite, and dimethylaminophenol.

Lund & Browder charts[1]

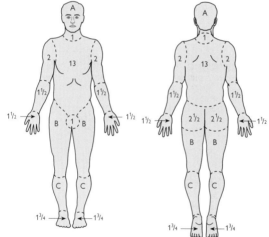

Relative percentage of body surface area affected by growth

Area	Age	0	1	5	10	15	Adult
A: half of head		$9\frac{1}{2}$	$8\frac{1}{2}$	$6\frac{1}{2}$	$5\frac{1}{2}$	$4\frac{1}{2}$	$3\frac{1}{2}$
B: half of thigh		$2\frac{3}{4}$	$3\frac{1}{4}$	4	$4\frac{1}{4}$	$4\frac{1}{2}$	$4\frac{3}{4}$
C: half of leg		$2\frac{1}{2}$	$2\frac{1}{2}$	$2\frac{3}{4}$	3	$3\frac{1}{4}$	$3\frac{1}{2}$

741

1 Accurate but time-consuming compared with the 'Rule of nines': arm: 9%; front of trunk 18%; head & neck 9%; leg 18%; back of trunk 18%; perineum 1%. This generally overestimates burn area (better than underestimating). It is even accurate for those <10 years old.

Hypothermia

Have a high index of suspicion and a low-reading thermometer. Most patients are elderly and do not complain, or feel, cold—so they have not tried to warm themselves up. In the young, hypothermia is usually either from cold exposure (eg near-drowning), or it is secondary to impaired level of consciousness (eg following excess alcohol or drug overdose).

Definition Hypothermia implies a core (rectal) temperature <35°C.

Causes In the elderly hypothermia is often caused by a combination of:
- Impaired homeostatic mechanisms: Usually age-related.
- Low room temperature: Poverty, poor housing.
- Disease: Impaired thermoregulation (pneumonia, MI, heart failure).
- Reduced metabolism (immobility, hypothyroidism, diabetes mellitus).
- Autonomic neuropathy (eg diabetes mellitus, Parkinson's).
- Excess heat loss (psoriasis). Cold awareness ↓ (dementia, confusion).
- ↑ exposure to cold (falls, especially at night when cold).
- Drugs (major tranquillizers, antidepressants, diuretics). Alcohol.

The patient Don't assume that if vital signs seem to be absent, the patient must be dead: Rewarm (see below) and re-examine. If T° <32°C, this sequence may occur: ↓BP → coma → bradycardia → AF → VT → VF. If T° >32°C, there may simply be pallor ± apathy.

Diagnosis Check oral or axillary T°. If ordinary thermometer shows <36.5°C, use a low-reading one PR. Is the rectal temperature <35°C?

Tests Urgent CMP, plasma glucose, and amylase. Thyroid function tests; CBC; blood cultures. Consider blood gases. The ECG may show J-waves or Osborn waves.

Treatment
- Ventilate if comatose or respiratory insufficiency.
- Warm IVI (for access or to correct electrolyte disturbance).
- Cardiac monitor (both VF and AF can occur during warming).
- Consider antibiotics for the prevention of pneumonia (p160). Give these routinely in patients over 65yrs with a temperature <32°C.
- Consider urinary catheter (to assess renal function).
- *Slowly rewarm.* Do not reheat too quickly, causing peripheral vasodilatation, shock, and death. Aim for a rise of ½°C/h. Old, conscious patients should sit in a warm room taking hot drinks. Thermal blankets may cause too rapid warming in old patients. The first sign of too rapid warming is falling BP.
- Rectal temperature, BP, pulse, and respiratory rate every ½h.

NB: Advice is different for victims of sudden hypothermia from immersion. Here, eg if there has been a cardiac arrest, and T° <30°C, mediastinal warm lavage, peritoneal or hemodialysis, and cardiopulmonary bypass (no heparin if trauma) may be needed.

Complications Arrhythmias (if there is a cardiac arrest continue resuscitating until T° >33°C, as cold brains are less damaged by hypoxia); pneumonia; pancreatitis; acute renal failure; intravascular coagulation.

Prognosis Depends on age and degree of hypothermia. If age >70yrs and T° <32°C then mortality >50%.

Before hospital discharge Anticipate problems. *Will it happen again? What is her network of support?* Review medication (could you stop tranquillizers?). *How is progress to be monitored?* Coordinate with physician/social worker.

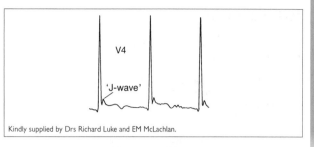
Kindly supplied by Drs Richard Luke and EM McLachlan.

Major disasters

Planning All hospitals have a detailed *Major Accident Plan*, but additionally the tasks of key personnel can be distributed on individual *Action Cards*.

At the scene Call the police; tell them to take command.

Safety: Is paramount—your own and others. Be visible (luminous mono-grammed jacket) and wear protective clothing where appropriate (safety helmet; waterproofs; boots; respirator in chemical environment).

Triage: Label RED if will die in a few mins if no treatment. YELLOW = will die in ~2h if no treatment; GREEN = can wait. (BLACK = dead).

Communications: Are essential. Each emergency service will dispatch a control vehicle and will have a designated officer for liaison. Support medical staff from hospital report to the medical safety officer—he is usually the first doctor on the scene: His job is to assess then communicate to the receiving hospital the number and severity of casualties, to organize resupply of equipment and to replace fatigued staff. He must resist temptation to treat casualties as this compromises his role.

Equipment: Must be portable and include: Intubation and cricothyrotomy set; intravenous fluids (colloid); bandages and dressings; chest drain (+flutter valve); amputation kit (when used, ideally 2 doctors should concur); drugs—*analgesic:* Morphine; *anesthetic:* Ketamine 2mg/kg IV over >60s (0.5mg/kg is a powerful analgesic without respiratory depression); limb splints (may be inflatable); defibrillator/monitor; ± pulse oximeter.

Evacuation: Remember: With immediate treatment on scene, the priority for evacuation may be reduced (eg a tension pneumothorax— RED—relieved can wait for evacuation—becomes YELLOW), but those who may suffer by delay at the scene must go first. Send any severed limbs to the same hospital as the patient, ideally chilled—but not frozen.

At the hospital a 'major incident' is declared. The *first receiving* hospital will take most of the casualties; the *support* hospital(s) will cope with overflow and may provide mobile teams so that staff are not depleted from the first hospital. A control room is established and the medical coordinator ensures staff have been summoned, nominates a triage officer, and supervises the best use of inpatient beds and ICU/operating room resources.

Blast injury may be caused by domestic (eg gas explosion) or industrial (eg mining) accidents or by terrorist bombs. Death may occur without any obvious external injury (air emboli). Injury occurs in 6 ways:

1 **Blast wave** A transient (milliseconds) wave of overpressure expands rapidly producing cellular disruption, shearing forces along tissue planes (submucosal/subserosal hemorrhage) and re-expansion of compressed trapped gas—bowel perforation, fatal air embolism.

2 **Blast wind** This can totally disrupt a body or cause avulsive amputations. Bodies can be thrown and sustain injuries on landing.

3 **Fragments** Penetration or laceration from blast fragments are by far the most common injuries. These arise from the bomb or are secondary, eg glass.

4 **Flash burns** These are usually superficial and occur on exposed skin.

5 **Crush Injuries:** Beware sudden death or renal failure after release.

6 **Psychological injury** Eg post-traumatic stress disorder.

Treatment Approach the same as any major trauma Rest and observe any suspected of exposure to significant blast but without other injury.

Index

750

Adult Basic Life Support HealthCare Provider Algorithm

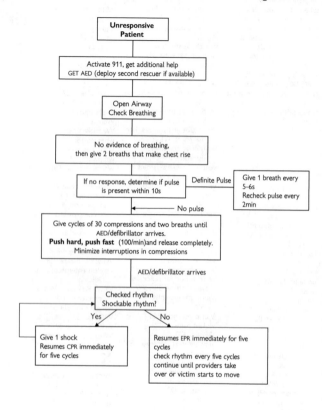

Management of Cardiac Arrest

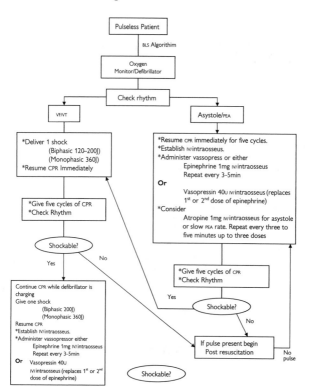

Ref: 2005 American Hearth Association Guidelines for CPR and ECC. *Circulation*, Vol 12, Issue 24 suppl, December 13, 2005. American Heart Association, 2005.

Supraventricular tachycardia

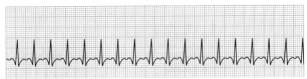

Adenosine
6mg initial dose; after 1–2min 12mg (may repeat 12mg dose x 1); give with 10mL NS flush (6–12 - 12)
Other drugs to consider for SVT include: amiodarone, metoprolol, digoxin, diltiazem, procainamide, or verapamil

Miscellaneous medications

Diphenhydramine
Allergic reaction—25–50mg IVP over secs
Hydrocortisone
100mg IVP over 30sec
Naloxone
0.4–2mg IVP q 2–3min; If patient on chronic opioid therapy (i.e. PCA), dilute 1mL (0.4mg/mL) in 9mL NS for a total volume of 10mL (0.04mg/mL). Administer 2mL dose (0.08mg) IV Push q2min until respirations >8/min.
Phenytoin
LD—15–20mg/kg; May NOT administer IV Push
Max rate of 50mg/min (25mg/min recommended)
Dilute each 1000mg (500mg in each drug box) w/100mL NS
NOTE: Fosphenytoin is not available in drug box

Reference: 2005 American Heart Association Guidelines for Cardiopulmonary Resuscitation and Emergency Cardiovascular Care. *Circulation* 2005; 112(Suppl IV)-19-IV-34.
Created by: W. Alvarez, PharmD, BCPS 3-1984 and H. Robinson, PharmD
Revised: 7/06

Ventricular Fibrillation Pulseless VT

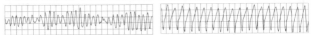

SHOCK @ 360J (Monophasic); 120 to 200J (Biphasic)
SHOCK @ 360J (Monophasic); 120 to 200J (Biphasic)
Epinephrine
1mg IVP q 3–5min THROUGHOUT entire duration of arrest
OR
May give 1 dose of Vasopressin
40 Units IVP over seconds (USE 2 VIALS) to replace the 1st or 2nd dose of epinephrine
SHOCK @ 360J
Amiodarone
300mg IVP over seconds; *May repeat with 150mg IVP over seconds if still in VF/pulseless VT after subsequent shock @360J*
OR
Lidocaine
1–1.5mg/kg; most of time given as 100mg and repeated if still shock refractory with at total Max of 3mg/kg (~300mg)
SHOCK @ 360J
Magnesium
1–2gm IVP undiluted over secs

If Pt awake (VT or Torsades *with a pulse*): 1–2gm diluted in 10mL given either as IVP over 1–2min (may be painful for patient) **OR** diluted in 50–100mL given over 5–60 minutes.

SHOCK @ 360J

NOTE: Procainamide is NOT an option due to prolonged administration time. Procainamide is not located in drug box.

ETT administration: Follow all meds with at least a 5mL 0.9% NaCl flush.
Patient should be vigorously ventilated.

NOTE: all doses 2–2.5 times the IV dose (except vasopressin)

Stable VT

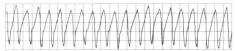

Amiodarone (may also be used or atrial fibrillation and atrial flutter)
150mg/100mL @ 600mL/hr 10min (15mg/min)

Drip: 450mg/250mL (conc = 1.8mg/mL) or 150mg/100mL
(conc = 1.5mg/mL) 1mg/min = 33mL/hr

OR

Lidocaine
1–1.5mg/kg; most of time given as 100mg and repeated if still shock refractory with at total Max of 3mg/kg (~300mg)
Drip: 2gm/250ml (conc = 8mg/mL); 2–4mg/min PREMIX IN PHARMACY 2mg/min = 15mL/hr

DRIPS for hypotension

Dopamine (will need 2 vials)
400mg/250ml (conc = 1600mcg/mL)
If pt weighs ~70kg, 5mcg/kg/min = 13mL/hr;
Suggested dose range = 5–25mcg/kg/min
May start @ 10mcg/kg/min

Norepinephrine (will need 2 ampules—do not filter)
8mg/250mL (conc = 32mcg/mL)
If pt weighs ~70kg, 0.15mcg/kg/min = 20mL/hr;
Suggested dose range = 0.01–2mcg/kg/min
May start @ 0.15mcg/kg/min (~10mcg/min)

Phenylephrine (will need 2 vials)
20mg/250mL (conc = 80mcg/mL)
If pt weighs ~70kg, 1mcg/kg/min = 53mL/hr
Suggested dose range = 0.5–4mcg/kg/min
May start @ 1mcg/kg/min (~70mcg/min)

Epinephrine (use 1mg/mL concentration to mix)
2mg/100mL (conc = 20mcg/mL)
If Pt weighs ~70kg, 0.1mcg/kg/min = 21mL/hr
Suggested dose range = 0.01–1mcg/kg/min
May start @ 0.1mcg/kg/min (~7mcg/min)

Naloxone 0.8–2mg ETT
Atropine 2mg ETT
Vasopressin 40 Units ETT
Epinephrine 2mg ETT (Use 1mg/mL concentration)
Lidocaine 2mg/kg (~200mg) ETT

PEA—Nonshockable

Epinephrine (given regardless of HR on monitor)

1mg IVP q 3–5min THROUGHOUT

OR

May give 1 dose of Vasopressin

40 Units IVP over seconds (USE 2 VIALS) to replace the 1st or 2nd dose of epinephrine

HR <60 (slow PEA):

Atropine 0.5–1mg IVP q 3–4min; Max of 0.04mg/kg (~4 syringes given)

Calcium Chloride (suspected HyperK+)

1gm IVP CENTRAL LINE PREFFERRED (lasts ~20min)

1amp = 1gm

Sodium Bicarbonate (suspected HyperK+, Acidosis)

50–100mEq IVP over 1min (1amp = 50mEq)

[NOT COMPATIBLE with Norepinephrine, Epinephrine, Dopamine, Phenylephrine, or calcium—Flush line pre/post administration]

Dextrose 50% (suspected HyperK+, hypoglycemia)

25gm (50ml) over 1min; use 16 gauge needle when drawing up. If giving for HyperK, then give prior to giving IV insulin.

Insulin (suspected HyperK+) 10 units IV Push given AFTER D50

*Alteplase (For suspected or known massive pulmonary embolism.
Massive PE Kit—IN ADULT PHARMACY SATELLITES ONLY)*

50mg IVP over 2min + heparin 5000 units (flush line between each), may repeat in 30min. **Note:** MIX AT BEDSIDE and remember to charge patient. If you are by yourself, have someone run to the pharmacy or run from the pharmacy with the kit.

Common Reversible Causes and treatment

Hypovolemia—NS wide open

Hypoxia—Oxygen

Hydrogen ion *(ACIDOSIS)*—Na Bicarb

Hyper-/hypokalemia—Trtmt for HyperK = Ca Cl, NaBicarb, D50% + IV Insulin

Hypoglycemia—Dextrose, glucagon (not in drug box)

Hypothermia—Warming blanket

Tablets—CaCl (CCB Toxicity), NaBicarb (TCA Toxicity)

Tamponade, cardiac—Pericardiocentesis (60mL syr w/18-g pinal needle - 3½")

Tension pneumothorax—Chest tube

Thrombosis, coronary (ACS)—Reteplase or PTCA

Thrombosis, pulmonary (embolism)—Massive PE Kit (Alteplase)

Trauma (hypovolemia)

Asystole—Nonshockable

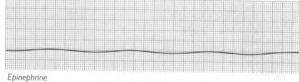

Epinephrine

1mg IVP q 3–5min THROUGHOUT

OR

May give 1 dose of Vasopressin

40 Units IVP over seconds (USE 2 VIALS) to replace the 1st or 2nd dose of epinephrine

Atropine (AFTER EPI)

1mg IVP q 3–5min; Max of 3mg

About the Oxford American Handbooks in Medicine

The Oxford American Handbooks are flexi-covered pocket clinical books, providing practical guidance in quick reference, note form. Titles cover major medical specialties or cross-specialty topics and are aimed at students, residents, internists, family physicians, and practicing physicians within specific disciplines.

Their reputation is built on including the best clinical information, complemented by hints, tips, and advice from the authors. Each one is carefully reviewed by senior subject experts, residents, and students to ensure that content reflects the reality of day-to-day medical practice.

Key series features

- Written in short chunks, each topic is covered in a two-page spread to enable readers to find information quickly. They are also perfect for test preparation and gaining a quick overview of a subject without scanning through unnecessary pages
- Content is evidence-based and complemented by the expertise and judgment of experienced authors
- Each Handbook takes a humanistic approach to medicine—it's more than just treatment by numbers
- A 'friend in your pocket'—the Handbooks offer honest, reliable guidance about the difficulties of practicing medicine and provide coverage of both the practice and art of medicine
- For quick reference, useful 'everyday' information is included on the inside covers
- Hard-wearing plastic covers, tough paper and built-in ribbon bookmarks—the Handbooks stand up to heavy usage
- Reader participation is encouraged by 'comments cards'